Comprehensive Women's Mental Health

Comprehensive Women's Mental Health

Edited by

David J. Castle
Chair of Psychiatry, St. Vincent's Hospital, Fitzroy, and Professor, The University of Melbourne, Melbourne, VIC, Australia

Kathryn M. Abel
Professor of Psychological Medicine and Director, Centre for Women's Mental Health, University of Manchester, Manchester, UK

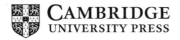
CAMBRIDGE
UNIVERSITY PRESS

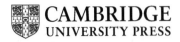

Shaftesbury Road, Cambridge CB2 8EA, United Kingdom

One Liberty Plaza, 20th Floor, New York, NY 10006, USA

477 Williamstown Road, Port Melbourne, VIC 3207, Australia

314–321, 3rd Floor, Plot 3, Splendor Forum, Jasola District Centre, New Delhi – 110025, India

103 Penang Road, #05–06/07, Visioncrest Commercial, Singapore 238467

Cambridge University Press is part of Cambridge University Press & Assessment,
a department of the University of Cambridge.

We share the University's mission to contribute to society through the pursuit of
education, learning and research at the highest international levels of excellence.

www.cambridge.org
Information on this title: www.cambridge.org/9781107622692

First published 2016

A catalogue record for this publication is available from the British Library

Library of Congress Cataloging-in-Publication data
Comprehensive women's mental health / edited by David J. Castle,
Kathryn M. Abel.
p. ; cm.
Includes bibliographical references and index.
ISBN 978-1-107-62269-2 (Paperback : alk. paper)
I. Castle, David J., editor.   II. Abel, Kathryn, 1961–, editor.
[DNLM: 1. Mental Disorders–etiology.   2. Women's Health.
3. Mental Disorders–therapy.   4. Socioeconomic Factors.
5. Women–psychology.   WM 140]
RC451.4.W6
616.890082–dc23   2015029629

ISBN   978-1-107-62269-2   Paperback

Contents

Contributors

Kathryn M. Abel
Centre for Women's Mental Health, University of Manchester, Manchester, UK

Jasmin Abizadeh
Reproductive Mental Health Program, BC Children's and Women's Hospital, Vancouver, Department of Psychiatry, University of British Columbia and BC Mental Health and Addiction Services, Provincial Health Services Authority, Vancouver, British Columbia, Canada

Roxane Agnew-Davies
Domestic Violence Training Ltd and School of Social and Community Medicine, University of Bristol, Bristol, UK

Nicholas B. Allen
Department of Psychology, University of Oregon, Eugene, OR, USA

Anthony P. Auger
Neuroscience Training Program and Department of Psychology, University of Wisconsin-Madison, Madison, WI, USA

Robert C. Baldwin
North Manchester General Hospital, Manchester, UK

Anna Barrett
Monash University, Melbourne, VIC, Australia and UNICEF

Annie Bartlett
Holloway Women's Prison and St. George's Hospital Medical School, London, UK

Dinesh Bhugra
Institute of Psychiatry, King's College London, London, UK

Anne Buist
The University of Melbourne, Austin Health and Northpark, Melbourne, VIC, Australia

Peter Carpenter
Avon and Wiltshire Partnership Mental Health Trust, Centre for Academic Mental Health, University of Bristol, Bristol, UK

Jessica Carty
Australian Centre for Posttraumatic Mental Health, The University of Melbourne, VIC, Australia

David J. Castle
St. Vincent's Hospital, Fitzroy and The University of Melbourne, Melbourne, VIC, Australia

Andrew M. Chanen
Orygen Youth Health Research Centre and Centre for Youth Mental Health, The University of Melbourne and Orygen Youth Health Clinical Program, Northwestern Mental Health, Melbourne, VIC, Australia

Michael C. Craig
Institute of Psychiatry, King's College London, London, UK

Mark Creamer
Australian Centre for Posttraumatic Mental Health, The University of Melbourne, Parkville, VIC, Australia

Eleanor Curran
St. Vincent's Hospital, Melbourne, VIC, Australia

Betsy Davis
Oregon Research Institute, Eugene, OR, USA

Timothy G. Dinan
Department of Psychiatry, University College Cork, Ireland

Dawn Edge
Centre for New Treatments and Understanding in Mental Health (CeNTrUM), Centre for Women's Mental Health, The University of Manchester, Manchester, UK

Alya Elmadih
Centre for Women's Mental Health, Institute of Brain Behaviour and Mental Health, University of Manchester, Manchester, UK

Emily Finch
South London and Maudsley NHS trust, Blackfriars Community Drug and Alcohol team, London, UK

Susan Fletcher
Australian Centre for Posttraumatic Mental Health, The University of Melbourne, Parkville, VIC, Australia

Sandra Flynn
University of Manchester, Manchester, UK

Jane Garner
Chase Farm Hospital, Enfield, UK

Fiona Gaughran
South London and Maudsley NHS Foundation Trust, National Psychosis Unit, Bethlem Royal Hospital, Kent and Department of Psychosis Studies, Institute of Psychiatry, Kings College London, London, UK

Ester di Giacomo
Institute of Psychiatry, King's College London, London, UK

Jill M. Goldstein
Department of Psychiatry, Harvard Medical School and Brigham and Women's Hospital, Boston, MA, USA

Heather Howell
Department of Psychiatry, Yale School of Medicine, New Haven, CT, USA

Naomi Humber
University of Manchester, Manchester, UK

John Kelly
Department of Psychiatry, University College Cork, Ireland

Bernice Knight
Avon and Wiltshire Partnership Mental Health Trust Centre for Academic Mental Health, University of Bristol, Bristol, UK

Melissa D. Latham
Department of Psychology, University of Oregon, Eugene, OR, USA

Nicola T. Lautenschlager
Academic Unit for Psychiatry of Old Age, St. Vincent's Health, Department of Psychiatry, The University of Melbourne, Melbourne, VIC, Australia

Susan W. Lehmann
Johns Hopkins School of Medicine, Baltimore, MD, USA

Serafino G. Mancuso
St. Vincent's Mental Health, Fitzroy, VIC, Australia

Sally Marlow
National Addiction Centre, Institute of Psychiatry, Psychology and Neuroscience, King's College London, London, UK

Shaila Misri
Reproductive Mental Health Program, BC Children's and Women's Hospital, Vancouver, Department of Obstetrics and Gynecology and Department of Psychiatry, University of British Columbia and BC Mental Health and Addiction Services, Provincial Health Services Authority, Vancouver, British Columbia, Canada

Cynthia A. Munro
Johns Hopkins School of Medicine, Baltimore, MD, USA

Arjun Nanda
Reproductive Mental Health Program, BC Children's and Women's Hospital, Vancouver, British Columbia, Canada

Carmine M. Pariante
Institute of Psychiatry, King's College London, London, UK

Andrea Phillipou
Department of Psychiatry, The University of Melbourne, and St. Vincent's Hospital, Melbourne, VIC, Australia

Peter V. Rabins
Division of Geriatric Psychiatry, Department of Psychiatry and Behavioral Sciences, Johns Hopkins University, Baltimore, MD, USA

Dheeraj Rai
Avon and Wiltshire Partnership Mental Health Trust, Centre for Academic Mental Health, University of Bristol, Bristol, UK

Margareta Reis
Department of Medical and Health Sciences, Clinical Pharmacology, Linköping University, Linköping and Laboratory Medicine, Clinical Chemistry, Skåne University Hospital, Lund, Sweden

Susan L. Rossell
Faculty of Health, Arts and Design, School of Health Sciences, Brain and Psychological Sciences Centre, Swinburne University, Hawthorn, VIC, Australia

Katherine Sevar
St. Vincent's Hospital, Melbourne, VIC, Australia

Jenny Shaw
University of Manchester, Manchester, UK

Lisa Sheeber
Oregon Research Institute, Eugene, OR, USA

Shubulade Smith
South London and Maudsley NHS Foundation Trust, Bethlem Royal Hospital and Department of Forensic and Neurodevelopmental Sciences, Institute of Psychiatry, Kings College London, London, UK

Nicky Stanley
School of Social Work, University of Central Lancashire, Preston, UK

Meir Steiner
Department of Psychiatry and Behavioural Neurosciences and Department of Obstetrics and Gynecology, McMaster University, Hamilton, Ontario, Canada

Katherine Thompson
Orygen Youth Health Research Centre and Centre for Youth Mental Health, The University of Melbourne, Melbourne, VIC, Australia

Simone N. Vigod
Department of Psychiatry, University of Toronto Adjunct Scientist, Institute for Clinical Evaluative Sciences, Toronto, Ontario, Canada

Darryl Wade
Australian Centre for Posttraumatic Mental Health, The University of Melbourne, Melbourne, VIC, Australia

Gilli Watson
Devon Partnership NHS Trust, Psychology and Psychological Therapies, Exeter, UK

Angelika Wieck
Manchester Mental Health and Social Care Trust and University of Manchester, Wythenshawe Hospital, Manchester, UK

Jennie Williams
Inequality Agenda Ltd, Faversham, Kent, UK

Kimberly A. Yonkers
Department of Public Health, Yale University, New Haven, CT, USA

Preface

This book provides a comprehensive overview of women's mental health. As editors, we were keen to ensure a broad international spread of authors and are delighted that so many luminaries in the field agreed to contribute. They have done a terrific job in bringing the science to the clinical arena, making this a book that should appeal both to researchers and clinicians.

We also wished to represent broad sociocultural aspects of women's lives alongside the biological, acknowledging how both remain pertinent to the aetiopathogenesis and manifestation of mental health maladies in women across the lifecycle. Integrating knowledge of the developmental phases of women's lives was also at the forefront of our minds when choosing topics and authors. Hence, the book weaves together these disparate yet essentially connected influences within and between each chapter. We trust this approach helps the reader by providing clear, coherent and clinically relevant signposts whilst retaining an appreciation of the complexity of the field.

The breadth of topics covered – from personality disorder to substance misuse, from anxiety to depression, bipolar disorder, psychosis and dementia – speaks to the comprehensive coverage of clinical topics. In addition, chapters, such as those dealing with domestic violence and women as carers, examine the sociocultural vulnerabilities and multifaceted roles that women play. In so doing, this book uniquely approaches women's mental health, starting from a point where women are considered within the context of their complex lives.

Treatment parameters are also comprehensively covered, again within a biopsychosocial framework. There is a strong emphasis on how treatments can be sensitive to the particular needs of women at particular stages of their lives.

We trust that this book will be an invaluable resource for anyone with an interest in understanding and helping women with mental health problems.

Surviving their lives
Women's mental health in context

Jennie Williams and Gilli Watson

Introduction

This chapter sets out a perspective on women and mental health that is radically different from that presented in the rest of the book: a book blatantly discussing mental health and mental illness. Here the reader is asked to understand women's psychological distress as evidence of their active struggle to survive lives shaped by abuse, exploitation, neglect and oppression. Evidence is presented to make the case that women's vulnerability to these experiences, and their efforts to survive them, are best understood within a framework that gives centrality to the existence of gender and other social inequalities. We aim to show that knowledge of these matters helps us to work well with women and to develop services for them that are acceptable and effective.

We begin with a reminder that social inequalities and hierarchies are still with us. Even in modern democracies where persistent efforts are made to extinguish inequalities, access to opportunities, rewards, power and status continue to be affected by the social categories to which we belong. Gender inequality is especially potent because of its centrality to identity and personal life; it also intersects with other systems of inequality including those founded on class, race, ethnicity, age and sexuality. The literature that explores the links between social inequalities and women's mental health is well-established and extensive, and is explored here under broad headings:

Risks and resources: This research focuses on social structural factors known to undermine or promote mental health and traces the ways gender and other social inequalities affect women.

Gender identity and socialisation: These matters have attracted the concern of researchers and clinicians for many decades. They draw attention to the detrimental effects of gender socialization on the ways women look after their own interests and cope with trauma, conflict and other challenges in their lives.

Ideologies: Social inequalities, especially gender, are sustained and hidden by ideologies that justify their existence and discourage their opposition. These systems of belief are woven into the fabric of society and tolerated as part of everyday life. So, when social inequalities cause mental health difficulties, it is difficult for people to make sense of what is happening and to find healthy ways forward. There is a persuasive body of research that shows that women and men's difficulties are likely to be compounded if they are given help from mental health services that are not gender-informed.

Survival: There is growing evidence that simply viewing women as victims of gender-based injustice and oppression is a partial account. There also needs to be acknowledgement of women's resilience and resistance to injustice, and especially their survival strategies, which frequently may be mislabeled abnormal or deviant behavior and disorders of personality.

Risks and resources

There is a wealth of evidence that alerts us to the risks embedded in women's lives that originate in systems of inequality. Some of these receive attention elsewhere in this book (e.g., Chapters 2, 3, 7, 17, 18). Selected for attention here are those that are commonplace and influential and that can usefully inform our work with women who have mental health needs.

Interpersonal violence and abuse
Gendered power relations

Gender inequality is perpetuated by processes that define women and men as different and that provide the justification and conditions for men to be accorded greater power, status and value than women. As Baker-Miller observes, "whenever one person or group has more power than the other(s) in a relationship, the danger of harm increases" (Baker-Miller 2008b, p. 375). Physical and sexual violence and abuse towards women and girls are common and often a covertly sanctioned means of expressing and maintaining dominance in family and community settings or of sustaining masculine identity (World Health Organization 2013a). Consequently, some of the most severe abuse of girls and women occurs within the most male-dominated families, subcultures and coercive contexts – including trafficking and gangs (McNeish and Scott 2014). So-called honor killing is an extreme example of this (Chesler 2010).

Gender inequality also underpins the commonly held belief that men should have their needs – including their sexual needs – met by women (Hill and Fischer 2001), including young women (Hlavka 2014); that what they do or want takes precedence over the needs of women; and that their prerogatives should not be questioned. Such a sense of entitlement, explicitly stated in widely accessible pornography (Office of the Children's Commissioner 2014), has been linked to rape, domestic violence, sexual abuse of children, sexual harassment and economic abuse.

A wealth of evidence also shows how women's lives, work and activities are systematically accorded less status and value than men's, the consequences of which are ameliorated or accentuated by the interactive effects of other aspects of a woman's life such as her class, ethnicity, age and sexual orientation. Femicide (World Health Organization 2012) is the most extreme form of gender-based devaluation and violence. This includes infanticide (World Health Organization 2011), which culminates in the far higher murder rate for female than male infants and is often linked to torture, mutilation, cruelty and sexual violence.

Scale of the problem

Findings about the prevalence of gender-based violence are readily available and can help us to gauge the scale of the problem and to think through the implications for mental health services. It is estimated that 35% of women worldwide have experienced either intimate partner violence or non-partner sexual violence in their lifetime (World Health Organization 2013a). On the basis of findings from the 2011/12 Crime Survey for England and Wales, it was estimated that 7% (1.2 million) of women had

experienced domestic abuse in the previous year (Women's Aid 2013) (see Chapter 14). Most recently, analysis of the Adult Psychiatric Morbidity Survey, a large scale general population study carried out in the UK (NatCen 2014), found that 1 in 25 of the population had experienced extensive physical and sexual violence, with an abuse history extending back to childhood. Women were 80% of this group, nearly all of whom had been assaulted by a partner. Half had been threatened with death. Most had been sexually abused as children and some severely beaten by a parent. Many had also been raped as an adult. While domestic violence, child sexual abuse, rape and sexual assault occur throughout and across societies, poverty and social divisions such as class and minority ethnic status also affect their prevalence (Humphreys 2007).

Implications for mental health

Much has been written about the processes that connect gendered violence and mental health and that differentiate it from post-traumatic stress disorder (PTSD) (van der Kolk, Roth et al. 2005). When a girl or woman experiences violence and abuse in a relational context that is complicit or indifferent to what is happening, then a common negative effect of this trauma is that she disconnects herself from others (Baker-Miller 2008b). Children experiencing abuse may believe they are responsible for their abuse – beliefs that are often fostered by abusers – and feel fearful, silenced, shamed and stigmatized. Childhood and adult abuse are major causes of the profound psychological and emotional difficulties that are subsequently diagnosed and labeled as pathologies (see also Chapter 17).

Research reviews (Chen, Murad et al. 2010, Cashmore and Shackel 2013) and landmark studies (Briere and Elliott 2003) provide strong confirmatory evidence that violence and abuse places mental health and personhood at risk, with effects that can be detected across most forms of adult distress and dysfunction (see also Chapter 17). Most recently, the UK Adult Psychiatric Morbidity Survey (NatCen 2014) identified a number of discrete groups of people with severe and sustained abusive experiences who experienced a wide range of distress and difficulties eligible for definition as psychosis, PTSD and eating disorders. For example, more than half of the people who had experienced the most relentless interpersonal trauma could be defined as clinically depressed or anxious – making them five times more likely than those with little experience of abuse to develop problems defined as a common mental health problem and 15 times more likely to have three or more such difficulties (NatCen 2014).

Confirmation that violent and abusive experiences are a predictor of subsequent psychological and emotional disorder and contact with mental health services is also provided by studies of clinical populations. An early study (Carmen, Ricker et al. 1984) found that almost half of the women using an inpatient service had histories of childhood sexual and physical abuse, findings that have continued to be replicated and elaborated (Chen, Murad et al. 2010). Abusive experiences are so highly prevalent as to be normative in the lives of women living in secure psychiatric services (Bland, Mezey et al. 1999). More recently, Abel et al. (2012) reviewed women in medium- and high-secure forensic mental health services in England and Wales. Over 90% of these women reported a history of childhood abuse (physical and sexual).

It is also important to be aware that women experiencing mental health problems are also at increased risk of violent victimization (Trevillion, Oram et al. 2013). Lifetime prevalence of violent victimization among women with serious mental problems may be as high as 97%; many of these women will have experienced multiple traumas (Goodman, Rosenberg et al. 1997). There is also consistency in the chronological ordering of experiences with histories of abuse, mental health problems and substance misuse generally preceding experience of homelessness, social exclusion and further revictimization (Fitzpatrick, Bramley et al. 2012).

Poverty

The relationship between poverty and mental health problems is one of the most well-recognized in psychiatric epidemiology (Wilkinson and Marmot 2003). It requires little imagination to identify the factors that can mediate this relationship, including living in poor housing in neighborhoods that do not offer a safe, cohesive community; worry over paying for essentials such as caring for children; poor diet; risk of exploitation at work; the psychological impact of racism; and negative and blaming attitudes toward the poor. People living in poverty who rely on the state also need to contend with the associated stigma of receiving benefits. Researchers report that "recipients often describe experiences of humiliation, dehumanization, denigration, depression and shame" (Belle and Doucet 2003, p. 108). Black and minority ethnic women living in persistent poverty are also at increased risk of victimization and of their mental health being affected by multiple traumas including sexual violence and abuse (Bryant-Jones, Ullman et al. 2010) (see also Chapter 2).

A substantial body of evidence supports the conclusion that the impact of social inequities on mental health is affected by the size of the gap between rich and poor, with the most unequal societies being the most toxic (Friedli 2009). Friedli (2009) comments: "For this reason, levels of mental distress among communities need to be understood less in terms of individual pathology and more as a response to relative deprivation and social injustice, which erode the emotional, spiritual and intellectual resources essential to psychological wellbeing" (p. iii). It is important, therefore, to be mindful that gender inequality means that many women have restricted access to money. To illustrate: figures for 2012 in the UK show that for every £1 a man takes home, a woman takes home 85p; and that 63% of people earning under £7 per hour (equivalent to ~$10 per hour) are women (Office for National Statistics 2013b). This pay gap persists because women tend to work in care-related services, work which is typically undervalued, underpaid and often part-time. This affects access to savings and pensions; women save considerably less than men and only 40% have adequate pension plans compared to 50% of men (Scottish Widows 2013).

Most at-risk of living in poverty are women who are lone parents, are older women, have disabilities (Macinnes, Aldridge et al. 2013) and are from ethnic minority groups (Kenway and Palmer 2007). Also included here are women living in nonpoor households where money is not distributed equally and where it is used by men to coerce and control their partner (NatCen 2014). There is also evidence (Byrne, Resnick et al. 1999) that women who live below the poverty line are at increased risk of violence and that physical and sexual assault increases the risk for poverty, divorce and unemployment (Goodman 2009). These dynamics, and the effects of these cumulative inequalities, are very evident in the backgrounds and life stories of women using mental health services (Goodman, Rosenberg et al. 1997, Goodman, Salyers et al. 2001, Williams, Scott et al. 2004).

Working lives
Paid work

Paid work provides a potential source of resilience for mental health through supporting self-esteem, a sense of identity and meaning, financial and emotional independence and social support. It can also be a source of overwork, conflict, dissatisfaction, insecurity, exploitation and harassment (MacDonald, Phipps et al. 2004). The impact of gender, ethnicity and other inequalities on the world of work means that women are more likely to experience the negative effects. Women continue to be concentrated in lower-skilled, part-time and lower-paid jobs than men, with less access to vocational training and education (TUC 2012). Those women whose lives are already most disadvantaged by social inequalities are most likely to experience the psychological disadvantages and least likely to experience the psychological advantages of paid work.

Unpaid work

Research consistently finds that men do less housework than women partners, and unsurprisingly, that women are less happy than men with this state of affairs. The most recent set of national UK statistics (Lanning, Bradley et al. 2013) found that women are continuing to spend more time on work within the home than men, regardless of income or whether they work full time. Women still carry the overwhelming burden of household tasks, even when they are cohabiting (Miller and Sassler 2012); this is particularly so after they have had children.

In terms of childcare, although there are indications that men are becoming more involved in the lives of their children (Fatherhood Institute 2011), data also suggest that there can be important differences in the quantity and nature of care provided by women and men even when women work full time (Craig 2006). Mothers give more time to childcare and are more likely to be alone with children, to multitask and to carry the overall responsibility for parenting.

Women also assume greater responsibility for caring for sick and incapacitated relatives, neighbors and friends than men – 58% of carers are female and women predominate in those groups with the heaviest commitments. They are also more likely to leave paid work in order to undertake care commitments (Carers UK 2012). While caring for others can be meaningful and intrinsically rewarding, it carries risks to mental health when it is associated with lack of social value, powerlessness, isolation, stress and poverty and when it is juggled with paid work outside the home (MacDonald, Phipps et al. 2004). The reader is

referred to Chapter 3 for a broader discussion of women's role as caregivers.

Embodied distress

Women's bodies also need to be understood in the context of social structure and constructions of gender. As discussed in Chapter 16, the connection between social value and physical appearance is particularly potent; research consistently finds that women have lower body satisfaction than men, regardless of age or ethnicity (Burrowes 2013a). Many women also attempt to control their lives and distress by controlling their bodies and what they eat; bodily disgust and disordered eating can add to these burdens (Bordo 2004) (see also Chapter 16).

Gender inequality and misogyny also affect women's experience of their reproductive lives, so that menstruation, fertility, childbearing and the menopause can become sources of disempowerment and distress (Ussher 2006). When women's embodied distress is named as, for example, psychosomatic, or eating disorders or self-harm, it becomes harder to detect the origins of this distress in gender and other inequalities and much easier to blame the woman herself. Wikund and colleagues (2014) remind us that we can avoid this trap by listening carefully to women's own narratives of their body-anchored responses and experiences within the context of their lives. This should include listening for experiences of violence and abuse in childhood and adulthood and to what women have to say about the effects of psychotropic medication they may have been prescribed (Jacobson 2014). The impact of psychotropic associated weight gain is discussed in more detail in Chapter 23.

Resources

Despite changes in the home and work roles for women and men over the last half century, women's restricted access to valued material and social resources continues to be a striking feature of gender relations in western countries. Women have less access to resources known to support and promote well-being, most notably physical and psychological safety, money, status and power. The effects of social inequalities on women's access to material, social and psychological resources are typically detrimental. An exception to this is their potential access to valued relationships with other women. Like members of any disadvantaged group, women are well-placed to seek support and value from each other.

It is well-documented that women's relationships with each other, both within (Watson, Scott et al. 1996, Burrowes 2013b) and outside (Giuntoli, South et al. 2011, Economic and Social Research Council 2013) mental health services, can be a source of therapeutic support. Opportunities to share experiences can enable women to see similarities among their difficulties, and to have their own experiences and feelings validated. This is particularly important when different diagnoses can make it difficult for women to find shared realities and commonalities with other women. Groups can help women to shift from believing their distress is a function of their personal abnormality and inadequacy to viewing it as an understandable reaction to the hardship, trauma and injustice in their lives. Importantly, groups can enable shared experiences of the injustices of racism, violence, abuse, loss, disadvantage and disappointment to be identified and named. Groups offer women a very different experience from that provided by their family networks: regular contact with a large family network does not necessarily lead to a higher level of well-being in women as it can place more obligations and burdens on them (Economic and Social Research Council 2013).

Socialization and identity

Gender socialization encourages women to develop characteristics and competencies in preparation for providing services to their families and society, which are compatible with a position of subordination. Ironically, there are indications that gender socialization has become increasingly robust as legislative barriers to equality have been removed. For example, babies are now enthusiastically color coded to remind everyone, especially the baby, of their gender (Eliot 2010). Shared understanding of what women are expected to be like include words such as empathic, emotionally expressive, deferential, dependent, passive, cooperative, able to multitask, mothers, attractive, warm, "nice" and ready to smile. Characteristics that can evoke disapproval, punishment and other negative responses towards women continue to include being too clever (except at school), ambitious, competitive, noisy, selfish, assertive, sleeping around, drinking heavily, being angry or violent, and being disinterested in or neglecting family life. Women continue to

be considered more irrational, incapable and incompetent than men – all characteristics that suggest that women are ill-suited to acting autonomously or to exercising power.

By contrast, men continue to be socialized to develop psychological characteristics that are consistent with the exercise of power (Seguino 2007, Connell 2011). The defining features of masculinity such as individualism, competition, acquisition, bravery and domination further the interests of global capitalism and nationalism, and when required, large numbers of men can be delivered to military life (Sjoberg and Via 2010). Although while shaping men's identities and lives in this way may serve the collective interests of some groups, this may be at considerable cost to the mental health of disadvantaged men, including Black and minority ethnic (BME) and working-class men who, along with the women and children in their lives, are held outside systems of power (Williams, Stephenson et al. 2014). The central requirement of hegemonic masculinity that is crucial for perpetuating the gender system – that men are strong, independent, heroic, winners and providers – has important mental health ramifications not least because of the link with interpersonal violence (Hearn and Whitehead 2006).

Being a 'good' woman

For many women, the dominant themes in their lived experience of inequalities are those of abandonment, abuse, disappointment, frustration and powerlessness. These experiences, which assault the self, can be a source of powerful emotions and distress including great sadness, shame, fear and rage. Yet, one of the injunctions that support the perpetuation of gender inequality is that women should not express rage or anger. In contrast, men are likely to be "authorized to be angry"; this anger is often associated with violence between men and from men towards women (Connell 2011, Williams, Stephenson et al. 2014). Angry women, on the other hand, are typically seen as a challenge to the gender system and to male dominance and may risk being viewed as bad or mad (van Wormer 2010). Too often mental health services medicate angry women and label them as problematic and personality disordered (Shaw 2005, Warne 2007, Ussher 2013). As Claire Allan (2011), a woman diagnosed as having borderline personality disorder, observes, "'inappropriate anger' is a classic symptom of a 'borderline personality.'"

The risk to women of being socialized to defer to men, to please men and to accommodate the wishes of others, is that they neglect their self and their needs and do not have a sense of their own entitlement. Jack (1991) called this "silencing the self." This can affect women's mental health and well-being in a number of ways. For example, a woman can feel that it is dangerous or disallowed to express anger or disappointment openly and instead express anger indirectly in covert ways that minimize the risk of conflict, hostility or backlash. Direct conflict is avoided when these well-documented, underground power processes (Smith and Siegel 1985) are used, but their success is contingent on the woman remaining silent about the causes of her distress, disappointment, loss or rage. Finally, gender expectations can also inhibit self-directed action so that a woman living in toxic circumstances may not feel entitled to look after her own interests (Grant, Jack et al. 2011).

Ideologies

The ideologies and relational processes that sustain systems of inequality, especially gender inequality, have far-reaching psychological implications. Although gender systems are shaped by culture and context, they are also consistently underpinned by expectations that women and men should differ in terms of personality, aptitudes, interests, responsibilities, rights and value. Women are positioned so that they have less access to resources, opportunities and decision-making power than men. Justifications and explanations for this are woven into the fabric of societies and daily life. Everyone – the privileged as well as disadvantaged – is enlisted in participating in systems and practices that sustain these inequalities: this is "normal life" (Fine 2010). Although dissenting and alternative realities exist and emerge from a range of sources, attempts to scrutinize and oppose inequality may be systematically challenged, discouraged or thwarted (Sidanius and Pratto 1999).

Ideologies, rules and practices may not only affect the mental health of individuals, but also the mental health services that try to meet their needs. Over the past four decades, important and powerful perspectives have emerged that view mental health services as no different from other social institutions in being shaped by ideologies that serve the interest of privilege and deflect attention from the existence of inequalities (Penfold and Walker 1984, Williams and Keating 2002). This is particularly manifest in the ways women's distress is defined and processed within mental health systems. The power to name is profound and is evident in the enduring emphasis on psychiatric diagnosis, individualized pathology and medicalized responses to social distress (Cutting and Henderson 2002, Warne 2007, Platform 51 2011). Diagnosing a mental illness such as a borderline or emotionally unstable personality disorder, bipolar disorder, depression, anorexia or psychosis is a serious misrepresentation of a woman's experience. The powerful connections between a woman's distress and her lived experience are severed and without these understandings, her rightful distress and associated struggles to survive are easily misunderstood as abnormal, dysfunctional, unhealthy, out of control or dangerous. It becomes easy to assume that there is something fundamentally wrong with her, rather than that something has gone badly wrong with her life.

Survival

If the illness model does not accurately reflect the processes at work in women's distress (Williams and Paul 2008), what are the alternatives? One important and viable approach that is consistent with the evidence presented here conceptualizes women with mental health needs as survivors of their lives. From this perspective, symptoms and feelings typically labeled as illness, pathologies and disorders of personality represent manifestations of the costs of inequalities for women and of their resilience in surviving these injustices. This perspective is supported by growing evidence that women do not respond to the trauma of abuse, exploitation, racism and oppression with passivity, but engage in an active struggle to survive physically and psychologically. Depression, hearing voices, somatization, dissociation, self-harm (Crowe 2004), eating distress, misusing alcohol, prescribed and non-prescribed drugs (Markoff, Reed et al. 2005, Bland, Mezey et al. 1999) are all common ways that women (and men) may manage unbearable feelings of terror, anger, fear, profound sadness, shame and loss when they have limited control and when they do not feel entitled to speak, or safe enough to do so (Briere and Elliott 2003, Baker-Miller 2008b, Larkin and Read 2008, Chen, Murad et al. 2010).

Gender-informed mental health provision and practice

Mental health services dominated by medical and other reductionist models are difficult contexts within which to meet the mental health needs of women, and indeed men. Furthermore, when staff are not trained and encouraged to think about the psychological implications of inequalities and power abuses, there is a heightened risk of re-traumatization. Nonetheless, the accumulating evidence base summarized earlier and the persistence of writers, clinicians and women service users is beginning to have a positive impact on policy, research and practice guidance. This is evident in work emerging from Australia (Kezelman and Stavropoulos 2012), the United States of America (APA 2007), the UK (Department of Health 2002, Itzin, Bailey et al. 2008, NHS England 2013, NHS Confederation 2014), as well as from some international bodies (World Health Organization 2013).

Innovations in service provision and practice have been stimulated by gender analysis of women's mental health, and achieved through service development and training interventions (Scott and Williams 2004, Read, Hammersley et al. 2007, Greater London Domestic Violence Project 2008, Nelson and Hampson 2008, Scott and McNeish 2008).

Service provision

Evidence that social inequalities and associated abuses of power are a root cause of mental health problems has helped identify processes of collaboration, mutuality and empowerment as defining characteristics of effective services for women. This is supported by evidence from a number of quarters. For example, it is well-recognized that service development should be shaped in collaboration with women who have experienced mental health difficulties and used mental health services (ReSisters 2002, Kalathil, Collier et al. 2011). Collaborative work in communities has also been shown to strengthen women's resilience through building relationships (Hartling 2008), providing trauma-informed peer support (Blanch, Filson et al. 2012) and groupwork (Watson, Scott et al. 1996, Ryan 2005, Burrowes 2013b).

Well-funded evaluation studies have an important contribution to make to developing services in this field. Research demonstrating the value of trauma-informed cognitive behavior therapy (CBT) in community settings (Cohen and Mannarino 2008) and of gender-informed service responses to women whose problems include substance misuse (Toussaint, VanDeMark et al. 2007) provide good examples. Gender-informed responses to women admitted to acute wards (Williams and Paul 2008, Judd, Armstrong et al. 2009) and with housing needs (Howard, Rigon et al. 2008) are advocated but need further support and evaluation. In recent years, there has also been specific guidance, including that led by government, that addresses domestic violence and its impact on women and young people (Humphreys, Houghton et al. 2008, Trevillion, Howard et al. 2012, NHS Confederation 2014); the importance of building links with developments in the domestic violence sector is now widely accepted. The reader is also referred to Chapter 14. Finally, there is recognition that effective responses to the complex needs of severely traumatized women requires trauma-informed commissioning (NHS England 2013) and collaborative, flexible commissioning between sectors and across agencies (NHS Confederation 2014).

Gender-informed mental health practice

The evidence presented in this chapter makes a strong case for concluding that mental health practitioners need to understand women's distress in the context of the complexity of their lives and with an appreciation of the ways gender, ethnicity and other social inequalities affect service responses to women. In short, they need to take a gender-informed approach to working with women. This includes being knowledgeable about the ways in which power abuses can shape the lives and mental health of diverse communities of women – for example, black and minority ethnic women (Edge and Rogers 2005), migrant and refugee women (Women's Therapy Centre 2009, Latif 2014), sexual minorities (Women's Resource Centre 2010), women with learning difficulties (Taggart, Mcmillan et al. 2008), women in prison (Marcus-Mendoza 2011), women whose psychological distress is linked to substance misuse (Markoff, Reed et al. 2005, Toussaint, VanDeMark et al. 2007, Covington 2008) and homelessness (St Mungo's 2014).

Mental health practice needs to be thoroughly grounded in knowledge and understanding of the workings of power in the context of largely Eurocentric, patriarchal mental health services. As mental health workers, we must develop an awareness of our use and misuse of power and privilege (Jordan, Kaplan et al. 1991, Baker-Miller 2008a, Jordan 2008) and of the boundaries of our relationships (Royal College of Psychiatrists 2007, Council for Healthcare Regulatory Excellence 2008). Mental health workers must actively avoid reproducing harmful dynamics in relationships where there is an imbalance of power, seeking instead to bring authenticity, mutual empathy and mutual empowerment to the relationship (Baker-Miller 2008a). Gender-informed practitioners enable women to feel safe to speak in their own voices about trauma and difficulties in their lives and to find safe ways to express anger, sadness and loss (Brown 2004). Working with women in these ways creates opportunities for them to strengthen their resilience in the face of oppression and abuse and find their path to recovery (Hartling 2008).

Unfortunately, as yet many mental health services are not capable of responding to women's distress in gender-informed ways. This is most evident in research exploring whether workers had tried to find out whether a woman client had experience of abuse and violence, information that is one of the keys to providing gender-informed care. While the majority of women service users (Feder, Hutson et al. 2006, Morgan, Zolese et al. 2010) and mental health workers (Hepworth and McGowan 2013) believe it is appropriate routinely to ask women about these matters, there is little evidence this is happening in practice (Scott and McNeish 2008, McLindon and Harms 2011, Hepworth and McGowan 2013). This is hardly surprising: most people working in the field of mental health have not been trained to work with the mental health consequences of abuse and violence; neither do they have access to the kinds of supervision and support they need to work safely as gender-informed practitioners. It is encouraging that the case

for change has been acknowledged (Department of Health 2010, NICE 2014) and that open-access web resources aimed at mental health practitioners have recently been made available to support better practice (www.scie.org.uk/publications/elearning/sexualhealth; www.e-lfh.org.uk/programmes/domestic-violence-and-abuse/trainer-resources). However, it seems unlikely that fundamental change will be achieved without corresponding developments in the curricula of courses used to prepare all mental health practitioners for their work. The body of evidence presented in this chapter, and elsewhere in this book, makes it clear that this should happen.

Conclusion

The approach to women's mental health that has been outlined here confronts us with the difficulties of redressing profound inequalities of power in society and in systems. It also reminds us that these inequalities have largely been unrecognized, ignored or underrepresented in mental health provisions. A social inequalities perspective alerts us to the fact that understanding effects of inequalities requires us to recognize that each of us derives varying amounts of privilege and penalty from the intersections of multiple systems of potential oppression. There is much to share and learn together. We need to strengthen our capacity and confidence to understand the connections between inequalities and mental health and our ability to have appropriate conversations with women about their lives, their experiences of injustice and power abuses and how it has made them feel. The value, benefit and efficacy of mental health services rests on their capacity to offer women the help they need to survive such systems in transformative ways that can justly be named as recovery.

References

Abel, K. M. et al. (2012). *The WEMSS Report: A clinical, economic and operational evaluation of the pilot for Women's Enhanced Medium Secure Services (WEMSS). Informing Secure Pathways for Women.* London, HMSO.

Allan, C. (2011). *As a person with borderline personality disorder, apparently I have no empathy.* London, Guardian.

American Psychological Association (2007). "Guidelines for psychological practice with girls and women." *American Psychologist* 62(9): 949–979.

Baker-Miller, J. (2008a). "Telling the truth about power." *Women & Therapy* 31(2–4): 145–161.

Baker-Miller, J. (2008b). "VI. Connections, disconnections, and violations." *Feminism and Psychology* 18: 368–380.

Belle, D. and J. Doucet (2003). "Poverty, inequality, and discrimination as sources of depression among U.S. women." *Psychology of Women Quarterly* 27(2): 101–113.

Blanch, A., B. Filson, D. Penney and C. Cave (2012). *Engaging women in trauma-informed peer support: A Guidebook.* National Center for Mental Health Services. Available at www.nasmhpd.org/docs/publications/EngagingWomen/

PeerEngagementGuide_ Color_REVISED_10_2012.pdf. Retrieved September 16, 2015.

Bland, J., G. Mezey and B. Dolan (1999). "Special women, special needs: A descriptive study of female Special Hospital patients." *Journal of Forensic Psychiatry* 10(1): 34–45.

Bordo, S. (2004). *Unbearable weight: Feminism, western culture, and the body: Tenth anniversary edition.* London, University of California Press.

Briere, J. and D. M. Elliott (2003). "Prevalence and psychological sequelae of self-reported childhood physical and sexual abuse in a general population sample of men and women." *Child Abuse & Neglect* 27: 1205–1222.

Brown, L. S. (2004). "Feminist paradigms of trauma treatment." *Psychotherapy: Theory, Research, Practice, Training* 41(4): 464–471.

Bryant-Jones, T., S. E. Ullman, Y. Tsong, S. Tillman and K. Smith (2010). "Struggling to survive: Sexual assault, poverty and mental health outcomes for Black American women." *American Orthopsychiatric Association* 80(1): 61–70.

Burrowes, N. (2013a). *Body image – a rapid evidence assessment of the literature: A project on behalf of the Government Equalities Office.* London, Government Equalities Office. www.gov.uk/government/ uploads/system/uploads/ attachment_data/file/202946/ 120715_RAE_on_body_image_ final.pdf. Retrieved July 1, 2014.

Burrowes, N. (2013b). *The courage to be me. Evaluating group therapy with survivors of rape and sexual abuse.* NB Research Ltd on behalf of Portsmouth Abuse and Rape Counselling Service. Available at www.nb-research.co.uk/index.php/ projects-2/.

Byrne, C. A., H. S. Resnick, R. Kilpatrick, D. G. Best and B. E. Saunders (1999). "The socioeconomic impact of interpersonal violence on women." *Journal of Consulting and Clinical Psychology* 67(3): 362–366.

Carers UK (2012). *Facts about carers 2012: Policy Briefing.* London, Carers UK. www.hscf.org.uk/sites/ default/files/article_attachments/ Facts_about_carers_2012.pdf. Retrieved June 10, 2014.

Carmen, E. H., P. P. Ricker and T. Mills (1984). "Victims of violence and psychiatric illness." *American Journal of Psychiatry* 141(3): 378–383.

Cashmore, J. and R. Shackel (2013). "The long-term effects of child sexual abuse." *Child Family Community Australia* 11: Available at http://cdn.basw.co.uk/upload/ basw_103914-103911.pdf.

Chen, L. P., M. H. Murad, M. L. Paras, K. M. Colbenson, A. L. Sattler, E. N. Goranson, M. B. Elamin, R. J. Seime, G. Shinozaki, L. J. Prokop and A. Zirakzadeh (2010). "Sexual abuse and lifetime diagnosis of psychiatric disorders: Systematic review and meta-analysis." *Mayo Clinic Proceedings* 10(85(7)): 618–629.

Chesler, P. (2010). "Worldwide trends in honor killings." *Middle East Quarterly* 17(2): 3–11.

Cohen, J. and A. P. Mannarino (2008). "Disseminating and implementing trauma-focused CBT in community settings." *Trauma Violence Abuse* 9(4): 214–226.

Connell, R. (2011). *Confronting equality: Gender, knowledge and global change.* Cambridge, Polity.

Council for Healthcare Regulatory Excellence (2008). *Learning about sexual boundaries between healthcare professionals and patients: A report on education and training.* London, Council for Healthcare Regulatory Excellence.

Covington, S. S. (2008). "Women and addiction: A trauma-informed approach." *Journal of Psychoactive Drugs Supplement* 5: 377–385. Available at www.stephanie covington.com/assets/files/ Covington%20SARC.pdf.

Craig, L. (2006). "Does father care mean fathers share? A comparison of how mothers and fathers in intact families spend time with children." *Gender & Society* 20(2): 259–281.

Crowe, M. (2004). "Never good enough – part 1: shame or borderline personality disorder?" *Journal Of Psychiatric And Mental Health Nursing* 11: 327–334.

Cutting, P. and C. Henderson (2002). "Women's experiences of hospital admission." *Journal of Psychiatric and Mental Health* 9: 705–712.

Department of Health (2002). *Women's mental health: Into the mainstream – strategic development of mental health care for women.* London, Department of Health. Available at http://webarchive .nationalarchives.gov.uk/+/www.dh .gov.uk/en/Consultations/ Closedconsultations/DH_4075478. Retrieved September 16, 2015.

Department of Health (2010). *Responding to violence against women and children – the role of the NHS: The report of the Taskforce on the Health Aspects of Violence Against Women and Children.* London, Department of Health. Available at www.health.org.uk/ media_manager/public/75/external-publications/Responding-to-violence-against-women-and-children%E2%80%93the-role-of-the-NHS.pdf.

Economic and Social Research Council (2013). *Mental health and social relationships.* Economic and Social Research Council. www.esrc.ac.uk/ _images/ESRC_Evidence_ Briefing_Mental_health_social_ rel_tcm8-26243.pdf. Retrieved June 10, 2014.

Edge, D. and A. Rogers (2005). "Dealing with it: Black Caribbean women's response to adversity and psychological distress associated with pregnancy, childbirth and early motherhood." *Social Science and Medicine* 61: 15–25.

Eliot, L. (2010). *Pink brain, blue brain: How small differences grow into troublesome gaps – and what we can do about it.* Oxford, OneWorld.

Fatherhood Institute (2011). *Fathers, mothers, work and family.* Fatherhood Institute. www .fatherhoodinstitute.org/2011/ fi-research-summary-fathers-mothers-work-and-family. Retrieved June 10, 2014.

Feder, G., M. Hutson, J. Ramsay and A. R. Taket (2006). "Women exposed to intimate partner violence: Expectations and experiences when they encounter health care professionals: A meta-analysis of qualitative studies." *Archives of Internal Medicine* 166(1): 22–37.

Fine, C. (2010). *Delusions of gender: The real science behind sex differences.* London, Icon.

Fitzpatrick, S., G. Bramley and S. Johnsen (2012). *Multiple exclusion homelessness in the UK: an overview of findings: Briefing paper no. 1.* Edinburgh, Heriot Watt University/ ESRC. Available at www.sbe.hw.ac .uk/documents/ MEH_Briefing_No_1_2012.pdf. Retrieved September 16, 2015.

Friedli, L. (2009). *Mental health, resilience and inequalities.* Geneva, World Health Organization.

Giuntoli, G., J. South, K. Kinsella and K. Karban (2011). *Mental health, resilience and the recession in Bradford.* York, Joseph Rowntree Foundation. www.jrf.org.uk.

Goodman, L. A., S. D. Rosenberg, K. T. Mueser and R. E. Drake (1997). "Physical and sexual assault history in women with serious mental illness." *Schizophrenia Bulletin* 23(4): 685–696.

Goodman, L. A., M. P. Salyers, K. T. Mueser, S. D. Rosenberg, M. Swartz, S. M. Essock, F. C. Osher, M. I. Butterfield and J. Swanson (2001). "Recent victimization in women and men with severe mental illness: Prevalence and correlates." *Journal of Traumatic Stress* 14(4): 615–632.

Goodman, L. A., K. F. Smyth, Borges, A. M. and Singer, R. (2009). "When crises collide: How intimate partner violence and poverty intersect to shape women's mental health and coping." *Trauma, Violence and Abuse Special Issue on the Mental Health Implications of Violence Against Women,* 10: 306–329.

Grant, T. M., D. C. Jack , A. L. Fitzpatrick and C. C. Ernst (2011). "Carrying the burdens of poverty, parenting, and addiction: Depression symptoms and self-silencing among ethnically diverse women." *Community Mental Health Journal* 47(1): 90–98.

Greater London Domestic Violence Project (2008). *Sane responses: Good practice guidelines for domestic violence and mental health services.* London, GLDVP. Available at www .avaproject.org.uk/our-resources/ good-practice-guidance–toolkits/ sane-responses-good-practice-guidelines-for-domestic-violence-and-mental-health-services-(2008). aspx.

Hartling, L. (2008). "Strengthening Resilience in a Risky World: It's All About Relationships." *Women & Therapy* 31(2–4): 51–70.

Hearn, J. and A. Whitehead (2006). "Collateral damage: Men's 'domestic' violence to women seen through men's relations with men." *Probation Journal* 53 (1): 38–56. Available at http://prb.sagepub .com/content/53/31/38.full.pdf +html.

Hepworth, I. and L. McGowan (2013). "Do mental health professionals enquire about childhood sexual abuse during routine mental health assessment in acute mental health settings? A substantive literature review." *Journal Of Psychiatric And Mental Health Nursing* 20(6): 473–483.

Hill, M. S. and A. R. Fischer (2001). "Does entitlement mediate the link between masculinity and rape-related variables? ." *Journal of Counseling Psychology* 48: 39–50.

Hlavka, H. R. (2014). "Normalizing sexual violence: Young women account for harassment and abuse." *Gender & Society* 28(337).

Howard, L., E. Rigon, L. Cole, C. Lawlor and S. Johnson (2008). "Admission to women's crisis houses or to psychiatric wards: Women's pathways to admission." *Psychiatric Services* 59(12): 1443–1449.

Humphreys, C. (2007). "A health inequalities perspective on violence against women." *Health and Social Care in the Community* 15(2): 120–127.

Humphreys, C., C. Houghton and J. Ellis (2008). *Literature review: Better outcomes for children and young people experiencing domestic abuse – directions for good practice.* Edinburgh, The Scottish Government.

Itzin, C., S. Bailey and A. Bentovim (2008). "The effects of domestic violence and sexual abuse on mental health." *Psychiatric Bulletin* 32: 448–450.

Jack, D. C. (1991). *Silencing the self: Women and depression.* Cambridge, MA, Harvard University Press.

Jacobson, R. (2014). "Psychotropic drugs affect men and women differently." *Scientific American Mind* 25(5): 114–115.

Jordan, J. V. (2008). "Learning at the margin: New models of strength." *Women & Therapy* 31(2–4): 189–208.

Jordan, J. V., A. G. Kaplan, J. Baker-Miller and I. P. Stiver, Eds. (1991). *Women's growth in connection: Writings from the Stone Centre.* New York, Guilford Press.

Judd, F., S. Armstrong and J. Kulkarni (2009). "Gender-sensitive mental health care." *Australasian Psychiatry* 17(2): 105–111.

Kalathil, J., B. Collier, R. Bhakta, O. Daniel, D. Joseph and P. Trivedi (2011). *Recovery and resilience: African, African-Caribbean and South Asian women's narratives of* recovering from mental distress. London, Mental Health Foundation. http://mentalhealth.org.uk/content/ assets/PDF/publications/ recovery_and_resilience.pdf. Retrieved June 20, 2014.

Kenway, P. and G. Palmer (2007). *Poverty Among Ethnic groups: How and why does it differ?* . York, Joseph Rowntree Foundation. www .poverty.org.uk/reports/ethnicity .pdf. Retrieved June 20, 2014.

Kezelman, C. and P. Stavropoulos (2012). *The last frontier: Practice guidelines for treatment of complex trauma and trauma-informed care and service delivery.* Kirribilli, New South Wales, Adults Surviving Child Abuse.

Lanning, T., L. Bradley, R. Darlington and G. Gottfried (2013). *Great expectations: exploring the promises of gender equality.* London, Institute for Public Policy Research.

Larkin, W. and J. Read (2008). "Childhood trauma and psychosis: Evidence, pathways, and implications." *Journal of Postgraduate Medicine* 54(5): 287–293.

Latif, Z. (2014). *The maternal mental health of migrant women.* London, A Race Equality Foundation, www.better-health.org.uk.

MacDonald, M., S. Phipps and L. Lethbridge (2004). "Taking its toll: the influence of Paid and unpaid work on women' s well-being." *Feminist Economics* 11(1): 63–94.

Macinnes, T., H. Aldridge, S. Bushe, P. Kenway and A. Tinson (2013). *Monitoring poverty and social exclusion.* York, Joseph Rowntree Foundation. www.jrf.org.uk/sites/ files/jrf/MPSE2013.pdf. Retrieved June 10, 2014.

Marcus-Mendoza, S. (2011). "Feminist therapy with incarcerated women: Practicing subversion in prison." *Women & Therapy* 34: 77–92.

Markoff, L. S., B. G. Reed, R. D. Fallot, D. E. Elliott and P. Bjelajac (2005). "Implementing trauma-informed alcohol and other drug and mental health services for women: Lessons learned in a multisite demonstration project." *American Journal of Orthopsychiatry* 75(4): 525–539.

McLindon, E. and L. Harms (2011). "Listening to mental health workers' experiences: Factors influencing their work with women who disclose sexual assault." *International Journal of Mental Health Nursing* 20: 2–11. Available at https://www.researchgate.net.

McNeish, D. and S. Scott (2014). *Women and girls at risk: Evidence across the life course.* London, LanKelly Chase Foundation. Available at www.lankellychase.org .uk/assets/0000/2675/ Women___Girls_at_Risk_- _Evidence_Review_040814.pdf.

Miller, A. M. and S. Sassler (2012). "The Construction of Gender Among Working-Class Cohabiting Couples." *Qualitative Sociology* 35(5): 427–446.

Morgan, J. F., G. Zolese, J. McNulty and S. Gebhardt (2010). "Domestic violence among female psychiatric patients: Cross-sectional survey." *The Psychiatrist* 11: 461–464. Available at www.avaproject.org.uk/ media/50832/dv%20prevalence% 20among%20psychiatric% 20patients.pdf.

NatCen (2014). *Violence, abuse and mental health in England: Preliminary evidence briefing.* London, NatCen.

Nelson, S. and S. Hampson (2008). *Yes you can! Working with survivors of childhood sexual abuse* (Second Edition). Edinburgh, The Scottish Government. Available at www.rapecrisisscotland.org.uk/ workspace/publications/ YesYouCan.pdf.

NHS Confederation (2014). *Violence and health and wellbeing boards: A practical guide for health and wellbeing boards.* London, HM Government. Available at www.nhsconfed.org/~/media/ Confederation/Files/Publications/ Documents/Violence_and_health_ and_wellbeing_boards.pdf. Retrieved September 16, 2015.

NHS England (2013). *Securing excellence in commissioning sexual assault services for people who experience sexual violence.* London, NHS England.

NICE (2014). *Domestic violence and abuse: How health services, social care and the organisations they work with can respond effectively.* National Institute for Health and Care Excellence. Available at www.nice.org.uk/guidance/ph50/ resources/guidance-domestic- violence-and-abuse-how-health- services-social-care-and-the- organisations-they-work-with-can- respond-effectively-pdf.

Office for National Statistics (2013b). *Patterns of pay: Results from the Annual Survey of Hours and Earnings, 1997 to 2012.* London, HMSO.

Office of the Children's Commissioner (2014). "*Basically ... porn is everywhere*" – *A Rapid Evidence Assessment on the effects that access and exposure to pornography has on children and young people.* London, Office of the Children's Commissioner. Available at www .childrenscommissioner.gov.uk/ publications/basically-porn- everywhere-rapid-evidence- assessment-effects-access-and- exposure. Retrieved September 16, 2015.

Penfold, P. S. and G. A. Walker (1984). *Psychiatric ideology and its functions. Women and the Psychiatric Paradox.* Milton Keynes, Open University Press.

Platform 51 (2011). *Checks and choices: Women and antidepressants.* London, Platform 51.

Read, J., P. Hammersley and T. Rudegeair (2007). "Why, when and how to ask about childhood abuse." *Advances in Psychiatric Treatment* 13: 101–110. Available at http://apt .rcpsych.org/content/113/102/101 .full.pdf+html.

ReSisters (2002). *Women Speak Out*. Leeds, ReSisters.

Royal College of Psychiatrists (2007). *Sexual boundary issues in psychiatric settings: College Report CR145*. London, Royal College of Psychiatrists.

Ryan, M., Nitsun, M., Gilbert, L. Mason, H. (2005). "A prospective study of the effectiveness of group and individual psychotherapy for women CSA survivors." *Psychology and Psychotherapy: Theory, Research and Practice* 78: 465–479.

Scott, S. and D. McNeish (2008). *Meeting the needs of survivors of abuse: Mental Health Trusts Collaboration Project. Overview of evaluation findings*. London, Department of Health/National Institute of Mental Health.

Scott, S. and J. Williams (2004). "Closing the gap between evidence and practice: the role of training in transforming women's services." In N. Jeffcote and T. Watson (eds.), *Working therapeutically with women in secure mental health settings*. London, Jessica Kingsley.

Scottish Widows (2013). *Women and Pensions Report. A journey through life and pensions*. Edinburgh, Scottish Widows. Availabe at www.scottishwidows.co.uk/documents/generic/2013_women_and_pensions_report.pdf.

Seguino, S. (2007). "Plus ça change? Evidence on global trends in gender norms and stereotypes." *Feminist Economics* 13(2): 1–28.

Shaw, C. (2005). "Women at the margins: A critique of the diagnosis of Borderline Personality Disorder." *Feminism & Psychology* 15: 483–490.

Sidanius, J. and F. Pratto (1999). *Social dominance: An intergroup theory of social hierarchy and oppression*. Cambridge, Cambridge University Press.

Sjoberg, L. and S. E. Via (2010). *Gender, war, and militarism: Feminist perspectives*. Santa Barbara, Praeger.

Smith, A. J. and R. F. Siegel (1985). "Feminist therapy: redefining power for the powerless." In L. B. Rosewater and L. E. A. Walker (eds.), *Handbook of Feminist Therapy*. New York, Springer.

St Mungo's (2014). *Rebuilding shattered lives: Getting the right help at the right time to women who are homeless or at risk*. London, St Mungo's.

Taggart, L., R. Mcmillan and A. Lawson (2008). "Women with and without intellectual disability and psychiatric disorders: An examination of the literature." *Journal of Intellectual Disabilities* 12(3): 191–211.

Toussaint, D. W, N. R. VanDeMark, A. Bornemann and C. J. Graeber (2007). "Modifications to the Trauma Recovery and Empowerment Model (TREM) for substance-abusing women with histories of violence: Outcomes and lessons learned at a Colorado Substance Abuse Treatment Center." *Journal of Community Psychology* 35(7): 879–894.

Trevillion, K., L. M. Howard, C. Morgan, G. Feder, A. Woodall and D. Rose (2012). "The response of mental health services to domestic violence: A qualitative study of service users' and professionals' experiences." *Journal of the American Psychiatric Nurses Association* 18(6): 326–336. Available at https://www.researchgate.net.

Trevillion, K., S. Oram and L. M. Howard (2013). "*Domestic violence and mental health.*" In L. Howard, G. Feder and R. Agnew-Davies (eds.), *Domestic violence and mental health*. London, RCP Publications.

TUC (2012). Women's pay and employment update: A public/private sector comparison. TUC. Available at www.tuc.org.uk/sites/default/files/tucfiles/womenspay.pdf. Retrieved June 9, 2014.

Ussher, J. (2006). *Managing the monstrous feminine*. Hove, Routledge.

Ussher, J. (2013). "Diagnosing difficult women and pathologising femininity: Gender bias in psychiatric nosology." *Feminism & Psychology* 23: 63–69.

van der Kolk, B. A., S. Roth, D. Pelcovitz, S. Sunday and J. Spinazzola (2005). "Disorders of extreme stress: The empirical foundation of a complex adaptation to trauma." *Journal of Traumatic Stress* 18(5): 389–399.

van Wormer, K. (2010). *Working with female offenders: A gender-sensitive approach* (p. 225–229). London, John Wiley.

Warne, T. (2007). "Bordering on insanity: Misnomer, reviewing the case of condemned women." *Journal of Psychiatric and Mental Health Nursing* 14: 155–162. Available at https://www.researchgate.net.

Watson, G., C. Scott and S. Ragalsky (1996). "Refusing to be marginalized: Groupwork in mental health services for women survivors of childhood sexual abuse." *Journal of Community and Applied Social Psychology* 6(5): 341–354.

Wiklund, M., A. Öhman, C. Bengs and E. Malmgren-Olsson (2014). "Living close to the edge: Embodied dimensions of distress during emerging adulthood." *Sage Open*, file:///D:/Documents/1.%20Chapter/REFERENCES/Wiklund%20-%20Embodied%20distress%20-%2014.pdf. Retrieved July 2, 2014 (April–June): 1–17.

Wilkinson, R. G. and G. Marmot, Eds. (2003). *Social determinants of health: The solid facts*. Geneva, World Health Organisation.

Williams, J. and F. Keating (2002). "The abuse of adults in psychiatric settings." In N. Stanley, J. Manthorpe and B. Penhale (eds.), *Institutional abuse: Perspectives across the life course*. London, Routledge.

Williams, J. and J. Paul (2008). *Informed Gender Practice: Mental health acute care that works for women.* London, National Institute for Mental Health England. Available at www.nacro.org.uk/data/files/nacro-2008080100-98.pdf.

Williams, J., S. Scott and C. Bressington (2004). "Dangerous journeys: Women's pathways into and through secure mental health services." In N. W. Jeffcote and T. London (eds.), *Working therapeutically with women in secure settings.* London, Jessica Kingsley.

Williams, J., D. Stephenson and F. Keating (2014). "A tapestry of oppressions." *The Psychologist* 27(6): 406–409. Available at www.thepsychologist.org.uk/

archive/archive_home.cfm/volumeID_427-editionID_288-ArticleID_2525-getfile_getPDF/thepsychologist/0614will.pdf.

Women's Aid (2013). *Statistics about domestic violence: Incidence and prevalence of domestic violence.* London, Women's Aid.

Women's Resource Centre (2010). *Lesbian, bisexual and trans women's services in the UK: Briefing 11.* London, Women's Resource Centre, www.wrc.org.uk/lgbt.

Women's Therapy Centre (2009). *A toolkit providing guidelines and models of good practice.* London, Women's Therapy Centre.

World Health Organization (2011). *Preventing gender-biased sex*

selection: An interagency statement OHCHR, UNFPA, UNICEF, UN Women and WHO.* Geneva, WHO.

World Health Organization (2012). *Femicide.* Geneva, WHO.

World Health Organization (2013a). *Global and regional estimates of violence against women: Prevalence and health effects of intimate partner violence and non-partner sexual violence.* Geneva, WHO. Available at http://apps.who.int/iris/bitstream/10665/85239/1/9789241564625_eng.pdf?ua=1.

World Health Organization (2013b). *Responding to intimate partner violence and sexual violence against women: WHO clinical and policy guidelines.* Geneva, WHO.

Ethnic and cultural effects on mental healthcare for women

Dawn Edge and Dinesh Bhugra

Introduction

Gender plays a major role in cultural perceptions and likelihood of diagnosis in mental illness. For women, there is often a "double-jeopardy" at play. First, many psychiatric disorders are more common in women; second, women are predominantly the caregivers across cultures, adding further difficulty and demand to their lives. For Black and minority ethnic (BME) women, there are additional dimensions related to ethnic and racial status.

In this chapter, we begin by defining the key terms "ethnicity" and "culture" before exploring relationships between ethnicity, culture and women's mental health. Using an intersectional framework, we examine the greater prevalence of common mental disorders among women and the social, ethnic and cultural concomitants of their mental health. We conclude by examining implications for mental health practice, policy and research.

Ethnicity, race and culture

The terms "ethnicity," "race" and "culture" are frequently used synonymously and interchangeably in both psychiatric epidemiology and clinical practice. However, although related, there are important differences between these concepts.

Ethnicity is commonly used to denote a system in which "ethnic group" members identify and are identified on the basis of shared characteristics such as ancestry, language and political or ideological nationalism, which set them apart from other groups. Whilst closely associated and overlapping with "race," the concepts differ in that "race" refers to biologically inherited and physically differentiating characteristics, such as skin color. Therefore, although "race" is

sometimes used to highlight common genetic characteristics of all people, as in "the human race," the concept is usually deployed to emphasize perceived immutable, hierarchical differences between groups. In many cultures, skin color plays a significant role in people's social acceptance and ascribed social roles. Thus, skin color may be used as a shortcut, or cultural stereotyping, for attributing certain values and attitudes, which become further complicated by the gender of the individual.

Ethnicity is best self-ascribed (Smaje 1995). Individuals can choose the categories to which they belong and, depending on individual preference and context; ethnicity can be fixed or fluid, displayed or hidden, unlike visible phenotypic differences. In a mental health context, this is important as, despite scientific evidence for human homogeneity at a global level, the tendency to attribute hereditary causes to profound inequalities in mental health has proved stubbornly persistent (Fernando 2009). This is not to imply that biological differences do not exist. For example, in relation to physical health, there are a number of conditions that exclusively affect particular groups such as sickle cell anaemia in people of African descent and thalassemia amongst Mediterranean peoples. However, the relationship between ethnicity, culture and mental health, which is the focus of this chapter, is much less straightforward and far more highly contested. Mental illness is rooted both in the individual *and* in society – in biology *and* culture, giving rise to differing explanatory models; the understanding of which is fundamental for the provision, delivery and evaluation of effective mental healthcare (Bhui et al. 2002, Fernando 2009).

Race is a hegemonic construct. Widely deployed by colonizers in the nineteenth century, the term holds

---

Comprehensive Women's Mental Health, ed. David J. Castle and Kathryn M. Abel. Published by Cambridge University Press.
© Cambridge University Press 2016.

both biological and power connotations that allowed some groups to have power and control over others by virtue of perceived racial superiority. As a result of scientific discredit and social opprobrium of related terms "racist" and "racism," to some extent, "race" has been subsumed into the more sociopolitically acceptable "ethnicity" – a sociological and anthropologically derived concept (Fernando 2009). As people have become more mobile, whether through choice or forced migration, the result of globalization is that Western societies in particular are becoming increasingly multiracial/multiethnic. In these societies, especially Europe, North America and Australia, ethnicity, in the context of mental healthcare and research, gains salience as an important factor for identifying illness prevalence, estimating disease burden and understanding need as a basis for planning and service delivery, as well as tackling interethnic inequalities in access, provision and outcome.

"Culture" is a socially constructed concept. It may be understood as a system of ideas, values, beliefs and understandings or "ways of knowing" deployed by individuals in the context of specific social networks or relationships to order and create meaning in their interpersonal interactions (Littlewood 2001). These co-constructed meanings are not self-evident, but culturally coded, derived from shared "in group" knowledge, experience, beliefs and assumptions. Consequently, those unfamiliar with the cultural codes employed by any particular cultural group might have difficulty interpreting them. This is important in relation to mental health diagnosis and treatment in two important ways. First, services might be rendered inaccessible to potential users and their families who might have difficulty decoding service culture, which may be compounded by needing to overcome language barriers. Second, the inability of services to interpret cultural codes of ethnic minority patients can hinder effective diagnosis and care delivery on the part of practitioners thus contributing to patients and carers' dissatisfaction with services for those who gain entry.

It is important to acknowledge that individuals have multiple identities, which interact with other factors to influence their perspectives significantly. Therapeutic encounters between patients and health professionals are influenced by a range of factors such as the reason, place and expected outcome of the encounters (Rogers et al. 2001). For healthcare professionals, in addition to factors such as cultural and gender identities, place of training and place of work will shape development of professional cultural identities. When the patient's experience is explored through the lens of the "clinical culture," this may add a further complicating dimension to communication. For example, health professionals may be unaware of the effect of their "taken for granted" assumptions and interpretations on their interactions with patients. Perhaps more importantly, the individuals' cultural identities, gender, education, socioeconomic status and worldview contribute to social distance between parties on both sides of the therapeutic alliance (Fung & Lo 2012). (Also, see Chapter 1 for discussion of power in relationships.)

Almost two decades ago, Lloyd (1998) and colleagues reported that, in a study of African-Caribbeans consulting UK General Practitioners (GPs), there was little shared "understanding" between patient and physician as, despite using the same words, the meanings attributed to them differed between patient and practitioner causing dissatisfaction on the part of the patient and potential misdiagnosis by the GPs who were unaware of how comprehensively they had misinterpreted the interaction (Lloyd 1998). A recent study into the influence of race on doctors' decision-making in relation to diagnosing depression among African-Americans and African-Caribbeans in the UK, suggests little has changed (Adams et al. 2014). In these encounters, what is often overlooked is that it is not only the patient who has culturally specific, "culture-bound" ways of understanding and reporting mental illness. Practitioners, usually powerful members of the dominant culture, also have their own encoded ways of conceptualizing and reporting mental illness (Lipsedge & Littlewood 2006).

Neither cultures are fixed entities. Rather they are fluid, influencing their members and in turn being influenced by them. They are contextually responsive; constantly being reinvented and reinterpreted (Hall & Carter 2006). In this context, every emergent culture can be viewed as a strategic solution to a particular set of material circumstances. This can be seen in urban "ethnic colonies" at the heart of most major Western cities, which have emerged in response to the marginalization and exclusion of migrants. Instead of assimilation, many "South Asian," Chinese and Caribbean post-war settlers and their locally born children cluster together within tight-knit ethnic communities, organizing their lives according to the traditional values and norms of the countries from which they migrated.

Whilst there is some between-group variation, there is increasing evidence that living in areas of high ethnic density is protective of the mental health of some ethnic groups (Das-Munshi et al. 2010). In contrast, it appears that acculturation might increase their risk of mental illness (Morgan et al. 2010).

However, ethnic and cultural minorities come under pressure to integrate and adapt to what the majority society determines is acceptable. Different societies have adopted a variety of approaches. In the USA, for example, the notion of a "melting pot" has had a major impact on the identity of migrants; the UK regards itself as a "multi-cultural society" (Hall & Carter 2006). In Canada, the idea of a "rainbow nation" has been developed even though the tendency to homogenize minority groups persists (Fung & Lo 2012). In Australia, cultural classification has sometimes been on the basis of ability to speak English. Following the US example in terms of labeling ethnic groups, successive generations in the UK have adopted hyphenated identities such as "Black-British," "British-Pakistani" or "British South Asian" to indicate membership to both country of birth/residence and ancestry. These "hyphenated identities," which serve as ethno-cultural signifiers, also highlight inherent tensions in belonging to both dominant and minority cultures whose competing values and beliefs can be detrimental to individuals' mental health.

Resultant tensions and the potential for "culture confusion" or "cultural schizophrenia" might have profoundly negative effects on the mental health of ethnic minorities in general, and minority women in particular (Littlewood 2001). According to Hofstede (2001), cultures have various dimensions such as egocentric versus sociocentric, feminine/masculine, distance to the center of power, uncertainty avoidance and long- or short-term orientation. However, not all members of an egocentric culture are likely to be egocentric in the same way that not all members of sociocentric cultures are sociocentric (Hofstede 2001). Thus, therapeutic interactions must become more intricate and complex if they are to be effective in terms of cultural relevance. For example, it has been noted that egocentricity and a focus on individual rights, freedom and autonomy are central features of most contemporary Western cultures. However, in more sociocentric cultural traditions, such as South Asian and Chinese communities, egocentrism might be regarded not only as counter-cultural, but as deleterious to social relationships and the collective reciprocities inherent in kinship ties based on mutuality and security. In such communities, personal needs and freedom are usually subordinate to family and group loyalty (Mawani 2008). It has been postulated that sociocentric individuals, especially if they are isolated in egocentric cultures, without members of their cultures around them may experience certain psychiatric illnesses (Bhugra 2005, James et al. 2010). As cultural values and attribution influence illness models, thus determining what is regarded as illness (or not), and culturally sanctioned forms of help-seeking, this has important implications for service provision and individuals' ability to receive appropriate care (Brown et al. 2010, Edge & Rogers 2005).

In addition to cultural values, the potential for "culture clash" between "modern" and more "traditional" cultures as well as between individuals who may feel caught between two cultures appears inevitable (Bhugra et al. 2011). Evidence suggests this is more likely to be an issue for migrant women who may carry the responsibility not only for maintaining their own culture's values, but are also expected to impart these to their children whilst needing to modify their gender roles in line with the new cultures (Baya et al. 2008). This discrepancy between gender roles and gender role expectations might go some way to explaining some of the higher than expected rates of self-harm, suicide and para-suicide among South Asian women in the UK (Bhugra 2004).

Researching ethnicity, culture and women's mental health

Many psychiatric conditions have higher rates in different ethnic groups and cultures. A lack of space does not allow us to go into details here. For a helpful review see Kirkbride and Jones (2011). However, using research tools developed in Western societies to measure mental health variables across groups without acknowledging the potential for "category fallacy" in the resultant epidemiological data is problematic. Furthermore, understanding cultural variation is crucial if therapeutic encounters are to be engaging and fruitful (Venkatapuram 2011). It is beyond the scope of this chapter to explore the reasoning behind and the functions of psychiatric diagnosis. Suffice to say that, whilst diagnosis facilitates understanding of the health needs of populations, the "new epidemiology" must take into account multiple factors in making sense of individual experience (Venkatapuram 2011).

It has been argued that higher rates of mental illness in women might more accurately reflect the process of detection and diagnosis than the presence of illness (McMullen & Stoppard 2006, Stoppard 2000). This gains particular salience when dealing with women from minority backgrounds. From a social construction perspective, diagnosis results from the encounter between clinician and patient in which what counts as mental illness is negotiated within a wider social context (Rogers et al. 2001). This means that what is regarded as mental illness in any particular place or time is neither constant nor fixed, but rather is influenced by sociopolitical forces (Metzl 2009). Exploring the distinction between disease (which is pathology) and illness (which is the social expression of underlying distress and may or may not be directly related to pathology), it is important to recognize that onset of an illness cannot always be understood in terms of direct causation. A "web of causation" has been defined as a potential way forward (Joffe et al. 2012). This model indicates that a series of factors directly and indirectly affect the development of disease and its outcomes. Combined with cultural variations in idioms used to express distress (see Chapter 1), there arises a major challenge to researchers and clinicians alike for diagnosis and investigations in relation to the mental health of minority women.

Culturally influenced gender stereotypes of mental illness exist, providing a variety of images, labels, definitions and templates for conceptualizing what counts as normal or abnormal behavior, as mental illness (or not) and a related repertoire of behaviors ascribed to someone who is deeply distressed or disturbed. In this context, Scheff and colleagues have theorized that society operates according to "residual rules" (Scheff & Brown 2002). Whether an individual's residual rule breaking is referred to an "elder," to police or to psychiatrists can be determined by a number of factors, including resources, levels of tolerance in community and social distance between the rule breaker and agencies. Persons of lower social status, those with less supportive families or social networks and the most marginalized may be more likely to be labeled and responded to as if mentally ill when residual rule breaking becomes public (Metzl 2009). These factors influence whether or not unusual behaviors are categorized as psychiatric symptoms, deviance or something altogether different, such as a legitimate ethno-cultural or spiritual response. Even in the twenty-first century, women and ethnic minorities disproportionately occupy low-status,

low-power positions, which not only increases their vulnerability to mental illness and mental illness diagnosis, but also increases the risk of their responses to trauma, neglect and abuse being medicalized, criminalized or both (Cermele et al. 2001, Rogers et al. 2001) (See Chapter 1).

In this context, there is also often a discrepancy between what is expected of women with conflict between gender role expectations and women's own needs and expectations. Such discrepancies can cause emotional distress that may lead to psychiatric disorders (Bhugra et al. 2011). For ethnic minority women there are additional difficulties, which include experiences related to racism and misogyny in certain cultures that can exacerbate vulnerability to mental illness. However, social and cultural expectations that they prioritize the needs of their families and members of the wider community are further compounded by explanatory models of distress, thus impeding help-seeking – especially from formal mental health services, which might be regarded as socioculturally inappropriate (Edge & Mackian 2010). For example, where mental illness in general, and depression in particular, is seen as a valid response to life's "ups and downs," help is more likely to be sought from nonmedical sources if at all (Edge & Rogers 2005). Furthermore, minority women highlight the role community-level stigma plays in preventing them seeking help (Nadeem et al. 2007).

Nevertheless, in common with others, minority women seek help more readily both for themselves and others in comparison with men (Collins et al. 2008). However, in certain settings, help-seeking is heavily influenced by language barriers. Women may be accompanied to consultations by men who may choose to speak on their behalf. Sometimes children may be asked/expected to interpret for their mothers and sisters. This is both clinically and ethically questionable in all general medical consultations, but all the more problematic for psychiatric conditions – especially where sexual violence is a feature. These encounters might therefore create further tensions for women, exacerbating their distress and resulting in behaviours such as denial and avoidance. The result is that many ethnic minority women experiencing psychological distress fail to receive timely and appropriate diagnosis, care and treatment.

We now provide a brief overview of studies among minority women to illustrate some of these issues. To do so, we focus on three areas that are particularly germane for highlighting the problems specific to the mental health of minority women: depressive illness, gender-based violence and migration.

Depressive illness

The evidence on depression among minority women is inconsistent. For example, in relation to perinatal depression, the global prevalence is agreed to be around 15% (O'Hara & Swain 1996). However, this masks significant inter- and intra-ethnic differences. To illustrate, in a recent study among Israeli Arab women in northern Israel using the Edinburgh Depression Scale (EPDS) (Cox et al. 1994), 20.8% and 16.3% scored above threshold (EPDS $\geq$10) in the antenatal and postnatal periods respectively. Rates of postnatal depressive symptoms were significantly higher among Moslem compared with Druze women (19.0% vs. 13.4%; p = 0.01); higher than previously reported for Jewish Israeli women in the same region (Fisch et al. 1997), but considerably lower than among Arab Bedouin women (43% at the EPDS $\geq$10 and 26% $\geq$13) in southern Israel (Glasser et al. 2012).

As space precludes exploration of all minority groups, we contrast two visible minority groups to highlight sociocultural factors and likelihood of being diagnosed with depression and perinatal depression (see Edge 2011b for useful review of perinatal mental healthcare for minority ethnic women, highlighting shortcomings in service provision and the need for research among minority women, including white and "hidden" minorities such as Irish and traveling communities). In the UK, researchers report depression rates of 30% and above among British Pakistani mothers, which appears to take an atypical course with a tendency to become chronic and to be associated with both physical ill-health and other psychological problems (Gater et al. 2010). This may reflect alternative conceptualizations, explanatory models and expression including presentation with somatic symptoms caused by underlying psychological factors, which may not be picked up by mental health professionals.

South Asian women's social isolation, being overly controlled by their families and poor literacy are factors that have also been identified as potential contributors to increased risk of depression. In south India, in the region of Kerala, the literacy rate is over 98% among women, yet suicide rates are the highest in the Indian nation. This phenomenon has been linked to discrepancies between achievement and aspiration of highly educated women, many of whom find it difficult to find work or come under social pressure not to work after marriage (Government of India 2008). Discrepancy between women's aspirations and their lived experience as a potential trigger for depression is also implicated in findings from the UK that rates of depression among Pakistani and Bangladeshi migrant women become even higher when they start to speak English (Gask et al. 2011). However, this might not be indicative of increased prevalence *per se*. Rather, acquiring the ability to speak English provides women with the means of conceptualizing and expressing their feelings as depressive symptoms. Language acquisition for this and other migrant groups might afford better understanding of the healthcare system and increase women's likelihood of seeking help and receiving a diagnosis.

In contrast to South Asian women, who are stereotypically regarded as passive and therefore depression-prone, Black women are frequently seen as strong and aggressive, characteristics that are at odds with perceptions of depressed individuals (Edge & Rogers 2005). There is evidence that Black women internalize these views, often minimizing depressive symptoms or regarding them as a reasonable response to adversity (Beauboeuf-Lafontant 2008, Edge 2008). Consequently, these women reject depression as an existent condition among Black women, seeing it as a "White woman thing" and a sign of moral weakness (Edge 2007). This might at least partly account for low rates of diagnosed depression in Black women. It has long been noted that, in contrast to elevated rates of psychotic illness, depression rates among some Black and ethnic minority groups in the USA and UK are significantly lower than the majority communities (Williams et al. 2007). However, community-level screening in the UK (Nazroo & Sproston 2002) and research among Black women elsewhere indicates higher-than-average levels of depression and consequent untreated morbidity (Brown et al. 2010). For example, perinatal depression rates in excess of 25% have been reported among Black Brazilian (Da-Silva et al. 1998), South African (Lawrie et al. 1998) and Jamaican (Pottinger et al. 2009) women.

This growing body of evidence has led some commentators to suggest that, in addition to cultural and social barriers to help-seeking (Edge & Mackian 2010), low rates of diagnosed depression in Black women might also reflect diagnostic bias and diagnosticians' often unconscious but deeply held views about the association of certain categories of mental illness with particular groups of people. As rates of diagnosed depression among people of African descent do not reflect community levels (Sproston & Nazroo 2002), it has been suggested that clinicians' perceptions of depression as a white Western illness, requiring levels of introspection and emotional literacy available only to those occupying higher biological and social roles, precludes diagnosis in people of African descent (Metzl 2009). Instead, African Diaspora women may be regarded as more vulnerable to undifferentiated "primitive psychoses" coupled with a tendency towards violence, "conversion hysteria" or somatic disorders resulting from limited self-exploration and ability to express emotions linguistically and consequently less likely to be diagnosed with depressive illness.

In summary, Black women's mental health tends to receive little attention despite paradoxical findings of low rates of diagnosed depression and suicide despite higher rates of psychosocial risk. In contrast, there is increasing research into South Asian women's mental health, which has become synonymous with depression, suicide and self-harm. There is evidence that this might be because stereotypical views of Asian women as passive, insular and overcontrolled more readily equate with illnesses that are often regarded as resulting from "turning in on oneself." In contrast, Black women do not readily conform to the stereotypical picture of depression. This might have given rise to a belief among clinicians that Black women do not experience depression and/or self-harm. However, emerging evidence suggests that this is not the case. Not only do they experience high levels of undiagnosed and, therefore, untreated depression, they also have higher rates of self-harm than either White or South Asians, but may be less likely to receive psychiatric assessment (Cooper et al. 2010). Their absence from epidemiological data is a serious omission as research from the Caribbean suggests that suicidal behaviour and deliberate self-harm have raised serious public health concerns (Hutchinson et al. 2008).

Gender-based violence

Gender-based, interpersonal violence, although seen as a social problem, has important consequences for health (see Chapter 14). Evidence indicates that minority women are especially vulnerable to interpersonal violence. Rape and its traumatic sequelae have serious implications for women's mental health, often leading to depression, post-traumatic stress disorders (PTSD), other psychiatric disorders and problems with intimacy. In a US study, 31% of all rape victims developed PTSD. Nearly one-third (30%) of women who had been raped developed at least one major depressive episode in their lifetimes with a similar proportion (33%) reporting suicidal ideation (Kilpatrick 2000). These figures gain particular salience when related to women of color. For example, high rates of child sexual abuse (CSA: defined as incest, rape or sexual coercion before age 18) have been documented in community samples of Black women recruited from Boston (34.1%) and Chicago (65%). In adulthood, 22% of the Black women in the National Intimate Partner and Sexual Violence Survey (NISVS) reported that they had been raped at some point in their lives. The NISVS also revealed that 41% of Black women experienced some form of sexual coercion or unwanted sexual contact. These prevalence rates translate to an estimated 3.1 million Black rape victims and 5.9 million Black survivors of other forms of sexual violence. Persistent stereotypes of Black women's sexuality, rooted in slavery and colonialization and women's inability to pay for high-quality support, contributes to an unsympathetic service response thus deterring women from seeking help and increasing the likelihood of chronic mental health problems (West & Johnson 2013).

Intimate personal violence is multidimensional and incorporates narrow as well as broad definitions creating epidemiological data that are not entirely comparable. Narrow definitions produce lower rates and broader definitions higher rates. A World Health Organisation (WHO) multination study from 15 centers in 10 countries, reported that life time prevalence of physical or sexual violence for ever-partnered women varied from 15% to 71% (WHO 2013). A 12-month prevalence rate varied from 4% to 54%. Among ever-partnered women in the population rates of physical violence varied from 4% in Japan to 49% in Peru (Howard et al. 2013). As the research in this area is still emerging, the correlates of gender-based violence and ethnic minority status are yet to be theorized. However, forced and arranged marriages, social isolation (especially when coupled with language barriers), low socioeconomic and educational status, which make women more vulnerable to being controlled by men, are likely to be among crucial factors. For women from collectivist cultures, where patriarchal ideology emphasizes the dominant role of the husband or father and subordination of individual views or needs in favor of family/kinship ties, women may be understandably reluctant to disclose intimate partner and/or sexual violence – especially as doing so risks ostracism and stigma not only for women but also their children and extended families (Mason & Hyman 2008). Accordingly, good practice suggests that partners, friends and family members should not be used for interpretation when these women access services (NICE 2014). Wherever possible, professional female interpreters should be used and information and educational leaflets should be available in both relevant languages and non-language-based formats (Agnew-Davies 2013, Trevillion & Agnew-Davies 2013). Also see Chapter 14.

Female genital mutilation (FGM) is common practice in many non-Western cultures and specifically affects women from minority backgrounds. Most Western societies are ill-equipped to deal either with the act or the process by which it is brought about, for example, girls being taken abroad to undergo FGM. Although there are no robust epidemiological data, the available evidence suggests that the scale of the problem is significant. In the UK, a Department of Health–funded project reported that, in 2001, there were almost 66,000 women living in England and Wales who had undergone FGM with a further estimated 16,000 girls under the age of 15 at high risk (Dorkenoo et al. 2001). In the absence of good quality evidence, the long-term impact of FGM cannot be estimated although anecdotal evidence suggesting potential problems with both physical and psychological aspects of childbirth such as increased vulnerability to perinatal mental illness and women being retraumatized. FGM is a reflection of social attitudes to sex and female sexuality among some cultural groups. In these cultures, it is not uncommon for women also to undergo hymen reconstruction in order to be perceived to be virgins at the time of marriage. This process further distorts evidence of the true extent of sexual violence against women including the possibility that many of these women may have been raped or be victims of incest (WHO 2013). Research is urgently needed better to elucidate the scale of the problem, understand the impact on women and girls, and inform appropriate service development and delivery.

Trafficking also particularly affects minority refugee and asylum-seeking women. Accurate data for rates of psychiatric illness among affected women are not available as women who have been trafficked are often underrepresented in studies. The problems they face are still not fully understood but it is clear that trafficking, forced prostitution, sexual abuse and being rendered stateless can all lead to a range of psychiatric problems. These factors contribute to poor mental health, which WHO cites as the dominant and persistent adverse health effect of human trafficking. Specific psychological sequelae include depression, PTSD, anxiety disorders, increased risk of suicide and somatic conditions including disabling physical pain and dysfunction. Additionally, there is increased risk of co-morbidity among victims of sex-trafficking. Forced or coerced use of drugs and alcohol as a means of controlling individuals and increasing profits is frequently reported, and victims might use drugs and alcohol as means of coping with being trafficked (WHO 2012).

Chandra (2011) points out that increasing numbers of women are migrating and it is likely that migration itself has a differential effect on women compared to men. She describes specific mental health difficulties for domestic workers in various countries that may lead to exploitation – physical and sexual – and enforced cultural isolation. Furthermore, disparity between aspiration and achievement may well affect their self-esteem and increase risk of depression.

Sexual and other forms of gender-based violence and exploitation affect all women. However, Black and ethnic minority women are particularly vulnerable. Although all women who have experienced violence, including rape and being trafficked, will have some difficulties in common; assessment and intervention needs to take cultural aspects into account. Women should be interviewed in private with a female chaperone, if necessary. Clinical assessment should include thorough questioning about financial independence, support networks, confidants and views about family honor as these will provide insight into the kinds of help and support that affected women are likely to find acceptable. Ideally, specifically trained, culturally competent therapists and appropriate services should be commissioned to meet the particular needs of women affected by gender-based violence. See also Chapter 14.

Migration

At the outset, it is important to acknowledge the heterogeneity of migrants. Whilst some migrants enter new countries by choice and/or active recruitment by others on the basis of their skills and expertise, others are forced to do so by economic or political circumstances in their country of origin. Still others are transported as victims of trafficking. In a 2004 study of independent and sponsored migrants to Quebec, Canada, half the respondents cited the political situation in their countries as the primary reason for migration (Rousseau & Drapeau 2004). Minority women, who might have less choice in the decision to migrate because of the patriarchal nature of their countries of origin, might experience migration as a form of trauma, thus making them vulnerable to mental health problems, depression and anxiety in particular. Women who become refugees or asylumseekers face additional stresses as a result of their migration status (or lack thereof), which means they have limited or no access to the services, rights and legal protections afforded to members of the majority population or settled migrants. Language barriers and lack of awareness of the cultural customs and norms of the countries to which they have migrated contribute to social isolation, increased vulnerability to mental health problems and challenges in accessing services (Mawani 2008).

Additionally, women's central role in maintaining family and kinship networks, including pressure to send money home and to sponsor others to join them, whilst raising their children without access to the support of extended families can be extremely stressful. Women report that these stresses negatively impact their marital relationships, especially where there are financial worries and/or women become the chief or only sources of family income, which generates tensions from reversal of gender-based roles within their culture. The possibility of divorce and family breakdown represent further stressors for women with pressure to remain in situations that are detrimental to their mental health for fear this would bring shame, stigma and potential financial ruin to their families (Chandra 2011).

Not surprisingly, women in these circumstances report lack of support (practical and emotional) and the absence of a close, confiding relationship; these are known triggers of common mental disorders such as anxiety and depression, perinatal depression in particular. For some women, their experience takes the form of "cultural bereavement" – grieving for the loss of home and shared cultural identity, which have been shown to be protective of mental health (James et al. 2010). In this context, women report facing "triple jeopardy" of belonging to marginalized communities, namely, experiencing racism, sexism and discrimination on the basis of their migrant status (Ardiles et al. 2008). The social exclusion and discrimination that both settled and migrant women face may be exacerbated by low socioeconomic status resulting from under/unemployment, low self-esteem and a sense of hopelessness emanating from perceived lack of control and powerlessness with deleterious consequences for their mental health (Mawani 2008). Clearly, these factors do not operate in isolation but overlap and intersect with each other in ways that increase minority women's vulnerability to onset of mental illness.

Ethnicity, culture and women's mental health: intersectional perspectives

The relationship between gender, ethnicity, culture and mental health is complex and multifaceted. "Intersectionality" affords a theoretical framework for examining these intersections in the specific context of minority women's mental health. Rooted in feminist and critical race theory, "intersectionality" is frequently embraced by both anti-racist and feminist scholars. Emerging in the last decades of the twentieth century, with its focus on problematizing and ultimately rejecting simple race/gender binaries, intersectionality became a powerful tool for examining and theorizing the multidimensional ways in which ethnicity and gender interact to shape Black women's experiences (Nash 2008). From a politico-theoretical perspective, intersectionality also acknowledges the existence of (multiple) socially constructed identities and seeks to understand the mechanisms by which their interaction shapes experiences of exclusion, oppression and subordination (Collins 2000). This is particularly germane for BME women who are so often "othered" by the experience of multiple forms of oppression and marginalization (Egharevba 2001, Ladson-Billings 2000).

Adopting an intersectional standpoint to scholarship and clinical research facilitates a shift away from a-contextual examinations of unidimensional variables towards alternative methodologies and ways of seeing (Christians et al. 2000) that allow more meaningful examination and understanding of the dynamic processes that influence individuals' lived experiences. Intersectionality encourages and enables scholars to go beyond epidemiology and other positivist approaches, actively seeking meanings beyond numeric values and "variables" such as "ethnicity" and "gender" in order to examine their impact on individuals and the various spheres that they inhabit. Intersectionality is therefore a useful heuristic for exploring the interrelationship between ethnicity, culture and women's mental health.

Examining the UK's two most researched ethnic minorities in relation to mental health, it appears that persistent stereotypes within psychiatry place Black Caribbean men and South Asian women in a binary position where the former are seen as being "out of control" and the latter as "private and too controlled" (Littlewood 2001). UK mental health service delivery and related research among Black Caribbeans, therefore, tends to focus on men and on conditions that are associated with dangerousness such schizophrenia and psychosis (Henderson et al. 2014). Mental health professionals' stereotyping of Caribbeans as "Big-Black-and-dangerous" (Ferguson 1993) means that resources are directed towards coercive interventions for men in secondary and tertiary care with relatively little attention being paid to addressing the mental health needs of Black and other minority women in primary care (Kotecha 2008).

Such perceptions might partly account for the large volume of research into perinatal depression among South Asian women. In terms of clinical practice and diagnosis, cultural perceptions and the available evidence base might sensitize practitioners to becoming alert to the possibility of perinatal depression among South Asian women, but not in Black and other minority groups (Edge 2010a, b). Specifically, Primary Care Physicians/General Practitioners (GPs) and others may regard contextual factors as influential and thus may be more likely to rely on judgments about coping and the extent to which social roles differentially affect women's mental state. This in itself may be influenced by stereotypical expectations of Black and other minority ethnic women and this may partly explain contrasting very high and low rates of depression diagnosis in such individuals despite similar psychosocial risks.

An intersectional approach is crucial, if we are to arrive at a more nuanced understanding of the differential impact of risk factors for individuals and groups of women and take these into account when developing and delivering mental health services. For example, whilst most migrant women might experience discrimination, the impact is likely to differ greatly. Racism might be experienced on three levels: institutional, personal and internalized. From this standpoint, not all minority women will experience institutional racism, the "differential access to goods, services, and opportunities of society by race" (Jones 2000), some will be shielded by factors such as skin color (for example, women migrating between European countries or North America), high socioeconomic status, education and language proficiency – factors that might also facilitate cultural understanding and acceptance by the majority population.

Indeed, although in the minority, being White Western in most non-Western countries affords women a higher status than similar women in their native countries. In contrast, minority women (particularly of African and Asian descent) are more likely to occupy low-status positions when they migrate. Lower socioeconomic status coupled with ethnocultural identities linked to the social determinants of mental illness (such as poverty and social isolation) not only place them at potentially increased risk of mental illness, but also serve as barriers to accessing care and treatment from statutory services. As a consequence, minority women's mental health provision in primary care is often delivered via voluntary sector agencies, services that rarely have long-term, sustainable funding. In times of financial constraint, these services are especially vulnerable. This is particularly deleterious to the mental health of minority women whose socioeconomic status means they are more likely than other groups to need mental health services. However, perceptions and negative experiences of services coupled with internalized racism and potential language barriers might create/reinforce fear and mistrust of mainstream mental health services (Edge 2011a, Henderson et al. 2014), rendering them inaccessible to ethnic minority women.

Conclusions

Hofstede (2001) postulates that cultures have 5 separate dimensions. For the purposes of the present chapter, we focus on his dimension of masculine and feminine cultures. Masculine cultures suggest that men in these cultures are more interested in earnings and career advancement whereas women see friendly atmosphere, position security, cooperation and physical conditions in their workplace as more important. Using such a "masculinity index" as a measure of national differences, he found that the role men play in high masculine index settings is very different from that played by women. These settings have higher stress, and a belief in individual decisions and work is very central, whereas in low masculine index settings almost the opposite is true. Thus, unemployment and gender role expectations will impact the mental health of minority men and women differently. In high masculine index societies, there is a strong gender differentiation in the social-ization of children thus perpetuating the gender roles. Both boys and girls may learn to be ambitious (Hof-stede 2001, p. 306), but the opportunities for girls to develop and achieve their ambitions are more limited. In these societies and cultures, family is important and traditional marriage concepts mean that mar-riages occur early and may well be arranged. There are also key differences in the work situations and behaviors, thereby creating (a sense of) male control. Thus, when women from such cultures migrate to less masculine cultures their behavior may change, creating a conflict with their male coun-terparts. In addition, there are clear religious and sexuality related differences. Such differences can therefore contribute to social expectations for women to behave in particular ways thereby creating addi-tional stress.

There is no doubt that women can and do play a significant role in identifying distress among family members and seeking help for them, tending to ignore their own needs. This perspective was high-lighted in the seminal work of Brown and Harris (1978) on depression. They found that women's psy-chological distress was often underreported because caring responsibilities meant women lacked time to seek help on their own behalf and/or were more likely to put the help-seeking needs of others above their own (Brown and Harris 1978), perhaps increasing duration of untreated illness among themselves.

Implications for policy and practice

I. Overall psychopathology must be seen in the context of cultural and gender roles and gender-role expectations. For example, among South Asian women in the UK, rates of depression are significantly higher and attempted suicide between the ages of 18–24 have been shown to be nearly 3 times those of their British counterparts. Culture-conflict is thought to play a significant role. Conflict may arise between families and women who are beginning to individuate and develop their own identities, identities that are not necessarily "traditional" or close to those held by their parents or other key members of their communities. Among migrant women, cultural bereavement may be noted, which reflects losses of place, people and property. These factors must be taken into consideration when commissioning and delivering women's mental healthcare in multicultural settings. Failure to do so might not mean only that some women fail to receive the care and treatment they need; services might also inadvertently create/reinforce perceptions of institutional racism in mental healthcare.

II. Academics, policy makers and services need to take cultural and ethnic phenomena into account when considering causation. This may mean reviewing overall rates of pathology in a population where cultural differences may be seen as "causing cultural variation" in rates and diagnoses. A major shift in clinical management and understanding also needs to occur so that the concept of a "web of causation" as described earlier is considered, rather than single factor etiological models.

III. Acknowledging and seeking to understand, the different effects of intersections between ethnicity, gender, culture and other mediating factors is fundamental to delivering services capable of meeting the needs of the range of women in a multicultural society. Such nuanced understanding in service design and delivery would not only affect the mental health of the visible minority women (those who stand out by virtue of skin color or dress), but is also important for 'hidden' minorities. For example, white Irish and European women might 'look like' the majority communities, but may have very different cultural beliefs and practices that contribute to the maintenance and restoration of their mental health. A key concern in this context is the role of spirituality and religion. This may often become 'pathologized' within mainstream mental health services. Ethnic minority communities in Western societies tend to have higher rates of religious adherence than the majority population; therefore, fostering alliance with major religious groups might be an effective means both of delivering mental health education and low-level interventions (such as counseling) in nonthreatening, accessible environments, as well as reducing the stigma in these communities, which represents a major barrier to women accessing care and treatment.

IV. "Culturally competent care" has been an aspiration for many mental health service commissioners and providers. Given the number of ethnic groups and increasing rates of interracial relationships, it may be time to rethink this strategy. Whilst it is crucial that services acknowledge variation in presentation and need, a move towards cultural awareness and developing

"culturally capable" care might prove a more attainable goal. By "cultural-capability," we mean that practitioners should develop the skills and confidence to ask culturally relevant questions and to work with communities to take greater responsibility for managing their mental health. Various approaches such as developing cultural brokers, cultural liaison services and community interpreters have been adopted by organizations like the Centre for Addiction and Mental Health (CAMH) in Canada.

V. Whatever strategy is adapted, the most important message for service delivery is ensuring that the service user and her family are at the core of healthcare delivery with service providers taking individual cultural values into account.

References

Adams, A., Vail, L., Buckingham, C. D., Kidd, J., Weich, S. & Roter, D. (2014) Investigating the influence of African American and African Caribbean race on primary care doctors' decision making about depression. *Social Science & Medicine* 116, 161–168.

Agnew-Davies, R. (2013) Identifying domestic violence experienced by mental health service users. In *Domestic violence and mental health* (Howard, L., Feder, G. & Agnew-Davies, R., eds.). RCPsych Press, London, pp. 29–48.

Ardiles, P., Dennis, C-L. & Ross, L. (2008) Postpartum depression among immigrant women. In *Working with immigrant women: Issues and strategies for mental health professionals* (Guruge, S. & Collins, E., eds.). CAMH, Toronto.

Baya, K., Simich, L. & Bukhari, S. (2008) Women at the centre of changing families: A study of Sudanese women's resettlement experiences. In *Working with immigrant women: Issues and strategies for mental health professionals* (Guruge, S. & Collins, E., eds.). CAMH, Toronto, pp. 157–176.

Beauboeuf-Lafontant, T. (2008) Listening past the lies that make us sick: A voice-centered analysis of strength and depression among Black women. *Qualitative Sociology* 31, 391–406.

Bhugra, D. (2004) *Culture and self-harm.* Psychology Press, Hove.

Bhugra, D. (2005) Cultural identities and cultural congruency: A new model for evaluating mental distress in immigrants. *Acta Psychiatrica Scandinavica* 111, 84–93.

Bhugra, D., Wojcik, W. & Gupta, S. (2011) Cultural bereavement: Culture shock and culture conflict – adjustment and reaction. In *Migration and mental health* (Bhugra, D. & Gupta, S., eds.). Cambridge University Press, Cambridge, pp. 139–148.

Bhui, K., Fenton, S., Grewal, I., Karlsen, S., Lloyd, K., Nazroo, J., O'Connor, W. & Sproston, K. (2002) *Ethnic differences in the context and experience of psychiatric illness: A qualitative study.* The Stationery Office, London, p. 1.

Brown, G. & Harris, T. (1978) *Social origins of depression: A study of psychiatric disorder in women.* Tavistock Publications, London.

Brown, J. S., Casey, S. J., Bishop, A. J., Prytys, M., Whittinger, N. & Weinman, J. (2010) How black African and white British women perceive depression and help-seeking: A pilot vignette study. *International Journal of Social Psychiatry.* OnlineFirst, published on March 2, 2010 as doi:2010.1177/0020764009357400.

Cermele, J. A., Daniels, S. & Anderson, K. L. (2001) Defining normal: Constructions of race and gender in the DSM-IV Casebook. *Feminism & Psychology* 11, 229.

Chandra, P. (2011) Mental health issues related to migration in women. In *Migration and mental health* (Bhugra, D. & Gupta, S., eds.). Cambridge University Press, Cambridge, pp. 209–219.

Christians, C. G., Denzin, N. K. & Lincoln, Y. S. (2000) Ethics and politics in qualitative research. In *Handbook of qualitative research.* Sage Publications, Inc, Thousand Oaks, CA, pp. 133–157.

Collins, E., Shakya, Y. B., Guruge, S. & Santos, E. J. (2008) Services for women: Access, equity and quality. In *Working with immigrant women: Issues and strategies for mental health professionals* (Guruge, S. & Collins, E., eds.). MH, Toronto.

Collins, P. H. (2000) *Black feminist thought: Knowledge, consciousness, and the politics of empowerment.* Routledge, New York.

Cooper, J., Murphy, E., Webb, R., Hawton, K., Bergen, H., Waters, K. & Kapur, N. (2010) Ethnic differences in self-harm, rates, characteristics and service provision: Three-city cohort study. *The British Journal of Psychiatry* 197, 212–218.

Cox, J., Cox, J. & Holden, J. (1994) Origins and development of the 10-item Edinburgh Postnatal Depression Scale. In *Perinatal Psychiatry: Use and misuse of the Edinburgh Postnatal Depression Scale.* Gaskell, London.

Da-Silva, V. A., Moraes-Santos, A. R., Carvalho, M. S., Martins, M.L.P. & Teixeira, N. A. (1998) Prenatal and postnatal depression among low income Brazilian women. *Brazillian Journal of Medical and Biological Research*, 31(6), 799–804.

Das-Munshi, J., Becares, L., Dewey, M. E. & Prince, M. J. (2010) Understanding the effect of ethnic density on mental health: Multi-level investigation of survey data from England. *British Medical Journal*, 341, c5367.

Dorkenoo, E., Morison, L. & Macfarlane, A. (2001) *A statistical study to estimate the prevalence of female genital mutilation in England and Wales.* Foundation for Women's Health, Research and Development (FORWARD); The London School of Hygiene and Tropical Medicine; The Department of Midwifery, City University, London.

Edge, D. (2007) Is perinatal depression a 'white woman thing'? In *Challenges for midwives* (vol. 2) (Richens, Y., ed.). Quay Books, London, pp. 183–200.

Edge, D. (2008) "We don't see Black women here": An exploration of the absence of Black Caribbean Women from clinical and epidemiological data on perinatal depression in the UK. *Midwifery* 24, 379–389.

Edge, D. (2010a) Falling through the net — Black and minority ethnic women and perinatal mental healthcare: Health professionals' views. *General Hospital Psychiatry* 32, 17–25.

Edge, D. (2010b) Perinatal mental health care for black and minority ethnic (BME) women: A scoping review of provision in England. *Ethnicity and Inequalities in Health and Social Care* 3, 24–32.

Edge, D. (2011a) "It's leaflet, leaflet, leaflet then 'see you later'" – Black Caribbean women's perceptions of perinatal mental healthcare in the UK. *British Journal of General Practice* 61, 256–262.

Edge, D. (2011b) *Perinatal mental health of Black and minority ethnic women: A review of current provision in England, Scotland and Wales.* Department of Health, London.

Edge, D. & Mackian, S. (2010) Ethnicity and mental health encounters in primary care: Help-seeking and help-giving for perinatal depression among Black Caribbean women in the UK. *Ethnicity & Health* 15, 93–111.

Edge, D. & Rogers, A. (2005) "Dealing with it": Black Caribbean women's response to adversity and psychological distress associated with pregnancy, childbirth, and early motherhood. *Social Science and Medicine* 61, 15–25.

Egharevba, I. (2001) Researching an-"other" minority ethnic community: Reflections of a black female researcher on the intersection of race, gender and other power positions on the research process. *International Journal of Social Research Methodology* 4, 225.

Ferguson, G. (1993) Editorial: Big, black and dangerous. *Community Psychiatric Nursing Journal*, 4–5.

Fernando, S. (2009) Inequalities and the politics of "race" in mental health. In *Mental health in a multi-ethnic society – a multidisciplinary handbook* (Fernando, S. & Keating, F., eds.). Routledge, London, pp. 42–57.

Fisch, R. Z., Tadmor, O. P., Dankner, R. & Diamant, Y. Z. (1997) Postnatal depression: A prospective study of its prevalence, incidence and psychosocial determinants in an Israeli sample. *Journal of Obstetrics and Gynaecological Research* 23, 547.

Fung, K. & Lo, T. (2012) Culturally competent practice and management of mental health in primary care. In *Collaborative mental health: An advanced manual for primary care professionals* (Khenti, A., Sapag, J. C., Mohamoud, S. & Ravindran, A., eds.). CAMH, Toronto, pp. 29–48.

Gask, L., Aseem, S., Waquas, A. & Waheed, W. (2011) Isolation, feeling "stuck" and loss of control: Understanding persistence of depression in British Pakistani women. *Journal of Affective Disorders* 128, 49–55.

Gater, R., Waheed, W., Husain, N., Tomenson, B., Aseem, S. & Creed, F. (2010) Social intervention for British Pakistani women with depression: Randomised controlled trial. *The British Journal of Psychiatry* 197, 227–233.

Glasser, S., Tanous, M., Shihab, S., Goldman, N., Ziv, A. & Kaplan, G. (2012) Perinatal depressive symptoms among Arab women in northern Israel. *Matern Child Health Journal* 16, 1197–1205.

Government of India (2008) *Kerala Development Report Planning Commission*, New Dehli.

Hall, S. P. & Carter, R. T. (2006) The relationship between racial identity, ethnic identity, and perceptions of racial discrimination in an Afro-Caribbean descent sample. *Journal of Black Psychology* 32, 155–175.

Henderson, C., Williams, P., Gabbidon, J., Farrelly, S., Schaumann, O., Hatch, S., Thornicroft, G., Bhugra,

D. & Clement, S. (2014) Mistrust of mental health services: ethnicity, hospital admission and unfair treatment. In *Epidemiology and psychiatric science*. Cambridge University Press, Cambridge.

Hofstede, G. (2001) *Culture's consequences*. Sage, Thousand Oaks, CA.

Howard, L., Feder, G. & Agnew-Davies, R. (2013) *Domestic violence and mental health*. RCPsych Press, London.

Hutchinson, G., Bruce, C. & Simmons, V. (2008) Increasing incidence of admissions to a general hospital for deliberate self-harm in Trinidad. *West Indian Med Journal* 57, 346–351.

James, C., Este, D., Thomas, W. B., Benjamin, A., Lloyd, B. & Turner, T. (2010) *Race and well-being*. Fernwood Publishing, Halifax & Winnipeg.

Joffe, M., Gambhir, M., Chadeau-Hyam, M. & Vineis, P. (2012) Causal diagrams in systems epidemiology. *Emerging Themes in Epidemiology*, 9 (1), doi: 10.1186/1742-7622-9-1.

Jones, C. (2000) Levels of racism: A theoretical framework and a gardener's tale. *American Journal of Public Health* 90, 1212–1215.

Kilpatrick, D. G. (2000) *The mental health impact of rape*. National Violence Against Women Prevention Research Center, Medical University of South Carolina, South Carolina.

Kirkbride, J. & Jones, P. (2011) Epidemiological aspects of migration and mental illness. In *Migration and mental health* (Bhugra, D. & Gupta, S., eds.). Cambridge University Press, Cambridge, pp. 15–43.

Kotecha, N. (2008) Black and minority ethnic women. In *Mental health in a multi-ethnic society: a multidisciplinary handbook* (Fernando, S. & Keating, F. eds.). Routledge, London: pp. 58–70

Ladson-Billings, G. (2000) Racialised discourses and ethnic epistemologies. In *Handbook of qualitative research – second edition* (Denzin, N. & Lincoln, Y., eds.). Sage Publications, Inc., Thousand Oaks, CA.

Lawrie, T. A., Hofmeyer, G. J., de Jager, M. & Berk, M. (1998) Validation of the Edinburgh Postnatal Depression Scale on a cohort of South African women. *South African Medical Journal* 88, 1340–1344.

Lipsedge, M. & Littlewood, R. (2006) *Aliens & Alienists: Ethnic minorities and psychiatrists*. Taylor & Francis, London.

Littlewood, R. (2001) "Culture" in the field of race and mental health. In *Health and ethnicity* (Macbeth, H. & Shetty, P., eds.). Taylor & Francis, London, pp. 209–222.

Lloyd, K. (1998) Ethnicity, social inequality, and mental illness. *British Medical Journal* 316, 1763–1770.

Mason, R. & Hyman, I. (2008) Intimate partner violence among immirant and refugee women. In *Working with immigrant women: Issues and strategies for mental health professionals* (Guruge, S. & Collins, E., eds.). CAMH, Toronto, pp. 279–300.

Mawani, F. N. (2008) Social determinants of depression among immigrant and refugee women. In *Working with immigrant women: Issues and strategies for mental health professionals* (Guruge, S. & Collins, E., eds.). CAMMH, Toronto, pp. 67–87.

McMullen, L. M. & Stoppard, J. M. (2006) Women and depression: A case study of the influence of feminism in Canadian psychology. *Feminism Psychology* 16, 273–288.

Metzl, J. M. (2009) *The protest psychosis: How schizophrenia became a Black disease*. Beacon Press, Boston.

Morgan, C., Charalambides, M., Hutchinson, G. & Murray, R. M.

(2010) Migration, ethnicity, and psychosis: Toward a sociodevelopmental model. *Schizophrenia Bulletin* 36, 655–664.

Nadeem, E., Lange, J. M., Edge, D., Fongwa, M., Belin, T. & Miranda, J. (2007) Does stigma keep poor young immigrant and U.S.-born Black and Latina women from seeking mental health care? *Psychiatry Serv* 58, 1547–1554.

Nash, J. C. (2008) Re-thinking intersectionality. *Feminist Review* 89, 1–15.

Nazroo, J. & Sproston, K. (2002) *Introduction: Ethnic Minority Psychiatric Illness Rates (EMPIRIC)* (Sproston, K. & Nazroo, J., eds.). The Stationery Office, London, p. 9.

NICE (2014) *Domestic violence and abuse: How health services, social care and the organisations they work with can respond effectively. Issued: NICE public health guidance 50*. National Institute for Health & Care Excellence (NICE), London.

O'Hara, M. & Swain, A. (1996) Rates and risk of postpartum depression – a meta-analysis. *International Review of Psychiatry* 8, 37–54.

Pottinger, A. M., Trotman-Edwards, H. & Younger, N. (2009) Detecting depression during pregnancy and associated lifestyle practices and concerns among women in a hospital-based obstetric clinic in Jamaica. *General Hospital Psychiatry* 31, 254–261.

Rogers, A., May, C. & Oliver, D. (2001) Experiencing depression, experiencing the depressed: The separate worlds of patients and doctors. *Journal of Mental Health* 10, 317.

Rousseau, C. & Drapeau, A. (2004) Premigration exposure to political violence among independet immigrants and its association with emotional distress. *Journal of Nervous and Mental Disease* 192, 852–856.

Scheff, T. J. & Brown, P. (2002) Schizophrenia as ideology. In

Radical psychology. Tavistock, London, p. 46.

Smaje, C. (1995) *Health, 'race' and ethnicity: Making sense of the evidence.* King's Fund Institute, London.

Sproston, K. & Nazroo, J. (2002) *Ethnic minority psychiatric illness rates in the community (EMPIRIC) Quantitative Report. National Centre for Social Research on behalf of DoH,* The Stationery Office, Norwich.

Stoppard, J. M. (2000) *Understanding Depression-Feminist Social Constructionist Approaches.* Routledge, London.

Trevillion, K. & Agnew-Davies, R. (2013) Interventions for mental health service users who experience domestic violence. In *Domestic violence and mental health* (Howard, L., Feder, G. & Agnew-Davies, R., eds.). RCPsych Press, London, pp. 64–77.

Venkatapuram, S. (2011) *Social justice.* Polity Press, Cambridge.

West, C. & Johnson, K. (2013) *Sexual violence in the lives of African American women.* National Resource Center on Domestic Violence, Harrisburg, PA.

WHO (2012) *Understanding and addressing violence against women:*

Human trafficking. World Health Organisation (WHO), Geneva.

WHO (2013) *Responding to intimate partner violence and sexual violence against women.* World Health Organization (WHO), Geneva.

Williams, D. R., Gonzalez, H. M., Neighbors, H., Nesse, R., Abelson, J. M., Sweetman, J. & Jackson, J. S. (2007) Prevalence and distribution of Major Depressive Disorder in African Americans, Caribbean Blacks, and Non-Hispanic Whites: Results from the National Survey of American Life. *Archives of General Psychiatry* 64, 305–315.

Chapter

3

Women as caregivers

Peter V. Rabins

Throughout the world, women are the primary providers of care and support to the chronically ill. Caregiving, defined as providing support to an individual who could not live independently without that care, is divided into formal care, where payment is given as a professional to provide care, and informal, where payment is not provided. This chapter will focus on nonprofessionals, who are usually relatives or close friends. The terms caregiver and carer will be used interchangeably to refer to the person providing this care and support.

In most parts of the world, at least 70–80% of carers are female. For people of older age, relatives are their most common carers. Children, daughters and daughters-in-law are most common, followed by spouses, then by other relatives such as nieces. For children, carers are most commonly mothers and when the family is a lone parent family, the overwhelming majority of parents again are mothers rather than fathers. This pattern appears common throughout developed and less developed world economies, although it is more gendered the less well-developed the economy. Within families one person is often the primary provider, but shared provision of care is also common.

Those requiring caregiving range across the life span from infants to the very old. The rapid rise in life expectancy over the past century in developed countries and the more recent rise in developing countries means that there will be a significant increase in the number of caregivers for dependent elders. Declining birth rates in many countries suggests a dearth of available family carers in future decades at the same time as government resources for supporting such care are being challenged.

Caregiving implies a broad range of activities. These include the provision of physical care, health monitoring, emotional support, financial support, medical decision making, out-of-home placement decisions and environmental modification. Caregiving often occurs in the context of family relationships and the conceptualization varies significantly by cultural and ethnic background. Nonetheless, there are generalizations that seem true across many groups and many different circumstances (Murray et al., 1999).

The increasing participation of women in the formal workforce has increased the challenges that women face in being the primary providers of caregiving services because the dual expectations at work and in caregiving increase time pressure and emotional stress (Odanker, 1990). The fragmentation and shrinking of family size has further increased the multiple demands placed on female carers. Neither of these trends has been accompanied by a changing expectation in most cultural groups that women be the primary care providers.

Challenges of caregiving

Emotional distress. A large literature worldwide has demonstrated that women who are carers have higher rates of emotional distress than matched noncarers. Rates vary, but are often two to three times higher in caregivers, meaning that 20–40% of carers are experiencing emotional distress related to their caregiving role (Brodaty & Arasaratnam, 2012). However, the vast majority of these studies depend on nonrepresentative samples of those providing care because they have identified study participants who volunteered to participate in a survey, are members of a disease-related organization, or responded to an advert or poster seeking participants. The very few representative samples find significantly lower rates of distress (Piercy et al., 2013).

Comprehensive Women's Mental Health, ed. David J. Castle and Kathryn M. Abel. Published by Cambridge University Press.
© Cambridge University Press 2016.

The term "depression" is often used to describe the emotional distress associated with caregiving, but most studies use scales that measure symptoms associated with depression or demoralization. Fewer than half, and often much less than half, of persons in such studies who are described as "depressed" meet criteria for clinical or major depression. Rather, they report higher levels of general distress, low energy, discouragement and social isolation.

A small body of literature compares female to male carers. Again, such studies have the flaw of comparing two groups that are differentially selected. Most male caregivers have "volunteered" for the role; on the other hand, a significant proportion of women have taken on the role because it is expected societally or culturally, because of their position in the family, because of proximity to the ill person, or because of a felt obligation. The common finding that female carers have higher rates of emotional distress than males might reflect the fact that the factors leading a person to become the identified caregiver are different for females and males (Fitting et al., 1986). (See Chapter 1 on gendered social roles.)

Other associated adverse outcomes. Some studies have found adverse health and longevity outcomes in caregivers (Schulz & Beach, 1999). Most report adverse effects on social well-being. Many women carers are either working in a paid job at the same time as they are the identified carer or report that they have had to stop working or limit their paid work because of the caregiving role. These paid work/caregiving dilemmas are much more common in female than male caregivers (Odanker, 1990).

Correlates of adverse outcomes. Correlates of negative outcomes in caregivers are similar to those for poorer emotional well-being in the community at large. Social isolation, low availability of social supports, a feeling that no alternative is available, a self-reported lack of meaning related to the caregiving role, and fewer available economic and support resources are common correlates of emotional distress in caregivers. The few studies that have examined personality characteristics have found that individuals who experience more emotional distress in general (sometimes referred to as "neuroticism") are at greater risk of emotional distress when in the caregiving role. An extensive literature has examined coping styles in relationship to emotional state during caregiving. There are no widely consistent findings, but carers who use problem solving approaches may do better than those who use emotion-focused coping styles (Tschanz et al., 2013).

Help for carers

More than 50 trials demonstrate the efficacy of caregiver interventions in reducing carer emotional distress (Brodaty & Arasaratnam 2012). The preponderance of evidence demonstrates that interventions broadly categorized as either emotional support-based and information-based both improve caregiver outcomes. Few studies combine the two, but those that have done so tend to support the idea that the combination might be more efficacious. A meta-analysis of non-pharmacological studies for neuropsychiatric symptoms of dementia by Brodaty and Arasaratnam (2012) identified 23 well-designed studies, 16 of which were randomized clinical trials. Their findings for this specific disorder can likely be generalized to caregiving more broadly. They identified six general categories of studies: skills training, education, activity planning, environmental design, caregiver support and self-care. While there are no population-based effectiveness trials, this strong efficacy trial database demonstrates that we know how to help caregivers deliver better care and to do better emotionally, at least for the 6–12 month follow-up period of most trials.

Positive outcomes

A small literature has identified positive outcomes associated with caregiving. About one-third of carers report predominantly positive emotional experiences associated with caregiving. A few studies have found that carers tend to report a mix of adverse and positive outcomes (Carbonneau, 2010).

In addition, longitudinal studies tend to demonstrate that caregivers of persons with chronic progressive illnesses such as dementia and Parkinson Disease do not do worse over time with respect to mental health outcomes, even though the disease and the symptoms suffered by the ill person are progressing (Rabins et al., 1990). This suggests that many caregivers are resilient and find ways to adapt emotionally to a circumstance that becomes physically and sometimes emotionally more demanding. Some studies demonstrate that those caregivers who use available resources, including social agencies, other family members and friends, and religious and spiritual services, have better emotional outcomes than those who either do not use or do not have available such resources. Factors associated with better outcomes and resilience include maintaining social contact with others, extraversion, having social supports available and the ability to attribute meaning to the caregiving situation (Rabins et al., 1990). At present there are no prospective trials demonstrating that targeting high-risk individuals can prevent depression in caregivers.

Caregivers of children with disabilities are also primarily women. They experience rates of emotional distress comparable to carers of people with dementia and benefit from similar interventions (Raina et al. 2005).

Summary

The number of dependent persons requiring caregiving services is likely to continue to rise over the coming decades and the proportion of elders who will require such care is likely to rise faster than the projected population increase because the elderly will be a greater proportion of the population and the prevalence of dementia is concentrated in this group. Women provide the majority of caregiving throughout the world and this is likely to continue, even though women are becoming more involved in the formal workforce in most countries. There is a strong evidence base that programs providing help to women caregivers improve both their care provision and their quality of life whether the recipient is young or old. The challenges of providing such support at a population level have yet to be surmounted.

References

Brodaty, H., & Arasaratnam, C. (2012). Meta-analysis of nonpharmacologic interventions for neuropsychiatric symptoms of dementia. *American Journal of Psychiatry* 169:946–953.

Carbonneau, H. (2010). Development of a conceptual framework of positive aspects of caregiving in dementia. *Dementia* 9:327–353.

Fitting, M., Rabins, P., Lucas, M. J., & Eastham, J. (1986). Caregivers for dementia patients: A comparison of husbands and wives. *Gerontologist* 26:248–250.

Gillick, M. R. (2013). The critical role of caregivers in achieving patient-centered care. *JAMA* 310:575–576.

Murray, J., Schneider, J., Banerjee, S., & Mann, A. (1999). Eurocare: A cross-national study of spouse carers for people with Alzheimer disease: II-A qualitative analysis of the experience of caregiving. *Int Psychogeriatrics* 14:662–667.

Odanker, S. Z. (1990). Family caregivers and a changing society: The effects of employment on caregiver stress. *Fam Community Health* 12:58–70.

Piercy, K. W., Fauth, E., Norton, M. C., Pfister, R., Corcoran, C. D., Rabins, P. V., Lyketsos, C., & Tschanz, J. T. (2013). Predictors of dementia caregiver depression in a population: The Cache County Dementia Progression Study. 68:921–926.

Rabins, P. V., Fitting, M. D., Eastham, J., & Fetting, J. (1990) The emotional impact of caring for the chronically ill. *Psychosomatics* 31:331–336.

Raina, P., O'Donnell, M., Rosenbaum, P., Brehout, J., Walther, S. D., Russell, D., Swinton, M., Zhu, B., & Wood, E. (2005). The health and well-being of caregivers of children with cerebral palsy. *Pediatrics* 115: e626–636.

Schulz, R., & Beach, S. R. (1999). Caregiving as a risk factor for mortality. *JAMA* 282:2215–2219.

Tschanz, J. T., Piercy, K., Corcoran, C. D., Fauth, E., Norton, M. C., Rabins, P. V., Tschanz, B. T., Deberard, M. S., Snyder, C., Smith, C., Lee, L., & Lyketsos, C. G. (2013). Caregiver coping strategies predict cognitive and functional decline in dementia: The Cache County dementia progression study. *Am J Geriatr Psychitr* 21:57–66.

Maternal caregiving, oxytocin and mental illness

Kathryn M. Abel and Alya Elmadih

Introduction

A healthy environment in which a new infant can thrive and develop to its full potential requires a number of elements. Shelter, warmth and adequate nutrition are considered fundamental aspects of such a milieu. More recently, increasing importance has been accorded to the emotional and cognitive environment into which an infant is born. Indeed, the emotional tie of a mother to her infant, the "bond," is especially important to ensure infant survival; the facial features and other physical and behavioral characteristics of human babies do an important job of ensuring that adults approach the "immobile infant" and provide him or her with essential protective care to survive.

Disruptions in this caregiving environment can have long-lasting effects on the resilience of an individual through his or her life. This chapter provides an overview of the science behind maternal caregiving behavior in both animals and humans. It focuses on the role of the hormone oxytocin in parenting behavior before considering briefly how mental illness might affect parenting capacity and interventions that might improve child outcomes.

Maternal caregiving behavior or maternal sensitivity

Because mothers are still the preeminent caregiver to both infants and children across sexually dimorphic species, we consider maternal sensitivity and maternal caregiving behavior as the most important parental exposure for offspring. However, it is important to acknowledge that mothers live in a context of greater or fewer resources and supports and our approach is keen to avoid misattribution of blame or responsibility for adverse offspring outcomes. The outcomes that have been linked to maternal care behavior and early life experience are also importantly associated with many complex characteristics within the wider family and social environment and individual temperament within the child him or herself. However, here we focus knowingly on maternal effects.

Survival of a species critically depends on a broad repertoire of parental behaviors designed to sustain each infant through an extensive period of dependency, thereby contributing to long-term health (Sroufe, 2000). Although such behaviors are likely to have been highly conserved through evolution, they show marked variation within species. In rodents, these variations in maternal caregiving behaviors (MCBs) show intergenerational stability (Champagne et al., 2003) and influence development of the neural substrates that underlie phenotypic behaviors and stress responses in offspring (Francis et al., 1999; Liu et al., 1997). Rodent offspring of mothers providing low levels of maternal care show heightened stress reactivity, less novelty seeking, poorer responses to novel environments and greater fearful behaviors overall. Similarly, in humans, levels of maternal caregiving vary and are distributed in a bell shape among the population. Differing levels of caregiving capacity in human mothers also relates to differing levels of stress reactivity and attachment security in their children. Children of healthy mothers who were nevertheless grouped by a measure of maternal sensitivity show differences in behavioral and stress responses at 4 and 9 months (Ghera et al., 2006); adults who experienced poor parental relationships show abnormalities of striatal dopamine binding (Pruessner et al., 2004).

Comprehensive Women's Mental Health, ed. David J. Castle and Kathryn M. Abel. Published by Cambridge University Press.
© Cambridge University Press 2016.

It is now increasingly recognized that the degree to which a mother responds appropriately, and in a timely way, to her infant's behavioral cues is a pivotal aspect of a healthy early environment and has become known as "maternal sensitivity" (Ainsworth,1978; NICHD, 1999; Warren & Simmens, 2005). Maternal sensitivity plays an important role in supporting the infant's secure attachment formation and social functioning as well as in the infant's self-regulation and subsequent development of its emotional and cognitive systems and its language competences (NICHD 1999; Warren & Simmens 2005; Bakermans-Kranenburg et al. 2003; Bigelow et al. 2010; Crosnoe et al. 2010; Pearson et al. 2011). Maternal sensitivity represents a pattern of behavior that provides the infant with its primary social experience. In the absence of a parent who is able to respond sensitively to the child's signals, there is a greater risk of maltreatment (Milner, 1993, 2003) and harsher parenting (Joosen et al., 2012). Better understanding of what underpins capacity for sensitive maternal care, and what predicts deviance from it, is crucial in developing interventions to protect children and promote healthy lives.

Oxytocin and the origins of maternal sensitivity

Research in rodents and other mammals (including humans) has highlighted the importance of the hormone oxytocin (OT) to facilitate the onset and maintenance of maternal behavior (Insel, 1990; Champagne et al., 2001, 2003, 2007; Champagne, 2008; Numan & Stolzenberg, 2009; Swain et al., 2014). Broadly, greater levels of this hormone in women have been linked to greater sensitivity of maternal caregiving (Feldman et al., 2012). OT is a nonapeptide hormone synthesized mainly by the magnocellular neurons of the supraoptic (SON) and paraventricular (PVN) nuclei of the hypothalamus (Lee et al., 2009) and to a lesser extent from the spinal cord and bed nucleus of stria terminalis (BNST) (Carter & Murphy, 1989; Gimpl & Fahrenholz, 2001). A range of brain regions receive OT projections (Ross & Young, 2009), explaining the wide distribution of this hormone in the brain (Feldman et al., 2011). Parturition, distension of the cervix, suckling, social recognition and pair bonding might all act as stimuli for OT release (Lee et al., 2009). Depending on the stimulus, stored OT is released episodically from the posterior pituitary into the blood and the brain (Gimpl & Fahrenholz, 2001).

Effects of oxytocin

In addition to its classical action facilitating milk ejection in *mammary tissues* through the "let-down" reflex (Gimpl & Fahrenholz., 2001), OT also acts on the *uterus* to facilitate myometrial contractility and parturition (Fuchs et al., 1995). OT is increasingly known to have an effect on behaviors related to social affiliation. In humans, such effects include enhancing *feelings of trust*, possibly by minimizing amygdala activation to fear, specifically anticipated social fear (Baumgartner et al., 2008; Meyer-Lindenberg., 2008) and increases *social memory* and *face recognition* (Lee et al., 2009), possibly through increased eye gaze to faces (Gimpl & Fahrenholz, 2001). OT works in a reciprocal way with the hypothalamic-pituitary-adrenal axis (HPA), which mediates stress responses (Dabrowska et al., 2011) and, therefore, exhibits an *anxiolytic effect* (antistress effect) by reducing the level of stress hormones in both humans (Legros, 2001) and rats (Stachowiak et al., 1995; Numan & Woodside, 2010). This antistress effect also facilitates the initiation of breastfeeding (Uvnas-Moberg, 1998) and *affiliation* (social bonding) between individuals (Grippo et al., 2007).

The connection of OT with the brain's dopaminergic "reward" system facilitates its role in romantic *pair bonding* (Williams et al., 1992) by the initiation of *sexual behavior* and *sexual maturity* (Kow & Pfaf, 1998). Similarly, this connection with a reward system also helps the reinforcement of the infant's value to his or her mother (Cardinal et al., 2002) and, consequently, mother-infant bonding (Galbally et al., 2011). Here, we focus on the crucial role that OT plays in mediating *parental behavior* in animals (e.g. Champagne at al., 2001, 2007; Champagne, 2008) and humans in particular (Feldman et al., 2007; Gordon et al., 2010; Atzil et al., 2011).

Oxytocin and maternal behavior in animals

Unlike human studies, animal studies can examine the role of OT in maternal behavior *directly*. A pioneering study on alloparental behavior (i.e., nurturing behavior that develops towards fostered pups) showed that 42% of virgin female rats injected with OT displayed a full range of maternal behavior (grooming, crouching over pups, licking pups, nest building and pup retrieval) towards foster pups within 2 hours of OT administration. Conversely, none of the saline or vasopressin-treated virgin rats displayed these behaviors (Pedersen

& Prange, 1979). This effect of OT on maternal behavior is dose-dependent: higher doses of OT elicit a greater range of maternal responses (Pedersen et al., 1982). More recently, higher levels of OT receptor (OTR) density were found in brains of virgin female prairie voles that displayed alloparental behavior compared to those who ignored or attacked pups (Olazabal & Young, 2006). Administration of an OTR antagonist into the brain of these prairie voles prevented expression of alloparental behaviors towards fostered pups (Olazabal & Young, 2006) and reduced postpartum maternal behaviors to own pups (van Leengoed et al., 1987).

During pregnancy and parturition, and when nursing, changes in the brain's OT levels and OTR have been reported to occur in the female rat brain (Lee et al., 2009; Landgraf et al 1991; Meddle et al., 2007) to facilitate the formation of a bond between mother and offspring (Leng et al., 2008). Similar changes in OT expression are seen in the PVN and SON of postpartum female prairie voles (Wang et al., 2000), rabbits (Caba et al., 1996) and in the olfactory bulb of ewes at parturition (Levy et al., 1995). Recent development of genetic "knockout" experiments using mice with a deletion in either the OT or OTR gene have supported the previous findings in relation to the role of OT (Lee et al., 2009). OT knockout (OTKO) and OTR knockout (OTRKO) mice were more aggressive, showing more infanticidal (i.e., kills pups) behavior than control mice in the same environment (Ragnauth et al., 2005).

Cross-generational transmission of maternal behavior in animals

The quality of maternal care that an animal experiences influences the future quality of care provided to its own offspring (cross-generational transmission) (Francis et al., 1999; Champagne & Meaney, 2007; Champagne, 2008), in part because animals adopt the same OT profile as their own rearing mothers (Champagne, 2008). In the seminal cross-fostering studies of Frances Champagne's group, the biological females of "low" licking and grooming arched-back nursing (LG-ABN) mothers were reared by "high" LG-ABN foster-mothers and were reported to show similarly high levels of LG-ABN (seen by their foster-mothers) when they become adult themselves and handled their own pups (Francis et al., 1999). By contrast, the biological offspring of high LG-ABN mothers who were cross-fostered to "low" LG-ABN foster-mothers showed

similarly *low* levels of LG-ABN as their foster-mothers when they reared their own pups. High licking and grooming mothers showed high-density brain OTR like their high licking and grooming foster-mothers (Champagne, 2008). This suggests that maternal affiliative care induces non-genomic (epigenetic) changes in OTR expression in brain areas related to maternal motivation and behavior such as the medial preoptic area, the lateral septum, and the BNST in high LG-ABN lactating rats (Francis et al., 2000). Epigenetic changes in offspring gene expression are believed to follow changes in DNA-methylation (Francis et al., 2002; see Chapter 5).

It is likely that the effects on offspring stress reactivity and physiology (alluded to earlier) from the quality of maternal care received are also mediated via epigenetic mechanisms (see Champagne & Meaney, 2007). In rodents, for example, offspring of high LG mothers showed an increase in the expression of glucocorticoid receptors in the hippocampus (Zhang & Meaney, 2010) and decreases in HPA axis responses to stress, which enhance learning and memory ability (Liu et al., 1997). This underscores how maternal care and the OT system interact to shape offspring reward and stress pathways (Feldman et al., 2011). It also points to the importance that stress likely plays in development by stimulating plastic responses to stressors and greater capacity.

Oxytocin and parental behavior in humans

Expression and distribution of OT in the brain and its link to maternal behavior shows substantial variation across species (Ross & Young, 2009) and, recently, researchers have begun to explore the role of OT in human parenting behavior. Two studies examined OT in women during pregnancy and the early postpartum period. The first study (N = 62) examined the relationship between maternal plasma OT levels during the first trimester (T1), third trimester (T2) and the first postpartum month (T3) and the mother's self-reported attachment to her fetus (using the Maternal Fetal Attachment Scale [MFAS]) in the third trimester (Levine et al., 2007). Interestingly, while OT levels were not found to be correlated with MFAS score among the whole sample, significantly higher MFAS scores were found among women who showed a steady increase in plasma OT across all time points compared to women who showed other profiles. The second study examined the same cohort at the same time points (Feldman et al., 2007). In this study, maternal behaviors (gaze, vocalization, touch and affect) were observed during unstructured play in the first postpartum month. Mothers were interviewed to assess levels of attachment representation towards their infants, preoccupation and infant checking behaviors. Maternal plasma OT levels measured prenatally (T1) and postnatally (T3) were significantly correlated with maternal behavior, attachment representation and infant checking behavior. Furthermore, high plasma OT at T1 predicted the amount of (postpartum) maternal behavior, suggesting that OT plays a role in the quality and quantity of maternal behavior in humans in the early postpartum period. Both Levine et al. (2007) and Feldman et al. (2007) found high stability of plasma OT levels across assessments within each individual woman. This lends support to the validity of using plasma OT to assess central OT in women.

In the first study to examine plasma OT levels in mothers *and* fathers, Gordon et al. (2010) studied 80 couples during the 2nd and 6th postpartum months. At each visit, plasma OT was obtained from both parents and interactions between each of the parents and their infants were videotaped and coded for parental affectionate behaviors (i.e., infant-focused speech, vocalization and affectionate touch) and stimulatory behaviors (i.e., tactile stimulation and object presentation). An overall increase in plasma OT levels was observed throughout the study period, with plasma OT levels of mothers and fathers positively correlated at both assessments. Plasma OT was specifically positively correlated with *affectionate* parenting behavior in mothers and to *stimulatory* parenting behavior in fathers, suggesting gender differences in OT's role in parenting.

Feldman et al. (2010a) measured salivary OT in 112 mothers and fathers (not couples) when their infants were 4 to 6 months. OT measurements (plasma and salivary) were again positively correlated with affectionate parenting behavior in women and to stimulatory parenting behavior in fathers. Atzil et al. (2011) rated 23 mothers for synchronous behavior ("episodes when mother and infant coordinate their positive social engagement") and intrusive behavior ("inappropriate responses from mother") with 4-to-6-month-old infants through observing play interaction. Plasma OT levels positively correlated with maternal-infant synchronous behavior (N = 13) but not with intrusive behavior (N = 10). More sensitive,

micro-analytic, assessment of maternal behavior was used in our recent study (Elmadih et al., 2014), where maternal plasma OT was assessed in 30 mothers who occupied opposite extremes of observed maternal sensitivity: 15 "high-sensitivity mothers" and 15 "low-sensitivity mothers" (taken from a population based sample of 105 mothers) at 7 to 9 months postpartum. Baseline and post mother-infant interaction plasma OT were significantly higher in low-sensitivity mothers (N = 14) than high-sensitivity mothers (N = 15). This implies *greater* stress responses to the demands of caring for an infant, or past deficiencies in own parenting relationship (see following section). In this context, OT may be acting to reduce stress and anxiety in mothers with relatively low sensitivity; this is consistent with studies that suggest a role for OT in stress regulation in women (Turner et al., 2002; Marazziti et al., 2006; Taylor et al., 2006, 2010; Tabak et al., 2011).

Oxytocin and own perceived parenting experience

Using the Adult Attachment Interview, Strathearn et al. (2009) assessed attachment representations of 61 pregnant women with their own mothers. At 7 months postpartum, plasma OT was examined before and following mother-infant play (physical and mirror-based) in 15 women with secure attachment and 15 with insecure-avoidant attachment with own mother. Although baseline plasma OT did not differ between secure and insecure mothers, mothers with secure attachment showed significantly higher post-interaction OT levels than mothers with insecure attachment. However, this difference disappeared when the interaction was mirror-based instead of physical, suggesting that the link between mother's own attachment experience and her OT profile might not be constant and probably subjected to modulation by other factors related to mode of social interaction. Gordon et al. (2008) measured plasma OT of 45 women and men who were not parents; their perceived bonding with their own parents was assessed using the Parental Bonding Instrument (PBI). Plasma OT levels were positively correlated with PBI parental care scores (maternal and paternal care).

In summary, earlier studies suggested a clear positive link between plasma OT level and favorable perceived bonding with own parents, while recent studies find a more complex relationship. In the first study to explore the relationship between OT and different human attachment relationships among parents, Feldman et al. (2011) used self-report measures to assess attachment with own parents as well as with a romantic partner among 71 mothers and 41 fathers. Relationship with own infant was also observed through interactive play at 4 to 6 months. Plasma, salivary and urinary OT levels were measured before and after 15 minutes play interaction with infants. Parents who were more synchronous with their infants in affective expression showed higher plasma and salivary OT levels than "low"-synchrony parents, supporting previous findings that link OT to more positive parenting behavior (Feldman et al., 2007; Gordon et al., 2010). However, among mothers, post-interaction urinary OT (which was not correlated with plasma or salivary OT) was positively correlated with anxiety in romantic attachment (i.e., relationship with partner), self-reported parenting stress and interactive stress (i.e., proportion of time when the infant shows negative reactivity while the mother tries to reengage her/him during "observed" interactive play). This is consonant with our recent findings (Elmadih et al., 2014) that low-sensitivity mothers show positive correlation between own maternal overprotection (assessed using PBI) and plasma OT (baseline and post mother-infant interaction). However, among high-sensitivity mothers, no such relationship was found between maternal plasma OT and perceived bonding with own parents.

In summary, OT appears to be an indicator of social affiliation (Feldman et al., 2007, 2010a, b), but it might also be a "signal" for the need to affiliate with others (Tabak et al., 2011; Taylor et al., 2006, 2010). The OT system may have an "openness" to early social experience, with higher OT receptor density found with enriched, early parenting environment (Champagne, 2008). Numan and Woodside (2010) suggest that OT serves a dual role in maternal behavior: it increases maternal motivation and decreases stress and anxiety. The latter effect may aid the mother in coping with difficult circumstances related to infant care. In the human literature, different study methods, such as differences in the postpartum stage of the mother-infant dyad and the ways in which mothers are classified, may differentially "tap into" one or other of these separable aspects of OT involvement in maternal caregiving behavior.

Oxytocin and social relationship stress in women

In a study assessing stress in partnership among 85 adults in stable relationships (62% women and 38% men), plasma OT was significantly positively correlated with relationship distress in women (while plasma vasopressin correlated with relationship distress in men) (Taylor et al., 2010). The same research group also reported that, among 73 post-menopausal women, plasma OT was negatively correlated with the relationship to their own mother and to their partner and marginally significantly in relation to their best friend (Taylor et al., 2006). Similarly, Tabak et al. (2011) reported a positive correlation between plasma OT levels and post-conflict (with partner, a relative or a friend) anxiety and decreased levels of forgiveness among 35 women. This positive relationship may relate to known antianxiety and antistress effect of OT (Numan & Woodside, 2010) where OT is released in stressful situations to moderate stress responsiveness (Marazziti et al., 2006). Elevation of OT in response to stress in women (including mothers) might be confined to relationship distress and interpersonal difficulties rather than general stress. This is suggested by the unsuccessful efforts to increase OT through laboratory stress induction using "Trier Social Stress Test" (Ditzen et al., 2007). In addition, with the exception of the "antistress" effect, most behavioral and physiological effects induced by OT can be blocked by administration of OT antagonist, suggesting a different receptor or mechanism (Uvnas-Moberg, 1998). Thus, the pathways by which OT mediates effects on stress and on social affiliation may be different (Taylor et al., 2010). This suggests a dual role for OT in prosocial behaviors; while OT increases as a result of affiliative contact, it also increases as a "signal for *demand to affiliate* with others, as the relationship is threatened" (Taylor et al., 2010). Maternal sensitivity is a construct that requires a reciprocal interactive relationship between a mother and her infant and, just as with other affiliative relationships, is likely to encounter difficulties.

Breastfeeding in humans as a proxy measure for maternal oxytocin

Studies also examine the relationship between maternal care and breastfeeding, where breastfeeding is used as a proxy for elevated plasma OT level. Feldman and Eidelman (2003) observed 86 mothers of premature infants for M-I interaction prior to hospital discharge. At 37 weeks, those who expressed substantial amounts of milk (more than 75% of infant nutrition) exhibited more maternal postpartum affectionate touch. In the other study, nine breastfeeding mothers and eight formula-feeding mothers were assessed for maternal sensitivity at 3 to 4 months, observed though interaction during feeding (Kim et al., 2011). Breastfeeding mothers showed higher sensitivity ratings compared to formula-feeding mothers. Neither of these studies provides direct evidence for the role of oxytocin in human maternal behavior. The first study (Feldman & Eidelman, 2003) was among premature infants who tend to interact less than full-term infants (Muller-Nix et al., 2004). Mothers perceive premature infants as fragile, which promotes overprotection (directiveness) in the interaction, which tends to counter sensitive responsiveness (Singer et al., 1999). Many recent studies reporting differences in plasma OT responses between mothers found no significant differences between breastfeeding and nonbreastfeeding mothers (Feldman et al., 2007).

The cross-generational transmission of behavior via oxytocin in humans

Feldman et al. (2010b) replicated their previous study with a smaller sample of 55 mothers and fathers (not couples) and 4-to-6-month-old infants. Interaction was coded for parent behavior (gaze, affect, vocalization and touch) and infant behavior (gaze, affect, vocalization and touch) and rated as two composites: affect synchrony and infant social engagement. Similar to their earlier findings (Feldman et al., 2010a), a positive correlation was reported between parental plasma OT levels following interaction and parental behavior. Interestingly, parent and infant OT levels correlated positively with each other, providing evidence for the role of OT in mediating transgenerational behavior in humans, equivalent to that reported in the rodent literature (Francis et al., 2000; Champagne et al., 2007).

Deviation from healthy parental caregiving in humans

In animals, the natural variation in the quality of maternal caregiving behavior (e.g., licking and grooming of pups and pup approach) has been linked to differences in the maternal brain; changing the biology of female primates (e.g., rodents) has been shown to alter how a mother responds to her infants. Despite wide recognition of the importance of maternal sensitivity to infant emotional, behavioral, cognitive and social outcomes, little is known about the neurocognitive mechanisms and neurobiology underpinning maternal sensitivity in humans and the causes of deviation in caregiving remain unknown.

Many things affect sensitivity, including past abuse, deprivation and mental illness (e.g., Elmadih et al., 2014; Swain et al., 2014). In clinical states like depression, affective and cognitive deficits disrupt the ability to recognize, process and respond to emotions (Harmer et al., 2011). Similar neurocognitive models may apply to variation in maternal sensitivity (perhaps particularly maternal insensitivity to infant distress). Thus, a mother's capacity to respond to her infant may depend on how well she recognizes and regulates emotions in general; or, on how well she copes with stress, such as crying infants. This is important because maternal sensitivity to infants involves many different cognitive and social abilities and if there is a problem in a brain pathway controlling one of them, maternal sensitivity may be affected. This means that poor sensitivity in one mother may stem from problems in a different brain pathway from that in another. For example, some mothers, like those with anxiety and related mood disorders, may be oversensitive to negative emotions, such as infant crying; they would require help with this aspect of interaction to improve sensitive caregiving. Other mothers, such as those with schizophrenia or associated deficits in social cognition, like Asperger's, may find it difficult to recognize infant emotions and to distinguish a distressed infant from a happy one. Better understanding of the brain differences that are linked with deviation in maternal sensitive caregiving may help us find solutions to difficult problems such as child maltreatment or neglect and lead to more effective treatments in at-risk families (see Swain et al., 2014).

Effects of maternal depression and anxiety on infant caregiving

Here, we consider the most common psychological difficulties experienced by new mothers, that is, maternal depression and maternal anxiety disorders.

Depressive states tend to make a person less emotionally available, but there are a range of processes that become distorted in the context of a depressive episode (Harmer et al., 2011; Elliott et al., 2011). For a new mother, this may manifest itself in difficulty recognizing and interpreting emotions in infant facial expressions, which can be rather subtle relative to the "bigger" displays of facial expression of emotion in adults; she may also find it hard to respond promptly to her infant's emotional cues (Kemppinen et al., 2006; Numan, 2006; Tronick & Reck, 2009), perhaps especially if there is distraction or psychomotor retardation.

Healthy mothers generally derive a feeling of great reward and satisfaction from interaction with their infants. By contrast, ill mothers might lack such reward and, indeed, might experience greater levels of anxiety or stress from a social interaction that they find difficult to gauge or manage, making sensitive responsiveness more challenging (Kemppinen et al., 2006). Depressive mood symptoms, even subclinically, hinder maternal sensitivity (Sidor et al., 2011). The mechanisms underlying poor parenting in nonclinically depressed mothers remain unclear; whether they are related to the effect of symptoms that impair communication of emotions between mother and infant (Blumberg, 1980; see Tronick & Reck, 2009) or to other unfavorable factors that coexist with depressive mood (e.g., poverty, lack of social supports and marital difficulties) remains to be determined (Tronick & Reck, 2009). A recent study suggested that effects of poverty on child brain development "are mediated by caregiving and stressful life events which imply that attempts to enhance early caregiving should be a focused public health target for prevention and early intervention" (Luby et al., 2013).

Most of the studies that examine the effects of mood on maternal sensitivity do so among clinically depressed samples (e.g. Murray et al., 1996); only a few studies consider community (nonclinical) samples (e.g., Mills-Koonce et al., 2008; Sidor et al., 2011). Among these community sample studies, significant correlations have been reported between higher postnatal maternal depression scores and lower maternal sensitivity (Campbell et al., 2007; Mills-Koonce et al., 2008). Mothers reporting more chronic symptoms of depression (through 36 months) were found to score the least on sensitivity rating compared with healthy controls (NICHD, 1999). Other studies of healthy populations also showed increases in depression scores among mothers who showed low parental care or high parental overprotection (Hill et al., 2001; Avagianou & Zafiropoulou, 2008). Apart from the comorbidity between depression and anxiety (Pollack, 2005), evidence suggests that anxiety on its own might decrease the mother's perceptual difficulties and lead to less engagement (Blumberg, 1980) and less sensitive engagement with her infant (Nicol-Harper et al., 2007). In a study that examined self-regulation in toddlers, women who reported symptoms of anxiety scored significantly lower than healthy controls on maternal sensitivity (Feldman & Klein, 2003).

Among the few studies that were unable to demonstrate a relationship between depression and maternal sensitivity, some methodological differences should be noted. For example, a recent study by Sidor et al. (2011) examined maternal postpartum depressive symptoms among a nonclinical sample of 106 women (using the Edinburgh Postnatal Depression Scale [EPDS]), while maternal sensitivity was observed (using the CARE-index). Although they did not find a correlation between maternal sensitivity and mood symptoms, their sample was chosen as a socially deprived sample (poverty, alcoholism, etc.), which might confound such a relationship.

> **Box 4.1 Special considerations for maternal caregiving**
>
> **Infants with congenital malformations**
> Psychological responses to a child born with a congenital abnormality are as varied as the degree of abnormality and disability. Responses are, of course, very varied even to infants with similar malformations, but often constitute components of grief reactions to the "loss of the expected infant." Parents may experience numbness and inability to accept abnormality, guilt, disgust, poor attachment or rejection of the infant. Alternatively, they may simply find it extremely challenging to soothe a disabled child who may be suffering in ways undetectable to the parent. Depending on the degree to which the child requires physical support, some parents cope by becoming absorbed in practical care and over-involved in parenting to the exclusion of other activities or relationships. Rates of depression and maltreatment are increased in the context of infant congenital abnormalities. Parents need information provided in a considerate manner by experienced clinical staff, as well support to understand their

Box 4.1 *(cont.)*

own limits and the child's prognosis and to manage feelings that may fluctuate unpredictably and unmanageably.

Mothers with learning disability

Better care means more women with learning disability are becoming pregnant and having children. Depending on the nature of the maternal condition, children will not necessarily have a learning disability or congenital syndrome. Support needs to be provided within a multidisciplinary context, where the degree of intellectual disability and the amount of external supports available to the woman are taken into consideration in decision making. If the woman has a partner with intellectual disability (as is relatively common), presence of institutional support is likely, especially if there is comorbid psychiatric illness such as psychosis, which is more common in the context of intellectual disability. In any case, every opportunity to support the woman to care for her own child should be provided before considering social care.

Interventions to support parenting

Parent-centered interventions

Most children whose mothers have a mental illness do not develop lasting attachment difficulties or developmental problems in later life. For clinicians working with maternal distress and mental illness, it is extremely important to reassure mothers that the evidence suggests most children are very resilient and to challenge such stigmatizing paradigms, which are likely to discourage parents, perhaps especially mothers with mental illness, from help-seeking and gaining the supports they need to be able to continue to care for their own children.

Some circumstances, however, are particularly likely to expose children to risk. For example, mothers with severe affective disorder and addiction disorders (also see Chapter 15; Webb et al., 2007), especially when paired with high levels of family deprivation. Risk to children from parental substance and alcohol addiction is well-recognized in the UK and United States and the Family Drug and Alcohol Courts have been established and shown to help prevent family breakdown and to promote successful abstinence by parents (Harwin et al., 2014).

For the 20% of mothers in the general population who have relatively poor maternal sensitivity, the situation is more complex. The presence of associated risk factors is very important in assessing risk-to-child outcomes. Factors that have traditionally been considered include maternal age, the number of children being looked after, parental supports including partner and family, and parent trauma or unresolved attachment status. In the context of prolonged or severe maternal mental health problems or diagnosed disorders, children are vulnerable to developing insecure or disorganized attachments to caregivers primarily when these additional risk factors are also present. Although most children are remarkably resilient; in spite of adverse circumstances, they manage to develop a secure attachment and appear to be protected from the adverse developmental outcomes associated with having an ill parent (Wan & Green, 2009 for review). More recently, conceptualizations of individual susceptibility are promoting the notion that a mother who is susceptible to stress and mental illness, or a child who is susceptible to maternal illness or stress, may also be a mother or child who is amenable to successful outcomes from parenting interventions (Bakermans Kranenburg & van Ijzendoorn, 2015).

Altering early infant attachment has become a focus of interventions aiming to encourage resilience and prevent subsequent problems. Attachment-based parenting interventions, therefore, aim to improve the quality of maternal caregiving behavior and thereby enhance the mother's sensitivity to her child's cues at a behavioral level. A variety of methods has been used; one of the more effective involves the use of video feedback with the mother watching her own infant interaction with the therapist (e.g., Juffer et al., 2008). There is little evidence on the efficacy of such interventions for mothers with mental illness (Wan et al 2008b), but such methods have been effective in a range of vulnerable groups, for example, low-socioeconomic, high-deprivation families (Bakermans-Kranenburg et al., 2003).

Evidence suggests that the key element in any intervention to improve parenting is through altering sensitivity and more modern approaches are beginning to recognize the need to support sensitive maternal behavior across a range of contexts, encompassing routine care situations as well as exploratory and stressful situations (Cassidy et al., 2005). This may be particularly relevant for mothers with a mental illness who may find it particularly difficult to care for a crying or distressed infant, however benign the source of the infant's apparent distress. Such work is usually started when children are infants or toddlers although other family and parent-focused interventions have been used in families with older children and adolescents.

Parent training interventions, like Triple P or Incredible Years/Dinosaur Schools, have tended to be educational and behavioral, often dealing with "problem children" or "coercive parenting." Although many have involved one-to-one guidance, a purely behavioral intervention may only be effective in some mothers. For example, mothers with unresolved attachment issues with respect to their own parents may be less likely to show improved sensitivity (Moran et al., 2005), while those with more social support may be more likely to show improvements (Guttentag et al., 2006). This notion is supported by evidence from animal populations discussed earlier where naturally occurring variation in maternal sensitivity charts distinct patterns of mothering, each associated with a specific bio-behavioral profile in mother and offspring (see Champagne & Curley, 2010).

Furthermore, little is known about the cognitive or neurobiological mechanisms underlying poor maternal care or individual mother/infant susceptibility to environmental adversity. Understanding these elements requires more research; gaps in understanding how individual (infant/mother) temperament, (maternal/infant) susceptibility and cognitive deficits are associated with poor outcomes may explain why interventions targeted at improving parenting through improved sensitivity, though promising, have shown inconsistent findings and generally small effect sizes (Bakermans-Kranenburg et al., 2003; Wan et al., 2008a; Bakermans-Kranenburg & van IJzendoorn, 2015).

Child-centered interventions

Evidence suggests that, unlike the concerns addressed by service- and parent-centered interventions, many children have a much broader range of worries and basic living needs related to the unpredictability of severe parental mental illness, which attachment-based interventions do not seek to address (Bee et al. 2013, 2014). Health-related quality of life is a key outcome that is only beginning to be widely considered in children, let alone children with ill

parents often caring for their parent. The concerns these children have may include how to manage a parent's deterioration in mental state, lack of understanding about how symptoms arise or what they mean, worries about dealing with adult services and adult service providers, concerns about being a carer and about staying well themselves. Interventions to date have not been tailored to this type of need, but have tended to focus on parental diagnosis. However, discussions about specific difficulties encountered by children with mentally ill parents suggests an understanding of how they can manage stress and cope with a set of circumstances is required, rather than anything more specific to a diagnosis. Many problems are also likely to be common for children's experience across different parental diagnoses. This broader perspective outside the diagnostic categories also reflects well-recognized research from *Children of Sick Parents* (Rutter, 1966), which suggested that problems encountered by children are not specific to parental diagnosis, but in the main relate to psychosocial factors. The recent National Society for the Prevention of Cruelty to Children (NSPCC) preliminary evaluation of its Family SMILES intervention also found that practitioners did not consider there was a need to tailor intervention to parental diagnosis. Instead, children said they wanted individual support and more information about their parent's mental illness; practitioners considered it an opportunity for young people to understand the range of mental health problems, to share experiences of stigma/reluctance to talk about it and to "normalize" their experiences. Young people said they benefited from hearing about each other's experiences and did not view the differences in parental diagnoses as a barrier.

In spite of the recognized growing need, our recent comprehensive systematic review (Bee et al., 2014) found there were no contemporary interventions with a sufficiently robust evidence base that adequately addressed health-related quality of life or the broader needs of children of parents with severe mental illness. Of those that displayed promise, both KidsTime (Wolpert et al., 2014) and Family SMILES demonstrated good acceptability and feasibility in this group, but both have yet to be formally evaluated. Family SMILES has shown some promising interim results from its nonrandomized, controlled sampling. Such models now require further development with stakeholders in order to create child-centered interventions for improved health-related quality of life that can be feasibly embedded across social and health services. The aim of such interventions should not be to treat the mental illness of the parent; rather it should be to enhance the experience of children in the context of living with severe parental mental illness thereby improving the quality of the child's life, their well-being and their resilience.

Conclusions

In humans, we lack a deep understanding of neurobiological mechanisms underpinning maternal caregiving behavior, concepts of individual resilience and susceptibility and impairments of parenting ability. This represents a potentially important obstacle to change: If neurobiological heterogeneity means more than one pathway leads to poor maternal sensitivity or high individual susceptibility then different "subgroups" may have different intervention needs and different outcomes. Identifying problems in specific maternal brain areas or in infant temperament could therefore provide important new targets for innovative treatments or make existing treatments work better.

In animal models, there is pretty good evidence that high oxytocin concentrations in a mother promotes maternal care behavior. Little is known about how it affects maternal caregiving in healthy or in low-sensitivity human mothers, whatever the cause of poor sensitivity. Little is known about how changing brain OT levels in mothers relates to OT and/or attachment in infants or how infant temperament affects this relationship. Understanding the neurobiology of poor maternal sensitivity and how it affects individual human infants may increase the likelihood that interventions improve sensitivity and promote understanding of effects on infant outcomes (e.g., brain development). Future studies should aim to evaluate the effect of variation in maternal caregiving / maternal sensitivity on infant neurodevelopment and to assess the effect of parenting intervention to change child neurodevelopmental outcomes.

Finally, the broader quotidian needs of children living with parental mental illness have been neglected. Newer initiatives across Europe and other parts of the world may begin to tackle this problem. Involving them as key stakeholders may give these "hidden children" the much-needed voice to express their difficulties and needs and help to create resilience and coping within their highly stressful childhood landscapes.

References

Ainsworth, M. D. S., Blehar, M. C., Waters, E. & Wall, S. (1978). *Patterns of attachment: A psychological study of the strange situation.* Hillsdale, NJ: Erlbaum.

Atzil, S., Hendler, T. & Feldman, R. (2011). Specifying the neurobiological basis of human attachment: Brain, hormones, and behavior in synchronous and intrusive mothers. *Neuropsychopharmacology* 36, 1–13.

Avagianou, P. A. & Zafiropoulou, M. (2008). Parental bonding and depression: Personality as a mediating factor. *International Journal of Adolescent Medicine and Health* 20, 261–269.

Bakermans-Kranenburg, M. J. & van IJzendoorn, M. H. (2015). The hidden efficacy of interventions: Gene×environment experiments from a differential susceptibility perspective. *Annual Review of Psychology* 3(66), 381–409.

Bakermans-Kranenburg, M. J., van IJzendoorn, M. H. & Juffer, F. (2003). Less is more: Meta-analyses of sensitivity and attachment interventions in early childhood. *Psychological Bulletin* 129, 195–215.

Baumgartner, T., Heinrichs, M., Vonlanthen, A., Fischbacher, U. & Fehr, E. (2008). Oxytocin shapes the neural circuitry of trust and trust adaptation in humans. *Neuron* 58, 639–650.

Bee, P., Berzins, K., Calam, R., Pryjmachuk, S. & Abel, K. M. (2013). Defining quality of life in the children of parents with severe mental illness. A preliminary stakeholder-led model. *PLOS One* 8(9), doi: 10.1371/journal.pone.0073739.

Bee, P., Bower, P., Byford, S., Churchill, R., Calam, R., Stallard, P., Pryjmachuk, S., Berzins, K.,

Cary, M., Wan, M. & Abel, K. (2014). The clinical-effectiveness, cost-effectiveness and acceptability of community-based interventions aimed at improving or maintaining quality of life in children of parents with serious mental illness; a systematic review. *Health Technology Assessment* 18(8), 1–250. doi: 10.3310/hta18080.

Bigelow, A. E, et al. (2010). Maternal sensitivity throughout infancy: Continuity and relation to attachment security. *Infant Behavior and Development* 33, 50–60.

Blumberg, N. L. (1980). Effects of neonatal risk, maternal attitude, and cognitive style on early postpartum adjustment *Journal of Abnormal Psychology* 89, 139–150.

Caba, M., Silver, R., Gonzalez-Mariscal, G., Jimenez, A. & Beyer, C. (1996). Oxytocin and vasopressin immunoreactivity in rabbit hypothalamus during estrus, late pregnancy, and postpartum. *Brain Research* 720, 7–16.

Campbell, S. B., Matestic, P., von Stauffenberg, C., Mohan, R. & Kirchner, T. (2007). Trajectories of maternal depressive symptoms, maternal sensitivity, and children's functioning at school entry. *Developmental Psychology* 43, 1202–1215.

Cardinal, R. N., Parkinson, J. A., Hall, J. & Everitt, B. J. (2002). Emotion and motivation: The role of the amygdala, ventral striatum, and prefrontal cortex. *Neuroscience & Biobehavioral Reviews* 26, 321–352.

Carter, D. A. & Murphy, D. (1989). Independent regulation of neuropeptide mRNA level and poly (A) tail length. *Journal of Biological Chemistry* 264, 6601–6603.

Cassidy, J., Woodhouse, S. S, Cooper, G., Hoffman, K., Powell, B. & Rodenberg, M. (2005). Examination of the precursors of infant attachment security: Implications for early intervention and intervention research. In: Berlin, L. J., Amaya-Jackson, L. & Greenberg, M. T. (eds.) *Enhancing early attachments: Theory, research, intervention, and policy*. New York: Guilford Press, pp. 34–60.

Champagne, F. A. (2008). Epigenetic mechanisms and the transgenerational effects of maternal care. *Frontiers in Neuroendocrinology* 29, 386–397.

Champagne, F. A. & Curley, J. P. (2010). Maternal care as a modulating influence on infant development. In: Blumberg, M. S., Freeman, J. H. & Robinson, S. R. (eds.) *Developmental and comparative neuroscience: Epigenetics, evolution & behavior*. Oxford, UK: Oxford University Press, p. 323–341.

Champagne, F., Diorio, J., Sharma, S. & Meaney, M. J. (2001). Naturally occurring variations in maternal behavior in the rat are associated with differences in estrogen-inducible central oxytocin receptors.

Proceedings of the National Academy of Sciences of the United States of America 98, 12736–12741.

Champagne, F. A., Francis, D. D., Mar, A. & Meaney, M. J. (2003). Variations in maternal care in the rat as a mediating influence for the effects of environment on development. *Physiology & Behavior* 79, 359–371.

Champagne, F. A. & Meaney, M. J. (2007). Transgenerational effects of social environment on variations in maternal care and behavioral response to novelty. *Behavioral Neuroscience* 121, 1353–1363.

Crosnoe, R., Leventhal, T., Wirth, R. J., Pierce, K. M. & Pianta, R. C.; NICHD Early Child Care Research Network. (2010). Family socioeconomic status and consistent environmental stimulation in early childhood. *Child Development* 81, 972–987.

Dabrowska, J., Hazra, R., Ahern, T. H., Dong Guo, J., McDonald, A. J., Mascagni, F., Muller, J. F., Young, L. J. & Rainnie, D. G. (2011). Neuroanatomical evidence for reciprocal regulation of the corticotrophin-releasing factor and oxytocin systems in the hypothalamus and the bed nucleus of the stria terminalis of the rat: Implications for balancing stress and affect. *Psychoneuroendocrinology* 36, 1312–1326.

Ditzen, B., Neumann, I. D., Bodenmann, G., Von Dawans, B., Turner, R. A., Ehlert, U. & Heinrichs, M. (2007). Effects of different kinds of couple interaction on cortisol and heart rate responses to stress in women. *Psychoneuroendocrinology* 32, 565–574.

Elliott, R., Zahn, R., Deakin, J. FW. & Anderson, I. M. (2011). Affective cognition in mood disorder. *Neuropsychopharmacology* 36, 153–182.

Elmadih, A., Wan, M. W., Numan, M., Elliott, R., Downey, D. & Abel, K.

M. (2014). Does oxytocin modulate variation in maternal caregiving in healthy new mothers? *Brain Research* 1580, 143–150.

Feldman, R. (2012). Oxytocin and social affiliation in humans. *Hormones and Behavior* 61, 380–391.

Feldman, R. & Eidelman, A. I. (2003). Direct and indirect effect of breast milk on neurobehavioural and cognitive development of premature infants. *Developmental Psychobiology* 43, 109–119.

Feldman, R., Gordon, I., Schneiderman, I., Weisman, O. & Zagoory-Sharon, O. (2010a). Natural variations in maternal and paternal care are associated with systematic changes in oxytocin following parent-infant contact. *Psychoneuroendocrinology*. 35, 1133–1141.

Feldman, R., Gordon, I. & Zagoory-Sharon, O. (2010b). The cross-generation transmission of oxytocin in humans. *Hormones and Behavior* 58, 669–676.

Feldman, R., Gordon, I. & Zagoory-Sharon, O. (2011). Maternal and paternal plasma, salivary, and urinary oxytocin and parent–infant synchrony: Considering stress and affiliation components of human bonding. *Developmental Science* 14, 752–761.

Feldman, R. & Klein, P. S. (2003). Toddlers' selfregulated compliance to mothers, caregivers, and fathers: Implications for theories of socialization. *Developmental Psychology* 39, 680–692.

Feldman, R., Weller, A., Zagoory-Sharon, O. & Levine, A. (2007). Evidence for a neuroendocrinological foundation of human affiliation: Plasma oxytocin levels across pregnancy and the postpartum period predict mother-infant bonding. *Psychological Science* 18, 965–970.

Francis, D. D., Champagne, F. C. & Meaney, M. J. (2000). Variations in maternal behaviour are associated with differences in oxytocin receptor levels in the rat. *Journal of Neuroendocrinology* 12, 1145–1148.

Francis, D., Diorio, J., Liu, D. & Meaney, M. J. (1999). Nongenomic transmission across generations of maternal behavior and stress responses in the rat. *Science*, 268 (5442), 1155–1158.

Francis, D. D., Young, L. J., Meaney, M. J. & Insel, T. R. (2002). Naturally occurring differences in maternal care are associated with the expression of oxytocin and vasopressin (V1a) receptors: Gender differences. *Journal of Neuroendocrinology* 14, 349–353.

Fuchs, A. R., Fields, M. J., Freidman, S., Shemesh, M. & Ivell, R. (1995). Oxytocin and the timing of parturition. Influence of oxytocin receptor gene expression, oxytocin secretion, and oxytocin-induced prostaglandin F2a and E2 release. *Advances in Experimental Medicine and Biology* 395, 405–420.

Galbally, M., Lewis, A. J., Ijzendoorn, M. V. & Permezel, M. (2011). The role of oxytocin in mother-infant relations: A systematic review of human studies. *Harvard Review of Psychiatry* 19, 1–14.

Ghera, M. M., Hane, A. A., Malesa, E. E. & Fox, N. A. (2006). The role of infant soothability in the relation between infant negativity and maternal sensitivity. *Infant Behavior and Development* 29, 289–293.

Gimpl, G. & Fahrenholz, F. (2001). The oxytocin receptor system: Structure, function, and regulation. *Physiological Reviews* 81, 629–683.

Gordon, I., Zagoory-Sharon, O., Leckman, J. F. & Feldman, R. (2010). Oxytocin and the development of parenting in humans. *Bilological Psychiatry* 68, 377–382.

Gordon, I., Zagoory-sharon, O., Schneiderman, I., Leckman, J. F., Weller, A. & Feldman, R. (2008). Oxytocin and cortisol in romantically unattached young adults: Associations with bonding and psychological distress. *Psychophysiology* 45, 349–352.

Grippo, A. J., Gerena, D., Huang, J., Kumar, N., Shah, M., Ughreja, R. & Carter, C. S. (2007). Social isolation induces behavioral and neuroendocrine disturbances relevant to depression in female and male prairie voles. *Psychoneuroendocrinology* 32, 966–980.

Guttentag, C. L. et al. (2006). Individual variability in parenting profiles and predictors of change: Effects of an intervention with disadvantaged mothers. *Journal of Applied Developmental Psychology* 27, 349–369.

Harmer, C. J. et al. (2011). Efficacy markers in depression. *Journal of Psychopharmacology* 25, 1148–1158.

Harwin, J. et al. (2014). Final Report of the Evaluation of the Family Drug and Alcohol Court Pilot. www .brunel.ac.uk/__data/assets/pdf_file/ 0007/366370/FDAC_May2014_ FinalReport_V2.pdf

Hill, J., Pickles, A., Burnside, E., Byatt, M., Rollinson, L., Davis, R. & Harvey, K. (2001). Child sexual abuse, poor parental care and adult depression: Evidence for different mechanisms. *British Journal of Psychiatry* 179, 104–109.

Insel, T. (1990). Oxytocin and maternal behavior. In N. A. Krasnegor & R. B. Bridges (eds.), *Mammalian parenting: biochemical, neurobiological and behavioral determinants*. New York: Oxford University Press, 260–280.

Joosen, K. J., Mesman, J., Bakermans-Kranenburg, M. J. & van IJzendoorn, M. H. (2012). Maternal sensitivity to infants in various settings predicts harsh discipline in toddlerhood. *Attachment & Human Development* 14, 101–117.

Juffer, F., Bakermans-Kranenburg, M. J. & van IJzendoorn, M. H.(2008). *Promoting positive parenting: An attachment-based intervention.* Lawrence Erlbaum.

Kemppinen, K., Kumpulainen, K., Raita-Hasu, J. & Moilanen, I. (2006). The continuity of maternal sensitivity from infancy to toddler age. *Journal of Reproductive and infant Psychology*, 24, 199–212.

Kim, P., Feldman, R., Mayes, L. C., Eicher, V., Thompson, N., Leckman, J. F. & Swain, J. E. (2011). Breastfeeding, brain activation to own infant cry, and maternal sensitivity. *Journal of Child Psychology and Psychiatry* 52, 907–915.

Kow, L. M. & Pfaf, D. W. (1998). Mapping of neural and signal transduction pathways for lordosis in the search for estrogen actions on the central nervous system. *Behavioural Brain Research* 92, 169–180.

Landgraf, R., Neumann, I. & Pittman, Q. J. (1991). Septal and hippocampal release of vasopressin and oxytocin during late pregnancy and parturition in the rat. *Neuroendocrinology* 54, 378–383.

Lee, H. J., Macbeth, A. H., Pagani, J. H. & Young, W. S. 3rd. (2009). Oxytocin: The Great Facilitator of Life. *Progress in Neurobiology* 88, 127–151.

Legros, J. J. (2001). Inhibitory effect of oxytocin on corticotrope function in humans: Are vasopressin and oxytocin ying-yang neurohormones? *Psychoneuroendocrinology* 26, 649–655.

Leng, G., Meddle, S. L. & Douglas, A. J. (2008). Oxytocin and the maternal brain. *Current Opinion in Pharmacology* 8, 731–734.

Levine, A., Zagoory-Sharon O., Feldman R. & Weller, A. (2007). Oxytocin during pregnancy and early postpartum: Individual patterns and maternal–fetal attachment. *Peptides* 28, 1162–1169.

Levy, F., Kendrick, K. M., Goode, J. A., Guevara-Guzman, R. & Keverne, E. B. (1995). Oxytocin and vasopressin release in the olfactory bulb of parturient ewes: Changes with maternal experience and effects on acetylcholine, gamma-aminobutyric acid, glutamate and noradrenaline release. *Brain Research* 669, 197–206.

Liu, D., Diorio, J., Tannenbaum, B., Caldji, C., Francis, D. & Freedman, A. (1997). Maternal care, hippocampal glucocorticoid receptors, and hypothalamic-pituitary-adrenal responses to stress. *Science* 277, 1659–1662.

Luby, J., Belden, A., Botteron, K., et al. (2013). The Effects of Poverty on Childhood Brain Development The Mediating Effect of Caregiving and Stressful Life Events. *The Journal of the American Medical Association Pediatrics*, doi:10.1001/jamapediatrics.2013.3139.

Marazziti, D., Dell'Osso, B., Baroni, S., Mungai, F., Catena, M., Rucci, P., Albanese, F., Giannaccini, G., Betti, L., Fabbrini, L., Italiani, P., Del Debbio, P., Lucacchini, A. & Dell'Osso, L. (2006). A relationship between oxytocin and anxiety of romantic attachment. *Clinical Practice and Epidemiology in Mental Health* 28, doi:10.1186/1745-0179-2-28.

Meddle, S. L., Bishop, V. R., Gkoumassi, E., van Leeuwen, F. W. & Douglas, A. J. (2007). Dynamic changes in oxytocin receptor expression and activation at parturition in the rat brain. *Endocrinology* 148, 5095–5104.

Meyer-Lindenberg, A. (2008). Impact of prosocial neuropeptides on human brain function. *Progress in Brain Research* 170, 463–470.

Mills-Koonce, W. R., Gariepy, J. L., Sutton, K. & Cox, M. J. (2008). Changes in maternal sensitivity across the first three years: Are mothers from different attachment dyads differentially influenced by depressive symptomatology? *Attachment & Human Development* 10, 299–317.

Milner, J. S. (1993). Social information-processing and physical child-abuse.

Clinical Psychology Review 13, 275–294.

Milner, J. S. (2003). Social information processing in high-risk and physically abusive parents. *Child Abuse and Neglect* 27, 7–20.

Moran, G. et al. (2005). Maternal unresolved attachment status impedes the effectiveness of interventions with adolescent mothers. *Infant Mental Health Journal* 26, 231–249.

Muller-Nix, C., Forcada-Guex, M., Pierrehumbert, B., Jaunin, L., Borghini, A. & Ansermet, F. (2004). Prematurity, maternal stress and mother-child interactions. *Early Human Development and Psychopathology* 79, 145–158.

Murray, L., Fiori-Cowley, A., Hooper, R. & Cooper, P. (1996). The impact of postnatal depression and associated adversity on early mother-infant interactions and later infant outcome. *Child Development* 67, 2512–2526.

NICHD. (1999). Chronicity of maternal depressive symptoms, maternal sensitivity, and child functioning at 36 months. *Developmental Psychology* 35, 1297–1310.

Nicol-Harper, R., Harvey, A. G. & Stein A. (2007). Interactions between mothers and infants: Impact of maternal anxiety. *Infant Behavior and Development* 30, 161–167.

Numan, M. (2006). Hypothalamic neural circuits regulating maternal responsiveness toward infants. *Behavioral and Cognitive Neuroscience Reviews* 5, 163–190.

Numan, M. & Stolzenberg, D. S. (2009). Medial preoptic area interactions with dopamine neural systems in the control of the onset and maintenance of maternal behavior in rats. *Frontiers in Neuroendocrinology* 30, 46–64.

Numan, M. & Woodside, B. (2010). Maternity: Neural mechanisms, motivational processes, and physiological adaptations.

Behavioral Neuroscience 124, 715–741.

Olazabal, D. E. & Young, L. J. (2006). Oxytocin receptors in the nucleus accumbens facilitate "spontaneous" maternal behavior in adult female prairie voles. *Neuroscience*, 559–568.

Pearson, R. M., Heron, J., Melotti, R., Joinson, C., Stein, A., Ramchandani, P. G. & Evans, J. (2011). The association between observed non-verbal maternal responses at 12 months and later infant development at 18 months and IQ at 4 years: A longitudinal study. *Infant Behavior and Development* 34, 525–533.

Pedersen, C. A., Ascher, J. A., Monroe, Y. L. & Prange, A. J. Jr. (1982). Oxytocin induces maternal behavior in virgin female rats. *Science* 216, 648–650.

Pedersen, C. A. & Prange, A. J. Jr. (1979). Induction of maternal behavior in virgin rats after intracerebroventricular administration of oxytocin. *Proceedings of the National Academy of Sciences of the United States of America* 76, 6661–6665.

Pollack, M. H. (2005). Comorbid anxiety and depression. *Journal of Clinical Psychiatry* 66, 22–29.

Pruessner, J. C., Champagne, F., Meaney, M. J., Dagher, A. (2004). Dopamine release in response to a psychological stress in humans and its relationship to early life maternal care: A positron emission tomography study using [11C] Raclopride. *The Journal of Neuroscience* 24(11), 2825–2831.

Ragnauth, A. K., Devidze, N., Moy, V., Finley, K., Goodwillie, A., Kow, L. M., Muglia, L. J. & Pfaff, D. W. (2005). Female oxytocin gene-knockout mice, in a semi-natural environment, display exaggerated aggressive behavior. *Genes, Brain, and Behaviour* 4, 229–239.

Ross, H. E. & Young, L. J. (2009). Oxytocin and the neural mechanisms regulating social cognition and affiliative behavior.

Frontiers in Neuroendocrinology 30, 534–547.

Rutter, M. (1966). *Children of sick parents: An environmental and psychiatric study* (Institute of Psychiatry, Maudsley Monographs No. 16). London: Oxford University Press.

Sidor, A., Kunz, E., Schweyer, D., Eickhorst, A. & Cierpka, M. (2011). Links between maternal postpartum depressive symptoms, maternal distress, infant gender and sensitivity in a high-risk population. *Child and Adolescent Psychiatry and Mental Health* 5.

Singer, L. T., Salvator, A., Guo, S., Collin, M., Lilien, L. & Baley, J. (1999). Maternal psychological distress and parenting stress after the birth of a very low-birth-weight infant. *Journal of the American Medical Association* 281, 799–805.

Sroufe, L. (2000). Early relationships and the development of children. *Infant Mental Health Journal* 21, 67–74.

Stachowiak, A., Macchi, C., Nussdorfer, G. G. & Malendowicz, L. K. (1995). Effects of oxytocin on the function and morphology of the rat adrenal cortex: In vitro and in vivo investigations. *Research in Experimental Medicine* 195, 265–274.

Strathearn, L., Fonagy, P., Amico, J. & Montague, P. R. (2009). Adult attachment predicts maternal brain and oxytocin response to infant cues. *Neuropsychopharmacology* 34, 2655–2666.

Swain, J. E., Kim, P., Spicer, J., Ho, S. S., Dayton, C. J., Elmadih, A. & Abel, K. M. (2014). Approaching the biology of human parental attachment: Brain imaging, oxytocin and coordinated assessments of mothers and fathers. *Brain Research*. doi: 10.1016/j.brainres.2014.03.007.

Tabak, B. A., McCullough, M. E., Szeto, A., Mendez, A. J. &

McCabe, P. M. (2011). Oxytocin indexes relational distress following interpersonal harms in women. *Psychoneuroendocrinology* 36, 115–122.

Taylor, S. E., Gonzaga, G. C., Klein, L. C., Hu, P., Greendale, G. A. & Seeman S. E. (2006). Relation of oxytocin to psychological stress responses and hypothalamic-pituitary-adrenocortical axis activity in older women. *Psychosomatic Medicine* 68, 238–245.

Taylor, S. E., Saphire-Bernstein, S. & Seeman, T. E. (2010). Are plasma oxytocin in women and plasma vasopressin in men biomarkers of distressed pair bond relationships? *Psychological Science* 21, 3–7.

Tronick, E. & Reck, C. (2009). Infants of depressed mothers. *Harvard Review of Psychiatry* 17, 147–156.

Turner, R. A., Altemus, M., Yip, D. N., Kupferman, E., Fletcher, D., Bostrom, A., Lyons, D. M. & Amico, J. A. (2002). Effects of emotion on oxytocin, prolactin, and ACTH in women. *Stress* 5, 269–276.

Uvnas-Moberg, K. (1998). Oxytocin may mediate the benefits of positive social interaction and emotions. *Psychoneuroendocrinology* 23, 819–835.

Van Leengoed, E., Kerker, E. & Swanson, H. H. (1987). Inhibition of postpartum maternal behaviour in the rat by injecting an oxytocin antagonist into the cerebral ventricles. *Journal of Endocrinology* 112, 275–282.

Wan, M. & Green J. (2009). The impact of maternal psychopathology on child-mother attachment. *Archives of Women's Mental Health* 12, 123–134.

Wan, M. W., Moulton, S. & Abel, K. M. (2008a). What interventions might improve the relationships of mothers with schizophrenia with their children? A Review. *Archives of Women's Mental Health* 11(3), 171–179.

Wan, M. W., Warren, K., Salmon, M. & Abel, K. M. (2008b). Patterns of maternal responding in postpartum mothers with Schizophrenia. *Infant Behavior and Development* 31, 532–538.

Wang, Z. X., Liu, Y., Young, L. J. & Insel, T. R. (2000). Hypothalamic vasopressin gene expression increases in both males and females postpartum in a biparental rodent. *Journal of Neuroendocrinology* 12, 111–120.

Warren, S. L. & Simmens, S. J. (2005). Predicting toddler anxiety, depressive symptoms: Effects of caregiver sensitivity on temperamentally vulnerable children. *Infant Mental Health Journal* 26, 40–55.

Webb, R., Pickles, A., Appleby, L., Mortensen, P. B. & Abel, K. M. (2007). Death by unnatural causes during childhood and early adulthood in offspring of psychiatric inpatients. *The Journal of the American Medical Association Psychiatry* 64, 345–352.

Williams, J. R., Catania, K. C. & Carter, C. S. (1992). Development of partner preferences in female prairie voles (Microtus ochrogaster): The role of social and sexual experience. *Hormones and Behaviors* 26, 339–349.

Wolpert, M., Hoffman, J., Martin, A., Fagin, L. & Cooklin, A. (2014). An exploration of the experience of attending the Kidstime programme for children with parents with enduring mental health issues: Parents' and young people's views. *Clinical Child Psychology and Psychiatry* 1359104514520759.

Zhang, T. Y. & Meaney, M. J. (2010). Epigenetics and the environmental regulation of the genome and its function. *Annual Review of Psychology* 61, 439–466.

Chapter

5

Genetic, epigenetic and gene-environment interactions
Impact on the pathogenesis of mental illnesses in women

Anthony P. Auger

Biological sex and brain pathology

The developmental programming of neuronal function within the human brain is influenced by the interplay of genes and the environment. An illustration of the critical importance of how the environment shapes neuronal development is that while all cells share the same genetic material, the maturation and functional role of neurons is dictated by the immediate environment. Importantly, perturbations during critical periods of brain development when neurons are sensitive to environmental influences can profoundly affect the overall health and well-being of an individual. While subtle differences in an individual's gene × environmental early experiences, including upbringing, can contribute to mental health risk later in life, they can also result in resilience to mental disorders. Perhaps one of the more intriguing biological factors that can increase one's resilience or risk to mental ill health is biological sex as defined by typical chromosomal sex. While biological sex can influence the development of peripheral tissues that are sensitive to chromosomal and hormonal differences, the brain is also exquisitely sensitive to some of these same influences, albeit at a more subtle level where it is challenging to observe physical differences. As a result of these differences, it is likely that biological sex can influence the occurrence, severity and age of onset in a number of neuropsychiatric disorders. Sex differences are well recognized in Alzheimer's disease, schizophrenia, Rett syndrome and autism spectrum disorders (ASD); however, the mechanisms associated with these sex differences remain unclear. Nonetheless, studies suggest biological sex contributes to an individual's risk or resilience to neuropsychiatric disorders across a lifespan and many such childhood disorders, such as autism and attention deficit hyperactivity disorder (ADHD), show greater prevalence in boys than girls. Understanding the biology controlling sexual differentiation of the developing brain may provide important clues (see Chapter 7) and *gene × environment × sex* interactions should be strongly considered when investigating etiology and course of mental health disorders (Figure 5.1).

Sex differences in brain

Many of the sex differences in some brain regions are organized during perinatal brain development. Sex differences are observed at a variety of levels and their functional impact on mental health risk remains to be clarified. Many regions involved in endocrine or reproductive function are sexually differentiated during development. The sexually dimorphic nucleus of the preoptic area (SDN-POA) has been consistently reported to be around 2–4 times larger in male compared to female rats (Gorski et al., 1978). Interestingly, in humans an analogous region has also been found to be larger in men than women. Analysis of four different cell groups, referred to as the Interstitial Nuclei of the Anterior Hypothalamus (INAH 1–4), indicated INAH-3 was around 2–3 times smaller in women than men. INAH-3 is similar to the SDN in rodents (Allen et al., 1989). While sex differences in size of this structure have been well characterized, in rodents it seems likely to inhibit female sexual behavior. Other regions also larger in volume in males include the bed nucleus of the stria terminalis and regions of the

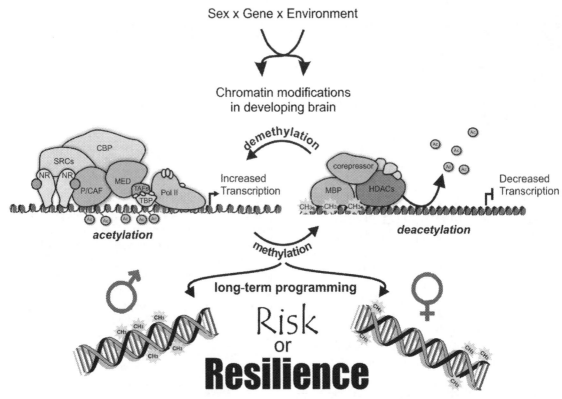

Figure 5.1 Sexual differentiation of the epigenome may underlie some sex differences in mental health risk or resilience. Several converging mechanisms program sex differences in the epigenome, such as sex chromosomes, hormones and environmental cues. These converging factors result in sex differences in the levels of epigenetic factors, such as cAMP response element binding protein-binding protein (CBP) and gene repressor molecules, such as methyl-binding protein (MBP) and corepressors, as well as in DNA methylation patterns. Sex differences in the epigenome may change the way neurons respond to environmental stressors. Therefore, epigenomic sex differences may underlie sex differences in risk and resilience to neurological and psychiatric disorders induced by environmental or genetic perturbations.

amygdala (Hines et al., 1992). The functional role of these areas is complex; the amygdala is increasingly recognized for its role in social cognition and socio-emotional processing. In contrast, the anteroventral periventricular nucleus (AVPV) is 2–3 times larger in women (Bleier et al., 1982) where this region of the brain is important in regulating the surge of luteinizing hormone that occurs in a healthy menstrual cycle and stimulates follicle maturation.

Other sexually dimorphic brain structures include the arcuate nucleus (Ciofi et al., 2006), ventromedial hypothalamus (Matsumoto and Arai, 1986) and substantia nigra pars compacta (Dewing et al., 2006). These structures play a major role in typical neuroendocrine functioning as well as in modifying both reproductive and nonreproductive behaviors; perturbations to the biological processes that produce these key sex dimorphisms may yield measurable differences in mental health risk between the sexes.

Therefore, it is important to understand the biological underpinnings of brain sexual differentiation.

Genetic contributions to sexual differentiation of brain

Numerous brain sex differences have been described in a variety of species, including humans, nonhuman primates, avian and rodent. Many of these differences manifest as varying degrees of difference in neuronal structure or function so there is no such thing as a recognizable "female brain" or "male brain"; rather, subtle but key differences can occur between the sexes in specific regions throughout the brain. Many are related to neuroendocrine systems associated with reproduction; neuroendocrine events can have an important impact on a wide variety of behaviors through widespread steroid receptor expression throughout the brain. Some brain sex differences may have the effect of reducing overt sex differences in neuronal functioning. That is, sex differences in gonadal hormone levels differentially affect brain cells in women and men, and some sex differences in brain may exist in order to "compensate" for these hormonal differences.

Sexual differentiation of the brain is influenced by a variety of processes, including genetic, hormonal and environmental factors (Lonstein and Auger, 2009; McCarthy and Arnold, 2011; Auger and Auger, 2011). Sexual differentiation of the brain mainly results from differences in gonadal steroid hormone exposure dictated by chromosomal sex. Gonadal differentiation is initiated by the sex-determining region Y (*Sry*) gene located on the Y chromosome. Following gonadal sex determination, testicular testosterone is released during a critical period of perinatal development and further differentiates female from male physiology, including the brain. Upon access to the brain, testosterone is converted into estradiol and dihydrotestosterone. While androgens are known to produce some brain sex differences, estradiol exposure is responsible for the most salient sex differences within brain estradiol during early perinatal development.

It is important to note that some level of estradiol exposure is necessary for the active feminization of the female brain. That is, interfering with the actions of estradiol during female brain development can further separate the female brain from that of males and disrupt normal female processes within brain (Lonstein and Auger, 2009). This indicates that some level of estradiol action within the developing female brain is necessary to produce typical levels of female sexual behavior and reproductive function. Interestingly, some regions within the female brain can produce local levels of estradiol that equal male levels (Amateau et al., 2004), which indicates the existence of biological pathways that induce neurosteroid synthesis within the female brain and may eliminate sex differences in estradiol exposure. The importance of estradiol action in female brain on other behavioral or physiological outcomes remains to be elucidated.

Regulation of steroid hormone transcription at the genome

While differences in steroid hormone exposure are important for brain sexual differentiation, hormones ultimately alter cell differentiation by binding to a variety of receptors, but most predominantly to steroid/nuclear receptors located within the cytoplasm or nuclear component of a cell. Steroid hormones are also known to bind to receptors located within the cell membrane; however, less is known about the importance of this pathway in differentiating female from male brain.

Nuclear receptors are well-categorized transcription factors that act upon the genome and provide for a molecular pathway by which environmental signals can act upon the genome to elicit brief or lasting changes in neuronal or gene function. Following binding, the hormone-bound steroid receptor forms a dimer complex with another steroid-bound receptor. This dimer complex then binds to a response element located within the promoter region of a vast number of target genes. The steroid receptor-bound complex initiates the recruitment of a variety of co-regulatory proteins and other transcriptional factors to the genome that results in alterations in the rate of gene transcription (Tetel et al., 2009). Proteins that bind steroid receptors to increase gene transcription are called co-activators and those that typically decrease gene transcription are called co-repressors (Auger and Jessen, 2009; Tetel et al., 2009). Therefore, regulating the cellular content of co-regulatory proteins provides for an additional pathway by which steroid hormones or other environmental signals can influence brain differentiation. Indeed, altering the expression of co-regulatory proteins can have profound and lasting consequences on sexual differentiation of juvenile and adult social and reproductive behaviors (Auger and Jessen, 2009). It remains to be fully determined how the expression of co-regulatory proteins is regulated within the developing or adult brain.

Importantly, the functional consequences of steroid receptor action at the genome can be both transient and lasting. Some of the more profound cellular changes that are initiated by steroid receptor action at the genome are alterations of cell number, migration patterns, phenotypical differentiation, as well as morphological differentiation of brain cells (Lonstein and Auger, 2009). Another mechanism by which brief changes in steroid hormones can produce lasting consequences on brain function throughout an organism's lifespan is by modifying the epigenome (McCarthy et al., 2009; Auger et al., 2010). Steroid receptor-induced epigenetic modifications provide an additional mechanism by which cells can store a "memory" of hormone exposure, as well as other endogenous or environmental experiences, at the level of the genome. As steroid hormones are extremely sensitive to subtle environmental changes, steroid receptor-sensitive neuroepigenetic processes provide for a signaling pathway by which environmental cues can influence brain development. Neuroendocrine differentiation of the brain, therefore, provides a useful model to study lasting epigenetic mechanisms that may affect mental health.

Hormone-induced male brain differentiation

While the developing brain can be considered bipotential with regard to sex, numerous developmental factors, such as hormones, chromosomes and the environment, can shift the developmental organization of the brain towards a male-typical phenotype. As discussed, many sex differences are observed at the level of neuronal density within some regions. Most data indicate that size differences in structural elements result from estradiol-induced neuronal protection from cell death, such as that occurring within the SDN. That is, programmed cell death within this region occurs due to reduced gonadal steroid hormone exposure. As human females have significantly lower levels of gonadal hormone exposure during the first few days of life, there is a dramatic increase in cell death within this region compared to males. Importantly, males castrated on the day of birth show increased cell death that resembles a female pattern. Likewise, in an adjacent region, the bed nucleus of the stria terminalis is also larger in males. In a similar process, the reduced gonadal hormone exposure in females or males castrated during the first week of life results in a dramatic increase in cell death. In contrast, females have a larger AVPV. Within this region, steroid hormone exposure induces cell death. Therefore, exposure to male-typical steroid hormone levels during early brain development results in dramatic alterations in cell number, and the mechanism by which this occurs is region dependent.

Exposure to male-typical steroid levels during brain development also results in phenotypic differentiation of neurons and glia (Mong et al., 1999). Indeed, steroid hormones alter the shape and the number of synaptic processes in a variety of brain regions. Perhaps some of the most robust phenotypic differences are within the vasopressin system (De Vries and Simerly, 2002). Males have more

vasopressin-expressing cells compared to females in amygdala and BST. These differences are mainly the result of steroid hormone exposure, although a small portion may be a result of direct chromosomal differences that are independent of gonadal hormone exposure (De Vries et al., 2002). As hormones elicit profound neurochemical and phenotypic changes in developing brain, it can be said that steroid hormones direct reorganization of neuroendocrine-sensitive systems throughout brain. Once such mechanisms are set in motion, any perturbations to these systems during active reorganization could produce maladaptive processing. It could be that the male brain is at greater risk of neurodevelopmental disorder as a result of "more active" reorganization of brain by steroid hormones. By contrast, as female brain development is subject to "default programming" relative to male brain differentiation, so the effect of endogenous or exogenous insults may have less impact.

Hormone-induced female brain differentiation

While hormonal differentiation of male brain has been extensively studied, less is known about the active differentiation of female brain. Female brain is considered "the default" but many mechanisms contribute to active organization of the female brain during development, including steroid hormone levels. Indeed, a number of reports indicate that disruption in estrogen exposure during development can have a lasting impact on female sexual behavior and brain morphology (Lonstein and Auger, 2009). In rats, ovariectomy during the first week of life reduces adult female sexual behavior. Furthermore, disrupting expression of estrogen receptor alpha in the first few days of life reduces the volume of the SDN (McCarthy et al., 1993). These data are supported by the findings that localized brain regions in females may be producing estradiol at male-like levels during development (Amateau et al., 2004). It is also likely that females produce male-like levels of estradiol within some brain regions in order to reduce sex differences that may occur through high circulating hormone levels in males. Combined, these data suggest that some level of estradiol exposure is necessary for typical female brain development. It is not known how disruptions in neurosteroid synthesis during female brain development affects adult neuropathology, and there remains a critical lack of research into the mechanisms behind female brain development.

A case for epigenetic programming in sexual differentiation of brain

Some of the cellular consequences of steroid hormone exposure can be nongenomic. Most of what we know about steroid hormone action results from modifications of chromatin structure and therefore is "epigenetic" in nature. The emergence of epigenetics explained how cells with the same genotype could produce different phenotypes. Conrad Waddington is credited with the origins of epigenetics. Its definition has evolved over the decades to include transgenerational epigenetic phenomena; here, we define epigenetics as a change to chromatin that may result in altered gene transcription efficiency (Auger and Auger, 2011). In the case of steroids, hormone-induced chromatin modifications allow for a mechanism by which cells can store a "memory" of hormone exposure and a biological mechanism by which environmental signals can alter gene expression. These alterations can be either lasting or brief, without the requirement of being passed on through cellular division. They include numerous modifications to both DNA and histones. Many epigenetic modifications result in subtle reorganization of chromatin structure resulting in subtle or profound effects on gene transcription.

Sexual differentiation of brain is mainly regulated by exposure to gonadal hormones during perinatal development. While exposure to gonadal hormones may be brief, the consequences may be long-lasting and represent an excellent model to study epigenetic programming of brain function. Indeed, reducing expression of proteins involved in histone modification, such as steroid receptor coactivater 1 (SRC-1) or cAMP response element binding protein-binding protein (CBP), disrupts sexual differentiation of behavior and brain morphology (Auger et al., 2000; Auger et al., 2002).

Numerous chromatin modifications have been identified: one of the more exciting alterations to DNA is through methylation of cytosine residues by a DNA methyltransferase (DNMT). Methylation of cytosine residues occurs mostly near guanine (CpG); however, cytosines can also be methylated near thymine (CpT), adenine (CpA), as well as other cytosines (CpC). Although it is unclear what the functional effects of methylation are at non-CpG sites, methylation of CpG sites has been found to have a profound impact on gene transcription. While CpG methylation itself can influence gene transcription, methylated CpGs appear to serve as a recognition site for methyl-binding proteins. Upon binding, methyl-binding proteins may recruit a co-repressor complex that ultimately brings in histone deacetylases that remove acetyl groups from histone tails. Decreasing acetylation of histones restores a positive charge, leading to chromatin condensation and reduced gene transcription. Therefore, changes in methylation of certain 5'-CpN-3' sites may have profound consequences on gene transcription.

While some DNA methylation patterns in the adult brain are actively maintained by a hormonal signal, therefore reversible (Auger and Auger, 2013; Auger et al., 2011), it is the relative stability of other methylation patterns that have led scientists to propose this as a mechanism for how early environmental influences can have lasting effects on gene expression. While some of these consequences may be minor, others may underlie differences in an individual's risk or resilience to a disorder.

Epigenetic risk or resilience

Epigenetic mechanisms provide an explanation of how a cellular signalling pathway can ensure a lasting difference in gene expression. As we progress towards understanding biological determinants of mental illness, we are finding associations of aberrant methylation patterns associated with psychiatric disorders. These methylation patterns may underlie symptoms of illness, and provide a potential explanation for increased risk of pathology. That is, if reduced activity of a particular signalling pathway confers risk for disorder, then the epigenetic markings that produced aberrations in that signalling pathway may be a critical factor conferring that risk. Some of these differences in epigenetic signatures may result from environmental perturbations, while others may result from naturally occurring sexual differentiation of the brain. Specifically, data indicate that during neonatal brain development, females and males may exhibit different methylation patterns as a result of testosterone exposure within the promoter regions of important molecules influencing brain development (Ghahramani et al., 2014; Kurian et al., 2010). Some of the sex differences in methylation patterns during brain development result in differential expression of genes and in differences in how cells respond to environment.

X chromosome confers resilience

Rett syndrome is a pervasive developmental disorder marked by impaired speech and social interactions, repetitive motor movements and seizures. Recently, it was found that disruptions in expression or function of methyl-CpG-binding protein 2 (MeCP2) occurs in over 90% of cases (Amir et al., 1999). As MeCP2 is an X-linked gene, Rett syndrome is primarily seen in females. Indeed, mutations in MeCP2 are usually embryonically lethal for males.

Interestingly, aberrant MECP2 promoter hypermethylation was also reported to occur in post-mortem tissue from individuals diagnosed with autism, suggesting that proper "dosing" of MeCP2 is important in a variety of autism-spectrum disorders. In women, one of their two X chromosomes is randomly inactivated by epigenetic mechanisms to correct for proper chromosomal dosage. In women, therefore, mutations on one X chromosome may be inactivated in some cells (including brain), creating mosaicism. Thus, female brain may be mosaic for a mutation; however, as males have no such "backup X chromosome," mutations will have consequences for all cells that require that gene for proper functioning (Figure 5.2). If the gene is important enough for survival, males may die from X chromosomal mutations. Nonlethal examples of mutations located on the X-chromosome include genes responsible for red and green cone cells, which is why men are more likely to be color-blind than women. Women would need to inherit two mutated copies for color blindness to occur.

Sex differences in epigenomic factors confer resilience in women

Sex chromosomal differences can contribute to mental health risk or resilience and sex differences in epigenetic factors may also underlie sex-differentiated mental health risk (Kigar and Auger, 2013; Jessen and Auger, 2011). We have observed sex differences in expression levels of a variety of epigenetic factors involved in brain development and juvenile social interactions. In particular, levels of MeCP2 were found to be higher in newborn female rats in amygdala and the hypothalamus; this is no longer apparent during the second week of life in developing rat brain (Kurian et al., 2007). We hypothesized that the lower level of MeCP2 expression at birth may put males at increased risk of developing symptoms inherent to MeCP2-related disorders. To test this concept, we transiently reduced levels of MeCP2 using small interfering (si)RNA targeted to MeCP2 within the developing amygdala during the first three days of life. We then assessed the impact on juvenile social play behavior, a sexually dimorphic behavior in which males play at higher levels (Auger and Olesen, 2009) and are sensitive to perturbations to epigenetic factors during brain development (Auger et al., 2010). Transient reduction of MeCP2 levels in amygdala had profound lasting consequences on juvenile social play behavior in males, but not females (Kurian et al., 2008). Specifically, MeCP2 siRNA-infused males engaged in less juvenile social play behavior; as this behavior is highly

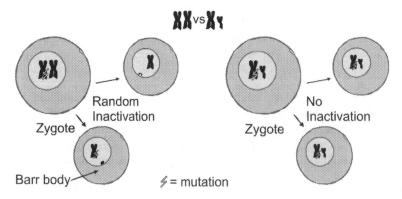

Figure 5.2 Chromosomal sex and X inactivation may be a contributing factor to female mental health resilience. As females have two X chromosomes, one of the X chromosomes is randomly inactivated by epigenetic mechanisms to correct for proper chromosomal dosage. As such, mutations on the X chromosome in females may be randomly inactivated in some brain cells. This creates a female brain that is mosaic for the mutation. As males have no additional X chromosome, mutations on the X chromosome will have consequences for all cells.

reward driven, reduction of MeCP2 may have induced social anhedonia in male, but not female rats who appear somewhat resilient to MeCP2-induced alterations at least in respect of juvenile social play behavior. Additionally, transient reductions of MeCP2 using siRNA in the developing amygdala resulted in lasting reduction of AVP expression in male, but not female rats (Forbes-Lorman et al., 2012). These data suggest that the male juvenile brain is more sensitive to neonatal perturbations in amygdala MeCP2 expression. It remains to be fully elucidated why females appear to be more resilient to perturbations in amygdala MeCP2 expression. It may be that females have higher background MeCP2 expression; alternatively, they may be able to compensate for perturbations in MeCP2 expression through activation of a compensatory MeCP2 allele on the X chromosome.

Epigenetic differences have been associated with a number of mental health and neuropsychiatric disorders, including Alzheimer's disease, schizophrenia and depression. Interestingly, sex differences in gene methylation patterns have been reported in patients diagnosed with schizophrenia and bipolar disorder (Mill et al., 2008; Connor and Akbarian, 2008). WNT1, part of the Wnt signalling pathway, is hypermethylated in women diagnosed with psychosis. Nuclear Receptor Related 1 protein (NURR1), also known as NR4A2 (nuclear receptor subfamily, group A, member 2), is also reported to be hypermethylated in women with schizophrenia. NURR1 is suggested to protect dopamine cells from inflammation. Hypermethylation of NURR1 could lead to inflammation-induced cell death of dopamine cells within female brain. Whether these differences occur as a result of psychosis or are predictors of psychosis is unclear. It is also unclear why epigenetic markings are different between the sexes, but epigenetic factors during brain development may contribute to explanations of sex differences in vulnerability to mental health and neurodevelopmental risk (Kigar and Auger, 2013; Jessen and Auger, 2011).

Converging lines of research indicate that female brain may express higher levels of proteins involved in blunting the actions of gonadal steroids during postnatal development. Newborn female brain expresses higher levels of DNMT3a (Kolodkin and Auger, 2011), MeCP2 (Kurian et al., 2007) and nuclear corepressor 1 (NCoR) (Jessen et al., 2010). If differences in early-life gonadal hormone exposure can increase susceptibility to psychopathology, then the female brain may be more resilient to gonadal hormone-induced mental health risk during perinatal brain development as it is exposed to lower levels of these steroids than male brain. That is, heightened gonadal exposure may induce differentiation into male brain, and perturbations during this differentiation period may yield increased psychopathological risk. Indeed, reducing levels of NCoR within neonatal amygdala results in impaired male-typical juvenile social interactions in males, but not females (Jessen et al., 2010). Thus, epigenetic mechanisms that reduce the impact of gonadal hormone exposure during brain development in females may also influence increased mental health risk observed in males.

Gene × environment × sex interactions on mental health risk

Chromosomal sex is well-recognized to confer risk of psychiatric and neurodevelopmental risk; less well-known is that subtle alterations in the genome may also confer risk in a sex-specific manner. For example, protection against alcohol dependence is associated with single nucleotide polymorphisms (SNP; SNP rs279871) in men with positive life events, but not in women (Perry et al., 2013). Polymorphisms of the oxytocin receptor gene (SNP rs53576) also seem to show sex-differentiated effects of negative environment. Specifically, women are affected by negative environments regardless of genotype, whereas genotype appears to influence how men respond to negative social environments (Lucas-Thompson and Holman, 2013). Brain-derived neurotrophic factor (BDNF) Val66Met polymorphism appears to confer resilience to childhood maltreatment in exposed boys but not girls (Min et al., 2013). Not only can alterations in genetic material affect how one responds to environmental stressors in a sex-specific manner, but subtle differences in gene sequences can also lead to increased susceptibility to neuropathology. For example, an SNP within the reelin gene (SNP rs7341475) is associated with increased schizophrenia risk in women only (Shifman et al., 2008; Liu et al., 2010). These data indicate that subtle alterations in gene sequence can confer risk to mental health in a sex-dependent way. Therefore, it is likely that subtle differences in the episexome may also confer risk to mental health disorders in a sex-specific manner.

Genetic, epigenetic and gene-environment interactions

Neuroepigenetics is an exciting new scientific field. As it matures, it will no doubt yield further understanding about how environmental effects can program lasting changes in gene expression and influence neuronal functioning. More importantly, it will elucidate how environmental-induced modifications to chromatin structure contribute to mental health risk. During brain development, sex chromosomes and differences in gonadal hormone exposure differentiate a female into a male brain. These subtle differences not only result in sex differences in neuroendocrine functioning and behavior between women and men, but may result in sex differences in resilience and risk to neuropsychiatric outcomes. Indeed, an additional X chromosome influences the occurrence of Rett syndrome and may also affect prevalence of other disorders. Sex differences in mutations within the DNA code can also influence how women and men differentially respond to environmental stressors. As epigenetic mechanisms are being implicated in numerous neurological or psychiatric disorders, it is not surprising that sex differences in epigenetic mechanisms may be a contributing factor to an individual's mental health risk.

Sex must also be considered when attempting to understand gene × environment interactions in disease; thus, brain sex differences will influence how one responds to environmental cues, and environment can also produce sex differences in the epigenome, for example through sex differences in mother-offspring interactions (Kurian et al., 2010). Intriguingly, sex differences in epigenetic factors may result in female resilience to developmental disorders that occur preadolescence: as discussed, boys are more at risk for childhood neurodevelopmental disorders like ADHD and autism, developmental language delay, dyslexia and dyspraxia and cognitive disability associated with obstetric complications (Abel and Allin 2015). Many of the sex differences in brain appear to be due to hormones acting on chromatin structure (Auger and Auger, 2013; Kigar and Auger, 2013). Therefore, epigenetic differences induced by early gonadal steroid exposure or those implicated in X inactivation are likely to contribute to female resilience to neurodevelopmental adversity.

References

Abel, K. M. & Allin, M. (2015) Placental programming & neurodevelopmental outcomes. In: *Placenta and neurodisability*, 2nd Edition, (Baker, P., & Sibley, C., eds.). London, UK: The MacKeith Press.

Allen, L. S., Hines, M., Shryne, J. E., & Gorski, R. A. (1989) Two sexually dimorphic cell groups in the human brain. *Journal of Neuroscience* 9:497–506.

Amateau, S. K., Alt, J. J., Stamps, C. L., McCarthy, M. M. (2004) Brain oestradiol content in newborn rats: sex differences, regional heterogeneity, and possible de novo synthesis by the female telencephalon. *Endocrinology* 145:2906–2917.

Amir, R. E., Van, de Veyver, I. B., Wan, M., Tran, C. Q., Francke, U., & Zoghbi, H. Y. (1999) Rett syndrome is caused by mutations in X-linked MECP2, encoding methyl-CpG-binding protein 2. *Nature Genetics* 23:185–188.

Auger, A. P., & Auger, C. J. (2011) Epigenetic turn ons and turn offs: Chromatin reorganization and brain differentiation. *Endocrinology* 152:349–353.

Auger, A. P., & Jessen, H. M. (2009) Corepressors, nuclear receptors, and epigenetic factors on DNA: a tail of repression. *Psychoneuroendocrinology* 34 Suppl 1:S39–S47.

Auger, A. P., Jessen, H. M., & Edelmann, M. N. (2010) Epigenetic organization of brain sex differences and juvenile social play behavior. *Hormones and Behavior* 3:358–363.

Auger, A. P., & Olesen, K. M. (2009) Brain sex differences and the organisation of juvenile social play behaviour. *Journal of Neuroendocrinology* 21:519–525.

Auger, A. P., Perrot-Sinal, T. S., Auger, C. J., Ekas, L. A., Tetel, M. J., & McCarthy, M. M. (2002) Expression of the nuclear receptor coactivator, cAMP response element-binding protein, is sexually dimorphic and modulates sexual differentiation of neonatal rat brain. *Endocrinology* 143:3009–3016.

Auger, A. P., Tetel, M. J., & McCarthy, M. M. (2000) Steroid receptor coactivator-1 (SRC-1) mediates the development of sex-specific brain morphology and behavior. *Proceedings of the National Academy of Sciences, USA* 97:7551–7555.

Auger, C. J., & Auger, A. P. (2013) Permanent and plastic epigenesis in neuroendocrine systems. *Frontiers in Neuroendocrinology* 34(3):190–197.

Auger, C. J., Coss, D., Auger, A. P., & Forbes-Lorman, R. M. (2011) Epigenetic control of vasopressin expression is maintained by steroid hormones in the adult male rat brain. *Proceedings of the National Academy of Sciences, USA* 108:4242–4247.

Bleier, R., Byne, W., & Siggelkow, I. (1982) Cytoarchitectonic sexual dimorphisms of the medial preoptic and anterior hypothalamic areas in guinea pig, rat, hamster, and mouse. *Journal of Comparative Neuroogyl* 212:118–130.

Ciofi, P., Leroy, D., Tramu, G. (2006) Sexual dimorphism in the organization of the rat hypothalamic infundibular area. *Neuroscience* 141:1731–1745.

Connor, C. M., & Akbarian, S. (2008) DNA methylation changes in schizophrenia and bipolar disorder. *Epigenetics* 3:55–58.

De Vries, G. J., Rissman, E. F., Simerly, R. B., Yang, L. Y., Scordalakes, E. M., Auger, C. J., Swain, A., Lovell-Badge, R., Burgoyne, P. S., Arnold, A. P. (2002) A model system for study of sex chromosome effects on sexually dimorphic neural and behavioral traits. *Journal of Neuroscience* 22:9005–9014.

De Vries, G. J., & Simerly, R. B. (2002) Anatomy, development, and function of sexually dimorphic neural circuits in the mammalian brain. In: *Hormones, brain and behavior* (Pfaff, D. W., Arnold, A. P., Etgen, A. M., Fahrbach, S. E., & Rubin, R. T., eds.), pp. 137–191. San Diego: Academic Press.

Dewing, P., Chiang, C. W., Sinchak, K., Sim, H., Fernagut, P. O., Kelly, S., Chesselet, M. F., Micevych, P. E., Albrecht, K. H., Harley, V. R., & Vilain, E. (2006) Direct regulation of adult brain function by the male-specific factor SRY. *Current Biology* 16:415–420.

Forbes-Lorman, R. M., Rautio, J. J., Kurian, J. R., Auger, A. P., & Auger, C. J. (2012) Neonatal MeCP2 is important for the organization of sex differences in vasopressin expression. *Epigenetics* 7:230–238.

Ghahramani, N. M., Ngun, T. C., Chen, P. Y., Tian, Y., Krishnan, S., Muir, S., Rubbi, L., Arnold, A. P., De Vries, G. J., Forger, N. G., Pellegrini, M., & Vilain, E. (2014) The effects of perinatal testosterone exposure on the DNA methylome of the mouse brain are late-emerging. *Biology of Sex Differences* 5:8.

Gorski, R. A., Gordon, J. H., Shryne, J. E., & Southam, A. M. (1978) Evidence for a morphological sex difference within the medial preoptic area of the rat brain. *Brain Research* 148:333–346.

Hines, M., Allen, L. S., & Gorski, R. A. (1992) Sex differences in subregions of the medial nucleus of the amygdala and the bed nucleus of the stria terminalis of the rat. *Brain Research* 579:321–326.

Jessen, H. M., & Auger, A. P. (2011) Sex differences in epigenetic mechanisms may underlie risk and resilience for mental health disorders. *Epigenetics* 6:857–861.

Jessen, H. M., Kolodkin, M. H., Bychowski, M. E., Auger, C. J., & Auger, A. P. (2010) The nuclear receptor corepressor has organizational effects within the developing amygdala on juvenile social play and anxiety-like behavior. *Endocrinology* 151:1212–1220.

Kigar, S. L., & Auger, A. P. (2013) Epigenetic mechanisms may underlie the aetiology of sex differences in mental health risk and resilience. *Journal of Neuroendocrinology* 25:1141–1150.

Kolodkin, M. H., & Auger, A. P. (2011) Sex difference in the expression of DNA methyltransferase 3a (DNMT3a) in the rat amygdala during development. *Journal of Neuroendocrinology* 7:577–583.

Kurian, J. R., Bychowski, M. E., Forbes-Lorman, R. M., Auger, C. J., & Auger, A. P. (2008) Mecp2 organizes juvenile social behavior in a sex-specific manner. *Journal of Neuroscience* 28:7137–7142.

Kurian, J. R., Forbes-Lorman, R. M., & Auger, A. P. (2007) Sex difference in mecp2 expression during a critical period of rat brain development. *Epigenetics* 2:173–178.

Kurian, J. R., Olesen, K. M., & Auger, A. P. (2010) Sex differences in epigenetic regulation of the estrogen receptor-alpha promoter within the developing preoptic area. *Endocrinology* 151:2297–2305.

Liu, Y., Chen, P. L., McGrath, J., Wolyniec, P., Fallin, D., Nestadt, G., Liang, K. Y., Pulver, A., Valle, D., & Avramopoulos, D. (2010) Replication of an association of a common variant in the Reelin gene (RELN) with schizophrenia in Ashkenazi Jewish women. *Psychiatry Genetics* 20:184–186.

Lonstein, J. S., & Auger, A. P. (2009) Perinatal gonadal hormone influences on neurobehavioral development. In: *Handbook of behavioral and comparative neuroscience* (Blumberg, M., Freeman, J., & Robinson, S., eds.), pp. 424–453. New York: Oxford University Press.

Lucas-Thompson, R. G., & Holman, E. A. (2013) Environmental stress, oxytocin receptor gene (OXTR) polymorphism, and mental health following collective stress. *Hormones and Behavior* 63:615–624.

Matsumoto, A., & Arai, Y. (1986) Male-female difference in synaptic organization of the ventromedial nucleus of the hypothalamus in the rat. *Neuroendocrinology* 42:232–236.

McCarthy, M. M., & Arnold, A. P. (2011) Reframing sexual differentiation of the brain. *Nature Neuroscience* 14:677–683.

McCarthy, M. M., Auger, A. P., Bale, T. L., De Vries, G. J., Dunn, G. A., Forger, N. G., Murray, E. K., Nugent, B. M., Schwarz, J. M., Wilson, M. E. (2009) The epigenetics of sex differences in the brain. *Journal of Neuroscience* 29:12815–12823.

McCarthy, M. M., Schlenker, E. H., Pfaff, D. W. (1993) Enduring consequences of neonatal treatment with antisense

53

oligodeoxynucleotides to estrogen receptor messenger ribonucleic acid on sexual differentiation of rat brain. *Endocrinology* 133:433–439.

Mill, J., Tang, T., Kaminsky, Z., Khare, T., Yazdanpanah, S., Bouchard, L., Jia, P., Assadzadeh, A., Flanagan, J., Schumacher, A., Wang, S. C., & Petronis, A. (2008) Epigenomic profiling reveals DNA-methylation changes associated with major psychosis. *American Journal of Human Genetics* 82:696–711.

Min, J. A., Lee, H. J., Lee, S. H., Park, Y. M., Kang, S. G., Chae, J. H. (2013) Gender-specific effects of brain-derived neurotrophic factor Val66Met polymorphism and childhood maltreatment on anxiety. *Neuropsychobiology* 67:6–13.

Mong, J. A., Glaser, E., & McCarthy, M. M. (1999) Gonadal steroids promote glial differentiation and alter neuronal morphology in the developing hypothalamus in a regionally specific manner. *Journal of Neuroscience* 19:1464–1472.

Perry, B. L., Pescosolido, B. A., Bucholz, K., Edenberg, H., Kramer, J., Kuperman, S., Schuckit, M. A., & Nurnberger, J. I., Jr. (2013) Gender-specific gene-environment interaction in alcohol dependence: the impact of daily life events and GABRA2. *Behavior Genetics* 43:402–414.

Shifman, S., Johannesson, M., Bronstein, M., Chen, S. X., Collier, D. A., Craddock. N. J., Kendler, K. S., Li, T., O'Donovan, M., O'Neill, F. A., Owen, M. J., Walsh, D., Weinberger, D. R., Sun, C., Flint, J., & Darvasi, A. (2008) Genome-wide association identifies a common variant in the reelin gene that increases the risk of schizophrenia only in women. *PLoS Genetics* 4:e28.

Tetel, M. J., Auger, A. P., & Charlier, T. D. (2009) Who's in charge? Nuclear receptor coactivator and corepressor function in brain and behavior. *Front Neuroendocrinology* 30:328–342.

Chapter

6

Developmental disorders in girls
Focus on autism spectrum disorders

Bernice Knight, Peter Carpenter and Dheeraj Rai

Autism spectrum disorders

Autism spectrum disorders (ASD) are neurodevelopmental disorders classically characterized by qualitative impairments in reciprocal social interaction, communication, restricted interests and repetitive and stereotyped patterns of behaviors.

The term autism spectrum disorder, only recently included in the Diagnostic and Statistical Manual (DSM-5), includes conditions classified as childhood autism, Asperger syndrome and other conditions classified as pervasive developmental disorders in DSM-IV and the International Classification of Diseases (ICD-10). In this chapter, we use the term autism interchangeably with ASD.

The reported prevalence of ASD has markedly increased over the past few decades. Fewer than 1 in 2000 children were estimated to have these disorders in the 1980s although recent population-based studies report a prevalence of 1% or greater of the child (Baird et al., 2006; Centers for Disease Control and Prevention, 2012; Idring et al., 2012; Kim et al., 2011) and adult (Brugha et al., 2011) population.

ASDs appear to be underrepresented in females in clinical as well as epidemiological studies. This gender bias has been evident since the earliest descriptions of autism (Asperger, 1944; Kanner, 1943). The male: female ratio in the various studies ranges from 2:1 to 9:1 (Baird et al., 2006; Baron-Cohen et al., 2009; Brugha et al., 2011; Idring et al., 2012; Kim et al., 2011; Lord et al., 1982; Mattila et al., 2011; Wing, 1981). The studies also point to the possibility that women and girls with autism exhibit relatively higher rates of coexisting intellectual disability (ID) than men and boys with autism (Lord et al., 1982; Volkmar et al., 1993; Wing, 1981). The differences in the sex ratios observed across studies

may be linked to differing methods of case-finding, diagnostic methods and definition of ASD; varying levels of ASD severity; and different proportions of individuals with co-occurring intellectual disability. However, a male preponderance of ASD is a consistent finding across studies and fits with the male preponderance in all neurodevelopmental disorders.

Despite much research, the reason(s) why ASD may be relatively underrepresented in females are not yet fully understood. In this chapter, we present an overview of the various possibilities that have been proposed to explain this phenomenon, and their implications for women with autism.

Diagnostic tools for ASD are geared towards identifying boys

There is increasing awareness amongst professionals that girls with ASD are probably being underdiagnosed, and this may, in part, reflect gender differences observed. A diagnosis of ASD is commonly made using structured assessments and the process involves a detailed developmental history, coupled with clinical observation. Commonly used instruments include the Autism Diagnostic Observation Schedule (ADOS) (Lord et al., 1989), the Autism Diagnostic interview – Revised (ADI-R) (Lord et al., 1994) and the Diagnostic Interview for Social and Communication Disorders (DISCO) (Wing et al., 2002), amongst others. Three recent studies have found that in the absence of other symptoms, such as intellectual disability or behavioral problems, girls with similar level of autistic symptoms are less likely to receive this diagnosis (Constantino et al., 2010; Dworzynski et al., 2012; Russell et al., 2010).

It is notable that the assessment tools do not assume any baseline differences between the genders

Comprehensive Women's Mental Health, ed. David J. Castle and Kathryn M. Abel. Published by Cambridge University Press.
© Cambridge University Press 2016.

and that the diagnoses of autism are made against absolute impairments. Gender-sensitive scales are not in routine use and it is therefore possible that the instruments used to ascertain ASD better capture the male manifestations of autism-like features, leading to underdiagnosis in girls (Kopp and Gillberg, 2011).

The defining features of autism are more likely to be observed in boys

Hans Asperger, in his detailed descriptions of four children whose presentation would later be used to describe "Asperger syndrome" stated (in German) that "autism is an extreme variant of male intelligence and characteristics" (Asperger, 1944). This notion has been further extended and researched as the "extreme male brain" theory of autism, which is expanded upon later in this chapter.

Before discussing autism, it would be useful to note that girls and boys are different in their development, behavior and preferences (also see Chapters 5 and 8 on social constructs and women's mental health). Typically, the social development of boys is known to be slower than that of girls. Socio-cognitive abilities that show a female superiority include the ability to read nonverbal communications signals (such as body posture and facial expression), language development and empathizing. All of these developmental domains are relevant to autism.

Female and male roles from an evolutionary perspective

Female and male gender roles may also be discussed from an evolutionary perspective. The two genders have been thought to have different requirements from social relationships for bringing up offspring to continue their bloodline (Geary, 1998). Women have thus been described as needing to place more value on reciprocal social relationships than men, while their relationships with other women should be more consistently communal. Women also typically exhibit greater empathy, nurturing, intimacy and emotional support, probably enabling a more stable social environment in which to bring up children. In contrast, men's relationships with each other may be more outcome-orientated, aiming to manipulate their environment. Reproductive success for early humans may have relied on domination of others, so social relationships may have been relatively disadvantageous for men.

Cognitive bias in female and male brains

Baron-Cohen has postulated that there is a cognitive gender bias in the human brain: women's brains are biased towards "empathizing," while men's are biased towards "systematizing." Women and men are therefore considered to be fundamentally different in their approach to the world because of these natural cognitive biases (Baron-Cohen, 2002). "Empathizing" can be described as the attribution of mental states to others, with an appropriate affective response to the other's mental state. To support this theory, Baron-Cohen reviewed a range of studies supporting women's superior ability to empathize (Baron-Cohen, 2002). According to these, girls and women displayed:

- less rough play;
- more concern for fairness through sharing and turn-taking;
- greater sharing of emotional distress with their friends;
- better inference of what others are thinking;
- greater sensitivity to facial expressions and preference for faces;
- more value in relationships;
- less psychopathic personality disorders, less aggression and less murder;
- more cooperative speech and conversations that have greater emotional expression; and
- better language development.

Conversely, the "systematizing" brain (anecdotally more prevalent in men), has a preference for data gathering and correlating variables with outcomes in order to devise a system of prediction. With that comes an understanding of how systems work through the formation of rules. Evidence to support this included (Baron-Cohen, 2002):

- preference for mechanical toys;
- adult occupational preferences in maths, physics, engineering and construction that are more systems-based;
- better constructional abilities;
- better attention to relevant detail;
- better map reading and rotational judgment;
- more precise neurological motor movements; and
- more advanced understanding of systems.

These observations led to the "extreme male brain" theory of autism (Baron-Cohen, 2002).

The extreme male brain theory of autism

According to the extreme male brain theory, people with autism show impaired empathizing on objective tests that is consistently poorer than in healthy males who are already less empathic on objective testing than healthy females. Furthermore, they also found superior systematizing, using proxy tests and observations that were already more advanced in healthy men compared to healthy women. Some evidence in favor of this hypothesis is outlined in this chapter, although some authors have questioned its validity (Jordan-Young, 2010). For instance, Jordan-Young (2010) argues that scientific research exploring causal relationships between sex and a disorder are wrong to assume a unidirectional relationship initiated by biological sex. Instead, brain structure and function should be thought of as resulting from an entangled interplay between social, biosocial and biological mechanisms that cannot be properly investigated without taking these multidirectional relationships into account. However, the predominant extreme male brain theory implies that women who develop autism are more divergent from healthy women (in brain and behavior) than men with autism are from healthy men.

Camouflage and social mimicry

As children grow up they tend to copy the actions of people they hold in esteem. When a child (or adult) with high-functioning autism tries to "pass as normal," they may do so by copying others. Women with autism seem to be more practiced at this social mimicry and, as a result perhaps, their social deficits can appear subtler. It has been suggested that girls with autism may use intellectual abilities rather than natural intuition for such interaction with others. For instance, they may do so by learning to observe and imitate social interactions (Attwood, 2007). It is interesting to note that high-functioning women and girls with autism have been shown to display relatively less autistic behavior during interpersonal interaction, despite having more reported autistic traits and sensory deficits (Lai et al., 2011). A recent population-based study found that men with higher levels of social cognition difficulties were more likely to have coexisting impairments in facial emotion recognition, but this was not observed for women, possibly suggesting that girls with autistic features may be able to compensate for their covert deficits in emotion recognition (Kothari et al., 2013).

The social camouflage just described may be aided in females with higher intellectual capacity – and they may be more skilled than those with a lower IQ at compensating for their qualitative difficulties in social interaction. They may require a greater severity of autistic symptoms or intellectual impairment before being diagnosable with an autism spectrum disorder. This observation is also in keeping with the hypothesis that women want to interact socially more than men and that, in those with ASD, this may be achieved through their intellectual skills rather than any "social instinct." Finally, this observation is also consistent with the possibility that ASD may be more likely to be suspected in women with a coexisting intellectual disability.

Girls with autism may, therefore, be harder to recognize during clinical assessment, as they appear more able to learn how to act in a social setting, such as using appropriate affect and gestures during a clinical interview.

Restricted and stereotyped patterns of interests and behavior

In normal early childhood, self-stimulation such as rocking, spinning and other repetitive behaviors is common. However, these are usually suppressed as the child develops in keeping with social norms. Children who are less aware or less bothered by the perceptions of others (typically children with ASD) may be less likely to suppress this self-stimulatory behavior. Some studies have indicated that stereotypic behaviors and interests are more pronounced in males with autism than females (Bolte et al., 2011). A recent systematic review and meta-analysis of 20 studies found no major gender differences between social and communication behaviors but reported that repetitive and stereotyped behaviors were observed less commonly in girls with ASD (Van Wijngaarden-Cremers et al., 2014). This, combined with the ability to camouflage social deficits, may make it harder for professionals to be able to identify autism in girls.

If women with ASD are keener than men with ASD to mask their deficits, then one might expect them to show fewer of these self-stimulatory behaviors when in the company of others. Clinical experience also suggests that the preoccupations and interests of women tend to differ from that of men.

In women, preoccupations tend to be more people and socially orientated. Preoccupations such as the psychology of others or animals are not uncommon. In these cases, it is the intensity and dominance of the interest rather than its peculiarity that may enable recognition of an autism spectrum disorder.

Other potential indicators of an ascertainment bias against females

Boys are also more likely to display externalizing problem behaviors such as aggression and hyperactivity, whereas girls may display more internalizing behaviors such as depression and anxiety or passive forms of demand avoidance (Werling and Geschwind, 2013). The finding of a greater prevalence of intellectual disabilities in girls with ASD may have biological explanations as noted in the following section, but may also be an indicator of ascertainment bias. In other words, girls with autism who also have intellectual disabilities may come to the attention of clinicians more easily. This possibility is supported by a recent study from South Korea that found a relatively lower male:female ratio where cases were ascertained using population screening rather than measured diagnoses (Kim et al., 2011). Some recent epidemiological studies also note that the male:female ratios decline from 5:1 at age 8 to 2:1 as the follow-up time is extended into adulthood, accounting for a delayed recognition of females (Idring et al., 2012).

Biological mechanisms

Although ascertainment bias may explain some of the sex differences observed, it is unlikely to be a complete explanation for these consistently observed phenomena, and biological mechanisms are likely to be important. Gender differences are apparent in normal and pathological human development, as well as brain functioning, and may therefore contribute to ASD in a variety of ways (Institute of Medicine et al., 2001). It is now increasingly acknowledged that ASDs constitute a group of conditions caused by several different and individual conditions (Lai et al., 2014; Levy et al., 2009). These may all affect the same final common pathway in the brain, and go on to cause individuals to present with autistic features (Gillberg and Coleman, 2000). Some recent advances and findings in relation to sex differences in autism are summarized next.

Genetic explanations

It is now well known that autism spectrum disorders are highly heritable. However, despite over 35 years of scrutiny since the first twin studies of autism were published (Folstein and Rutter, 1977), there is still much to learn about the precise genetic etiology of ASD (Rutter, 2005). It is accepted that multiple genetic factors, including genes that are passed down from parents, may predispose individuals towards developing ASD. There are a number of possible genetic mechanisms that may explain the apparently lower prevalence of ASD in girls and women.

One of the first factors examined in relation to this was the possibility that autism is an X-linked condition whereby females, who have two X chromosomes, could be protected from the deleterious effects of mutations on one of them through compensatory transcription from the other, intact X chromosome (Werling and Geschwind, 2013). Although there is little evidence to suggest that significant proportions of cases of autism are X-linked disorders (in the Mendelian sense), the chromosomal complement may modulate the risk (Werling and Geschwind, 2013).

Females have two X chromosomes: one maternal and one paternal copy. Males always inherit their single X chromosome from their mother and a Y chromosome from their father. A mechanism called "imprinting" silences one copy of the X chromosome in women, to prevent an excess of gene products. After studying autism in women with Turner's syndrome (XO), Skuse (2000) reported that those who developed autism had predominantly inherited their intact X chromosome from the mother. This led to the hypothesis that there may be a "protective gene" that is only expressed by the paternally inherited X chromosome (Skuse, 2000). The genetic code for this gene may be silenced when it is transmitted by a mother and is switched on when transmitted by a father. (See Figure 6.1.) By virtue of possessing a "protective locus" that is expressed from the paternally derived X chromosome, girls may have a higher threshold for expression of ASD features that would be uniformly impaired in both genders with an ASD predisposition. Despite this presenting a compelling argument, no specific genes have been located on the human X chromosome that behave in such a manner.

There has been much discussion about the possibility that girls have inherent biological protection

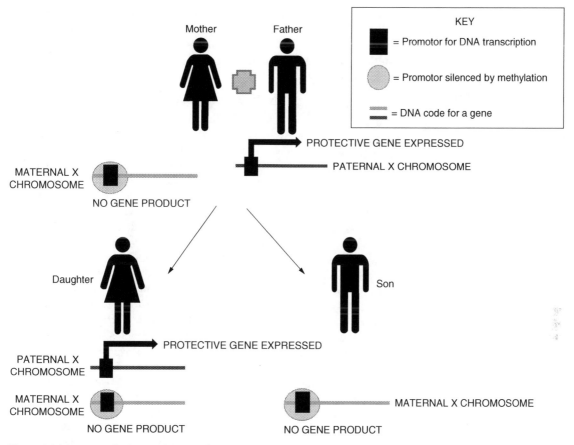

Figure 6.1 Inheritance of a theoretical imprinted protective ASD gene on the X chromosome

or resilience against developing symptoms associated with autism, having a higher threshold for displaying the symptoms compared to boys. This would imply that girls require a *greater* number of heritable genetic mutations in order to display the *same* level of ASD symptomatology as boys (Jacquemont et al., 2014; Werling and Geschwind, 2013). One recent study examining the "resilience argument" reported that girls with more quantitative autistic trait impairments than boys had more autistic features within their families (Robinson et al., 2013). There is also increasing evidence of the sex-specific penetrance of heritable loci (proportion of individuals with a genetic mutation experiencing clinical symptoms), as well as de novo (spontaneous) genetic insults. A reexamination of genome-wide association studies found new genetic markers that were not detected when sex-specificity was ignored (Lu and Cantor, 2012). Two recent studies reported that de novo Copy

Number Variations (expansions in the genetic code) associated with ASD were larger and more functionally disruptive when present in females compared to males (Gilman et al., 2011; Levy et al., 2011).

Hormonal effects

Many sex differences are developmentally organized, and then activated or revealed by the action of adult hormones (McCarthy et al., 2012). Hormones such as testosterone, estrogen and oxytocin (Chapter 4, 8), levels of which differ between sexes, are potential biomarkers for gender differences observed in ASD (Knickmeyer and Baron-Cohen, 2006; Schwarz et al., 2011).

Testosterone is made first in the fetal testes at about 9 weeks gestation; otherwise small amounts cross the placenta from the mother in both sexes. At 12–18 weeks, sex differences in serum testosterone are highest and sexual differentiation in the brain usually occurs, probably reflecting an important period for masculinization of the brain (Knickmeyer and Baron-Cohen, 2006). Small amounts of ovarian hormones are additionally required for active feminization of the female brain. It is understood that androgens organize male-type brain circuitry regardless of the genetic sex. If androgens were responsible for the development of autism, they would likely act via points of developmental sensitivity such as cognitive brain systems that are androgen-sensitive. Women with autism could be subjected to the masculinizing effect of more androgen-related molecules such as male sex hormones, usually present in small amounts in females. This hypothesis is supported by findings that women with autism have higher rates of androgen-related medical conditions such as polycystic ovarian syndrome (Ingudomnukul et al., 2007), late onset menarche (Knickmeyer et al., 2006b) and elevated serum testosterone levels with masculinized physical features (Schwarz et al., 2011). Furthermore, girls with congenital adrenal hyperplasia, characterized by an excess of steroid hormones, have been reported to have higher levels of autistic traits than their unaffected sisters (Knickmeyer et al., 2006a).

It has also been suggested that testosterone could drive male-specific ASD risks (Auyeung et al., 2009; Auyeung et al., 2010; Baron-Cohen et al., 2005). Instead of testosterone "causing" ASD, it could reduce a cognitive resilience factor, such as the ability to develop social communication skills. One longitudinal study suggested that variations in fetal testosterone are related to social cognition and attentional focus in typically developing children (Knickmeyer and Baron-Cohen, 2006). Preliminary evidence suggesting that sensitivity to prenatal sex steroid influence (indexed by second-and-fourth-finger length ratio) may be relevant for regions of the brain, such as anterior cingulate cortex and extrastriate cortex, could support the extreme male brain theory of autism (Lai et al., 2013).

Oxytocin and vasopressin are two neuropeptide hormones under scrutiny for their potential role in ASD (Carter, 2007; Francis et al., 2014). Both these hormones are known to be associated with social and repetitive behaviors (Carter, 2007). Oxytocin is involved in bonding, romantic attachment and other "pro-social" behaviors (Chapter 4). It influences social and repetitive behaviors in women and men (Kirsch, 2010). Furthermore, oxytocin administration has been shown to reduce repetitive behaviors temporarily in adults with ASD (Hollander et al., 2003) and to enhance social functioning. However, the evidence

behind oxytocin as causative agent in ASD is inconclusive; it may be considered as one of several potentially relevant biomarkers which show sex-specificity with unclear clinical significance (Schwarz et al. 2011).

Neurobiological differences

Understanding gender differences in the brains of clinical populations with ASD remains limited by the focus of published research papers in predominantly male samples. It is increasingly highlighted that conclusions from studies including only one sex should not be extrapolated to another (Zucker and Beery, 2010). Innovative neuroimaging studies are beginning to elucidate underlying neurobiological influences on ASD (Philip et al., 2012; Via et al., 2011). Studies that examine the brains of women and men separately support possible differential risk and protective mechanisms that may lead to their development (Lai et al., 2013). Recent research using structural magnetic resonance imaging (MRI) examined whether neuroanatomy of ASD was different in female and male brains, and if neuroanatomical features fit predictions from the "extreme male brain" theory of ASD (Lai et al., 2013). They found that the neuroanatomy of ASD differed between females and males in a way that could not have occurred by chance and that atypical brain areas in females with ASD, in both grey and white matter, suggested neural "masculinization." Lai et al (2013) also concluded that males with ASD showed gender-incoherence, representing possible "feminization" of the brain. However, this study included only participants with average or above-average IQ, meaning they cannot be generalized to all people with ASD. Furthermore, the differences could not be correlated with cognitive profiles, so do not explain how they might be causally linked to ASD. As well as gross anatomical differences, there may also be gender differences at the cellular level (e.g., in size, number of branches, parts of neurons, or distribution of neurotransmitters) and in variations of fiber connections between neurocognitive systems. Such investigations will be possible with future technological advances.

Implications for the gender disparities in girls

It is increasingly clear that girls with ASD may be missed by parents, teachers and clinicians, and receive the diagnosis relatively later than boys (Cheslack-Postava and Jordan-Young, 2012). It has been argued that girls with ASD are also often misdiagnosed with other mental health conditions. As a result, they do not often get adequate help or support for their ASD-specific needs. Low self-esteem, depression, vulnerability to relationship predators and abusive relationships have been reported in clinical settings (Attwood, 2007).

Children usually intrinsically fear strangers and learn social rules about interacting with others from a young age. Developing women will normally learn social rules about consensual sexual relationships as they progress through childhood and adolescence. Women with ASD may be more vulnerable to abuse both as children and adults, because they do not develop an understanding of social cues and rules in the same way. However, although girls with learning disability are well-recognized as being vulnerable to abuse (see Chapter 14), very little is known about the prevalence of sexual abuse in individuals with ASD. Clinical experience suggests that women with ASD have a high rate of adverse sexual experiences, even as children. Early life experiences of abuse will affect their expectations and understanding of sexual relationships later in life. For example, a woman who has been the victim of sexual abuse may have difficulty negotiating consensual sexual relationships in the future and understanding that she has the right to say no; if she has ASD, she may also lack the social skills to divert a predator. A developing personality is invariably harmed by childhood sexual abuse. Self-image may be distorted, often making the development of stable, reciprocal relationships even more challenging.

It is often suggested that women with ASD display increased masculine behavior and interests, and this may further contribute to social disadvantage faced by such women (Bejerot et al. 2012). Departure from gender norms in women with ASD may also place them at greater risk of social stigma as well as relationship difficulties. Bullying is reportedly more prevalent in girls with ASD, especially in childhood as female peer groups are more prone to psychological bullying, which may be less obvious to others (Baron-Cohen, 2002). Because they may be less well understood by others, girls with ASD may also be more likely to face discrimination. Girls may employ avoidance strategies, such as being well-behaved and polite, so as not to draw attention to themselves and to prevent social exclusion. The fact that girls may be able to camouflage their deficits may lead to symptoms being missed by parents as well as teachers. Women with ASD may only notice that they are different once they reach adulthood, and perhaps when they have children of their own. At this time, their mothering skills may be called into question, further worsening their self-esteem.

Conclusions

Girls and women are less likely to be diagnosed with ASD than boys and men. This may in part be related to a true protective effect of the biological differences between them. But it is increasingly acknowledged that underrecognition may also contribute. A delayed or misdiagnosis may have important implications and lead to poor outcomes for girls. There is still much to be learned about female presentations of autism, the explanations for this difference and how best they might access genuinely holistic and gender-specific care.

References

Asperger, H. (1944). Die "Autistischen Psychopathen" im Kindesalter. *Archiv fur Psychiatrie und Nervenkrankheiten*, 76–136.

Attwood, T. (2007). *The complete guide to Asperger's syndrome*. London, UK: Jessica Kingsley Pub.

Auyeung, B., Baron-Cohen, S., Ashwin, E., Knickmeyer, R., Taylor, K. & Hackett, G. (2009). Fetal testosterone and autistic traits. *British Journal of Psychology* 100, 1–22.

Auyeung, B., Taylor, K., Hackett, G. & Baron-Cohen, S. (2010). Foetal testosterone and autistic traits in 18 to 24-month-old children. *Molecular Autism* 1, 11.

Baird, G., Simonoff, E., Pickles, A., Chandler, S., Loucas, T., Meldrum, D. & Charman, T. (2006). Prevalence of disorders of the autism spectrum in a population cohort of children in South Thames: the Special Needs and Autism Project (SNAP). *Lancet* 368, 210–215.

Baron-Cohen, S. (2002). The extreme male brain theory of autism. *Trends in Cognitive Sciences* 6, 248–254.

Baron-Cohen, S., Knickmeyer, R. C. & Belmonte, M. K. (2005). Sex differences in the brain: implications for explaining autism. *Science* 310, 819–823.

Baron-Cohen, S., Scott, F. J., Allison, C., Williams, J., Bolton, P., Matthews, F. E. & Brayne, C. (2009). Prevalence of autism-spectrum conditions: UK school-based population study. *British Journal of Psychiatry* 194, 500–509.

Bejerot, S., Eriksson, J. M., Bonde, S., Carlstrom, K., Humble, M. B. & Eriksson, E. (2012). The extreme male brain revisited: gender coherence in adults with autism spectrum disorder. *British Journal of Psychiatry* 201, 116–123.

Bolte, S., Duketis, E., Poustka, F. & Holtmann, M. (2011). Sex differences in cognitive domains and their clinical correlates in higher-functioning autism spectrum disorders. *Autism* 15, 497–511.

Brugha, T. S., McManus, S., Bankart, J., Scott, F., Purdon, S., Smith, J., Bebbington, P., Jenkins, R. & Meltzer, H. (2011). Epidemiology of autism spectrum disorders in adults in the community in England. *Archives of General Psychiatry* 68, 459–465.

Carter, C. S. (2007). Sex differences in oxytocin and vasopressin: implications for autism spectrum disorders? *Behavioural Brain Research* 176, 170–186.

Centers for Disease Control and Prevention (2012). Prevalence of autism spectrum disorders – Autism and Developmental Disabilities Monitoring Network, 14 sites, United States, 2008. *MMWR Surveillance Summaries* 61, 1–19.

Cheslack-Postava, K. & Jordan-Young, R. M. (2012). Autism spectrum disorders: toward a gendered embodiment model. *Social Science & Medicine* 74, 1667–1674.

Constantino, J. N., Zhang, Y., Frazier, T., Abbacchi, A. M. & Law, P. (2010). Sibling recurrence and the genetic epidemiology of autism. *American Journal of Psychiatry* 167, 1349–1356.

Dworzynski, K., Ronald, A., Bolton, P. & Happe, F. (2012). How different are girls and boys above and below the diagnostic threshold for autism spectrum disorders? *Journal of the*

American Academy of Child & Adolescent Psychiatry 51, 788–797.

Folstein, S. & Rutter, M. (1977). Infantile autism: a genetic study of 21 twin pairs. *Journal of Child Psychology and Psychiatry* 18, 297–321.

Francis, S. M., Sagar, A., Levin-Decanini, T., Liu, W., Carter, C. S. & Jacob, S. (2014). Oxytocin and vasopressin systems in genetic syndromes and neurodevelopmental disorders. *Brain Research*, 1580, 199–218.

Geary, D. C. (1998). *Male, female: The evolution of human sex differences.* Washington, DC: American Psychological Association.

Gillberg, C. & Coleman, M. (2000). *The biology of the autistic syndromes.* London: Mac Keith.

Gilman, S. R., Iossifov, I., Levy, D., Ronemus, M., Wigler, M. & Vitkup, D. (2011). Rare de novo variants associated with autism implicate a large functional network of genes involved in formation and function of synapses. *Neuron* 70(5), 898–907. doi: 10.1016/j.neuron.2011.05.021.

Hollander, E., Novotny, S., Hanratty, M., Yaffe, R., DeCaria, C. M., Aronowitz, B. R. & Mosovich, S. (2003). Oxytocin infusion reduces repetitive behaviors in adults with autistic and Asperger's disorders. *Neuropsychopharmacology* 28(1), 193–198.

Idring, S., Rai, D., Dal, H., Dalman, C., Sturm, H., Zander, E., Lee, B. K., Serlachius, E. & Magnusson, C. (2012). Autism spectrum disorders in the Stockholm Youth Cohort: design, prevalence and validity. *PLoS One* 7, e41280.

Ingudomnukul, E., Baron-Cohen, S., Wheelwright, S. & Knickmeyer, R. (2007). Elevated rates of testosterone-related disorders in women with autism spectrum conditions. *Hormone and Behavior*, 51, 597–604.

Institute of Medicine, Committee on Understanding the Biology of Sex

and Gender Differences, Wizemann, T. M. & Pardue, M. L. (2001). *Exploring the biological contributions to human health: Does sex matter?* Washington, DC: National Academy Press.

Jacquemont, S., Coe, B. P., Hersch, M., Duyzend, M. H., Krumm, N., Bergmann, S., Beckmann, J. S., Rosenfeld, J. A. & Eichler, E. E. (2014). A Higher Mutational Burden in Females Supports a "Female Protective Model" in Neurodevelopmental Disorders. *American Journal of Human Genetics* 94, 415–425.

Jordan-Young, R. M. (2010). *Brain storm: The flaws in the science of sex differences.* Cambridge, MA: Harvard University Press.

Kanner, L. (1943). Autistic disturbances of affective contact. *Nervous Child* 2, 217–250.

Kim, Y. S., Leventhal, B. L., Koh, Y. J., Fombonne, E., Laska, E., Lim, E. C., Cheon, K. A., Kim, S. J., Kim, Y. K., Lee, H., Song, D. H. & Grinker, R. R. (2011). Prevalence of autism spectrum disorders in a total population sample. *American Journal of Psychiatry* 168, 904–912.

Knickmeyer, R. & Baron-Cohen, S. (2006). Fetal testosterone and sex differences in typical social development and in autism. *Journal of Child Neurology* 21, 825–845.

Knickmeyer, R., Baron-Cohen, S., Fane, B. A., Wheelwright, S., Mathews, G. A., Conway, G. S., Brook, C. G. & Hines, M. (2006a). Androgens and autistic traits: a study of individuals with congenital adrenal hyperplasia. *Hormones and Behavior* 50, 148–153.

Knickmeyer, R. C., Wheelwright, S., Hoekstra, R. & Baron-Cohen, S. (2006b). Age of menarche in females with autism spectrum conditions. *Developmental Medicine & Child Neurology* 48, 1007–1008.

Kopp, S. & Gillberg, C. (2011). The Autism Spectrum Screening

Questionnaire (ASSQ)-Revised Extended Version (ASSQ-REV): an instrument for better capturing the autism phenotype in girls? A preliminary study involving 191 clinical cases and community controls. *Research in Developmental Disabilities* 32, 2875–2888.

Kothari, R., Skuse, D., Wakefield, J. & Micali, N. (2013). Gender differences in the relationship between social communication and emotion recognition. *Journal of the American Academy of Child & Adolescent Psychiatry* 52, 1148–1157.

Lai, M. C., Lombardo, M. V. & Baron-Cohen, S. (2014). Autism. *Lancet* 383, 896–910.

Lai, M. C., Lombardo, M. V., Pasco, G., Ruigrok, A. N., Wheelwright, S. J., Sadek, S. A., Chakrabarti, B. & Baron-Cohen, S. (2011). A behavioral comparison of male and female adults with high functioning autism spectrum conditions. *PLoS One* 6, e20835.

Lai, M. C., Lombardo, M. V., Suckling, J., Ruigrok, A. N., Chakrabarti, B., Ecker, C., Deoni, S. C., Craig, M. C., Murphy, D. G., Bullmore, E. T. & Baron-Cohen, S. (2013). Biological sex affects the neurobiology of autism. *Brain* 136, 2799–2815.

Levy, D., Ronemus, M., Yamrom, B., Lee, Y. H., Leotta, A., Kendall, J., Marks, S., Lakshmi, B., Pai, D., Ye, K., Buja, A., Krieger, A., Yoon, S., Troge, J., Rodgers, L., Iossifov, I., & Wigler, M. (2011). Rare de novo and transmitted copy-number variation in autistic spectrum disorders. *Neuron* 70(5), 886–897. doi: 10.1016/j.neuron.2011.05.015.

Levy, S. E., Mandell, D. S. & Schultz, R. T. (2009). Autism. *Lancet* 374, 1627–1638.

Lord, C., Rutter, M., Goode, S., Heemsbergen, J., Jordan, H., Mawhood, L. & Schopler, E. (1989). Autism diagnostic observation schedule: a standardized observation of communicative and social behavior. *Journal of Autism and Developmental Disorders* 19, 185–212.

Lord, C., Rutter, M. & Le, C. A. (1994). Autism Diagnostic Interview-Revised: a revised version of a diagnostic interview for caregivers of individuals with possible pervasive developmental disorders. *Journal of Autism and Developmental Disorders* 24, 659–685.

Lord, C., Schopler, E. & Revicki, D. (1982). Sex differences in autism. *Journal of Autism and Developmental Disorders* 12, 317–330.

Lu, A. T. & Cantor, R. M. (2012). Allowing for sex differences increases power in a GWAS of multiplex Autism families. *Molecular Psychiatry* 17(2), 215–222. doi: 10.1038/mp.2010.127

Mattila, M. L., Kielinen, M., Linna, S. L., Jussila, K., Ebeling, H., Bloigu, R., Joseph, R. M. & Moilanen, I. (2011). Autism spectrum disorders according to DSM-IV-TR and comparison with DSM-5 draft criteria: an epidemiological study. *Journal of the American Academy of Child & Adolescent Psychiatry* 50, 583–592.

McCarthy, M. M., Arnold, A. P., Ball, G. F., Blaustein, J. D. & De Vries, G. J. (2012). Sex differences in the brain: the not so inconvenient truth. *Journal of Neuroscience*, 32, 2241–2247.

Philip, R. C., Dauvermann, M. R., Whalley, H. C., Baynham, K., Lawrie, S. M. & Stanfield, A. C. (2012). A systematic review and meta-analysis of the fMRI investigation of autism spectrum disorders. *Neuroscience & Biobehavioral Reviews* 36, 901–942.

Robinson, E. B., Lichtenstein, P., Anckarsater, H., Happe, F. & Ronald, A. (2013). Examining and interpreting the female protective effect against autistic behavior. *Proceedings of the National Academy of Sciences of the United States of America* 110, 5258–5262.

Russell, G., Ford, T., Steer, C. & Golding, J. (2010). Identification of children with the same level of impairment as children on the autistic spectrum, and analysis of their service use. *Journal of Child Psychology and Psychiatry* 51, 643–651.

Rutter, M. (2005). Aetiology of autism: findings and questions. *Journal of Intellectual Disability Research* 49, 231–238.

Schwarz, E., Guest, P. C., Rahmoune, H., Wang, L., Levin, Y., Ingudomnukul, E., Ruta, L., Kent, L., Spain, M., Baron-Cohen, S. & Bahn, S. (2011). Sex-specific serum biomarker patterns in adults with Asperger's syndrome. *Molecular Psychiatry* 16, 1213–1220.

Skuse, D. H. (2000). Imprinting, the X-chromosome, and the male brain: explaining sex differences in the liability to autism. *Pediatric Research* 47, 9–16.

Van Wijngaarden-Cremers, P. J., van, E. E., Groen, W. B., Van Deurzen, P. A., Oosterling, I. J. & Van der Gaag, R. J. (2014). Gender and age differences in the core triad of impairments in autism spectrum disorders: a systematic review and meta-analysis. *Journal of Autism and Developmental Disorders* 44, 627–635.

Via, E., Radua, J., Cardoner, N., Happe, F. & Mataix-Cols, D. (2011). Meta-analysis of gray matter abnormalities in autism spectrum disorder: should Asperger disorder be subsumed under a broader umbrella of autistic spectrum disorder? *Archives of General Psychiatry* 68, 409–418.

Volkmar, F. R., Szatmari, P. & Sparrow, S. S. (1993). Sex differences in pervasive developmental disorders. *Journal of Autism and Developmental Disorders* 23, 579–591.

Werling, D. M. & Geschwind, D. H. (2013). Sex differences in autism spectrum disorders. *Current Opinion in Neurology* 26, 146–153.

Wing, L. (1981). Sex ratios in early childhood autism and related conditions. *Psychiatry Research* 5, 129–137.

Wing, L., Leekam, S. R., Libby, S. J., Gould, J. & Larcombe, M. (2002). The Diagnostic Interview for Social and Communication Disorders: background, inter-rater reliability and clinical use. *Journal of Child Psychology and Psychiatry* 43, 307–325.

Zucker, I. & Beery, A. K. (2010). Males still dominate animal studies. *Nature* 465, 690.

Chapter

7

Pubertal development and the emergence of the gender gap in affective disorders
A developmental and evolutionary synthesis

Nicholas B. Allen, Melissa D. Latham, Anna Barrett, Lisa Sheeber and Betsy Davis

The emergence of gender differences in affective disorders during adolescence

Perhaps the most robust finding in psychiatric epidemiology is that the rate of unipolar depression is higher among women than it is among men (Weissman et al., 1996; see also Chapter 19). Studies from the 1970s to the 1990s consistently found that women were nearly twice as likely as men to experience case-level depression diagnoses (McGrath et al., 1990; Kessler et al., 1994; Nolen-Hoeksema, 1990; Weissman & Klerman, 1977). More recent studies report an odds ratio of 1.5 (Kessler et al., 2005; Romans et al., 2007), indicating that, even if the gender gap is narrowing over time, the female excess is a robust finding. Indeed, the female preponderance in depression holds true across a variety of cultures and racial/ethnic groups (Gater et al., 1998; Kuehner, 2003). Furthermore, studies of nonclinical depressed mood states have shown that women experience more symptoms during episodes of depressed mood than do men (Wilhelm et al. 1998; Romans et al., 2007). Although studies have generally found that there are not gender differences in depression in prepubescent children, by 15 years of age girls are twice as likely as boys to have experienced a major depressive episode (e.g., Hankin et al. 1998). This places the gender disparity in depressive disorders firmly within the domain of developmental psychopathology, and specifically those developmental processes associated with early adolescence. An understanding of the developmental processes that underlie the emergence of this gender difference may have implications for understanding vulnerability to depression throughout the life cycle.

While anxiety disorders have also been shown to be more common in females (Yonkers & Gurguis, 1995; see also Chapter 18), there is comparatively less research on the causes and developmental pattern of gender differences in anxiety. Lewinsohn and colleagues (1998) found that retrospective reports of anxiety disorders indicated that the gender gap in such disorders emerges much earlier in life than it does in depression; by age 6, girls are twice as likely as boys to have experienced an anxiety disorder. Given that the early emergence of anxiety disorders is thought to be a marker of risk for later depressive disorder (Parker et al., 1999),the gender gap in anxiety may be a developmental precedent for the gender disparity in depressive disorders that emerges in adolescence. In what follows, we concentrate explicitly on depression and depressive disorders.

The gender gap: fact or artifact?

Before examining theories to account for the gender difference in the prevalence of depression, it is important to establish that the female preponderance is not artifactual. Two major reporting artifacts have been cited as potentially contributing to the reported gender gap in depression – a help-seeking artifact, and a recall artifact. The *help-seeking artifact* refers to a perceived reticence in males to seek treatment or advice for depressive symptoms, which could explain the preponderance of females seeking treatment. However, in a worldwide epidemiological survey for the World Health Organization, Weissman et al. (1996) found that the rates of depression identified in community samples were in accord with those reported from primary care settings. More recently, Kuehner (2003) came to the same conclusion through a systematic review of the literature. The *recall artifact* postulates that women's recall is biased in favor of past negative affective states, and thus women report a higher rate of lifetime depression. Kuehner (1999) conducted a controlled test of this by comparing women and men's reports of depressive symptomatology during a depressive episode, and their recall of these symptoms six months later. He found no recall artifact: there was no sex difference in the differential between the reported severity of symptoms at times one and two, and Kuehner's more recent systematic review of the literature also concluded that this artifact could not explain gender disparities in mood disorders (Kuehner, 2003).

A third suggested artifact is that the higher rate of sexual abuse and rape experienced by girls and young women accounts for subsequent depression rates, although it is worth noting that this does not constitute an artifact *per se*, but rather a potential etiological explanation for the gender difference in mood disorders. Kessler (2000) did find that, after rape and sexual trauma were controlled for in a population database, the gender difference in a first episode of depression was halved. However, when traumatic experiences more likely to be experienced by men were also controlled for, the female preponderance was restored. Findings such as these suggest that the increased prevalence of depression in females is not due to artifact (but see Chapter 1).

Theories of the emergence of the gender gap during early adolescence

The gender intensification hypothesis

The *gender intensification hypothesis* (Hill & Lynch, 1983; Wichstrom, 1999) suggests that gender role orientations become more differentiated between the sexes over the adolescent years, as a result of exacerbated gender socialization pressures during this time. For women, these pressures, both direct and in the form of social learning, are primarily thought to occur through observation of their parents' marital relations, which emphasize lesser public power and greater responsibility for the domestic sphere and care as part of the female gender role (Obeidallah et al., 1996), and through the socializing effects of parenting behaviors (Sheeber et al., 2002). The hypothesized effect of these socialization experiences

is the promotion of assumptions that emphasize collectivity, and a lower sense of self-esteem amongst women. These tendencies, in turn, contribute to the increase in depressive symptoms in women. The consequence of this intensified gender stereotyping, according to these theorists, is that deficits in self-efficacy and instrumentality (i.e., the belief that one can take action to influence personally important outcomes), reflected in low levels of traditionally masculine personality characteristics, may place young adolescent girls at higher risk for depression through greater exposure to experiences that promote learned helplessness (Obeidallah et al., 1996).

One important source of socialization experiences is parenting behaviors throughout childhood and adolescence. Based on reviews of clinical and developmental literature, Hops (Hops et al., 1990; Hops, 1992, 1996) posited two pathways by which parents may inadvertently increase their daughter's risk for depressive symptomatology and disorder. First, familial socialization processes may serve to normalize and encourage girls' expression of depressive-like behaviors (e.g., sadness; self-derogation). Indeed, there is some evidence that girls may be differentially socialized to display depressive behaviors during childhood. In a review of parental socialization of emotion, Eisenberg and colleagues (1998) found that, although parents do not typically report reacting differently to girls' and boys' emotional displays, observational data suggest that there are indeed differences, "albeit perhaps less than one might expect." In particular, a series of studies indicated that parents put more pressure on boys to control their emotions and "unnecessary" crying. Block (1983) reported that parents were quicker to respond to crying in girls than in boys. Parents' meta-messages about the acceptability of emotional expressions are apparently clear to children in that boys expect their parents to disapprove of their expression of sadness more so than girls (Fuchs & Thelen, 1988).

Parents' reactions to children's negative emotions may also provide them with gender-differentiated strategies for regulating negative affect. Although the data are limited, some evidence suggests that boys may be encouraged to use distraction and problem-solving more so than are girls (Eisenberg et al., 1998). In fact, one study indicated that school-age children expected fathers to respond to boys' emotional expressions with problem-solving and mothers to respond to girls' by focusing on feelings (Dino et al., 1984). Maternal encouragement of emotional expression in response to a stressor was also found to mediate the path from sex to depression by age 15 (Cox et al., 2010). Similarly, in a review of the origins of ruminative coping styles, Nolen-Hoeksema (1998) indicates that failure to teach girls active coping strategies for dealing with negative affect contributes to their greater use of ruminative styles of responding to depressed moods. Further, she suggests that, to the extent girls are told they are naturally emotional, they may have lower expectations that their behavior can influence their affective experiences. A recent study on gender and coping styles supported this, indicating that coping style accounted for 36% of the variance in a sample of 14- to 18-year-olds, and that girls were more likely to use ruminative coping, which in turn significantly predicted depressive symptoms. On the other hand, males were more likely to use problem-solving and distraction coping, which accounted for the protection against depression that has been attributed to masculine traits, as discussed later in this chapter (Li et al., 2006).

Second, differential parental reinforcement of gender-typic behaviors may lead girls to display less instrumental and more relationship-focused behaviors, both of which are related to theoretically derived and empirically supported risk factors for depression. Huston (1983) reported that girls receive more encouragement for dependency and affectionate behavior. They are also reported to receive more support for nurturant play (Ruble et al., 1993) (also see Chapter 1). Interestingly, Block (1983) reported that in Baby X studies, in which infants are "assigned" a gender (i.e., the same baby is labelled a "boy" and a "girl" in interactions with different participants), adults provided more reinforcement for nurturant play when the baby is said to be a girl. Such evidence is compelling in that Baby X studies control for gender differences in children's actual behavior.

On a related theme, evidence suggests that mothers encourage girls more than boys to have concern for others, to share and to behave prosocially (see Keenan and Shaw, 1997 for a review). However, recent literature has suggested that girls and boys do not actually differ in their levels of prosocial behavior, but instead in how those prosocial behaviors are manifested. A brief longitudinal study indicated that the same parenting behaviors and parental attributions for prosocial behavior led to more feminine (compassionate) prosocial behaviors in preschool girls, and to more masculine (agentic) prosocial behaviors in preschool boys (Hastings et al., 2007). However, the rates of prosocial behavior overall between girls and boys did not differ. Parents may be less attentive to girls' assertive behavior (Kerig et al., 1993), and may also impede the development of girls' sense of mastery by limiting their activities and freedom. In a 1983 review of the literature, it was reported that mothers were more likely to give unnecessary assistance to girls than to boys, and were more likely to reward frustration with physical comfort (Block, 1983).

There is also modest evidence that girls have lower self-evaluations of their own efficacy and that such evaluations are related to depressive symptomatology (Avison & McAlpine, 1992; Ohannessian et al., 1999). In an older review, Ruble and colleagues (1993) found that preadolescent girls tended to report lower expectations for success, more maladaptive attributions for success and failure, and poorer self-esteem than age-matched boys. Though gender differences did not emerge in all of these older studies reviewed by Ruble and colleagues, the direction of effects was consistent when gender differences were observed. It is important, however, to remain cognizant of the likelihood that disturbances in perceived self-competence may be sequelae rather than causes of depressive symptomatology. Hence, two longitudinal 17–18-year-old studies by Cole and colleagues (1998, 1999) suggest that children's underestimates of their own competence emerge as a function of depressive symptomatology and that controlling for depression eliminates the observed gender differences in estimation of competencies.

Thus, although these older data suggest that parents' early gender-differentiated socialization of children's emotional and social behaviors may have an effect on children's ability and motivation to regulate emotion, large gaps remain in the literature. In particular, these largely cross-sectional studies do not provide evidence of current gender differences or that such parental behaviors are predictors rather than consequences of children's sex-typed behaviors. For example, if girls display more sadness and boys more anger, it would be reasonable to hypothesize that parents' tendency to discuss sadness with girls and anger with boys emerged consequent to the children's behavioral propensities. Similarly, it is not clear whether parents' tendency to be more emotion-focused in response to young girls' emotions and more problem-focused in response to young boys does not reflect girls' earlier verbal and emotional development (Keenan & Shaw, 1997). An important caveat is that the research discussed herein focuses on parents' responses to children's normative emotional expressions. Though we consider it reasonable to construe depressive symptomatology as being at one end of a continuum that includes normative affective expression, the connection between early socialization of depressive-like behaviors and subsequent depressive functioning remains speculative.

In a meta-analysis of research dating from the 1950s to 1990, Lytton and Romney (1991) concluded that, although there is modest evidence of parental encouragement for sex-typed activities, overall the evidence does not support differences in parental restrictiveness or encouragement of either achievement or dependency as a function of child gender. Hence, it appears that the evidence for the shaping of differential activities for girls and boys is stronger than that for other areas of gender-socialization. Additionally, a more recent longitudinal study that examined intensification of gender roles at the beginning of adolescence found that, although masculinity did predict lower levels of depression among both girls and boys, no difference in masculine traits was found between the sexes. Thus, the finding did not account for the higher rates of depression in girls (Priess et al., 2009).

Limitations of the gender intensification hypothesis

Aside from the limited number and lack of contemporary studies that would allow strong causal inferences to be drawn regarding socialization and the emergence of the gender gap in mood disorders, there is also some literature that is inconsistent with this hypothesis. Studies documenting the trajectories of children's own gender role concepts have shown that the rigidity of children's gender stereotypes tends to *lessen* as adolescence approaches. These studies have also found that boys are likely to labor under more rigid self-imposed sex-types than girls (Banerjee & Lintern, 2000). Furthermore, gender intensification theorists cite the emergence of the gender gap at adolescence as support for their argument; however, as will be discussed below, the onset of the gender difference in depression is not predicted by age as such, but rather by the pubertal status of the individual (Angold et al., 1999). If female depression is a consequence of a broad societal pressure applied to girls when they reach a certain age or stage of schooling, this should not be the case.

Another problematic finding with regards to gender intensification theories of adolescent depression is that the rates of female depression have not markedly lessened over the last 50 years (Weissman et al., 1996). While the feminist movement has yet to yield true gender equality, it is clear that the status and opportunities that adolescent girls may expect at present far outstrip those available 50 years ago. Gender intensification theories would logically predict that a rise in the financial and social power of women would be accompanied by a commensurate fall in depression onset at that developmental stage where the assumption of adult female roles is hypothesized to be paramount to adolescent girls' sense of self-worth and efficacy. This matter, however, may not be as straightforward as it first appears. Thus, if the socialization of female roles in terms of reduced instrumentality and increased sensitivity to social relationships has not changed fundamentally over time, then the increased opportunity for women and girls may actually increase the gap between their behavioral repertoire and the demands placed on them. Nevertheless, the lack of change in the gender gap in rates of depression over a period of dramatic historical change in the type and range of roles socialized in young women does seem puzzling if gender socialization is the key process driving this phenomenon.

Another contradiction within these theories is their heavy emphasis on the timing of gender intensification as a corollary to the timing of the emergence of the gender gap in affective disorders. As noted earlier, social learning and gender typing have been shown to begin in the first few years of life. If identification with a feminine stereotype is as strongly linked to depression as some of these theorists suggest, the finding that the rates of depression in prepubertal children are equal between genders is counterintuitive (Gelman et al., 2004). A more sophisticated version of the gender intensification hypothesis posits that what is socialized in girls during childhood are reductions in instrumentality and increased experiences of helplessness and dependency (see earlier; Sheeber et al., 2002). These socialization experiences then constitute a diathesis that interacts with the developmental demands of early adolescence to create greater risk for depression in females. However, even this very plausible view of the role of socialization pressures during adolescence needs to explain what it is about the developmental demands of early adolescence that is specifically associated with the emergence of depressive disorders in vulnerable females (as opposed to, say, anxiety where gender differences are seen much earlier in life; Lewinsohn et al., 1998).

Finally, although the degree of gender gap in depressive disorders is unevenly distributed, such that women in disadvantaged sectors of society (e.g., women of color, women living in poverty, single mothers and those with less than a high school education) are disproportionately affected (Everson et al., 2002), the fact that the gender gap is also reliably observed in more privileged social groups casts doubt on the validity of a theory which posits membership of a devalued social group as the primary causative influence on depression.

Gender roles and individual differences in personality and emotion

An alternative possibility posits that there are more fundamental gender differences in affective functioning that may place females at greater risk for affective disorders, and that these differences are reflected in gender divergences in personality and emotional functioning. Indeed, investigations into developmental changes in gender identity often use self-report measures of traits traditionally thought to be more characteristic of males than females or *vice versa*. In the Personal Attributes Questionnaire, for example, the "masculine" item endorsements include: *independent, active, competitive, making decisions easily, self-confident, not giving up easily,* and *standing up well under pressure* (Spence et al. 1974). The finding that high scores on these traits are protective against depression certainly seems to be robust (e.g., Hoffman et al., 2004), although given that a number of these items overlap with depressive symptoms (e.g., difficulty making decisions, low self-confidence, hopelessness, and poor resilience) these associations may be, in part, tautological.

Indeed, the assumption that these are inherently masculine traits may need reevaluation. When these traits are considered in their own right, decoupled from their description as "masculine," the argument becomes circular, in claiming that, for example, low self-confidence leads to depression, which is in part indexed by low self-confidence (Barrett & White, 2002). In addition, several recent studies suggest that "feminine" traits do not predict depression at all, but "masculine" traits are predictive of lower levels of depression, specifically in adolescence (Priess et al., 2009; Li et al., 2006). For example, Priess and colleagues suggest that, based on these and other findings (e.g., Wichstrom, 1999) perhaps the framing of

masculinity and femininity should be rethought to be more synonymous with female versus male traits, which show secular changes over time with the changing social environment/landscape.

One way to reframe the relationship between gender roles and depressive phenomena is by taking into account the correlation between sex role inventory scores and broader personality traits. For example, Francis and Wilcox (1998) found that high scores on the masculinity scale of the Bem Sex Role Inventory (Bem, 1974) were associated with low neuroticism and high extraversion, whereas high scores on femininity were associated with high neuroticism. Neuroticism is a temperament trait that may place individuals at higher risk for depression and anxiety, and is also reliably found to be higher in females (Fanous et al., 2002). O'Shea (2002, cited in Parker & Brotchie, 2004) found that, although adolescent girls did record higher neuroticism scores than boys, high neuroticism was a strong predictor of first onset depression, regardless of gender. In fact, adjustment for neuroticism greatly attenuated the gender differential in first onset depression in this sample. This suggests that it may be neuroticism, rather than gender role *per se*, that confers risk for depression, although this still begs the questions as to why female gender and typical female gender role descriptions are associated with higher levels of neuroticism.

A second way to conceptualize traits that place one at risk for depression is to examine the relationships between negative emotionality (related to neuroticism), approach (related to positive emotionality) and effortful control. As early as childhood, effortful control is more characteristic of females, whilst approach is more characteristic of males. Negative emotionality tends to be higher in females, especially after the onset of adolescence (Martel, 2013). Of these broad characteristics, there is evidence that negative emotionality is a general marker of risk for psychopathology and that low approach is related to internalizing disorders such as depression. These sex differences may contribute to the larger subset of females at risk for depression (Martel, 2013). The author emphasizes, however, that these are broad group differences and that there are females and males who exhibit the opposite genders' average pattern of traits and are thus at risk for a different psychopathology presentation than the larger subset of their gender (Martel, 2013).

With respect to measures of emotion, there is some evidence for gender differences across a range of emotional processes (i.e., emotion perception, reactivity, regulation and experience), although negative findings are also reported (Barrett et al., 1998). Most of these studies have used self-report measures, which are open to language, retrospective and stereotype biases, as noted earlier (Fischer, 2000; Fugate et al., 2009). A recent review by Whittle and colleagues (2011) found that these sex differences in emotionality are not limited to self-report methodologies, but are also observed in brain measures derived from neuroimaging studies of emotional processes. Specifically, they found evidence that women recruit different neurocircuitry to men during perceptual emotion processing, which may, in some cases, lead to more accurate or faster processing, although in others may result in overreactivity. Also, while it appears that women show greater neural activation during reactivity to a range of negative emotional stimuli (particularly involving the amygdala), men show greater activation during reactivity to negative emotional stimuli that signal cues of dominance. A growing number of imaging studies also suggest that women and men use different strategies to downregulate negative emotions, and that these strategies might be mediated by different neural circuitry. Further, some research suggests that men may engage in more efficient automatic or unconscious emotion regulation when exposed to emotional stimuli, which may result from greater integration of cognitive and emotional neural circuits. Finally, sex differences in neural activity associated with reactivity to positive emotional stimuli appears to depend on the type of positive emotion and the stimulus modality. Overall, this review suggests that sex differences in emotional processes that are likely to confer greater risk for affective disorders are also evident in methodologies that directly measure neural processes that are outside of volitional control (hence ruling out a role for reporting and other self-report biases).

Pubertal development and the diathesis for affective disorder

The relevance of pubertal changes to the developmental examination of the gender gap lies primarily in the potential role of hormonal changes at puberty as catalytic agents for the development of depression in those women placed at risk by temperamental predisposition. Angold and colleagues (1999) reported that the transition to Tanner stage III (an index of body shape change and pubertal stage) of puberty predicted the increase in rates of DSM-IV unipolar depression in girls, exerting a much-larger effect than chronological age. This supports the view that changes in rates of depression at adolescence are specifically related to the physical and physiological changes of puberty, rather than to broad psychosocial factors common to girls at a particular stage of adolescence. However, it does not rule out the possibility that societal pressures are the primary precipitators of depression, but are prompted not by age but by the visible manifestations of puberty. This problem was later clarified by the addition of hormonal variables into the model (Angold et al., 1999), which eliminated the effect of morphological status, strongly implicating the effects of estrogen in the development of depression in adolescent girls.

Importantly, there are considerable individual differences in the timing and rapidity of pubertal development (Ellis, 2004; Mendle et al., 2010), with the timing of puberty (i.e., the timing of changes in pubertal status relative to peers) being found to be the most consistent pubertal predictor of vulnerability to adolescent onset depression and other poor outcomes during adolescence (Mendle et al., 2010). Specifically, early onset of puberty has consistently been associated with depressive symptoms in girls (Graber et al., 1997; Kaltiala-Heino et al., 2003). The literature for boys is more mixed, with different studies finding that earlier or later onset of puberty (and some finding that both early and late onset) is associated with depressive symptoms and disorders (Graber, 2009).

At puberty, hormonal levels begin to fluctuate cyclically over a broader spectrum in girls than in boys. Estrogen in particular is recognized as playing an important role in mediating female sensitivity to stress. Estrogen apparently acts as an anxiolytic, and thus the cyclical withdrawal of estrogen that occurs shortly prior to menstruation may be analogous to the physiologic effects of anxiolytic withdrawal, creating a greater sensitivity in menstruating women to the anxiogenic and depressogenic effects of negative life events. At the onset of puberty for men, on the other hand, the increase of testosterone has been suggested to have a protective effect against depression and anxiety, although it tends to increase aggressive and risk-taking behaviors (Seeman, 1997).

It is important to note that the cyclical release and withdrawal of estrogen alone is not suggested to be the causative factor for the sudden increase in the incidence of depressive episodes in adolescent girls. Rather, this cycle is thought to result in a biological "kindling" that increases the stress reactivity of at-risk individuals to negative life events. In this respect, negative perceptions of gender role expectations or a socialized limitation in the behavioral repertoire of women may indeed come into play as proximal risk factors, but are regarded as precipitants of the development of mood disorder in girls who are, by virtue of temperament and biology, already at risk. In other words, the interaction of temperament and hormonal change may create a vulnerability diathesis upon which social factors may act as a catalyst to generate gender difference in rates of depression.

In support of the putative interaction between pubertal estrogen changes and negative life events, Brooks-Gunn and Warren (1989) found that, while the increase in pubertal estrogen levels accounted for 4% of variance in increased negative affect reported by 100 adolescent white girls, the joint contributions of estrogen rise and negative life events accounted for only 17% of the variance. It would appear that the onset of puberty sensitizes young women to the stress of negative life events, and possibly desensitizes young men, via the protective influence of testosterone. Prepubertal girls and boys tend to show similar correlations between number of life stressors and depressive affect. However, after the onset of puberty, the relationship between stress and negative affect strengthens for young women, and declines almost to elimination in young men (Angold et al., 1999).

Pubertal brain development, emotional processes and risk for mood disorders

The body of research reviewed earlier suggests that both the stage and timing of puberty affect emotional and behavioral dysregulation, and consequently vulnerability to mental health problems. However, the mechanisms underpinning these effects are still poorly understood (Ge & Natsuaki, 2009). Hormonal changes of puberty may be associated with changes in dysregulated affect and (perhaps) vulnerability to affective psychopathology, but evidence of the direct hormonal effects is mixed (Graber, 2009). Rather, it is the action of these hormones on the development of social, cognitive and affective systems in the *brain*

(and the resultant psychological changes) that may be most likely to explain puberty-related trends in the emergence of symptoms. Recent reviews have made it clear that we still lack a full understanding of the relationship between pubertal processes and brain development (Blakemore et al., 2010).

The principle focus of studies of adolescent brain development has been on age-related changes (e.g., Giedd et al., 1999), although based on findings such as peaks in gray matter density that seem to coincide with timing of puberty onset (Blakemore et al., 2010) some researchers have suggested that brain developmental patterns align better with pubertal development rather than age *per se* (Peper et al., 2011). Brain regions associated with reward processing (i.e., mesolimbic circuitry mediating reward-related behavior) are densely innervated by gonadal steroid receptors. Several pubertal hormones are considered neurosteroids, as they are centrally converted or synthesized de novo by the brain. These and other neurosteroids are thought to play a role in regulating neurotransmitter systems associated with affective and social responsiveness, including dopamine, serotonin, endogenous opioids, oxytocin and vasopressin (Epperson et al., 1999). Furthermore, gonadal steroids have their own direct effects on affective processes (McEwen, 2001). Thus, although the main function of pubertal changes may be to increase sensitivity to sexual stimuli and increase sexual motivation (Sisk & Foster, 2004), there is also evidence that increases in affective reactivity reflect a more general reorientation to social and emotional aspects of the environment, and this may in turn result in heightened vulnerability to emotional and behavioral disorders (Nelson, et al., 2005).

Importantly, although there is informative animal work regarding the links between puberty and brain structure and function, as noted earlier relatively little is known about this relationship in humans (Blakemore et al., 2010). Recently, a small number of adolescent MRI studies have investigated, in more detail, the relationships between brain structure and function, gender and hormones that change at puberty. For example, a structural MRI study by Peper and colleagues (2009a) reported an association between testosterone levels and global gray matter density in males (but not in females): females showed a negative association between estradiol levels and both global and regional gray matter density. Neufang and colleagues (2009) found a positive relationship between pubertal stage and gray matter volume in the amygdala, and a negative relationship between these measures and hippocampal volume, regardless of gender. In addition, females showed a positive relationship between estrogen levels and limbic gray matter, whilst males showed a negative relationship between testosterone and parietal cortex gray matter volume. Finally, Goddings et al. (2014) recently reported that pubertal development is significantly related to structural volume in a range of brain regions (i.e., amygdala, hippocampus and corpus striatum including the nucleus accumbens, caudate, putamen and globus pallidus) in both sexes.

Trajectories of white matter development also differ as a function of pubertal hormones (Peper et al., 2009 a,b; Perrin et al., 2008, 2009). For example, Herting and colleagues (2012) found pubertal development to be associated with patterns of white matter structure in the insula, and, in boys, testosterone predicted white matter integrity in sexually dimorphic regions as well as whole-brain white matter; in girls, estradiol showed a negative relationship with white matter. These findings all suggest a significant role for puberty, distinct to that of chronological age, in sex differences in structural brain development during early adolescence. The implications of these puberty-related sex differences in brain development for behavior and mental health are yet to be determined.

Forbes and colleagues (2010) found that individuals with more advanced pubertal maturation exhibited less striatal and more medial prefrontal reactivity to reward; further, testosterone was positively correlated with striatal reactivity in boys during reward anticipation and negatively correlated with striatal reactivity in girls and boys during reward outcome. Goddings and colleagues (2012) examined both social and basic emotions in early adolescent girls. They found that increased hormone levels (independent of age) were associated with higher left anterior temporal cortex (ATC) activity during social emotion processing. This latter finding is particularly important as it suggests that the effects of pubertal development may be somewhat specific to social cognitive brain function, which may be relevant given the strong link between social processes and vulnerability to depression.

Few published studies have directly investigated whether the association between mental health symptoms and pubertal processes might be mediated by neurobiological variables. Whittle and colleagues (2012) examined the relationship between pubertal

timing, brain structure and depressive symptoms during early adolescence. This study revealed that a larger volume of the pituitary gland, a key component of the hypothalamic-pituitary-gonadal (HPG) and hypothalamic-pituitary-adrenal (HPA) axes, mediated the relationship between early pubertal timing and depressive symptoms in female and male adolescents. These findings are consistent with neurobiological mechanisms being responsible for the link between exposure to pubertal hormones and depressive symptoms in adolescents.

In conclusion, there are good reasons to suspect that pubertal hormonal changes affect social, cognitive and affective systems in the brain, and that the resultant psychological changes might be critical mediators of the relationship between pubertal development and the emergence of symptoms of mental disorder during early adolescence. However, the extant human literature on the relationship between pubertal processes and brain development remains preliminary and far more work is needed to describe the biological and psychosocial mechanisms that underlie these developmental effects fully.

Pubertal change and interpersonal stressors

An alternative account of the relationship between pubertal development and affective disorders is suggested by examining whether the relation between pubertal hormone changes and depression in women is mediated by negative life events. In this respect, it is notable that the majority of stressors preceding the onset of adolescent depression are interpersonal (Cyranowski et al., 2000). Consistent with this observation, it has been proposed that the relationship between the quality of family relationships and depressive symptoms may be stronger for females than males (Kavanagh & Hops, 1994). During adolescence, females tend to gain independence more slowly from their families (Huston & Alvarez, 1990) and have relationships that are both more disclosing and more conflictual with their parents than do males (Noller, 1994; Montemayor, 1983). Many older studies using self-report measures found a stronger negative correlation between cohesive and supportive family relationships and depressive symptoms amongst girls than boys (Avison & McAlpine, 1992; Rubin et al., 1992; Slavin & Rainer, 1990; Windle, 1992), although a study by Sheeber and colleagues (1997), which included observational as well as self-report measures of family functioning, reported that the relationship between family functioning and depression was equivalent for females and males. This suggests that the stronger link between family processes and depression amongst females may be primarily determined by the way depressed states affect female *perceptions* of the family environment rather than objectively observable features.

The correspondence between the findings of a specific association between interpersonal stress and risk for depression on the one hand, and the evidence of increased affiliative proclivities amongst women (both as compared to men and after menarche) on the other, led Cyranowski and colleagues (2000) to examine potential biological substrates for female affiliative behavior. Nonhuman mammal research has strongly implicated the hypothalamic neuropeptide oxytocin in affiliative and caregiving behaviors (Depue & Lenzenweger, 2001; see also Chapter 8). Oxytocin transmission is thought to be regulated by estrogen and progesterone levels, giving rise to the idea of a hormonally driven pubertal increase in affiliative proclivity in females (Cyranowski et al., 2000). The review by Gordon and colleagues (2011) suggests that reproductive hormones, including testosterone and estradiol, potentiate the release of oxytocin. This potential connection between pubertal development and an increase in biologically controlled sensitivity to social stressors allows for a synthesis of psychosocial, biological and stress-response precipitants to adolescent onset depression, with the important caveat that the role of oxytocin in human female affiliative behavior is yet to be fully understood. Oxytocin plays a role in many complicated reproductive behaviors, including the formation of social (not just sexual) bonds (Lee et al., 2009). Although the formation of affiliative networks is in itself a protective factor against depression, the increased desire and need for these relationships, as well as the burden of increased care-taking within relationships, may mean that affiliative failures form potent stressors for girls who are temperamentally at risk, as has been emphasized by recent evolutionary models of depression.

An evolutionary synthesis of pubertal influences on vulnerability to affective disorders

Many theorists have argued that depressed states are most essentially related to reductions of positive affect (anhedonia being a key defining feature), and that the regulators of positive affect are embedded in *social* cognition and behavior (e.g., Allen & Badcock, 2003; Gilbert, 1989, 1992; Gotlib & Hammen, 1992; Joiner & Coyne, 1999; Watson, 2000). Critical to a functional or evolutionary view of depression is the proposition that there are various biological processes that guide individuals to enact certain social or interpersonal roles, including gender roles. There are many clues in the research literature to suggest that social processes (both in terms of social cognition and interpersonal behaviors) play a critical role in the etiology and maintenance of depressed states in both genders. Critical empirical observations here include findings demonstrating that depression is often precipitated by interpersonal events (as noted earlier), and that interpersonal processes often mediate the exacerbation or resolution of depressive episodes (Joiner et al., 1999). Stressful interpersonal contexts are amongst the most reliable antecedents of depressed states (e.g., Kendler et al., 2003; Monroe et al., 1999) and certain interpersonal behaviors, such as excessive reassurance seeking, are strong and specific predictors of risk for depression (Joiner & Metalsky, 2001).

An evolutionary model has been proposed to explain why there is such a close link between social cognition, social behavior and depressive phenomena. The *social risk* hypothesis of depression (Allen & Badcock, 2003) suggests that depressed mood (i.e., downregulation of positive affect and confident engagement with the world) evolved to facilitate a risk-averse approach to social interaction in situations where individuals perceive their social resources (e.g., status, affection, friendship, power) to be at critically low levels. Thus, whereas positive affect encourages engagement in a range of activities, most especially social ones, reduced positive affect discourages such engagement. In this sense, depressed mood was, in the evolutionary past, a defensive-protective strategy designed to reduce such activities, especially those with uncertain payoffs.

There are, in fact, a whole range of social activities and social roles wherein people have to make decisions about how costly or risky it is to develop or maintain the relationships, taking into consideration the possibility that others might not want to develop or maintain such a relationship in return. Clearly roles are coconstructed between self and other(s) and attempts to develop or maintain a role relationship is not without risks and potential costs.

For example, cooperating in a group of exploitative individuals might mean they benefit at one's expense, and competing for status and access to resources with others who are more powerful might elicit attacks or rejections. Thus it is important that individuals evaluate risks against benefits in whatever goal or role they are pursuing.

The social risk hypothesis suggests that depressed mood evolved as a salient mediator between estimates of social risk and social behavior. In other words, positive moods will fall when people evaluate that they have suffered a defeat or rejection that forces a reappraisal of their roles pursuits. This risk-assessing/mood-regulating mechanism affects social-perceptual processes such that the individual becomes hypersensitive to indications of social risk. In the area of social behavior, the mechanism affects both communicative behavior (signaling in order to reduce threats and to elicit safe forms of support) and resource acquisition behaviors (a general reduction in behavioral propensities towards high-risk social investments that may result in interpersonal conflict or competition). Recently, a team empirically tested this hypothesis using structural equation modelling to examine the relationships between the different components of the social risk hypothesis. They found support for defeat, social comparison and attachment as predictors of depression, and that depression predicted interpersonal sensitivity and submission (Dunn, et al., 2012). It is interesting to note that work on self-esteem has also conceptualized a similar process called a "sociometer," which monitors others' reactions and alerts individuals to the possibility of social exclusion (Leary et al., 1995).

Sexual selection and vulnerability to depression

Buss (1995) has proposed that sexual selection defines the domains in which the sexes have faced different adaptive challenges and, therefore, should explain those psychological sex differences that appear to exist at a species-wide level. The primary theory of the differential selective pressures facing women and men is referred to as "Parental Investment Theory," and was originally proposed by Trivers (1972). The central idea of parental investment theory is that, in mammals, including humans, the *minimal* requirements for successful reproduction differ dramatically between the sexes. For males, only the sex act and the contribution of easily replenished sperm are required; whereas for females there is a long period of gestation (and its associated limitations and vulnerabilities), along with intensive care of offspring during infancy and childhood. This means that some of the fundamental reproductive-adaptive tasks facing each of the sexes are different: for females these tasks include identifying males who are able *and* willing to invest resources in her (especially during pregnancy) and their offspring (Buss, 1994, 1995); for males these tasks include gaining sexual access to females, identifying reproductively valuable females and ensuring paternity certainty.

Sexual selection has been used to understand the emergence of sex differences in a variety of areas of human behavior (e.g., Buss, 1994; Daly & Wilson, 1983; Geary, 1996; Symons, 1979). Particularly relevant to the arguments presented here is the conceptualization of gender differences in inhibitory control of behavior, presented by Bjorklund and Kipp (1996). These authors point out that parental investment theory not only predicts that women must be able to choose well-resourced and dependable partners, but that the consequences of abandonment in mating (and other) relationships are potentially more damaging to their inclusive fitness as compared to men, given the differences in resources required for each of the sexes to enter into new reproductive relationships.

Eibl-Eibesfeldt (1989) observed that the need for enhanced female social sensitivity may not have applied only to mating relationships, but that the social style of females has also provided the primary basis for the long-term stability of social groups. Indeed, given that the major reproductive task predicted for females by parental investment theory is to gain investment and protection for herself and her offspring, the quality and consistency of this investment has probably been more critical than from whom it is obtained. This would suggest that quality of social relationships in general (i.e., not simply mating relationships) is more critical for females than males. Consistent with this, Essock and colleagues (1985) have pointed out that women invest more energy in the initiation and maintenance of non-kin social support networks. Bjorklund and Kipp (1996) linked this investment to selective pressures to choose and maintain relationships carefully. Their review of the evidence is consistent with this assertion and indicates that females exhibit greater inhibitory control in social, cognitive and behavioral realms.

In short, the evolutionary challenges predicted by parental investment theory and evolutionary views of sex differences would require women to exercise greater caution in negotiating the social ecology than men. The view that gender differences in depression are related to sexual selection mechanisms is also consistent with the data indicating that depression is only more common in women during their reproductive years (Bebbington, et al., 1998). However, newer studies suggest this may not be the case (see Chapter 20).

Research on sex differences in social cognition has supported the prediction that women are more sensitive to the negative social implications of information. For instance, Ruble and colleagues (1993) reviewed the evidence and suggested that women are more susceptible than men to self-evaluative concerns, particularly negative behavioral and evaluative reactions to failure. Roberts and Nolen-Hoeksema (1994) have likewise found that women's self-evaluations were more reliant on the views of others than was the case for men. At a more general level, there are clear sex differences in being object-oriented versus people-oriented, with women showing a strong tendency to be more people-oriented (Geary, 1996; McGuiness, 1993). Clearly, according to the social risk hypothesis, greater sensitivity to (and processing of) feedback regarding social performance would be expected to result in more frequent activation of depressed states, given that depressed states are understood to be instigated by a perception of loss of social value.

Another aspect of the greater female dependence on relationships to achieve "fitness-enhancing" goals is that women may be more constrained than men from exiting relationships (even very unsatisfactory ones) without compromising their pursuit of important goals (McGuire & Troisi, 1998). This may result in situations of chronic social threat, which may provide signals that continually engage and escalate depressive mechanisms.

Conclusions

In sum, our evolutionary synthesis seeks to explain a number of key features of the gender gap in affective disorders. The social risk hypothesis (Allen & Badcock, 2003), when combined with predictions from evolutionary theory regarding social and cognitive differences between the sexes, predicts a greater

likelihood of depressed states amongst women that may be linked to evolved reproductive biology. Evolutionary theory predicts that women will be more likely to perceive social threats and make negative self-evaluations based on interpersonal feedback, and that this gender difference (which is predicted by parental investment theory) is, therefore, likely to emerge during reproductive phases of the lifespan. It is during these years that depression has been shown to be most common amongst women. This evolutionary synthesis, therefore, suggests that the emergence of the gender gap in depression at adolescence cannot be attributed solely, or even primarily, to the influence of gender socialization processes, but that these processes interact with prepotent, evolved gender differences to influence the emergence of the gender gap in mood disorders. The basic measures of femininity and masculinity that drive much of the gender socialization theory on this topic are confounded with known risk factors for depression (such as a past history of abuse or violence [see Chapter 5] or personality) and even depression itself. An alternative conceptualization of these characteristics suggests that they reflect variations of temperament, most particularly in measures of neuroticism or even subclinical depression. Neuroticism is then posited as a temperamentally anxiogenic and depressogenic trait, which may place some girls more at risk than others prior to the onset of puberty (but see Chapter 1). This trait vulnerability may be exacerbated by the cyclical withdrawal of estrogen after menarche.

Furthermore, it has been suggested that the hormonal and brain changes that occur as part of pubertal development directly contribute to heightened female sensitivity to social circumstances. This may be linked to evidence that interpersonal events provide the vast majority of precipitating life stressors before a first episode onset of depression in adolescents. Given the specific link between depressed states and perceptions of social threat predicted by evolutionary views, such as the social risk hypothesis, it is not surprising that these hormonal changes appear to be the strongest predictor of the emergence of gender differences in rates of depression (Angold et al., 1999).

We have attempted here to synthesize a range of disparate literatures into a more integrative view of the role of gender in depressive disorders. We believe this perspective may inform attempts at early intervention and prevention. Pubertal women represent one of the most clearly identified groups for indicated prevention and early intervention efforts in affective disorders. When gender is associated with other risk factors, such as exposure to abuse and violence (see Chapter 14), social disadvantage (Everson et al., 2002), early puberty (Graber et al., 1997) or past perinatal depression (Sheeber et al., 2002), cohorts at very high risk for the emergence of depressive symptoms and disorders can be identified. The design of these intervention strategies, however, needs to be informed by a sophisticated understanding of the interplay between these disparate processes: biological, socialization pressures, life events and individual differences. Indeed, we would emphasize that the evolutionary view we have proposed does not imply that biological processes have primacy, but rather points the way towards understanding how biology can interact profoundly with socialization experiences and life experiences to create a diathesis for affective disorder. This has also been emphasized by findings that have shown that pubertal timing in girls can be influenced by adverse life experiences, especially those associated with paternal investment (Belsky et al., 1991; Ellis, 2004). These perspectives open up new directions for both research and intervention in women and girls suffering from affective disorders.

References

Allen, N. B., & Badcock, P. B. T. (2003). The social risk hypothesis of depressed mood: Evolutionary, psychosocial, and neurobiological perspectives. *Psychological Bulletin*, 129, 887–913.

Angold, A., & Costello, E. J. et al. (1998). Puberty and depression: The roles of age, pubertal status and pubertal timing. *Psychological Medicine*, 28, 51–61.

Angold, A., Costello, E. J., Erkanli, A., & Worthman, C. M. (1999). Pubertal changes in hormone levels and depression in girls. *Psychological Medicine*, 29(5), 1043–1053.

Avison, W. R., & McAlpine, D. D. (1992). Gender differences in symptoms of depression among adolescents. *Journal of Health and Social Behavior*, 33(June), 77–96.

Banerjee, R., & Lintern, V. (2000). Boys will be boys: The effect of social evaluation concerns on gender-typing. *Social Development*, 9(3), 397–408.

Barrett, A. E., & White, H. R. (2002). Trajectories of gender role orientations in adolescence and early adulthood: A prospective study of the mental health effects of masculinity and femininity. *Journal of Health & Social Behavior*, 43(4), 451–468.

Barrett, L. F., Robin, L., Pietromonaco, P. R., & Eyssell, K. M., 1998. Are women the "More emotional" sex? Evidence from emotional experiences in social context. *Cognition & Emotion* 12(4), 555–578.

Bebbington, P. E., Dunn, G., Jenkins, R., Lewis, G., Brugha, T., Farrell, M., & Meltzer, H. (1998). The influence of age and sex on the prevalence of depressive conditions: Report from the National Survey of Psychiatric Morbidity. *Psychological medicine*, 28, 9–19.

Belsky, J., Steinberg, L., & Draper, P. (1991). Childhood experience, interpersonal development, and reproductive strategy: An evolutionary theory of socialization. *Child Development*, 62, 647–670.

Bem, S. L. (1974). The measurement of psychological androgyny. *Journal of Consulting & Clinical Psychology*, 42, 155–162.

Bjorklund, D. F., & Kipp, K. (1996). Parental investment theory and gender differences in the evolution of inhibition mechanisms. *Psychological Bulletin*, 120, 163–188.

Blakemore S. J. et al. (2010). The role of puberty in the developing adolescent brain *Human Brain Mapping* 31, 926–933.

Block, J. H. (1983). Differential premises arising from differential socialization of the sexes: Some conjunctures. *Child Development*, 54, 1335–1354.

Brooks-Gunn, J., & Warren, M. P. (1989). Biological and social contributions to negative affect in young adolescent girls. *Child Development*, 60(1), 40–55.

Buss, D. M. (1994). *The evolution of desire: Strategies of human mating.* New York: Basic Books.

Buss, D. M. (1995). Psychological sex differences: Origins through sexual selection. *American Psychologist*, 50, 164–168.

Cole, D. A., Martin, J. M., Peeke, L. A., Seroczynski, A. D., & Fier, J. (1999). Children's over- and underestimation of academic competence: A longitudinal study of gender differences, depression, and anxiety. *Child Development*, 70(2), 459–473.

Cole, D. A., Martin, J. M., Peeke, L. G., Seroczynski, A. D., & Hoffman, K. (1998). Are cognitive errors of underestimation predictive or reflective of depressive symptoms in children: A longitudinal study. *Journal of Abnormal Psychology*, 107(3), 481–496.

Cox, S. J., Mezulis, A. H., & Hyde, J. S. (2010). The influence of child gender role and maternal feedback to child stress on the emergence of the gender difference in depressive rumination in adolescence.

Developmental Psychology, 46(4), 842–852. doi:10.1037/a0019813

Cyranowski, J. M., Frank, E., Young, E., & Shear, K. (2000). Adolescent onset of the gender difference in lifetime rates of major depression. *Archives of General Psychiatry*, 57(1), 21–27.

Daly, M. & Wilson, M. (1983). *Sex, evolution, and behavior (Second edition)*. Boston: Willard Grant Press.

Depue, R. A. and Lenzenweger, M. F. (2001). A neurobehavioral dimensional model. In W. J. Livesley (Ed.), *Handbook of personality disorders: Theory, research, and treatment* (pp. 136–176). New York: Guilford Press.

Dino, G. A., Barnett, M. A., & Howard, J. A. (1984). Children's expectations of sex differences in parents' responses to sons and daughters encountering interpersonal problems. *Sex Roles*, 11(7–8), 709–717.

Dunn, J. C., Whelton, W. J., & Sharpe, D. (2012). Retreating to safety: Testing the social risk hypothesis model of depression. *Evolution and Human Behavior*, 33(6), 746–758. doi:10.1016/j.evolhumbehav. 2012.06.002

Eisenberg, N., Cumberland, A., & Spinrad, T. L. (1998). Parental socialization of emotion. *Psychological Inquiry*, 9(4), 241–273.

Eibl-Eibesfeldt, I. (1989). *Human ethology*. New York: Aldine de Gruyter.

Ellis, B. (2004). Timing of pubertal maturation in girls: An integrated life history approach. *Psychological Bulletin*, 130, 920–958.

Epperson, C. et al. (1999). Gonadal steroids in the treatment of mood disorders. *Psychosomatic Medicine*, 61, 676–697.

Essock Vitale, S. & Mcguire, M. T. (1985). Women's lives from an evolutionary perspective II: Patterns of helping. *Ethology and Sociobiology*, 6, 155–173.

Everson, S. A., Maty, S. C., Lynch, J. W., & Kaplan, G. A. (2002). Epidemiologic evidence for the relation between socioeconomic status and depression, obesity, and diabetes. *Journal of Psychosomatic Research*, 53, 891–895.

Fanous, A., Gardner, C., Prescott, C., Cancro, R., & Kendler, K. (2002). Neuroticism, major depression and gender: A population-based twin study. *Psychological Medicine*, 32, 719–728.

Fischer, A. H. (Ed.), 2000. *Gender and emotion: social psychological perspectives*. Cambridge: Cambridge University Press.

Forbes, E. E. et al. (2010). Healthy adolescents' neural response to reward: Associations with puberty, positive affect, and depressive symptoms. *Journal of the American Academy of Child and Adolescent Psychiatry* 49, 162–172.

Francis, L. J., & Wilcox, C. (1998). The relationship between Eysenck's personality dimensions and Bem's masculinity and femininity scales revisited. *Personality & Individual Differences*, 25(4), 683–687.

Fuchs, D., & Thelen, M. H. (1988). Children's expected interpersonal consequences of communicating their affective state and reported likelihood of expression. *Child Development*, 59(5), 1314–1322.

Fugate, J. M. B., Gouzoules, H., Barrett, L. F. 2009. Separating production from perception: Perceiver-based explanations for sex differences in emotion. *Behavioral and Brain Sciences* 32 (5), 394–395.

Gater, R., Tansella, M., Korten, A., Tiemens, B., Mavreas, V., Olatawura, M. (1998). Sex differences in the prevalence and detection of depressive and anxiety disorders in general health care settings. *Archives of General Psychiatry*, 55, 405–413.

Ge, X. & Natsuaki, M. N. (2009). In search of explanations for early pubertal timing effects on developmental psychopathology. *Current Directions in Psychological Science*, 18, 327–331.

Geary, D. C. (1996). Sexual selection and sex differences in mathematical abilities. *Behavioral and Brain Sciences*, 19, 229–284.

Gelman, S. A., Taylor, M. G., & Nguyen, S. P. (2004). Mother-child conversations about gender. *Monographs of the Society for Research in Child Development*, 69(1), vii–127.

Giedd, J. N., et al. (1999). Brain development during childhood and adolescence. *Nature Neuroscience*, 2, 861–863.

Gilbert, P. (1989). *Human nature and suffering*. Hove: Lawrence Earlbaum Associates.

Gilbert, P. (1992). *Depression: The evolution of powerlessness*. New York: Guilford.

Goddings, A.-L., Burnett Heyes, S., Bird, G., Viner, R. M., & Blakemore, S.-J. (2012). The relationship between puberty and social emotion processing. *Developmental Science*, 15(6), 801–811.

Goddings, A.-L., Mills, K. L., Clasen, L. S., Giedd, J. N., Viner, R. M., & Blakemore, S.-J. (2014). The influence of puberty on subcortical brain development. *NeuroImage*, 88(C), 242–251.

Gordon, I., Martin, C., Feldman, R., & Leckman, J. F. (2011). Oxytocin and social motivation. *Developmental Cognitive Neuroscience*, 1(4), 471–493. doi:10.1016/j. dcn.2011.07.007

Gotlib, I. H., & Hammen, C. L. (1992). *Psychological aspects of depression: Towards a cognitive interpersonal integration*. Chichester: John Wiley and Sons.

Graber, J. A. (2009). Pubertal and neuroendocrine development and risk for depression. In N. B. Allen & L. Sheeber (Eds.), *Adolescent emotional development and the emergence of depressive disorders.* Cambridge: Cambridge University Press.

Graber, J. A., Lewinsohn, P. M., Seeley, J. R., & Brooks-Gunn, J. (1997). Is psychopathology associated with the timing of pubertal development? *Journal of the American Academy of Adolescent and Child Psychiatry*, 36, 1768–1776.

Hankin, B. L., Abramson, L. Y., Moffitt, T. E., Silva, P. A., McGee, R., & Angell, K. E. (1998). Development of depression from preadolescence to young adulthood: Emerging gender differences in a 10-year longitudinal study. *Journal of Abnormal Psychology*, 107, 128–140.

Hastings, P. D., McShane, K. E., Parker, R., & Ladha, F. (2007). Ready to make nice: Parental socialization of young sons and daughters prosocial behaviors with peers. *The Journal of Genetic Psychology*, 168(2), 177–200.

Herting, M. M., Maxwell, E. C., Irvine, C., & Nagel, B. J. (2012). The impact of sex, puberty, and hormones on white matter microstructure in adolescents. *Cerebral Cortex*, 22(9), 1979–1992.

Hill, J. P., & Lynch, M. E. (1983). The intensification of gender-related role expectations during early adolescence. In J. Brooks-Gunn & A. C. Petersen (Eds.), *Girls at puberty: Biological and psychosocial perspectives* (pp. 201–228). New York: Plenum.

Hoffman, M., Powlshta, K., & White, K. (2004). An examination of gender differences in adolescent adjustment: The effect of competence on gender role differences in symptoms of psychopathology. *Sex Roles*, 50, 795–810.

Hops, H. (1992). Parental depression and child behaviour problems: Implications for behavioural family intervention. *Behaviour Change*, 9(3), 126–138.

Hops, H. (1996). Intergenerational transmission of depressive symptoms: Gender and developmental considerations. In C. Mundt, M. J. Goldstein, K. Hahlweg, & P. Fiedler (Eds.), *Interpersonal factors in the origin and course of affective disorders* (pp. 113–128). London: Gaskell/Royal College of Psychiatrists.

Hops, H., Sherman, L., & Biglan, A. (1990). Maternal depression, marital discord, and children's behavior: A developmental perspective. In G. R. Patterson (Ed.), *Depression and aggression in family interaction* (pp. 185–208). Hillsdale, NJ: Lawrence Erlbaum.

Huston, A. C. (1983). Sex-typing. In P. H. Mussen (Ed.), *Handbook of child psychology* (pp. 387–467). New York: Wiley.

Huston, A., & Alvarez, M. (1990). The socialization context of gender role development in early adolescence. In R. Montemayor, G. R. Adams et al. (Eds.) *From childhood to adolescence: A transitional period?* Advances in adolescent development: An annual book series, Vol. 2 (pp. 156–179). Thousand Oaks, CA: Sage Publications, Inc.

Joiner, T. E. & Coyne, J. C. (1999). *The interactional nature of depression: Advances in interpersonal approaches.* Washington DC: American Psychological Association.

Joiner, T. E., Jr., & Metalsky, G. I. (2001). Excessive reassurance seeking: Delineating a risk factor involved in the development of depressive symptoms. *Psychological Science*, 12(5), 371–378.

Kaltiala-Heino, R., Marttunen, M., Rantanen, P., & Rimpela, M. (2003). Early puberty is associated with mental health problems in middle adolescence. *Social Science & Medicine* 57, 1055–1064.

Kavanagh, K., & Hops, H. (1994). Good girls? Bad boys? Gender and development as contexts for

diagnosis and treatment. In T. H. Ollendick & R. J. Prinz (Eds.), *Advances in clinical child psychology* (pp. 45–79). New York: Plenum.

Kendler, K., Hettema, J., Butera, F., Gardner, C., & Prescott, C. (2003). Life event dimensions of loss, humiliation, entrapment, and danger, in the prediction of onsets of major depression and generalised anxiety. *Archives of General Psychiatry*, 60, 789–796.

Keenan, K., & Shaw, D. (1997). Developmental and social influences on young girls' early problem behavior. *Psychological Bulletin*, 121(1), 95–113.

Kerig, P. K., Cowan, P. A., & Cowan, C. P. (1993). Marital quality and gender differences in parent-child interaction. *Developmental Psychology*, (29), 931–939.

Kessler, R. C. (2000). *Gender differences in major depression: Epidemiological findings.* Washington, DC: American Psychiatric Publishing, Inc.

Kessler, R. C., Chiu, W. T., Demler, O., & Walters, E. E. (2005). Prevalence, severity, and comorbidity of 12-month DSM-IV disorders in the National Comorbidity Survey Replication. *Archives of General Psychiatry*, 62, 617–627.

Kessler, R. C., McGonagle, K. A., Zhao, S., Nelson, C. B., Huges, M., Eshman, S., Wittchen, H-U. & Kendler, K. S. (1994). Lifetime and 12-month prevalence of DSM-III-R psychiatric disorders in the United States. *Archives of General Psychiatry*, 51, 8–19.

Kuehner, C. (1999). Gender differences in the short-term course of unipolar depression in a follow-up sample of depressed inpatients. *Journal of Affective Disorders*, 56(2–3), 127–139.

Kuehner, C. (2003). Gender differences in unipolar depression: An update of epidemiological findings and possible explanations. *Acta Psychiatrica Scandinavica* 108, 163–174.

Leary, M. R., Tambor, E. S., Terdal, S. K., & Downs, D. L. (1995). Self-esteem as an interpersonal monitor: The sociometer hypothesis. *Journal of Personality and Social Psychology*, 68, 519–530.

Lee, H., Macbeth, A. H., Pagani, J. H., & Young, W. S. (2009). Oxytocin: The great facilitator of life. *Progress in Neurobiology*, 88(2), 127–51. doi:10.1016/j. pneurobio.2009.04.001

Lewinsohn, P. M., Gotlib, I. H., Lewinsohn, M., Seeley, J. R., & Allen, N. B. (1998) Gender differences in anxiety disorders and anxiety symptoms in adolescents. *Journal of Abnormal Psychology*, 107,109–117.

Li, C. E., DiGiuseppe, R., & Froh, J. (2006). The roles of sex, gender, and coping in adolescent depression. *Adolescence* 41(163), 409–415.

Lytton, H., & Romney, D. M. (1991). Parents' differential socialization of boys and girls: A meta-analysis. *Psychological Bulletin*, 109(2), 267–296.

Martel, M. M. (2013). Sexual selection and sex differences in the prevalence of childhood externalizing and adolescent internalizing disorders. *Psychological Bulletin*, 139(6), 1221–1259. doi:10.1037/a0032247

McEwen, B. S. (2001). Invited Review: Estrogens effects on the brain: Multiple sites and molecular mechanisms. *Journal of Applied Physiology*, 91, 2785–2801.

McGrath, E., Keita, G. P., Strickland, B. R., & Russo, N. F. (1990) *Women and depression: Risk factors and treatment issues*. Washington, DC: American Psychological Association.

McGuiness, D. (1993) Gender differences in cognitive style: Implications for mathematics performance and achievement. In L. A. Penner, G. M. Batsche, H. M. Knoff, & D. L. Nelson (Eds.), *The challenge of mathematics and science education: Psychology's response*.

Washington, DC: American Psychological Association.

McGuire, M. T. & Troisi, A. (1998). Prevalence differences in depression among males and females: Are there evolutionary explanations? *British Journal of Medical Psychology*, 71, 479–491.

Mendle, J. et al. (2010) Development's tortoise and hare: Pubertal timing, pubertal tempo, and depressive symptoms in boys and girls. *Developmental Psychology*, 46, 1341–1353.

Monroe, S. M., Rohde, P., Seeley, J. R., & Lewinsohn, P. M. (1999). Life events and depression in adolescence: Relationship loss as a prospective risk factor for first-onset of major depressive disorder. *Journal of Abnormal Psychology*, 108, 606–614.

Montemayor, R. (1983). Parents and adolescents in conflict: All of the families some of the time and some families most of the time. *Journal of Early Adolescence*, 3, 83–103.

Nelson, E. et al. (2005). The social re-orientation of adolescence: A neuroscience perspective on the process and its relation to psychopathology. *Psychological Medicine*, 35, 163–174.

Neufang, S., et al. (2009). Sex differences and the impact of steroid hormones on the developing human brain. *Cerebral Cortex*, 19, 464–473.

Nolen-Hoeksema, S. (1990). *Sex differences in depression*. Palo Alto, CA: Stanford University Press.

Nolen-Hoeksema, S. (1998). Ruminative coping with depression. In J. Heckhausen & C. S. Dweck (Eds.), *Motivation and self-regulation across the life span* (pp. 237–256). New York: Cambridge University Press.

Noller, P. (1994). Relationships with parents in adolescence: Process and outcome. In R. Montemayor & G. R. Adams et al. (Eds.), *Personal relationships during adolescence*. Advances in adolescent

development: An annual book series, Vol. 6 (pp. 37–77). Thousand Oaks, CA: Sage Publications, Inc.

Obeidallah, D. A., McHale, S. M., & Silbereisen, R. K. (1996). Gender role socialization and adolescents' reports of depression: Why some girls and not others? *Journal of Youth & Adolescence*, 25(6), 775–785.

Ohannessian, C. M., Lerner, R. M., Lerner, J. V., & von Eye, A. (1999). Does self-competence predict gender differences in adolescent depression and anxiety? *Journal of Adolescence*, 22, 397–411.

Parker, G. B., & Brotchie, H. L. (2004). From diathesis to dimorphism: The biology of gender differences in depression. *Journal of Nervous & Mental Disease*, 192(3), 210–216.

Parker, G., Wilhelm, K., Mitchell, P., Austin, M., Roussos, J., & Gladstone, G. (1999). The influence of anxiety as a risk to early onset depression. *Journal of Affective Disorders*, 52, 11–17.

Peper, J. S. et al. (2009a). Heritability of regional and global brain structure at the onset of puberty: A magnetic resonance imaging study in 9-year-old twin pairs. *Human Brain Mapping*, 30, 2184–2196.

Peper, J. S. et al. (2009b). Sex steroids and brain structure in pubertal boys and girls. *Psychoneuroendocrinology*, 34, 332–342.

Peper, J. S., Hulshoff Pol, H. E., Crone, E. A., & van Honk, J. (2011). Sex steroids and brain structure in pubertal boys and girls: A mini-review of neuroimaging studies. *Neuroscience*, 191, 28–37.

Perrin, J. S. et al. (2008). Growth of white matter in the adolescent brain: Role of testosterone. *Journal of Neuroscience*, 28, 9519–9524.

Priess, H. A., Lindberg, S. M., & Hyde, J. S. (2009). Adolescent gender-role identity and mental health: Gender intensification revisited. *Child Development*, 80(5), 1531–1544.

doi:10.1111/j.1467-8624.
2009.01349.x

Roberts, T. A., & Nolen-Hoeksema, S. (1994). Gender comparisons in responsiveness to other's evaluations in achievement settings. *Psychology of Women Quarterly*, 18, 221–240.

Romans, S. E., Tyas, J., Cohen, M. M., & Silverstone, T. (2007). Gender differences in the symptoms of major depressive disorder. *The Journal of Nervous and Mental Disease*, 195(11), 905–911. doi:10.1097/ NMD.0b013e3181594cb7

Rubin, C., Rubenstein, J. L., Stechler, G., Heeren, T., Halton, A., Housman, D., & Kasten, L. (1992). Depressive affect in "normal" adolescents: Relationship to life stress, family, friends. *American Journal of Orthopsychiatry*, 62(3), 430–441.

Ruble, D. N., Greulich, F., Pomerantz, E. M., & Gochberg, B. (1993). The role of gender-related processes in the development of sex differences in self-evaluation and depression. *Journal of Affective Disorders*, 29, 97–128.

Seeman, M. V. (1997). Psychopathology in women and men: Focus on female hormones. *American Journal of Psychiatry*, 154(12), 1641–1647.

Sheeber, L. B., Davis, B., & Hops, H. (2002). Gender specific vulnerability to depression in children of depressed mothers. In S. H. Goodman & I. H. Gotlib (Eds.), *Children of depressed parents: Mechanisms of risk and implications for treatment* (pp. 253–274).

Washington, DC: American Psychological Association.

Sheeber, L., Hops, H., Alpert, A., Davis, B., & Andrews, J. (1997). Family support and conflict: Prospective relations to adolescent depression. *Journal of Abnormal Child Psychology*, 25(4), 333–344.

Sisk, C. L., & Foster, D. L. (2004). The neural basis of puberty and adolescence. *Nature Neuroscience*, 7, 1040–1047.

Slavin, L. A., & Rainer, K. L. (1990). Gender differences in emotional support and depressive symptoms among adolescents: A prospective analysis. *American Journal of Community Psychology*, 18(3), 407–421.

Spence, J., Helmreich, R., & Stapp, J. (1974). The Personal Attributes Questionnaire: A measure of sex role stereotypes and masculinity-femininity. *Catalogue of Selected Documents in Psychology*, 4, 43–44.

Symons, D. (1979). *The evolution of human sexuality*. New York: Oxford University Press.

Trivers, R. L. (1972). Parental investment and sexual selection. In B. Campbell (Ed.), *Sexual selection and the descent of man: 1871-1971*. Chicago: Aldine.

Watson, D. (2000). *Mood and temperament*. New York: The Guilford Press.

Weissman, M. M., Bland, R. C., Canino, G. J., Faravelli, C., Greenwald, S., Hwu, H. G., et al. (1996). Cross-national epidemiology of major depression and bipolar disorder. *Journal of the American Medical Association*, 276(4), 293–299.

Weissman, M. M. & Klerman, G. L. (1977). Sex differences and the epidemiology of depression. *Archives of General Psychiatry*, 34, 98–111.

Whittle, S., Yücel, M., Lorenzetti, V., Byrne, M. L., Simmons, J. G., Wood, S. J., Pantelis, C., & Allen, N.B. (2012). Pituitary volume mediates the relationship between pubertal timing and depressive symptoms during adolescence. *Psychoneuroendocrinology*, 37, 881–891.

Whittle, S., Yücel, M., Yap, M. B. H., & Allen, N. B. (2011). Sex differences in the neural correlates of emotion: Evidence from neuroimaging. *Biological Psychology*, 87(3), 319–333.

Wichstrom, L. (1999). The emergence of gender difference in depressed mood during adolescence: The role of intensified gender socialization. *Developmental Psychology*, 35, 232–245.

Wilhelm, K., Parker, G., & Asghari, A. (1998). Sex differences in the experience of depressed mood state over fifteen years. *Social Psychiatry and Psychiatric Epidemiology*, 33, 16–20.

Windle, M. (1992). A longitudinal study of stress buffering for adolescent problem behaviors. *Developmental Psychology*, 28, 522–530.

Yonkers, K. A., & Gurguis, G. (1995). Gender differences in the prevalence and expression of anxiety disorders. In M. V. Seeman (Ed.), *Gender and psychopathology* (pp. 113–130). Washington, DC: American Psychiatric Press.

The effects of hormones on the female brain across the lifespan

Michael C. Craig, Ester di Giacomo and Carmine M. Pariante

Introduction

There are sex differences in the incidence of many neuropsychiatric disorders. For example, neurodevelopmental disorders (e.g., autism, attention deficit hyperactivity disorder) and alcohol dependence occur more commonly in males, whereas the incidence of Alzheimer's disease, anxiety disorders and depression is increased in females. The biological basis for these gender differences is still poorly understood but probably involves a complex interaction between genes, the environment and hormones on the brain across the lifespan. The aim of this chapter is to offer examples of clinical conditions in women where the link between psychopathology and hormonal changes are more clearly supported by the scientific evidence. Within this context, we shall also discuss how hormonal changes occurring during pregnancy are relevant not only for women's psychopathology but also for the transmission of psychopathology from one generation to the next.

The *in utero* environment

Sex hormones: Sex is defined by an individual's karyotype, which can be either XY (male) or XX (female). This chromosomal difference leads to differentiation of gonads into testes or ovaries, and associated changes in the hormonal milieu of the *in utero* environment. Human studies have reported a surge of testosterone from the fetal testes, at around the 6th week of pregnancy (Hughes, 2001), peaking between 12 and 18 weeks gestation (Finegan et al., 1989). This results in levels of testosterone at term that are 10 times higher than in females (de Zegher et al., 1992). In males, a second testosterone surge also occurs in the first 3 months after birth (Quigley, 2002). Recent studies suggest that the early testosterone peak(s) plays a significant role in subsequent sex differences in

behavioral phenotype and may predispose to sex differences in vulnerability to specific disorders, such as autism (Phoenix et al., 1959).

The *in utero* effects of testosterone exposure on neurotypical human brain development have been investigated in several ways. Studies in females with congenital adrenal hyperplasia (CAH), for example, have reported increased male-typical play behavior in childhood (Hines et al., 2004) and more aggression in adolescence and adulthood (Berenbaum and Resnick, 1997). Increased aggression has also been reported in girls of opposite, compared to same, sex twins (Cohen-Bendahan et al., 2005). In both cases, this has been attributed to increased testosterone exposure prenatally. A further approach has been to examine directly the relationship between fetal testosterone levels measured at amniocentesis and later behavior. Using this technique, studies have reported a relationship between fetal testosterone and sexually dimorphic behaviors. This has included a positive correlation between fetal testosterone and restricted interests at 48 months old (Knickmeyer et al., 2005) and mental rotation at age 7 (Grimshaw et al., 1995); and a negative correlation with vocabulary level at 24 months old (Lutchmaya et al., 2002a), eye contact at 12 months old (Lutchmaya et al., 2002b), quality of social relationships at 48 months old (Knickmeyer et al., 2005), and empathy at 6–8 years old (Chapman et al., 2006). Fetal testosterone levels have also been found to be positively associated with number of autistic traits (Auyeung et al., 2009, 2012). However, one of the main criticisms when interpreting the results of these studies is the potential confounding effect of the post-natal environment. Future studies are needed to analyze these putative effects closer to delivery. Also, brain-imaging studies are needed to clarify the biological basis of these effects. These suggestions are

---

Comprehensive Women's Mental Health, ed. David J. Castle and Kathryn M. Abel. Published by Cambridge University Press. © Cambridge University Press 2016.

also pertinent when considering studies into the effects of stress hormones on infant brain development.

Stress hormones: There is increasing evidence that prenatal maternal stress can have significant effects on specific aspects of the development of offspring (for review see Glover, 2011). Studies in rats, for example, have reported that maternal prenatal stress is associated with impaired cognitive and behavioral functioning in their progeny (Weinstock, 2001). Also, in nonhuman primates there is an association between prenatal stress and shorter attention span and irritability in their young (Schneider and Coe, 1993; Schneider et al., 1992; Schneider et al., 2002).

More recently, several prospective studies in humans have also reported that acute and chronic prenatal stress, including anxiety, depression and stressful life events, are associated with a significant increase in childhood emotional, behavioral and cognitive problems (Van den Bergh et al., 2005; Talge et al., 2007a; Austin et al., 2005; Mohler et al., 2006; Davis et al., 2004; Dieter et al., 2001). However, the longer-term effects of severe maternal antenatal stress on human psychopathology such as serious neurodevelopmental disorders (Talge et al., 2007b), including autism (Kinney et al., 2008b; Kinney et al., 2008a), attention deficit hyperactivity disorder (ADHD) (Van den Bergh and Marcoen, 2004; Wadhwa, 1998; O'Connor et al., 2003; Huizink et al., 2007) and conduct disorder (O'Connor et al., 2003; Huizink et al., 2007) is mixed (for review see Glover et al., 2009b). In the Avon Longitudinal Study of Parents and Children ($n=7,448$), the level of ADHD symptoms doubled from 5% to 10% in children born to mothers who had been most anxious during pregnancy (the top 15%) (O'Connor et al., 2002); however, the exposure variable was a cross-sectional self-report measure on one occasion antenatally at 18 weeks. Similarly, in the South London Child Development study, the rates of any psychopathology in adolescent offspring born from mothers who were depressed during pregnancy doubled from around 24% to 50% (Pawlby et al., 2011). In contrast, Class et al. (2011) examined a prospective population sample of over 3 million births and measured individual-level severe antenatal maternal stress. They found no increase in rates of any psychosis or affective disorder in offspring, but did find a moderately raised risk of offspring ADHD and autism spectrum disorder. Abel et al. (2014) also reported an increase in any psychopathology postnatally following severe antenatal

maternal stress. However, when they looked at postnatal events, severe maternal stress or suicide was associated with an increase in risk of later affective psychosis. Clearly prenatal stress does not affect all children, most of whom appear resilient to antenatal maternal psychological effects; there may be significant gene-environment interactions alongside such resilience mechanisms (Kim-Cohen et al., 2006).' Nevertheless, evidence is more robust in respect of maternal prenatal stress directly affecting children's subsequent cognitive development, although the biological basis to this is poorly understood.

A range of mechanisms has been invoked to explain such associations including epigenetic, immune and hormonal. Here, we confine ourselves to consideration of a hormonal mechanism. Genetic and epigenetic considerations are covered in Chapter 5. It has been suggested that the effect of maternal stress on the fetus is partly mediated by the transplacental transport of maternal stress hormones, particularly cortisol (Huizink et al., 2004). This suggestion is supported by some animal and human studies (Trautman et al., 1995), which report a significant association between prenatal maternal exposure to synthetic dexamethasone and increased anxiety and reduced memory and socialization of their children (Rayburn et al., 1997). The fetus is usually protected from maternal cortisol by a placental enzyme, 11ß-hydroxy steroid dehydrogenase Type II (11ß-HSD2), which converts maternal cortisol to inactive cortisone (Mairesse et al., 2007). However, recent studies in mice (Holmes et al., 2006), rats (Mairesse et al., 2007) and humans (Glover et al., 2009a) suggest that maternal stress may cause down-regulation of placental 11ß-HSD2, potentially allowing greater placental permeability to maternal cortisol, as well as other potentially relevant maternal factors such as cytokines and macrophages.

Animal studies suggest that maternal stress hormones, such as cortisol, may affect subsequent child behavior by modulating development of the limbic (social) brain system. Rodent and monkey offspring of prenatally stressed mothers, for example, have significant differences in the anatomy (Salm et al., 2004) and the function (Coe et al., 2003b) of limbic/para-limbic (including amygdala) and medial prefrontal cortical regions, which are densely populated with glucocorticoid receptors. Further, exogenous administration of the stress hormone corticosterone to pregnant rats and nonhuman primates significantly affects development of their infants' limbic system (Jutapakdeegul et al., 2010; Coe et al., 2003a). These findings are supported by a study in humans which reported an association between increased maternal prenatal cortisol levels and increased amygdala volume in later childhood (Buss et al., 2012) and reduced volume in prefrontal cortical brain regions, including orbitofrontal cortex (Buss et al., 2010). However, brain regions do not function in isolation – they form networks connected by white matter tracts. Two of the key paralimbic brain regions that are affected by prenatal maternal stress, the amygdala and prefrontal cortex, are connected by the uncinate fasciculus (UF). A recent study examined the effects of prenatal stress on this tract using DT-MRI (diffusion tensor magnetic resonance imaging) tractography; the authors found a significant correlation between self-reported prenatal maternal stress exposure and proxy measures of microstructural integrity of the right UF in children at age 6–9 (Sagari et al., 2014). These findings suggest that, in addition to prenatal stress modifying the neurodevelopment of the amygdala and prefrontal cortex, it also modifies the white matter that connects these regions (i.e., UF).

These studies are of great interest, but do not take into account the postnatal environment into which children exposed to maternal stress have been born. It is increasingly recognized that family-wide influences throughout childhood also play an important role in the cognitive and behavioral development of children. Thus, early prenatal maternal effects must interact with factors such as social class, maternal social supports, wealth and deprivation, family size and structure, as well as the quality of maternal caregiving (see Chapter 4). Following, we consider the particular experience of childhood trauma and its potential relationship to neuroendocrine development in children.

Trauma during childhood and neuroendocrine development

Cumulative prevalence rates for physical abuse in children have been estimated to range from 5–35%, with rates of 4–9% for severe emotional abuse, 15–30% for sexual abuse in girls (5–15% in boys), and 6–12% for neglect (Bick et al., 2012). Apart from the social relevance, this phenomenon has important biological implications: early childhood trauma has been reported to cast a "long shadow" effect on subsequent hormonal changes and risk of psychopathology, particularly for

mood and personality disorders (Bick et al., 2012; Heim et al., 2008; Duman, 2009). Cardiovascular, auto-immune, mental and neurodegenerative disorders are all reported to be more common among adults who report childhood abuse (Bick et al., 2012).

Biological mechanisms purported to explain these findings include hyperactivity of the hypothalamic pituitary adrenal (HPA) axis (Bick et al., 2012; Taylor et al., 2006; Cicchetti et al., 2011; De Bellis et al., 1994), and elevated immune system activity (Bick et al., 2012; Shirtcliff et al., 2009; Danese et al., 2007; Danese et al., 2008). These effects have consistently been reported in individuals reporting early trauma, abuse and neglect. Dysregulation of both the stress and immune axes are considered to be associated with risk of psychopathology and ill physical health in adults. Early life trauma may be particularly important as some suggest it may be more likely to have long-term neuroendocrine consequences because of the rapid neuroendocrine development that occurs in this period of life (Shirtcliff et al., 2009). Other psychological factors, such as excessive threat vigilance, poor social relationships, impaired self-regulation and unhealthy lifestyle (Miller et al., 2011) may also be important associations between childhood trauma and later psychopathology.

The reproductive years

Depression: It is important to emphasize that clinical and psychosocial risk factors probably play a more significant role than hormonal fluctuations in most women who suffer depression during the reproductive years. In particular, poor social supports, problematic or violent partner relationships, past poor maternal care (see Chapter 4) and childhood trauma, as well as other family history of psychiatric illness are important risk factors. However, increasing evidence suggests that fluctuations in the concentration of sex hormones across the reproductive years can also significantly influence risk of depression in some women. It has been proposed that this vulnerability represents a discrete nosological entity, sometimes referred to as "reproductive depression" (Payne et al., 2009).

Support for the concept of a reproductive depression includes the observation that, after controlling for relevant risk factors, and comparing with appropriate control groups, the incidence of unipolar depressive episodes doubles (Eberhard-Gran et al., 2002) and the rate of inpatient admissions triples in the first 3 months postpartum (Munk-Olsen et al., 2006; see Chapter 10). Furthermore, women with vulnerability to depressed mood associated with one period of hormonal fluctuation (e.g., premenstrual dysphoric disorder [PMDD]) are particularly vulnerable to depression at other times of hormonal fluctuation (e.g., postnatal and perimenopausal depression) (Bloch et al., 2000; Rubinow et al., 1998; Stewart and Boydell, 1993; Payne et al., 2007).

Additional support for the concept of reproductive depression is derived from family (Widholm and Kantero, 1971) and twin studies (Dalton et al., 1987; Kendler et al., 1992; Condon, 1993), which have reported that the heritability of PMDD is greater than 50% (Kendler et al., 1998) and that PMDD is associated with significant differences in single nucleotide polymorphisms modulating the alpha estrogen receptor (Huo et al., 2007). Similarly, unipolar, nonpsychotic, postnatal depression has been reported to have a heritability of 40% (Treloar et al., 1999) and a significant familial aggregation (particularly when it is narrowly defined as developing within 6 to 8 weeks post delivery) (Forty et al., 2006).

Cooper et al. (1995) describe a significantly greater risk of subsequent postnatal mood disorder in women whose incident mood disorder was also postnatal than in women who developed their first episode of depression outside of the peripartum. These data converge to suggest that some are exquisitely sensitive to "normal" reproductive hormonal fluctuation and may explain why early literature failed to find a link between hormonal levels in women and risk of illness.

In vulnerable women, iatrogenic induction of acute hormonal fluctuation has also been reported to trigger a recurrence of symptoms. For example, using a hormonal regime that involved acute suppression of ovarian function, then administration of high doses of estrogen and progesterone, followed by acute sex hormone withdrawal (i.e., modeling postnatal hormonal changes), a recurrence of depressive symptoms was triggered in women with a history of postnatal depression (Bloch et al., 2000). Importantly, these mood changes were not found in women without a prior history of postnatal depression, further supporting the notion that acute hormonal fluctuation may trigger depressive symptoms in only a specific subgroup of women.

In summary, the aforementioned studies support the suggestion that the concentration of sex hormones across the reproductive years can significantly influence depression in some women. Studies also suggest that fluctuations in sex hormones can act as significant triggers for schizophrenia and bipolar disorder in some women.

Schizophrenia and bipolar disorder: Women with schizophrenia have an increased vulnerability to relapse postpartum and around the time of menopause (Craig et al., 2005). Those with bipolar disorder have also been estimated to have greater than a 1 in 4 risk of relapse during the postpartum period (Jones and Craddock, 2001), particularly during the first 2 weeks (Heron et al., 2007). This risk doubles in those with a past history of severe postpartum psychosis or in bipolar women with a family history of postpartum psychosis (Jones and Craddock, 2001; Robertson et al., 2005). Familial (probably genetic) factors have been implicated in this postpartum susceptibility (Jones and Craddock, 2001) and linkage studies have reported the location of possible susceptibility genes (Jones and Craddock, 2007).

It has been suggested that this risk is modulated by estrogen and that women are protected from psychotic illness when estrogen levels are relatively high. This hypothesis has received support from a recent RCT of 100 acutely psychotic women. Those randomized to transdermal 17β-estradiol, combined with antipsychotic medication, reported significantly reduced positive and general psychopathological symptoms after 28 days, compared with women prescribed antipsychotic medication alone (Kulkarni et al., 2008). It may be that transdermal estrogen increased the bioavailability (i.e., plasma levels) of antipsychotic medication in treated women. Results of this pilot have yet to be replicated and it is not recommended that women or men with residual psychotic symptoms are treated with adjunctive hormonal therapy unless there are indications of sex hormone deficiency or a lack of ovulation.

In summary, sex hormones, particularly estrogen, may play a role in the expression of schizophrenia and other major mental illnesses during reproductively active years. The reader is also referred to Chapters 22 and 23.

The post-reproductive years

Memory: One of the most significant factors to have driven recent research into the effects of sex hormones on brain were early studies reporting that estrogen replacement therapy (ERT) reduced the risk of cognitive impairment and Alzheimer's Disease

(AD) in aging postmenopausal women. However, the direction of this risk may be critically dependent on a woman's age on starting ERT and the length of time postmenopause for which ERT is prescribed. It has been reported that ovariectomy in younger women (i.e., prior to menopause) significantly increases the risk for development of cognitive impairment and dementia in later life (Nee and Lippa, 1999; Rocca et al., 2007). This risk disappeared if women were prescribed ERT until at least 50 years of age (Rocca et al., 2007). The suggestion of a "critical period" during which ERT may be protective is consistent with many prospective observational studies that have reported that ERT reduced the risk of AD by up to 50%.

Conversely, a large multi-center randomized controlled trial, the Women's Health Initiative Memory Study (WHIMS), reported an *increased* risk of dementia in women *over 65 years old* randomized to treatment with estrogen (and medroxyprogesterone acetate [MPA]) versus placebo (Shumaker et al., 2003). In other words, in the WHIMS, women were only eligible to start ERT from the age of 65 if they had not received it before. The effects on cognitive risk were only significant in women randomized to conjugated estrogen (CEO) plus MPA rather than to CEO alone, suggesting that MPA (not CEO) may have negative effects on cognition. Also, both arms of the study were underpowered to analyze the risk of AD. In addition, it has been noted that during the period this study was undertaken (1990s and early 2000s), most women were approaching primary care for ERT to treat menopausal symptoms at much younger ages.

Mood: Longitudinal studies have reported that the perimenopause is associated with an increased risk of depression compared to both the premenopausal and postmenopausal periods (Bromberger et al., 2001; Freeman et al., 2004; Schmidt et al., 2004; Maartens et al., 2002; Chim et al., 2003). These findings have been replicated across a variety of cultures, and in both rural and urban settings (Jablensky et al., 1992; Castle and Murray, 1993). The precise role of sex hormones in the etiology of symptoms at this time remains unclear. However, reports into the efficacy of estradiol for the treatment of depressive disorders in perimenopausal women (Soares et al., 2001) indicates that further research is still needed.

Conclusions

There are a number of studies showing that hormonal changes are involved in the pathogenesis and the course of behavioral abnormalities that affect aspects of human experience as diverse as caregiving to a child or cognitive impairment in aging. Further research is needed to develop greater understanding of the molecular mechanisms through which hormonal changes may affect the brain and influence behavior as well as a better understanding of the ways in which environmental effects interact with mechanisms at the cellular and molecular level. The identification of therapeutic tools and preventive interventions that can translate a deeper scientific understanding into patient benefit lags some way behind. We hope that the next few years will bring these new and important developments to improve the lives of women and their families.

References

Abel, K. M., Heuvelman, H., Jorgensen, L., Wicks, S., Susser, E., Magnusson, C., Hallqvist, J., & Dalman, C. 2014. Does prenatal or childhood severe psychological stress increase the risk of subsequent psychosis? A Swedish national population cohort. *British Medical Journal*, 348:f7679.

Austin, M. P., Hadzi-Pavlovic, D., Leader, L., Saint, K. & Parker, G. 2005. Maternal trait anxiety, depression and life event stress in pregnancy: Relationships with infant temperament. *Early Human Development*, 81, 183–190.

Auyeung, B., Ahluwalia, J., Thomson, L., Taylor, K., Hackett, G., O'Donnell, K. J. & Baron-Cohen, S. 2012. Prenatal versus postnatal sex steroid hormone effects on autistic traits in children at 18 to 24 months of age. *Molecular Autism*, 3, 17.

Auyeung, B., Baron-Cohen, S., Ashwin, E., Knickmeyer, R., Taylor, K. & Hackett, G. 2009. Fetal testosterone and autistic traits. *British Journal of Psychology*, 100, 1–22.

Berenbaum, S. A. & Resnick, S. M. 1997. Early androgen effects on aggression in children and adults with congenital adrenal hyperplasia. *Psychoneuroendocrinology*, 22, 505–515.

Bick, J., Naumova, O., Hunter, S., Barbot, B., Lee, M., Luthar, S. S., Raefski, A. & Grigorenko, E. L. 2012. Childhood adversity and DNA methylation of genes involved in the hypothalamus-pituitary-adrenal axis and immune system: Whole-genome and candidate-gene associations. *Development and Psychopathology*, 24, 1417–1425.

Bloch, M., Schmidt, P. J., Danaceau, M., Murphy, J., Nieman, L. & Rubinow, D. R. 2000. Effects of gonadal steroids in women with a history of postpartum depression. *American Journal of Psychiatry*, 157, 924–930.

Bromberger, J. T., Meyer, P. M., Kravitz, H. M., Sommer, B., Cordal, A., Powell, L., Ganz, P. A. & Sutton-Tyrrell, K. 2001. Psychologic distress and natural menopause: A multiethnic community study. *American Journal of Public Health*, 91, 1435–1442.

Buss, C., Davis, E. P., Muftuler, T. L., Head, K. & Sandman, C. A. 2010. High pregnancy anxiety during mid-gestation is associated with decreased gray matter density in 6–9-year-old children. *Psychoneuroendocrinology*, 35, 141–153.

Buss, C., Davis, E. P., Shahbaba, B., Pruessner, J. C., Head, K. & Sandman, C. A. 2012. Maternal cortisol over the course of pregnancy and subsequent child amygdala and hippocampus volumes and affective problems. *Proceedings of the National Academy of Sciences of the United States of America*, 109, E1312-9.

Castle, D. J. & Murray, R. M. 1993. The epidemiology of late-onset schizophrenia. *Schizophrenia Bulletin*, 19, 691–700.

Chapman, E., Baron-Cohen, S., Auyeung, B., Knickmeyer, R., Taylor, K. & Hackett, G. 2006. Fetal testosterone and empathy: Evidence from the Empathy Quotient (EQ) and the "Reading the Mind in the Eyes" Test. *Social Neuroscience*, 1, 135–148.

Chim, H., Tan, B. H. I., Ang, C. C., Chew, E. M. D., Chong, Y. S. & Saw, S. M. 2003. The prevalence of menopausal symptoms in a community in Singapore. *Maturitas*, 41, 275–282.

Cicchetti, D., Rogosch, F. A. & Oshri, A. 2011. Interactive effects of corticotropin releasing hormone receptor 1, serotonin transporter linked polymorphic region, and child maltreatment on diurnal cortisol regulation and internalizing symptomatology. *Development and Psychopathology*, 23, 1125–1138.

Class, Q. A., Abel, K. M., Khashan, A. S., Rickert, M. E., Dalman, C., Larsson, H., Hultman, C. M., Langstrom, N., Lichtenstein, P., D'Onofrio, B. M. (2014). Offspring psychopathology following preconception, prenatal, and postnatal maternal bereavement stress, *Psychological Medicine*, 44(1), 71–84.

Coe, C. L., Kramer, M., Czeh, B., Gould, E., Reeves, A. J., Kirschbaum, C. & Fuchs, E. 2003a. Prenatal stress diminishes neurogenesis in the dentate gyrus of juvenile Rhesus monkeys. *Biological Psychiatry*, 54, 1025–1034.

Coe, C. L., Kramer, M., Czeh, B., Gould, E., Reeves, A. J., Kirschbaum, C. & Fuchs, E. 2003b. Prenatal stress diminishes neurogenesis in the dentate gyrus of juvenile rhesus monkeys. *Biological Psychiatry*, 54, 1025–1034.

Cohen-Bendahan, C. C., Buitelaar, J. K., van Goozen, S. H., Orlebeke, J. F. & Cohen-Kettenis, P. T. 2005. Is there an effect of prenatal testosterone on aggression and other behavioral traits? A study comparing same-sex and opposite-sex twin girls. *Hormones and Behavior*, 47, 230–237.

Condon, J. T. 1993. The premenstrual syndrome: A twin study. *British Journal of Psychiatry*, 162, 481–486.

Cooper, P. J. & Murray, L. 1995. Course and recurrence of postnatal depression: evidence for the specificity of the diagnostic concept. *British Journal of Psychiatry*, 166, 191–195.

Craig, M. C., Cutter, W. J., Norbury, R. & Murphy, D. G. M. 2005. X chromosome, estrogen and brain development, implications for schizophrenia. *In*: Keshavan, M., Kennedy, J. L. & Murray, R. (eds.) *Neurodevelopment and Schizophrenia*. London/New York: Cambridge University Press.

Dalton, K., Dalton, M. E. & Guthrie, K. 1987. Incidence of the premenstrual syndrome in twins. *British Medical Journal (Clinical Research Ed)*, 295, 1027–1028.

Danese, A., Moffitt, T. E., Pariante, C. M., Ambler, A., Poulton, R. & Caspi, A. 2008. Elevated inflammation levels in depressed adults with a history of childhood maltreatment. *Archives of General Psychiatry*, 65, 409–415.

Danese, A., Pariante, C. M., Caspi, A., Taylor, A. & Poulton, R. 2007. Childhood maltreatment predicts adult inflammation in a life-course study. *Proceedings of the National Academy of Sciences of the United States of America*, 104, 1319–1324.

Davis, E. P., Snidman, N., Wadhwa, P. D., Glynn, L. M., Schetter, C. D. & Sandman, C. 2004. Prenatal maternal anxiety and depression predict negative behavioral reactivity in infancy. *Infancy*, 6, 319–331.

de Bellis, M. D., Chrousos, G. P., Dorn, L. D., Burke, L., Helmers, K., Kling, M. A., Trickett, P. K. & Putnam, F. W. 1994. Hypothalamic-pituitary-adrenal axis dysregulation in sexually abused girls. *The Journal of Clinical Endocrinology and Metabolism*, 78, 249–255.

de Zegher, F., DeVlieger, H. & Veldhuis, J. D. 1992. Pulsatile and sexually dimorphic secretion of luteinizing hormone in the human infant on the day of birth. *Pediatric research*, 32, 605–607.

Dieter, J. N., Field, T., Hernandez-Reif, M., Jones, N. A., Lecanuet, J. P., Salman, F. A. & Redzepi, M. 2001. Maternal depression and increased fetal activity. *Journal of Obstetrics and Gynaecology*, 21, 468–473.

Duman, R. S. 2009. Neuronal damage and protection in the pathophysiology and treatment of psychiatric illness: Stress and depression. *Dialogues in Clinical Neuroscience*, 11, 239–255.

Eberhard-Gran, M., Eskild, A., Tambs, K., Samuelsen, S. O. & Opjordsmoen, S. 2002. Depression in postpartum and non-postpartum women: Prevalence and risk factors. *Acta Psychiatrica Scandinavica*, 106, 426–433.

Finegan, J. A., Bartleman, B. & Wong, P. Y. 1989. A window for the study of prenatal sex hormone influences on postnatal development. *The Journal of Genetic Psychology*, 150, 101–112.

Forty, L., Jones, L., Macgregor, S., Caesar, S., Cooper, C., Hough, A., Dean, L., Dave, S., Farmer, A., McGuffin, P., Brewster, S., Craddock, N. & Jones, I. 2006. Familiality of postpartum depression in unipolar disorder: Results of a family study. *American Journal of Psychiatry*, 163, 1549–1553.

Freeman, E. W., Sammel, M. D., Liu, L., Gracia, C. R., Nelson, D. B. & Hollander, L. 2004. Hormones and menopausal status as predictors of depression in women in transition to menopause. *Archives of General Psychiatry*, 61, 62–70.

Glover, V. 2011. Annual Research Review: Prenatal stress and the origins of psychopathology: An evolutionary perspective. *Journal of Child Psychology and Psychiatry*, 52, 356–367.

Glover, V., Bergman, K., Sarkar, P. & O'Connor, T. G. 2009a. Association between maternal and amniotic fluid cortisol is moderated by maternal anxiety. *Psychoneuroendocrinology*, 34, 430–435.

Glover, V., O'Connor, T. G. & O'Donnell, K. 2009b. Prenatal stress and the programming of the HPA axis. *Neuroscience Biobehavioral Reviews*, 35, 17–22.

Grimshaw, G. M., Sitarenios, G. & Finegan, J. A. 1995. Mental rotation at 7 years: Relations with prenatal testosterone levels and spatial play

experiences. *Brain and Cognition*, 29, 85–100.

Heim, C., Newport, D. J., Mletzko, T., Miller, A. H. & Nemeroff, C. B. 2008. The link between childhood trauma and depression: Insights from HPA axis studies in humans. *Psychoneuroendocrinology*, 33, 693–710.

Heron, J., Robertson Blackmore, E., McGuinness, M., Craddock, N. & Jones, I. 2007. No "latent period" in the onset of bipolar affective puerperal psychosis. *Archives of Women's Mental Health*, 10, 79–81.

Hines, M., Brook, C. & Conway, G. S. 2004. Androgen and psychosexual development: Core gender identity, sexual orientation and recalled childhood gender role behavior in women and men with congenital adrenal hyperplasia (CAH). *Journal of Sex Research*, 41, 75–81.

Holmes, M. C., Abrahamsen, C. T., French, K. L., Paterson, J. M., Mullins, J. J. & Seckl, J. R. 2006. The mother or the fetus? 11-hydroxysteroid dehydrogenase type 2 null mice provide evidence for direct fetal programming of behavior by endogenous glucocorticoids. *Journal of Neuroscience*, 26, 3840–3844.

Hughes, I. A. 2001. Minireview: Sex differentiation. *Endocrinology*, 142, 3281–3287.

Huizink, A. C., Dick, D. M., Sihvola, E., Pulkkinen, L., Rose, R. J. & Kaprio, J. 2007. Chernobyl exposure as stressor during pregnancy and behaviour in adolescent offspring. *Acta Psychiatrica Scandinavica*, 116, 438–446.

Huizink, A., Mulder, E. & Buitelaar, J. 2004. Prenatal stress and risk for psychopathology: Specific effects or induction of general susceptibility? . *Psychological Bulletin*, 130, 115–142.

Huo, L., Straub, R. E., Roca, C., Schmidt, P. J., Shi, K., Vakkalanka, R., Weinberger, D. R. & Rubinow, D. R. 2007. Risk for premenstrual dysphoric disorder is associated with genetic variation in ESR1, the

estrogen receptor alpha gene. *Biological Psychiatry*, 62, 925–933.

Jablensky, A., Sartorius, N. & Ernberg, G. 1992. Schizophrenia: Manifestations, incidence and course in different cultures. A World Health Organisation Ten-Country Study. *Psychological Medicine Monograph*, 20.

Jones, I. & Craddock, N. 2001. Familiality of the puerperal trigger in bipolar disorder: Results of a family study. *The American Journal of Psychiatry*, 158, 913–917.

Jones, I. & Craddock, N. 2007. Searching for the puerperal trigger: Molecular genetic studies of bipolar affective puerperal psychosis. *Psychopharmacology Bulletin*, 40, 115–128.

Jutapakdeegul, N., Afadlal, S., Polaboon, N., Phansuwan-Pujito, P. & Govitrapong, P. 2010. Repeated restraint stress and corticosterone injections during late pregnancy alter GAP-43 expression in the hippocampus and prefrontal cortex of rat pups. *International Journal of Developmental Neuroscience*, 28, 83–90.

Kendler, K. S., Karkowski, L. M., Corey, L. A. & Neale, M. C. 1998. Longitudinal population-based twin study of retrospectively reported premenstrual symptoms and lifetime major depression. *American Journal of Psychiatry*, 155, 1234–1240.

Kendler, K. S., Silberg, J. L., Neale, M. C., Kessler, R. C., Heath, A. C. & Eaves, L. J. 1992. Genetic and environmental factors in the aetiology of menstrual, premenstrual and neurotic symptoms: A population-based twin study. *Psychological Medicine*, 22, 85–100.

Kim-Cohen, J., Caspi, A., Taylor, A., Williams, B., Newcombe, R., Craig, I. W. & Moffitt, T. E. 2006. MAOA, maltreatment, and gene-environment interaction predicting children's mental health: New evidence and a meta-analysis. *Molecular Psychiatry*, 11, 903–913.

Kinney, D. K., Miller, A. M., Crowley, D. J., Huang, E. & Gerber, E. 2008a. Autism prevalence following prenatal exposure to hurricanes and tropical storms in Louisiana. *Journal of Autism and Developmental Disorders*, 38, 481–488.

Kinney, D. K., Munir, K. M., Crowley, D. J. & Miller, A. M. 2008b. Prenatal stress and risk for autism. *Neuroscience & Biobehavioral Reviews*, 32, 1519–1532.

Knickmeyer, R., Baron-Cohen, S., Raggatt, P. & Taylor, K. 2005. Foetal testosterone, social relationships, and restricted interests in children. *Journal of Child Psychology and Psychiatry, and Allied Disciplines*, 46, 198–210.

Kulkarni, J., de Castella, A., Fitzgerald, P. B., Gurvich, C. T., Bailey, M., Bartholomeusz, C. & Burger, H. 2008. Estrogen in severe mental illness: A potential new treatment approach. *Archives of General Psychiatry*, 65, 955–960.

Lutchmaya, S., Baron-Cohen, S. & Raggatt, P. 2002a. Foetal testosterone and vocabulary size in 18- and 24-month-old infants. *Infant Behavior and Development* 24, 418–424.

Lutchmaya, S., Baron-Cohen, S., Raggatt, P., Knickmeyer, R. & Manning, J. 2002b. Foetal testosterone and eye contact in 12-month-old infants. *Infant Behavior and Development*, 25, 327–335.

Maartens, L. W., Knottnerus, J. A. & Pop, V. J. 2002. Menopausal transition and increased depressive symptomatology: A community based prospective study. *Maturitas*, 42, 195–200.

Mairesse, J., Lesage, J., Breton, C., Breant B, Hahn, T., Darnaudery, M., Dickson, S. L., Seckl, J., Blondeau, B., Vieau, D., Maccari, S. & Viltart, O. 2007. Maternal stress alters endocrine function of the feto-placental unit in rats. *American Journal of Physiology-Endocrinology Metabolism*, 292, E1526–E1533.

Miller, G. E., Chen, E. & Parker, K. J. 2011. Psychological stress in childhood and susceptibility to the chronic diseases of aging: Moving toward a model of behavioral and biological mechanisms. *Psychological Bulletin*, 137, 959–997.

Mohler, E., Parzer, P., Brunner, R., Wiebel, A. & Resch, F. 2006. Emotional stress in pregnancy predicts human infant reactivity. *Early Human Development*, 82, 731–737.

Munk-Olsen, T., Laursen, T. M., Pedersen, C. B., Mors, O. & Mortensen, P. B. 2006. New parents and mental disorders: A population-based register study. *Journal of the American Medical Association*, 296, 2582–2589.

Nee, L. E. & Lippa, C. F. 1999. Alzheimer's disease in 22 twin pairs – 13-year follow-up: Hormonal, infectious and traumatic factors. *Dementia and Geriatric Cognitive Disorders*, 10, 148–151.

O'Connor, T. G., Heron, J., Golding, J., Beveridge, M. & Glover, V. 2002. Maternal antenatal anxiety and children's behavioural/emotional problems at 4 years. Report from the Avon Longitudinal Study of Parents and Children. *British Journal of Psychiatry*, 180, 502–508.

O'Connor, T. G., Heron, J., Golding, J. & Glover, V. 2003. Maternal antenatal anxiety and behavioural/emotional problems in children: A test of a programming hypothesis. *Journal of Child Psychology and Psychiatry*, 44, 1025–1036.

Pawlby, S., Hay, D., Sharp, D., Waters, C. S. & Pariante, C. M. 2011. Antenatal depression and offspring psychopathology: The influence of childhood maltreatment. *British Journal of Psychiatry: The Journal of Mental Science*, 199, 106–112.

Payne, J. L., Palmer, J. T. & Joffe, H. 2009. A reproductive subtype of depression: Conceptualizing models and moving toward etiology. *Harvard Review of Psychiatry*, 17, 72–86.

Payne, J. L., Roy, P. S., Murphy-Eberenz, K., Weismann, M. M., Swartz, K. L., McInnis, M. G., Nwulia, E., Mondimore, F. M., Mackinnon, D. F., Miller, E. B., Nurnberger, J. I., Levinson, D. F., Depaulo, J. R., Jr. & Potash, J. B. 2007. Reproductive cycle-associated mood symptoms in women with major depression and bipolar disorder. *Journal of Affective Disorders*, 99, 221–229.

Phoenix, C. H., Goy, R. W., Gerall, A. A. & Young, W. C. 1959. Organizing action of prenatally administered testosterone propionate on the tissues mediating mating behavior in the female guinea pig. *Endocrinology*, 65, 369–382.

Quigley, C. A. 2002. Editorial: The postnatal gonadotropin and sex steroid surge-insights from the androgen insensitivity syndrome. *The Journal of Clinical Endocrinology and Metabolism*, 87, 24–28.

Rayburn, W. F., Christensen, H. D. & Gonzalez, C. L. 1997. A placebo-controlled comparison between betamethasone and dexamethasone for fetal maturation: Differences in neurobehavioral development of mice offspring. *American Journal of Obstetrics & Gynecology*, 176, 842–850; discussion 850–851.

Robertson, E., Jones, I., Haque, S., Holder, R. & Craddock, N. 2005. Risk of puerperal and non-puerperal recurrence of illness following bipolar affective puerperal (post-partum) psychosis. *British Journal of Psychiatry: The Journal of Mental Science*, 186, 258–259.

Rocca, W. A., Bower, J. H., Maraganore, D. M., Ahlskog, J. E., Grossardt, B. R., de Andrade, M. & Melton III, L. J. 2007. Increased risk of cognitive impairment or dementia in women who underwent oophorectomy before menopause. *Neurology*, 69, 1074–1083.

Rubinow, D. R., Schmidt, P. J. & Roca, C. A. 1998. Estrogen-serotonin interactions: Implications for affective regulation. *Biological Psychiatry*, 44, 839–850.

Sagari, S., Craig, M. C., Dell'Acqua F., O'Connor, T. G., Catani, M., Deeley, Q., Glover, V. & Murphy, D. G. M. 2014. Prenatal stress and limbic-prefrontal white matter microstructure in children aged 6–9 years: A preliminary diffusion tensor imaging study. *The World Journal of Biological Psychiatry*, 15(4), 346–352.

Salm, A. K., Pavelko, M., Krouse, E. M., Webster, W., Kraszpulski, M. & Birkle, D. L. 2004. Lateral amygdaloid nucleus expansion in adult rats is associated with exposure to prenatal stress. *Brain Research. Developmental Brain Research*, 148, 159–167.

Schmidt, P. J., Haq, N. & Rubinow, D. R. 2004. A longitudinal evaluation of the relationship between reproductive status and mood in perimenopausal women. *The American Journal of Psychiatry*, 161, 2238–2244.

Schneider, M. L. & Coe, C. L. 1993. Repeated social stress during pregnancy impairs neuromotor development of the primate infant. *Journal of Developmental and Behavioral Pediatrics*, 14, 81–87.

Schneider, M. L., Coe, C. L. & Lubach, G. R. 1992. Endocrine activation mimics the adverse effects of prenatal stress on the neuromotor development of the infant primate. *Developmental Psychobiology*, 25, 427–439.

Schneider, M. L., Moore, C. F., Kraemer, G. W., Roberts, A. D. & Dejesus, O. T. 2002. The impact of prenatal stress, fetal alcohol exposure, or both on development: Perspectives from a primate model. *Psychoneuroendocrinology*, 27, 285–298.

Shirtcliff, E. A., Coe, C. L. & Pollak, S. D. 2009. Early childhood stress is associated with elevated antibody levels to herpes simplex virus type 1. *Proceedings of the National Academy of Sciences of the United States of America*, 106, 2963–2967.

Shumaker, S. A., Legault, C., Rapp, S. R., Thal, L., Wallace, R. B., Ockene, J. K., Hendrix, S. L., Jones, B. N., III, Assaf, A. R., Jackson, R. D., Morley Kotchen, J., Wassertheil-Smoller, S. & Wactawski-Wende, J. 2003. Estrogen plus progestin and the incidence of dementia and mild cognitive impairment in postmenopausal women: The Women's Health Initiative Memory Study: A randomized controlled trial. *Journal of the American Medical Association*, 289, 2651–2662.

Soares, C., Almeida, O., Joffe, H. & Cohen, L. 2001. Efficacy of estradiol for the treatment of depressive disorders in perimenopausal women: A double-blind, randomized, placebo-controlled trial. *Archives of General Psychiatry*, 58, 529–534.

Stewart, D. E. & Boydell, K. M. 1993. Psychologic distress during menopause: Associations across the reproductive life cycle. *International Journal of Psychiatry in Medicine*, 23, 157–162.

Talge, N. M., Neal, C. & Glover, V. 2007a. Antenatal maternal stress and long-term effects on child neurodevelopment: How and why? *Journal of Child Psychology and Psychiatry and Allied Disciplines*, 48, 245–261.

Talge, N. M., Neal, C. & Glover, V. 2007b. Antenatal maternal stress and long-term effects on child neurodevelopment: How and why? . *Journal of Child Psychology and Psychiatry*, 48, 245–261.

Taylor, S. E., Lehman, B. J., Kiefe, C. I. & Seeman, T. E. 2006. Relationship of early life stress and psychological functioning to adult C-reactive protein in the coronary artery risk development in young adults study. *Biological Psychiatry*, 60, 819–824.

Trautman, P. D., Meyer-Bahlburg, H. F. L., Postelnek, J. & New, M. I. 1995. Effects of early prenatal dexamethasone on the cognitive and behavioral development of young children: Results of a pilot study. *Psychoneuroendocrinology*, 20, 439–449.

Treloar, S. A., Martin, N. G., Bucholz, K. K., Madden, P. A. & Heath, A. C. 1999. Genetic influences on post-natal depressive symptoms: Findings from an Australian twin sample. *Psychological Medicine*, 29, 645–654.

van den Bergh, B. R. H. & Marcoen, A. 2004. High antenatal maternal anxiety Is related to ADHD symptoms, externalizing problems, and anxiety in 8- and 9-year-olds. *Child Development*, 75, 1085–1097.

van den Bergh, B. R., Mulder, E. J., Mennes, M. & Glover, V. 2005. Antenatal maternal anxiety and stress and the neurobehavioural development of the fetus and child: Links and possible mechanisms. A review. *Neuroscience & Biobehavioral Review*, 29, 237–258.

Wadhwa, P. 1998. Prenatal stress and life-span development. In: Friedman, H. S. (ed.) *Encyclopedia of mental health*. San Diego: Academic Press.

Weinstock, M. 2001. Alterations induced by gestational stress in brain morphology and behaviour of the offspring. *Progress in Neurobiology*, 65, 427–451.

Widholm, O. & Kantero, R. L. 1971. A statistical analysis of the menstrual patterns of 8,000 Finnish girls and their mothers. *Acta Obstet Gynecol Scand Suppl*, 14, Suppl 14:1–36.

Sexual, reproductive and antenatal care of women with mental illness

Angelika Wieck and Kathryn M. Abel

The burden of mental illness is increasing steadily across the world's people. And most of those with mental illness develop problems during their reproductive lives. This has several implications for mental health services. Deinstitutionalization, better care and use of fertility-preserving medication mean more women with mental illness and severe mental illness are becoming parents. It is estimated that 70% of people with mental illness are now parents and the latest systematic review from the UK finds 10% of women and 5% of men (over 4 million people) are parents with mental illness (SCIE 2009).

Women with the most chronic and enduring illnesses are particularly vulnerable. Unlike most healthy women, they may struggle managing their fertility and sexual choices: unintended conceptions are particularly common. Miller (1997) reported that women with schizophrenia show high rates of coerced sex, high-risk sexual behavior and little use of contraception, even if they do not wish to become pregnant.

Women with severe mental illness are also more likely to be single, have less education and income, which are factors associated with unplanned pregnancies. Current depression is also associated with a higher risk of unplanned pregnancies as shown in a recent national survey in Britain (Wellings et al., 2013). Women who do not intend to become pregnant may be less likely to take folic acid, stop drugs or alcohol, or stop smoking in early pregnancy. Women with mental illness taking psychotropic medications and second generation antipsychotics may be more likely to be obese or have a high prepregnancy BMI. All these factors make a pregnancy more risky even in the absence of maternal mental illness. Women with unintended pregnancies also tend to receive antenatal care later (Lindberg et al., 2014) so that screening and

management of physical illnesses may be delayed. In addition, making a decision about continuing with the pregnancy often poses difficult ethical and personal dilemmas and the experience of termination of a pregnancy, although not associated with an increased risk of mental ill health, can cause great distress.

Women with affective disorders who do not plan childbearing are more likely to discontinue their psychotropic medication abruptly on learning that they are pregnant (Roca et al., 2013; Viguera et al., 2007), which places them at a high risk of acute recurrences, especially if the illness is severe or unstable. Although women tend to stop the medication out of fear that it may harm their fetus, there is evidence that the risks are often overestimated. In their study of risk perception, Bonari et al. (2005) interviewed callers to a teratology information service who were taking antidepressant, antibiotics or gastric drugs. The risks were grossly overestimated for all three groups of medications, but particularly so for antidepressants. Encouragingly, evidence-based counselling improved the risk estimations (Bonari et al., 2005).

The rate of unplanned pregnancies in background populations has been reported to be 40% worldwide in 2012, with 47% for more developed and 39% for less developed countries (Sedgh et al., 2014). The annual rate of unplanned pregnancies per 1000 women aged 15–44 was 43–80 depending on the world region (Sedgh et al., 2014). This means that clinicians working in general adult psychiatry are likely to have several women on their case load every year who become pregnant unintentionally. For all of these reasons, it is essential that clinicians discuss family planning with all female patients who have a past or current mental illness and are planning a pregnancy or have childbearing potential.

Reproductive and sexual health

Women with mental illness show significantly worse physical health and related mortality outcomes compared with the general population. In spite of the greater longevity of women compared to men across the world, women with severe mental illness are doubly disadvantaged: they experience health inequalities as well as marked socioeconomic disadvantage by being female in society (Chapter 1). Poor sexual and reproductive health exacerbates the difficulties and can significantly affect their quality of life.

The sexual and reproductive health inequalities faced by women in mental health services represents an opportunity for mental health practitioners to reflect and improve their practice. In their review, Henshaw and Protti (2010) consider this aspect of women's health in detail. They recognize a broad range of problems such as the lack of attendance at screening for preventable cancers by mentally ill women and a greatly increased risk of preventable and treatable sexually transmitted infections (STIs) such as HIV, gonorrhoea and syphilis. STIs can have long-term consequences including neurological problems, pelvic inflammatory disease or even abdominal adhesions; they can result from unwanted or non-consensual and exploitative sex in mentally ill women, especially perhaps in women with severe or psychotic illness. The US NHANES III Survey of people with severe mental illness concluded that between 50–75% were sexually active in the previous year, with one-third reporting two or more partners and little or inconsistent condom use, whilst large numbers reported a history of injection drug use. Overall, data indicate that the severely mentally ill engage regularly in practices known to involve increased risk for HIV transmission.

Perhaps none of these figures will come as a surprise to experienced clinicians. The problem, however, is that most mental health professionals fail to appreciate the risks for their clients, and how these pervade the quality of their lives, for example risking HIV infection and long-term infertility. In order to do this, clinicians must understand the nature and extent of the problems women face and also the need to assess barriers within their own practice that prevent women accessing appropriate services for these areas of their health.

Most mental health practitioners are well able to take a sufficient history about reproductive and sexual health of women with mental illness under their care, and to access information on current good practice in fields outside their own. However, we and others find mental health nurses are still reluctant to talk with patients about sex or sexual practice; practitioners continue to complain about a lack of confidence to discuss and plan this aspect of care. High rates of sexual abuse in women in psychiatric care create a further layer of complexity (see also Chapters 14, 17). Unsurprisingly perhaps, many mental health professionals say they are not keen to ask about current or previous abuse, for fear of "opening a Pandora's box"; worse, they may question the validity of women's abusive experiences. Initially, the woman may simply require a trusted witness with whom to share her experience. Sexual abuse training to equip staff to better meet the needs of women – and men – survivors is now taking place in many mental health arenas. In the UK, this was supported nationally by the Implementation of Violence and Abuse Policy Programme by the late Professor Cathy Itzin; a history of violence or abuse is now routinely considered by many mental health teams. The UK Department of Health also supported development of an open access learning tool to support training of mental health professionals in sexual and reproductive health: www.scie.org.uk/publications/elearning/sexualhealth/index.asp. This contains simple advice about how to talk to patients about this aspect of their lives; many useful training exercises to download; tips on how to help women record their menstrual cycles accurately; when and who to refer for abnormalities of menstruation; how to manage disclosure of abuse; as well as advice about fertility planning.

Service and policy implications

To achieve better reproductive and sexual health for women in psychiatric care, the changes required are relatively straightforward, but they rely on an acceptance that these issues are the legitimate concern of mental health services. Sexual health is a key component of both mental and physical well-being. However, some mental health professionals may find it hard to see how this view relates to their core work. Breaking down the still prevalent mind/body dichotomy is key to the delivery of genuinely holistic, person-centered care. Seeing the links between a history of abuse, depression and irritable bowel syndrome is just one example of how this process can lead to more appropriate care pathways for symptomatic women.

Changes in both policy and practice are needed so that sexual and reproductive health of clients is recognised as part of mental health practitioners' core work. Without such acceptance, these topics will remain difficult to deal with for women and services alike. Accepting that a patient's sexuality and reproductive health are integral to their mental healthcare requires good working links with other clinicians in gynecology, obstetrics, genitourinary medicine, as well as with primary care practitioners. One cannot expect that new members of a mental health team could undertake intimate or sensitive interviews with women; rather this should be part of regular reviews and care planning.

Ideological shifts are needed not just for clinicians. Equally important is the organizational response by mental health service providers and policy makers. Sexual and reproductive health must be addressed within policies and training; sexual safety needs to be seen alongside physical safety. In recognition of this, the freely available e-learning resource mentioned earlier also seeks to raise awareness and improve knowledge among mental health practitioners and managers.

PRECONCEPTION COUNSELING AND CARE

Defining "preconception"

In the United States, the term preconception is used in a broad sense and includes all women of childbearing age. In fact, in response to a lack of progress in national pregnancy and infant outcomes and growing recognition of the role of women's health status before they conceive, the Centers for Disease Control launched the preconception care and health initiative (Johnson et al., 2006). This recommends a wide range of health promotion, screening and interventions for all women of reproductive age. In the UK, there are no comparable global health care recommendations, although general guidance does exist for planning a pregnancy aimed at health professionals and women themselves (National Institute for Health and Care Excellence, 2012). In this chapter a distinction is made between women who are planning a pregnancy and those who are not, but who have childbearing potential.

Preconception assessment

If a woman has a severe mental illness or an enduring milder illness and is planning a pregnancy, she should be referred to a secondary mental health service, preferably a specialist in perinatal mental health, for preconception advice (National Institute for Health and Care Excellence, 2014). The partner of the woman should be invited to the appointment. Because preconception counseling covers complex issues and requires a comprehensive approach, it is essential that sufficient time should be scheduled. Several clinic appointments may be required. Women should be given information that is clear, up to date and comprehensive and, wherever possible, written information should supplement the face-to-face discussions. She should be encouraged to ask for clarification if needed. It is good practice to copy the clinic letter to the patient. It is also essential that all discussions are clearly documented in the patient records.

A preconception assessment requires a careful review of the woman's psychiatric history. The accuracy of diagnosis is particularly relevant in this context because the use of medication or psychological treatments across the whole childbearing episode must be justified and appropriate. Areas of particular difficulty here are the differential diagnosis between bipolar affective disorder and emotionally unstable personality disorder, which require different treatment approaches. The course of the illness, including the number of episodes experienced, inpatient admissions and inter-episode symptom levels, should be established.

The clinician should assess what the woman's response has been to previous and current medications, her adherence to them, the side effects she experienced and what her preferred treatments are. Equally important is the history of psychological treatments, the quality of the therapy and her response to it. Other areas to explore carefully are her physical condition, her social history and current social situation, support from family, friends and neighborhood, any substance misuse, forensic history and her personal characteristics, such as resilience to stress. Should there be insufficient information, time should be invested in obtaining it from an informant and the services with which the patient was previously involved. A preliminary impression of any potential risks to a child should be formed. This should take into consideration any potential parenting problems as well as the woman's previous childcare history, the relationship with her partner, her social functioning and her wider social environment and supports.

A comprehensive and sensitive psychiatric assessment will not only aid clinical management, but also afford the woman an opportunity to reflect on what her own contributions could be to optimize the outcome of a future pregnancy. Although there are no studies, the experience of many specialists working in this area is that even women with severe mental illness and complex comorbidities can show considerable capacity for change in the desire to achieve the best possible outcome for their children.

Preconception advice and management

The woman should be informed about what is known about the effect of childbearing on her mental illness. In general, pregnancy does not protect from recurrences or new episodes of mental illness. In addition, childbirth is a powerful trigger particularly for bipolar recurrences, new bipolar onsets and the related condition of puerperal psychosis (see Chapters 10, 21). These illnesses typically have a sudden onset within two weeks of childbirth, a markedly fluctuating and rapidly deteriorating course, and are often extremely severe (Jones et al., 2014). An effect of childbirth on the course of schizophrenia and severe depression is also seen, albeit less dramatic (Munk-Olsen et al., 2006; Munk-Olsen et al., 2009). For many women, this means that not only the risks and benefits of taking psychotropic medication in pregnancy, but also the risks and benefits of not taking them, need to be carefully considered. Discussions and decisions will vary greatly between women according to their individual circumstances.

Optimization of nonpharmacological treatments

Nonpharmacological measures to improve maternal and fetal health should be optimized. The relapse prevention plan should be reviewed and updated with the woman. As needed, she should be offered a referral for dietary advice, a smoking cessation clinic or the community treatment team for substance misuse. The need for additional psychological treatment options should be assessed. Smoking cessation in pregnancy is most likely to require more than advice and the ability to attend a clinic in women with more severe mental illness. Personalizing a smoking cessation plan can reduce the rates of relapse.

Discussing the reproductive safety of psychotropic medication

The reproductive safety of psychotropic medication during pregnancy and lactation and prescribing

principles are addressed in Chapter 11. It should be emphasized that women who are planning a pregnancy should not be offered valproate or carbamazepine for the treatment of psychiatric disorders due to their fetotoxic potential (National Institute for Care Excellence, 2014; see Chapters 11, 21). Explaining reproductive medication risks to patients is difficult because of the considerable uncertainty of the evidence and conveying the magnitude in a way that is helpful for the patient. Rather than using percentages, the NICE guidelines (National Institute for Health and Care Excellence, 2007) recommend to use natural frequencies, that is, the actual number of pregnancies or children affected (e.g., 1:1,000) and to put the magnitude of the risk into the context of everyday life (e.g., the number of affected children of all those born in this hospital). The use of visual formats can help to convey the individual risk to the woman concerned.

The woman should be informed that, independent of psychotropic medication, 2–4/100 children are born with major congenital anomalies (Nelson & Holmes, 1989). Valproate increases the rate of several major congenital anomalies so that the overall risk of major congenital malformations (MCMs) is markedly increased. Other drugs, such as antidepressants or antipsychotics have been associated with structural defects in one or two particular organ systems and the risks are much smaller. The most common specific anomalies involve the cardiovascular system with a prevalence in the general population of about 1 in 100. In contrast, neural tube defects occur very rarely with an estimated incidence of 1 in 1000 deliveries worldwide (Mitchell et al., 2005). These conditions can lead to a varying degree of functional impairment, from mild to very severe. When quoting background figures, clinicians should also be aware that there can be variation due to regional, cultural and ethnic differences.

Medication and fertility

In the preconception counseling session, any possible effects of the woman's current psychotropic medication on her fertility should also be evaluated. If she is taking an antipsychotic drug with prolactin-elevating potential, the serum prolactin level should be measured, regardless of whether she has a regular menstrual cycle or not. Antipsychotic-induced hyperprolactinaemia can disrupt normal ovulation and cause subfertility or infertility despite the menstrual cycle appearing to be normal to the patient. Should she have drug-induced hyperpro-lactinaemia, her antipsychotic could be switched to a prolactin-sparing agent. The switch could be, for example, from risperidone, which has strong prolactin-raising properties to quetiapine, olanzapine or aripiprazole, which have no or only mild effects. If a woman has a history of a strongly preferential response to a prolactin-elevating antipsychotic, there are alternative options to switching the antipsychotic (Haddad & Wieck, 2004). These include the addition of a dopamine agonist, such as bromocriptine or cabergoline, or direct ovarian stimulation. To explore these options, an opinion from a gynecological endocrinologist should be sought.

Potential concerns about parenting competence

Many women with severe or complex mental illness are judged to parent their children successfully, particularly if they have access to social support (Abel et al., 2005). However, if there are any concerns that there will be significant difficulties in parenting, the clinician should raise the possibility with the patient that a referral may have to be made to social care once she is pregnant. Clinicians not experienced in this area may assume that this will damage their therapeutic relationship. Patients, however, often value clinicians talking about these issues openly if this is done with sensitivity. Even if the concerns are serious, it is important that the patient is reassured that she will be supported by mental health services no matter what she decides in regard to childbearing. Some clinicians may have strong preexisting feelings about women with severe forms of mental illness having children and this may cloud their clinical judgment (Coverdale et al., 2004). It is advisable in this situation to refer the patient for a second opinion.

The effectiveness and value of preconception counseling

Clinical experience suggests that few mental health professionals working in general adult psychiatry offer preconception advice (Abel & Rees, 2010). Women who are referred to a perinatal psychiatry clinic tend to have requested it themselves. It has not yet been systematically investigated whether women with severe mental illness find preconception counseling helpful and whether they improve outcome. In a recent uncontrolled retrospective study, the outcome of preconception counseling was investigated in women with bipolar disorder attending such a specialist perinatal psychiatry clinic (Wieck et al., 2010). Pharmacological recommendations and suggestions for a change in psychosocial management were followed by the referring clinician in most cases. In the 12 months after counseling, only 5/26 (19.2%) women experienced a mood episode that fulfilled DSM-IV criteria and all were treated as outpatients, suggesting that medication adjustments made in preparation of pregnancy did not destabilize the illness. It is possible that this favorable outcome arose because of selection bias. Further research is needed in this area.

THE CARE OF WOMEN WITH SEVERE MENTAL ILLNESS WHO HAVE CHILDBEARING POTENTIAL

Clinicians should discuss family planning issues with all women of childbearing potential who have a new, preexisting or past mental health problem (Abel & Rees, 2010; Henshaw & Protti, 2010). This should include how pregnancy and childbirth might affect a mental health problem, and how a mental health problem and its treatment might affect the woman, the fetus and the baby (National Institute for Health and Care Excellence, 2014). If the woman is not planning to become pregnant, her reproductive health and contraceptive status should be discussed and optimized, which may require consultation with her general practitioner or referral to a family planning clinic.

Family planning is frequently neglected in clinical practice, even if the woman is taking psychotropic medication that has teratogenic potential. Two studies have shown that when women of childbearing potential are prescribed ongoing or newly initiated medication with valproate, carbamazepine or lithium, basic childbearing aspects are addressed in less than half of all cases (Wieck et al., 2007; James et al., 2007). This area urgently requires improvement in clinical practice. A recent UK Department of Health initiative with the University of Manchester and University of Greenwich has developed an open access e-learning tool to support mental health professionals to address the particular reproductive and sexual health needs of their clients. This resource can be accessed freely via the following link: www.scie.org.uk/publications/elearning/sexualhealth/index.asp.

ANTENATAL CARE

The first appointment

On learning of her pregnancy, a woman with a severe past or current mental illness should be seen as soon as possible by a psychiatrist and, if possible, by a perinatal specialist. The NICE guidelines (National Institute for Health and Care Excellence, 2014) state that an assessment for treatment should take place within two weeks of referral. During the first pregnancy appointment, the clinician should check whether the woman is booked for antenatal care and refer her to the obstetric and midwifery service if necessary. It should be explained to the woman why it is important to inform antenatal staff about her mental illness and her permission should be sought. The current psychotropic medications that women are taking are often not known to antenatal staff and need to be communicated. This is essential for the sonographic assessment of the fetus, in particular for the structural ultrasound around 20 weeks gestation. If the woman is admitted for psychiatric inpatient treatment, close liaison is required with the midwifery and obstetric service.

The assessment and management should follow similar principles as for preconception patients. There is either no, little or inconsistent evidence specifically for the prevention or treatment of acute episodes in women with severe mental illness who are pregnant, and this applies to medication, psychological and psychosocial therapy and other interventions (National Institute for Health and Care Excellence, 2014; Dennis & Dowswell, 2013). In general, clinicians should allow their treatment approaches to be guided by the clinical effectiveness of interventions in nonpregnant populations.

Decisions about medication in pregnancy

The timing of fetal exposure to psychotropic drugs is of particular importance and should inform the earliest discussions with the patient and her family. For example, major developmental milestones for the gross development of the human heart span gestational week 6 to 10 (Dhanantwari et al., 2009) and any major structural anomalies are unlikely from the second trimester onwards. The central nervous system is sensitive to major structural defects from week 3 to 16, so that the risk of neural tube defects

is high during this window. Additionally, the central nervous system remains sensitive to drug exposure and minor structural defects and functional impairments can occur until birth and beyond (Rice & Barone, 2000; Moore, 1988). Valproate is a drug that continues to be toxic to predisposed children until birth and possibly beyond. This is the reason why the recent NICE guidelines (National Institute of Health and Care Excellence, 2014) state that valproate should not be offered to women during the entire pregnancy. Adverse effects that are known to arise from late pregnancy exposure to other psychotropic medication are unlikely to be a serious threat to the physical health of the newborn child. An exception is persistent pulmonary hypertension, which can occur after late SSRI exposure, although the complication is rare (see Chapter 11).

Untreated mental illness and outcomes

The consequences of not taking medication in pregnancy should also be discussed with the patient. The existing evidence on the effects of the maternal mental illness on obstetric and infant outcome is limited. Only a few studies have compared treated and untreated pregnant women with the same psychiatric disorder and have taken into account illness severity during pregnancy and confounding factors. On reviewing the literature, Hanley and Oberlander (2014) came to the conclusion that considerable evidence suggests that untreated or undertreated maternal mood disorders in pregnancy can increase the risk for preterm birth and low birth weight and alter neurobehavioral development in utero, although they acknowledged some variability exists among studies. Bodén et al. (2012) found that women with bipolar disorder, regardless of treatment with mood stabilizers, were at an increased risk of adverse pregnancy outcomes such as delivering a preterm infant. In addition, infants of untreated women were at increased risk of microcephaly and neonatal hypoglycemia whereas infants not exposed to mood stabilizers were not. Lin et al. (2010) reported that infants born to women with schizophrenia had low birth weight and small size for gestational age, irrespective of antipsychotic medication.

Discontinuing medication

If valproate, carbamazepine or lithium need to be discontinued, the question arises how quickly this should be done. In the case of valproate, NICE (National Institute for Health and Care Excellence, 2014) recommends to stop the medication, which can be replaced with an antipsychotic that has been shown to be effective in the acute or maintenance treatment of bipolar disorder. For lithium, a gradual withdrawal over four weeks is recommended in order to avoid rebound recurrences (National Institute for Health and Care Excellence, 2014). Should the decision be to discontinue antidepressants, tapering should follow local guidelines. Women should be informed that stopping the medication may not remove the risk of fetal malformations and that additional monitoring may be required (National Institute for Health and Care Excellence, 2014). If the woman is unsure whether she should continue with the pregnancy, she should be offered counseling.

Medication dose

Sometimes the dose of ongoing psychotropic medication, and in particular antidepressants and lithium, is lowered in the last few weeks before the expected delivery date in the attempt to avoid withdrawal or other neonatal effects. There is currently no evidence that this reduces neonatal symptoms, whilst it may increase the risks of recurrence for the mother. In the absence of any known benefit, it appears prudent to be guided by recommended dose ranges for the patient's condition and her own history of dose-response relationships.

Monitoring of mental health and nonpharmacological treatments

If any medication is stopped or changed, the woman's mental health should be monitored more closely, by symptom diaries, liaison with relatives and more frequent contacts with mental health professionals. If the woman requires psychological therapy, the intervention needs to be evidenced as effective for the woman's condition and delivered by a competent therapist. NICE (National Institute for Health and Care Excellence, 2014) recommends for pregnant women that talking therapy should commence within one month after initial assessment. In many services this means that pregnant women should be prioritized. Where waiting lists for psychological therapies are long, the intervention may begin only sometime after delivery when the time of greatest risk and benefit to the patient has passed.

Prevention of postnatal recurrences

Although the high risk of recurrences of severe mental illnesses after childbirth, and in particular bipolar disorder (see Chapters 10, 21), has been recognized for several decades, their prevention has received little attention in research. There are no randomized, double-blind placebo controlled trials using medication or other interventions. Lithium prophylaxis taken during pregnancy or immediately postpartum was effective in three series of women at risk of postpartum psychosis and in a small controlled trial of women with bipolar disorder (Bergink et al., 2012, Stewart, 1988; Stewart et al., 1991; Austin et al., 1992). Treatment with estrogens in the early postpartum period has produced conflicting results in two case series (Kumar et al., 2003, Sichel et al., 1995). Valproate was ineffective in one small controlled, but nonrandomized trial (Wisner et al., 2004).

Multidisciplinary and interagency working

In order to facilitate interagency working, face-to-face meetings with all involved health professionals should be arranged and scheduled in a timely manner. The number of meetings required depends on the complexity of the clinical scenario. As the core members of the team, the psychiatrist, the key community mental health professional, the named midwife as well as the health visitor should be invited. Depending on the individual needs of the patient, a clinical psychologist, housing officials, support workers from voluntary organizations and health professionals from specialist services, such as substance misuse, asylum seekers, HIV and domestic violence teams should be asked to join the group.

The team's careful analysis of the woman's changing needs for support in housing, building social contacts in the community and finances, will enable appropriate advice and help. The woman may also require support in making appropriate preparations for the new baby. The woman's attendance at antenatal clinic appointments and specialist health clinics should be facilitated. The team should revisit the relapse prevention plan in view of the potential for recurrences postnatally and rehearse an emergency intervention plan with the patient and relatives. It is useful for the patient to discuss with family and friends how they might support the woman to have rest periods after the birth and help with activities of daily living as well as the care of older children. Health visitors and community midwives will be able to assist with support services available in the local community. The indications for the postnatal involvement of other mental health services, such as the home treatment team or the local mother and baby inpatient unit, if available, should be discussed with the patient and any required referrals made.

Establishing a perinatal care plan

The team should summarize the overall care plan that has been agreed with the patient for the immediate perinatal period in one single document. This should be available several weeks before the expected delivery date, circulated among involved professionals and attached to the records the woman herself holds. It should detail her delivery plan, how long it is planned for her to stay on the ward, any current medication and postnatal dose changes, and therapeutic drug monitoring. It is particularly important to describe what has been discussed prenatally with the woman about breastfeeding if she is taking psychotropic medication, and to request, before any alternative advice is given to the woman, a discussion with the psychiatric team. If the woman is at risk of being unwell postnatally, psychiatric review before discharge is required. It is important to inform key professionals involved in her postnatal care that the woman has delivered and when she will be discharged.

Prebirth assessments by social care

If there are concerns about significant harm to the unborn or expected newborn resulting from the pregnant woman's behavior or social circumstances, a referral to children and families social services must be considered. Few mental health services (in England specifically) take into account the unborn child in their safeguarding policies (Mian & Wieck, 2014), but most Local Safeguarding Children Boards specify separate procedures. They usually recommend that a referral is initiated by the first health professional who identifies the risk in the pregnant woman. This may be the midwife or the mental health professional depending on local resources and service configurations. Referral criteria are similar to those for older children. In England, in addition to a likelihood of significant harm to this child by the mother or

another person in the household, the criteria usually include a history of a previous child having come to significant harm or having been removed as a result of the woman's parenting capacity, a previous child having died whilst in the care of either parent, domestic or interpartner violence (IPV) in a current relationship (Chapter 14), or a history of violence or sexual offense in either the woman or her partner. These criteria reflect the conclusions by Brandon et al. (2010) that the three background factors commonly associated with serious untoward incidents related to abuse or neglect of children are parental mental illness, violence and substance misuse. The ability of services to manage such difficult constellations of adversity are also likely to be significantly affected by local cultural and legal practices, such as whether or not IPV is illegal; these factors will have to be taken into account in determining management strategies for vulnerable new mothers.

Mental Health and Social Care – multiagency working

Successful safeguarding of the child in high-risk pregnant women is founded on separate assessments by health professionals and child social workers, but also joint work in the form of information-sharing between the agencies, listening to the views of the patient and her partner/family member, and finally coming to professional conclusions that have incorporated all available information and the views of others. This process, often led by child social workers (e.g., in the UK), frequently requires the mental health professional involved with the woman to attend meetings convened by social care. It is sometimes also helpful for the child social worker or equivalent to attend a meeting of the mental health team with the patient and her partner, to share information, clarify the prebirth assessment process and ensure that an appropriate plan is in place for the immediate perinatal period.

Professionals working in mental health in England, at least, have, like other health and social care professionals, a statutory responsibility to promote the welfare of children and protect them from harm as set out by the guidance of the Department of Education (2013). In a report on the progress of child protection practice in England, Lord Laming (2009) came to the conclusion that there are still significant deficiencies in working across all involved agencies. In practice, mental health professionals often find themselves in a conflict between maintaining a therapeutic relationship and contributing to proceedings that may result in the removal of the newborn child from the patient. Achieving a constructive balance can be a difficult dilemma for the individual practitioner and should be discussed within the team, with the supervisor or in peer group supervision.

Disclosure of patient information

Another frequent concern is the disclosure of information about patients in meetings or documents that are external to the mental health service. Precise guidelines vary locally but in Britain the general principle is that consent should be obtained from the patient for disclosure "unless there are overriding considerations" (Royal College of Psychiatrists, 2010). In England and Wales, the Children's Act (1989) states that the welfare of the child is paramount in deciding any question in relation to the child. Therefore, where there is doubt as to whether sharing information is necessary, the best interests of the welfare of the child should be the overriding principle (Royal College of Psychiatrists, 2010). If the woman has refused to give consent for disclosure and the child is at significant risk of harm the minimum necessary information may be provided (Royal College of Psychiatrists, 2010). If there is uncertainty, clinicians should seek advice from their supervisor or the confidentiality guardian in their health service. It is important to document the decision-making process about disclosure of sensitive patient information in her records.

Plans by children's social services for the immediate postnatal period

If the newborn is judged to be at risk of significant harm, there is frequently uncertainty for the mother and health professionals about actions that will be taken by children and families social services in the immediate postnatal period. The child social worker should be requested to inform all involved of their intended plans in writing, well in advance of the expected delivery date.

Conclusion

Helping women with mental illness fulfill healthy lives requires a range of different approaches and a truly holistic approach to care. We recognize that many mental health practitioners work in very challenging settings. The difficulties faced in such circumstances mean that prioritizing reproductive, sexual and pregnancy health may seem inappropriate. However, it is clear that far more can and should be done for women in this health domain if we are to support ill women to achieve better quality lives. Sexual health and sexual choices, reproductive health and reproductive choices are recognized human rights; their lack in people with especially severe mental illness further promotes the inequalities they experience across so many aspects of their lives. Better understanding and greater awareness of the problems by clinicians is the first step in creating healthier lives and reducing inequality.

References

Abel, K. M. & Rees, S. (2010). The reproductive and sexual health of women service users: what's the fuss? *Advances in Psychiatric Treatment*, 16, 279–289. doi: 10.1192/apt.bp.108.006635.

Abel, K. M., Webb, R. T., Salmon, M. P., et al. (2005). Prevalence and predictors of parenting outcomes in a cohort of mothers with schizophrenia admitted for joint mother and baby psychiatric care in England, *Journal of Clinical Psychiatry*, 66, 781–789.

Austin, M. P. (1992). Puerperal affective psychosis: is there a case for lithium prophylaxis? *British Journal of Psychiatry*, 161, 692–694.

Bennett, P. N. (1996). Use of monographs in drugs. In: Bennett, P. N. (Ed.), *Drugs and human lactation* (pp. 67–74). Amsterdam: Elsevier Science Publishers.

Bergink, V., Bouvy, P. F., Vervoort, J. S., et al. (2012). Prevention of postpartum psychosis and mania in women at high risk. *American Journal of Psychiatry*, 169, 609–615.

Bodén, R., Lundgren, M., Brandt, L., Reutfors, J., Andersen, M., & Kieler, H. (2012). Risks of adverse pregnancy and birth outcomes in women treated or not treated with mood stabilisers for bipolar disorder: population based cohort study. *BMJ*. Nov 8; 345, e7085. doi: 10.1136/bmj.e7085.

Bonari, L., Koren, G., Einarson, T. R., et al. (2005). Use of antidepressants by pregnant women: evaluation of perception of risk, efficacy of evidence based counseling and determinants of decision making. *Archives of Women's Mental Health*, 8, 214–220.

Brandon, M., Bailey, S., and Belderson, P. (2010) Building on the Learning from Serious Case Reviews: a two year analysis of child protection database notifications 2007–2009. London: Department for Education, DFE-RR040.

Children Act (1989). www.legislation .gov.uk/ukpga/1989/41/contents.

Coverdale, J. H., McCullough, L. B., Chervenak, F. A. (2004). Assisted and surrogate decision making for pregnant patients who have schizophrenia. *Schizophrenia Bulletin*, 30, 659–664.

Dennis, C. L. & Dowswell, T. (2013). Interventions (other than pharmacological, psychosocial or psychological) for treating antenatal depression. *Cochrane Database of Systematic Reviews*, 7, CD006795.

Department of Education (2013). Working together to safeguard children. A guide to inter-agency working to safeguard and promote the welfare of children. www .workingtogetheronline.co.uk/ documents/Working% 20TogetherFINAL.pdf

Dhanantwari, P., Lee, E., Krishnan, A., et al. (2009). Human cardiac development in the first trimester: a high-resolution magnetic resonance imaging and episcopic fluorescence image capture atlas. *Circulation*, 120, 343–351.

Haddad, P. M., & Wieck, A. (2004). Antipsychotic-induced hyperprolactinaemia: mechanisms, clinical features and management. *Drugs*, 64, 2291–2314.

Hanley, G. E., & Oberlander, T. F. (2014). The effect of perinatal exposures on the infant: antidepressants and depression. *Best Practice & Research Clinical Obstetrics & Gynaecology*, 28, 37–48.

Henshaw, C., & Protti, O. (2010) Addressing the sexual and reproductive health needs of women who use mental health services. *Advances in Psychiatric Treatment*, 16, 272–278.

Howard, L. M., Kumar, C., Leese, M., et al. (2002). The general fertility rate in women with psychotic disorders. *American Journal of Psychiatry*, 159, 991–997.

James, L., Barnes, T. R., Lelliott, P., et al. (2007). Informing patients of

the teratogenic potential of mood stabilizing drugs: a case note review of the practice of psychiatrists. *Journal of Psychopharmacology*, 21, 815–819.

Johnson, K., Posner, S. F., Biermann, J. et al. (2006). Recommendations to Improve Preconception Health and Health Care-United States. A Report of the CDC/ATSDR Preconception Care Work Group and the Select Panel on Preconception Care. Centers for Disease Control and Prevention, www.cdc.gov/MMWR/preview/ mmwrhtml/rr5506a1.htm, accessed Oct. 30, 2014.

Jones, I., Chandra, P. S., Dazzan, P., et al (2014). Bipolar disorder, affective psychosis, and schizophrenia in pregnancy and the postpartum period. *Lancet*, 384, 1789–1799.

Kumar, C., McIvor, R. J., Davies, T., et al. (2003). Estrogen administration does not reduce the rate of recurrence of affective psychosis after childbirth. *Journal of Clinical Psychiatry*, 64, 112–118.

Lin, H. C., Chen, I. J., Chen, Y. H., Lee, H. C., Wu, F. J. (2010) Maternal schizophrenia and pregnancy outcome: does the use of antipsychotics make a difference? *Schizophrenia Research*, 116, 55–60.

Lindberg, L., Maddow-Zimet, I., Kost, K., et al. (2014). Pregnancy intentions and maternal and child health: an analysis of longitudinal data in Oklahoma. *Maternal and Child Health Journal*, 19(5), 1087–1096.

Lord Laming (2009). *The protection of children in England: a progress report*. https://www.education.gov .uk/publications/.../HC-330.pdf. ISBN: 9780102958928.

Mian, S., & Wieck, A. (2014). *Safeguarding unborn children policies by Mental Health Trusts and Local Safeguarding Children Boards*. Poster abstract. Annual Perinatal Scientific Conference, London, November 20, 2014.

Miller, L. J. (1997). Sexuality, reproduction, and family planning in women with schizophrenia. *Schizophrenia Bulletin*, 23, 623–635.

Mitchell, L. E. (2005). Epidemiology of neural tube defects. *American Journal of Medical Genetics Part C: Seminars in Medical Genetics*, 135C(1), 88–94.

Moore, K. L. (1988). *Essentials of human embryology*. Toronto: B.C. Decker Inc.

Munk-Olsen, T., Laursen, T. M., Mendelson, T., et al. (2009). Risks and predictors of readmission for a mental disorder during the postpartum period. *Archives of General Psychiatry*, 66, 189–95.

Munk-Olsen, T., Laursen, T. M., Pedersen, C. B., et al. (2006). New parents and mental disorders: a population-based register study. *JAMA*, 296, 2582–2589.

National Institute for Health and Care Excellence (2007). Antenatal and postnatal mental health: clinical management and service guidance. Clinical guideline 045, guidance. www.nice.org.uk/cg045.

National Institute for Health and Care Excellence (2012). Pre-conception advice and management. http://cks .nice.org.uk/pre-conception-advice- and-management, accessed Oct. 20, 2014.

National Institute for Health and Care Excellence (2014). Antenatal and postnatal mental health: clinical management and service guidance. Clinical guideline 192, guidance. www.nice.org.uk/cg192.

Nelson, K., & Holmes, L. B. (1989). Malformations due to presumed spontaneous mutations in newborn infants. *New England Journal of Medicine*, 320, 19–23.

Rice, D., & Barone, S. Jr (2000). Critical periods of vulnerability for the developing nervous system: evidence from humans and animal models. *Environmental Health Perspectives*, 108 Suppl 3, 511–533.

Roca, A., Imaz, M. L., Torres, A., et al. (2013). Unplanned pregnancy and discontinuation of SSRIs in Pregnant women with previously treated affective disorder. *Journal of Affective Disorders*, 150, 807–813.

Royal College of Psychiatrists (2010). *Good psychiatric practice: confidentiality and information sharing. College Report CR160.* ISBN 978-1-904671-96-1. www.rcpsych.ac.uk/usefulresources/publications/collegereports/cr/cr160.aspx

SCIE (2009). e-Learning: Sexual, reproductive and mental health. www.scie.org.uk/publications/elearning/sexualhealth/

Sedgh, G., Singh, S., & Hussain, R. (2014). Intended and unintended pregnancies worldwide in 2012 and recent trends. *Studies in Family Planning*, 45, 301–314.

Sichel, D. A., Cohen, L. S., Robertson, L. M., et al. (1995). Prophylactic estrogen in recurrent postpartum affective disorder. *Biological Psychiatry*, 38, 814–818.

Stewart, D. E. (1988). Prophylactic lithium in postpartum affective psychosis. *Journal of Nervous and Mental Disease*, 176, 485–489.

Stewart, D. E., Klompenhouwer, J. L., Kendell, R. E., et al. (1991). Prophylactic lithium in puerperal psychosis. The experience of three centres. *British Journal of Psychiatry*, 158, 393–397.

Viguera, A. C., Whitfield, T., Baldessarini, R. J., et al. (2007). Risk of recurrence in women with bipolar disorder during pregnancy: prospective study of mood stabilizer discontinuation. *American Journal of Psychiatry*, 164, 1817–1824.

Wellings, K., Jones, K. G., Mercer, C. H., et al. (2013). The prevalence of unplanned pregnancy and Associated factors in Britain: findings from the third National Survey of Sexual Attitudes and Lifestyles (Natsal-3). *Lancet*, 382, 1807–1816.

Wieck, A., Kopparthi, S., Sundaresh, S., et al. (2010). One-year outcome after preconception consultation in women with bipolar disorder. *Journal of Clinical Psychiatry*, Jun; 71(6), 806.

Wieck, A., Rao, S., Sein, K., et al. (2007). A survey of antiepileptic prescribing to women of childbearing potential in psychiatry. *Archives of Women's Mental Health*, 10, 83–85.

Wisner, K. L., Hanusa, B. H., Peindl, K. S., et al. (2004). Prevention of postpartum episodes in women with bipolar disorder. *Biological Psychiatry*, 56, 592–596.

Mood, anxiety and obsessive compulsive disorders in pregnancy and the postpartum period

Phenomenology and epidemiology

Simone N. Vigod, Anne Buist and Meir Steiner

Introduction

Mental illness in pregnancy and postpartum has significant and potentially serious long-term consequences for a mother, her entire family, and in particular, for her infant (Grigoriadis, VonderPorten et al. 2013c). Perinatal mood and anxiety disorders are not culturally bound: they affect women in every society and from every socioeconomic background. The aim of this chapter is to increase awareness among healthcare providers about mood- and anxiety-related disorders in pregnancy and postpartum (the "perinatal" period). To achieve this goal, the chapter provides key information about the presentation of these disorders in the perinatal period, along with research about biological and psychosocial risk factors for illness.

Clinical presentations

Most psychiatric disorders can occur in the perinatal period, but mood and anxiety disorders are particularly common among women of reproductive age. Pregnancy is not protective against the development or recurrence of these disorders, and evidence suggests that the postpartum period is a time of increased risk for new-onset mood and anxiety problems. In particular, there is a risk of mood-related psychosis in the postpartum period, with women suffering from bipolar disorder at high risk. Further, there is a high risk of comorbidity with mood and anxiety disorders co-occurring (Grigoriadis, et al. 2011). In the 5th edition of the *Diagnostic and Statistical Manual of Mental Health Disorders* (DSM-5) mood and anxiety disorders are classified into five separate categories: Depressive disorders, Bipolar and related disorders, Anxiety disorders (including generalized anxiety disorder, panic disorder and social anxiety disorder), Obsessive-compulsive and related disorders, and Trauma and Stressor-related disorders (including adjustment disorder, acute stress disorder and post-traumatic stress disorder [PTSD]) (American Psychiatric Association, 2013). Mood and anxiety disorders occurring in pregnancy or postpartum are not classified as distinct disorders in the DSM-5. However, due to the distinct risks related to perinatal mood disorders, episodes of depressive and bipolar disorders occurring during this time are classified with the use of the specifier: "with peripartum onset." Specifically, the DSM-5 specifier indicates that "peripartum-onset" pertains only to episodes occurring in pregnancy or with onset in the first four weeks after delivery, although research suggests that risk is likely elevated throughout the first postpartum year. Perhaps because less work to date has focused on this area, the relationship to the perinatal period is not specified for anxiety, obsessive compulsive and trauma- and stressor-related disorders in the DSM-5. For a more general overview of these disorders in women, the reader is referred to Chapters 21 (bipolar disorder), 19 (depression), 18 (anxiety disorders) and 17 (PTSD).

Depressive and bipolar disorders

For depressive and bipolar disorders, the predominant symptom is a disturbance in mood. This disturbance can involve primarily low mood (depressive disorders)

---

or can also involve episodes of mania or hypomania with elevated or irritable mood (bipolar disorders). To be diagnosed with a depressive or bipolar disorder, a woman must also be experiencing marked impairment or change in psychosocial or interpersonal functioning. Women may also present with other mood disorders such as persistent depressive disorder (dysthymia), cyclothymic disorder, and adjustment disorder with depressed mood, with anxiety, or with mixed anxiety and depressed mood (the latter adjustment disorder category is fairly common); however, less is known about the pregnancy-specific epidemiology and impact of these disorders.

Pregnancy

Population-based studies have reported that the period prevalence of major depression in pregnancy ranges from 3.3 to 13%, and the risk does not appear to be lower than among nonpregnant women (Bennett, et al. 2004; Gavin, et al. 2005; Vesga-Lopez, et al. 2008; Banti, et al. 2011; Le Strat, et al. 2011). When other depressive disorders such as unspecified depressive disorder (minor depression) and persistent depressive disorder (dysthymia), or the presence of adjustment disorders with depressed mood are considered, higher rates are reported (between 9 and 25%). Although most studies have found that the risk of depression remains stable throughout pregnancy, some research has suggested that depressive symptoms are more prevalent in the third trimester of pregnancy, possibly related to the impact of anxiety about delivery and/or the physical symptoms of late pregnancy. Among women with bipolar disorder, almost 25% will experience a mood disturbance (mania or depression) during pregnancy, with depressive episodes predominating (Gavin, et al. 2005; Viguera, et al. 2011; Di Florio, et al. 2013). Risk factors associated with relapse of depression during pregnancy in women with bipolar disorder include younger age at onset, previous postpartum episodes, fewer children and being unmarried (Viguera, et al. 2011). Women with severe depressive and bipolar disorders are at high risk of relapse, particularly if the doses of psychotropic medications are lowered or stopped altogether early in pregnancy (Cohen, et al. 2006; Viguera, et al. 2007).

Postpartum

The "postpartum blues"

This is by far the most common of the mood changes related to postpartum, with as many as 80% of women experiencing some symptoms. It commonly occurs shortly after childbirth and resolves within the first few weeks postpartum. Symptoms may include transient low mood, emotional lability, crying and irritability. However, it can be distinguished from a major depressive episode by its transient nature and by the lack of severe symptoms such as persistent insomnia, thoughts of guilt or worthlessness and/or suicidal ideation. It is self-limiting, and does not require any treatment other than reassurance and support and is not considered a "mood disorder," but is mentioned here because of its possible biological link to significant mood changes later in the postpartum period (Edhborg 2008; Watanabe, et al. 2008; Reck, et al. 2009). It is thought that so many women experience these transient mood changes because of the impact of the rapid hormonal drop after childbirth on neurotransmitter systems involved in mood disorders (Doornbos, et al. 2008; O'Keane, et al. 2011). For example, it has been shown that binding of brain monoamine oxidase (MAO-A), which is responsible for the breakdown of monoamines in the synaptic cleft, is elevated postpartum (Sacher, Wilson et al. 2010). Why some women go on to develop major depression in the context of these changes, while others do not, is still being investigated, but some research supports the idea that genetic predisposition plays a role (Sanjuan, Martin-Santos et al. 2008).

Postpartum depression

Approximately 13% of women experience a major depressive episode in the first year postpartum. Estimates for postpartum depressive symptomatology differ depending on the timing of the measurement, the measurement tool (e.g., self-report scales versus diagnostic criteria), as well as whether unspecified depressive disorder is included in the estimates. Significant cultural and ethnic differences in rates are increasingly recognized (see Chapter 2). When only comparative studies assessing major depression are included, the period prevalence in the first 6–8 weeks postpartum appears to be significantly higher among postpartum versus nonperinatal women (Gorman, et al. 2004; Gaynes, et al. 2005; Kitamura, et al. 2006; Dietz, et al. 2007; Mota, et al. 2008). According to the DSM-5, mood disorder symptoms must have their onset late in pregnancy or within four weeks postpartum in order for the episode to qualify for the "peripartum-onset" specifier (American Psychiatric Association 2013). However, most clinicians and researchers prefer less stringent criteria when symptoms emerge in the first few months (Austin 2010; Jones & Cantwell 2010; Wisner, et al. 2010).

According to the DSM-5 definition, postpartum depression is not qualitatively different from other depressive illnesses, with low mood, energy and interest, as well as sleep and appetite disturbance. Although many women with postpartum depression do report these symptoms, the context of the postnatal period is often apparent in the manner in which the symptoms are manifested. There are common themes to women's experiences of childbirth and motherhood that separate perinatal depression from depression at other times. These themes may aid the clinician in better understanding the illness. In Beck's meta-synthesis of 18 qualitative studies in developed world samples on postpartum depression (Beck 2002), four common themes arose: incongruity between expectations and reality, spiraling downward, pervasive loss and making gains through acceptance of help. "Spiraling downward" refers to feelings of anxiety and anger, feeling overwhelmed, obsessive thinking and cognitive impairment. While these symptoms are common components of any depressive illness, in postpartum depression (PPD), they occur in response to specific triggers, including incongruence between the type of postpartum experience that was expected and that which occurred, isolation in dealing with one's feelings and the loss of former identities. These triggers occur very predictably to many women after childbirth.

It is also clear that self-harm and suicidal thoughts are common among women suffering from postpartum depression. In a large population-based sample in the United States, approximately 14% of women screened positive for having self-harm thoughts. Although the majority of these women had a diagnosis of major depressive disorder, with comorbid generalized anxiety disorder, approximately one-fifth had a diagnosis of bipolar disorder (Wisner, et al. 2013). In clinical samples, suicidal thoughts may be present in up to 60% of women with depression (Healey, et al. 2013). Although mothers overall tend to have lower rates of suicide than non-mothers (Appleby, et al. 1998), suicide in the first postpartum year remains a major cause of maternal mortality in developed countries (Oates 2003; Austin, et al. 2007; Palladino, et al. 2011).

It is important to highlight that most studies on postpartum depression prevalence have been conducted in Western societies, and recent research suggests that there is wide variability in reported prevalence across the world. A systematic review identified 143 studies in 40 countries across the world and found that reported prevalence of postpartum depression ranged from almost zero to approximately 60%. There were some countries where very low rates of postpartum depression were reported (e.g., Singapore, Malta, Malaysia, Austria and Denmark) whereas other countries reported very high rates (Brazil, Guyana, Costa Rica, Italy, Chile, South Africa, Taiwan and Korea) (Halbreich & Karkun 2006). It is hard to know whether the variability in reported postpartum depression rates is due to cultural differences in the way that symptoms are reported (i.e., symptoms are under- or over-reported in some areas depending on social and/or cultural factors), whether there are differences in the prevalence of risk factors across cultures (e.g., levels of social support, levels of economic deprivation, levels of life stress), or whether there is variability in biological vulnerability. However, these data suggest that postpartum depression exists in all cultures, though the contributing factors may vary from culture to culture. These differences will require consideration in management of perinatal depression, in particular, women immigrating from one culture to another may have issues specifically related to one – or both – of these cultures. Furthermore, Edge (2007) reported significant ethnic variation in the presentation of perinatal mood disorder in a UK sample, raising questions about the expression of ethnic differences within cultures.

Postpartum psychosis

Postpartum psychosis is the most concerning of the postpartum mood disorders, occurring in approximately 1 in 600 women. Evidence from studies of women with a history of bipolar disorder and women with history of postpartum psychosis suggest that there is a relationship between postpartum psychosis and bipolar disorder (Chaudron & Pies 2003). It is thought to be, in the majority of cases, a variant of bipolar disorder rather than a primary psychotic disorder, and is discussed in this section of the chapter. It should be noted, however, that there is an increased risk of postpartum relapse in women with primary psychotic disorders as well (Munk-Olsen, et al. 2006).

Postpartum psychosis tends to occur rapidly after delivery: usually within the first week or at the latest, the first month, postpartum. It can also occur at weaning, although this is a rare occurrence. The symptoms represent a striking change from a woman's usual personality, with confusion and clouding of consciousness considered to be classic presenting features (Ganjekar, et al. 2013). However, there is also evidence that hypomanic or manic symptoms such as elation, decreased need for sleep, increased goal-directed activity and hyper-talkativeness may precede the onset of psychosis (Heron, et al. 2008). Women may present with psychotic depression, paranoia, mania, schizophrenic symptoms or an organic-appearing presentation such as confusion. Psychotic thinking includes a break from reality, where the mother is no longer able to distinguish her thoughts from reality and may develop fixed false beliefs (delusions) about herself, her infant or others around her (Engqvist & Nilsson 2013).

Risk of a postpartum psychosis may be particularly increased for women with previously existing bipolar and psychotic illnesses if medication is stopped during pregnancy or the early postpartum period. Other risk factors are family history of psychiatric illness, especially bipolar affective disorder; there is some evidence that sleep deprivation could precipitate an episode in women with bipolar mood disorder (Sharma & Mazmanian 2003). Not all women who develop postpartum psychosis have a previous psychiatric history, though a family history of bipolar disorder is not uncommon. They are also at higher risk for developing a mood or psychotic disorder (usually bipolar disorder) at times unrelated to pregnancy (Nager, et al. 2013). The risk related to future pregnancies is very high, in the range of 50 to 60% (Robertson, et al. 2005; Blackmore, et al. 2013).

Women who present with postpartum psychosis require urgent psychiatric consultation, pharmacologic treatment and likely hospitalization, as well as ongoing support to optimize recovery (Heron, et al. 2012). Unfortunately, women with psychotic symptoms may have difficulty caring for their infants due to the thought disturbance and confusion that accompanies postpartum psychosis. They may also experience delusions that could increase the risk of harm to themselves or to their infants (Spinelli 2004). As such, ongoing comprehensive safety assessments should be conducted to ensure optimal safety of the mother and her infant, with education and engagement of family members (Doucet, et al. 2012).

Anxiety disorders

Both quantitative and qualitative studies have identified anxiety as one of the primary features of perinatal depression (Matthey, et al. 2003). The prevalence of anxiety symptoms in the postpartum period ranges from 14–20% (Figueiredo & Conde 2011; Dennis, et al. 2013). Perinatal anxiety often relates to the welfare of the infant, insecurity about one's parenting abilities, or being alone, and may or may not meet criteria for a diagnosis of an anxiety disorder. When anxious symptoms are present in the context of a depressive or bipolar disorder, DSM-5 has introduced a "with anxious features" specifier to the depressive or bipolar disorder diagnosis to reflect the frequency with which anxious symptoms are present. However, increasing attention has been focused on understanding the prevalence, incidence and impact of anxiety disorders themselves in the perinatal period.

Generalized Anxiety Disorder. Generalized anxiety disorder is characterized by excessive anxiety and worry about anticipated events or activities. Sufferers find it difficult to control the worry, to the extent that it interferes with their daily functioning in a meaningful way. Postpartum worries include themes related to finances, appearances and maintaining household duties, as well as those related to the infant's welfare (Ross & McLean 2006). By definition, symptoms are required to last at least 6 months before a diagnosis is made, such that it is rare for new-onset generalized anxiety to be diagnosed during the perinatal period. However, it is prevalent. In a study of nearly 3000 women, 9.5% had generalized anxiety disorder at some time during pregnancy but this decreased towards term (Buist, et al. 2011). This is higher than 12-month prevalence rates for anxiety of approximately 4% quoted in epidemiological studies for nonperinatal anxiety disorders (Meng & D'Arcy 2012).

Panic disorder. Panic disorder during the perinatal period can have a significant impact on functioning, including being confined to home and feeling that one is a burden to one's family. Panic can be especially problematic in pregnancy when panic symptoms precipitate and perpetuate concerns about the health of the fetus. In the postpartum period, women with panic disorder may experience increased isolation and loss of social support due to difficulty in leaving home or being in groups (Metz, Stump, et al. 1983; Beck 1998; Weisberg & Paquette 2002). In a systematic review, Ross and MacLean reported that the prevalence of panic disorder in pregnancy (1 to 3%) approximates that of nonpregnant women of reproductive age (Ross & McLean 2006; Guler, Sahin, et al. 2008). Some, but not all, studies report symptom worsening and/or high rates of relapse in subsequent pregnancies for women with preexisting panic disorder (Dannon, Iancu, et al. 2006; Guler, Koken, et al. 2008).

Specific phobias. Blood-injection injury phobia ("needle phobia") is common, affecting 7–8% of the population. Although the risk is not increased in pregnancy, this anxiety disorder has specific implications related to antenatal care, labor and delivery. Pregnant women experiencing this specific phobia have higher levels of depressive and anxious symptoms than their nonphobic counterparts (Lilliecreutz, et al. 2011).

Social phobia. Social phobia is also important to consider in the perinatal period, considering evidence that points to associations between maternal social phobia and infant responsiveness to strangers (de Rosnay, et al. 2006; Murray, et al. 2007). There have been few estimates of the prevalence of this disorder, but a clinic-based cross-sectional study estimated a prevalence of 0.5% in the postpartum period (Navarro, Garcia-Esteve et al. 2008).

Obsessive-compulsive disorder

The category of obsessive compulsive and related disorders in DSM-5 includes obsessive-compulsive disorder (OCD) itself as well as several other compulsive disorders (American Psychiatric Association 2013). With respect to the perinatal period, however, most research has been focused on obsessive-compulsive symptoms and OCD. Commonly, perinatal OCD symptoms are related to contamination obsessions as well as checking and ordering compulsions. In addition, obsessions and/or repetitive thoughts, including thoughts related to harming the infant, can occur (Uguz, et al. 2007; Uguz, et al. 2007; Speisman, et al. 2011). Obsessional thoughts are difficult to control, and are typically very distressing to the mother, as she has no desire to act on them. She may even exhibit avoidance behaviors in a compulsive manner (i.e., avoiding the baby to alleviate intrusive thoughts). Obsessional symptoms can be distinguished from postpartum psychotic symptoms where thoughts related to harming the infant are more likely to be ego-syntonic and to be part of a delusional system of fixed, false beliefs about the infant.

Similar to the anxiety disorders, many women experience obsessional symptoms during the postpartum period. These symptoms can be experienced in the context of a depressive disorder, but prospective studies suggest that OCD itself occurs in approximately 2–9% of new mothers (compared to 1–3% in the general population) (Sasson, et al. 1997; Uguz, et al. 2007; Zambaldi, et al. 2009). A recent meta-analysis of studies using diagnostic interviews to establish the prevalence of perinatal OCD found that the risk was higher in pregnancy than among non-pregnant women, and higher still in the postnatal period (risk ratio for perinatal versus nonperinatal OCD of 1.79) (Russell, et al. 2013). Several retrospective studies in clinical OCD populations suggest that at least one-third of women report increased symptoms postpartum (Sasson, et al. 1997; Uguz, et al. 2007; Forray, et al. 2010).

Trauma and stress-related disorders

Adjustment disorder. The essential feature of an adjustment disorder is a psychological response to an identifiable stressor or stressors that results in the development of clinical significant emotional or behavioral symptoms. The symptoms resolve within several weeks to months of the resolution of the stressor and the individual's symptoms do not meet criteria for another psychiatric disorder at any time point. Issues related to pregnancy, childbirth and parenting can sometimes be stressful, and this diagnosis may be appropriate when women do not meet criteria for a mood, anxiety, obsessive-compulsive or other trauma or stress-related disorder, but require supportive or other psychological treatment to alleviate symptoms.

Post-traumatic stress disorder and acute stress disorder. These disorders occur after exposure to a traumatic event. Symptoms of acute stress disorder are time-limited, resolving within 1 month from the event, whereas a diagnosis of post-traumatic stress disorder requires symptoms to last 1 month or longer. In both situations, individuals exposed to traumatic events may experience intrusive symptoms such as nightmares or flashbacks, avoid stimuli associated with the traumatic event, experience alterations in thinking or mood (e.g., distortions about causality of the event) and/or experience symptoms of arousal and reactivity related to the event (e.g., irritability, sleep disturbance, exaggerated startle response). These disorders can have significant impact on quality of life, on a mother's relationship to her infant, and on subsequent pregnancy and childbirth experiences

(Beck & Watson 2010). Increasingly, post-traumatic stress symptoms have been reported postnatally in response to traumatic aspects of the labor and delivery experience. In a large clinical sample (N=890 women), Boorman, et al. (2013) reported that almost 30% of women experienced birth as traumatic, although only 14% reported a significant emotional response (Boorman, et al. 2013). In another large clinical sample (N=1221), Soderquist et al. (2009) found that 13% of women met criteria for PTSD one month after childbirth. In a large U.S. national survey of 1373 women, Beck et al. (2011) reported a prevalence of 9% for PTSD, with 18% having at least some symptoms of the disorder. However, in another large clinical sample in Australia (N=933), the reported prevalence was only 1.2% at 4–6 weeks postpartum, and 3.1% at 12 and 24 weeks postpartum, after accounting for PTSD due to previous traumatic events and significant anxiety and depression during pregnancy (Alcorn, et al. 2010). These discrepant numbers indicate that more research is needed to clarify the prevalence of this disorder. However, fairly consistent risk factors have been identified across studies, including comorbid depression and severe fear of childbirth. Having to undergo unexpected, emergency obstetric procedures, negative interactions with staff, and feeling a loss of control over the labor and delivery situation have also been reported as potential risk factors (Olde, et al. 2006; Vythilingum 2010).

Differential diagnoses

In the care of any woman presenting with mood, anxiety, obsessive-compulsive or trauma and stressor-related disorders during pregnancy or postpartum, it is always important to ensure that another medical condition or substance use neither caused nor is contributing to the presenting psychiatric symptoms. Medical conditions to consider may include (but are not limited to) hypo- or hyper-thyroidism, vitamin B12 or iron-deficiency anemia (Bodnar & Wisner 2005; Bunevicius, et al. 2009b; Leung & Kaplan 2009; Kaplan, et al. 2012; Khalafallah & Dennis 2012; Leung, et al. 2013) and structural or functional neurological abnormalities. In particular, there is evidence that thyroid dysregulation is present in up to 10% of postpartum women and in some research elevated anti-thyroid antibodies were present in up to 19% of women with postpartum psychosis

(Bergink, et al. 2011). These studies suggest the prudence of assessing thyroid function in women with perinatal mood disorders (Pedersen, et al. 2007). Substances of abuse and dependence are also associated with psychiatric syndromes, and women should be screened for use of prescription and non-prescription substances.

Risk factors / etiology

Most researchers and clinicians agree that a complex, interactive etiological pathway involving biological, psychological and environmental factors is likely responsible for the development of depressive and anxiety disorders (Belmaker & Agam 2008). There is some empirical evidence that a biopsychosocial model accounts for symptoms of depression and anxiety in perinatal populations as well. For example, Ross et al. (2004) used structural equation modeling techniques to model relationships between biological (including hormonal) and psychosocial variables in the development of pre- and postnatal symptoms of depression and anxiety. In the model of prenatal mood, the biological variables had no relationship with symptoms of depression. Rather, they acted indirectly through their effects on psychosocial variables and symptoms of anxiety. These results were interpreted to suggest that biological vulnerability factors, including hormonal changes, determine the threshold at which psychosocial triggers, including lack of social support, will provoke symptoms of depression and anxiety in pregnancy. These same relationships, however, could not account for postpartum symptoms of depression and anxiety, possibly lending more support to the idea that biological variables may act independently of psychosocial variables during such times. As such, in any discussion of risk factors it is important to be mindful that the etiology of perinatal mood and anxiety disorders is complex, and to consider a competitive formulation for each individual woman.

Clinical and epidemiological risk factors

Most research related to psychosocial risk factors for perinatal psychiatric disorders has focused on perinatal depression. Three meta-analyses have been conducted on risk factors for postpartum depression, with the strongest factors being a previous history of depression, depression or anxiety in pregnancy, poor social support and significant life stressors

(O'Hara & Swain 1996; Beck 2002; Robertson, et al. 2004). The risk factors associated with postpartum depression likely apply to depression in pregnancy (Bunevicius, et al. 2009a) as well as to perinatal anxiety disorders (Schmied, et al. 2013). However, women with depression in pregnancy may be more likely than women whose depression develops postpartum to have a previous history of depression and/ or postpartum depression. In addition, psychosocial stressors appear to be even more commonly associated with depression in pregnancy than depression with postpartum onset (Altemus, et al. 2012).

Social support, stressful life events and other psychosocial risk factors. Lack of social support, and in particular, lack of support from an intimate partner, is associated with depressive and anxious symptoms during both pregnancy and in the postpartum period. In some recent research, the quality of the marital relationship has been shown to explain completely the variance of postpartum depression symptomatology (Akincigil, et al. 2010). Stressful life events may include financial or social stressors, interpersonal violence, obstetrical conditions and neonatal complications (Vigod, et al. 2010). A meta-analysis of partner violence concluded a 1.5-to-2-fold increase in risk of postpartum depression in women exposed to domestic violence (Beydoun, et al. 2012). These women experience anxiety and PTSD as well (Howard, et al. 2013). Negative experience of a previous birth has been associated with increased depressive symptoms and symptoms of post-traumatic stress in subsequent births (Rubertsson, et al. 2003; Beck & Watson 2010). Other psychosocial factors identified in meta-analyses as independently associated with postpartum depression include neuroticism, low self-esteem, single parenthood, unplanned pregnancy, low socioeconomic status, obstetrical complications and difficult infant temperament (O'Hara & Swain 1996; Beck 2002; Robertson, et al. 2004).

Biological mechanisms

Genetics and heritability. Family psychiatric history is an important predictor of both prenatal and postpartum mood disorders, leading some to suggest a genetic component to its etiology (Robertson, et al. 2004; O'Hara & McCabe 2013). Women with postpartum depression have a higher than expected proportion of first-degree relatives with a mood disorder. In addition, there is now evidence from at least three

independent studies that perinatal depression tends to cluster in families (Treloar, et al. 1999; Forty, et al. 2006; Murphy-Eberenz, et al. 2006). In these studies, having a sister who had suffered from PPD increased the risk that a woman would also suffer from PPD, particularly when the onset of the depression was between six and eight weeks postpartum. Additionally, genetic polymorphisms in the serotonin-gene-linked polymorphic region as well as in genes encoding MAO-A, and catechol-O-methyl-transferase (COMT) enzymes, glucocorticoid and type 1 corticotropin-relating hormone receptors gene variants, and estrogen receptor alpha have been identified that support the idea that some women may have a genetic predisposition to postpartum depression (Sanjuan, et al. 2008; Doornbos, et al. 2009; Engineer, et al. 2013; Pinsonneault, et al. 2013).

Hormones, neurotransmitters and the neuroendocrine system. During pregnancy, significant changes occur in several steroid and peptide hormones, including estrogen, progesterone, corticotrophin-releasing hormone, thyroid hormone, prolactin and oxytocin. However, it does not appear to be the absolute levels of any of these hormones that is important, rather the abrupt change in the hormonal milieu in predisposed, vulnerable women may be the trigger (Russell, et al. 2001; Pedersen, et al. 2007; Glover, et al. 2010; Meltzer-Brody, et al. 2011; Skrundz, et al. 2011; Gonzalez, et al. 2012; Mileva-Seitz, et al. 2013; Murgatroyd & Nephew 2013; Stuebe, et al. 2013). Levels of estrogen and progesterone, the main sex hormones, increase slowly but substantially during pregnancy with a relatively rapid drop to prepregnancy levels shortly after delivery (Fernandez, et al. 2013; Schiller, et al. 2013). It has been hypothesized that this rapid drop in hormone levels contributes to the preponderance of mood disorder that occurs particularly in the postpartum period (Ahokas, et al. 2001). This has biological plausibility given the known interplay between sex hormones and neurotransmitter systems involved in depression, notably serotonin and dopamine (Steiner, et al. 2003; Hall & Steiner 2013). Estrogen modulates changes in several neurotransmitter systems, including MAO-A and MAO-B, serotonin and norepinephrine. These, as well as Gamma-amino-butyric acid (GABA) and dopamine, have been studied in perinatal populations (Mileva-Seitz, et al. 2011; Mileva-Seitz, et al. 2012). Of note are the studies that suggest that pregnancy may be associated with a relative deficiency in these neurotransmitters, acting as a vulnerability to the onset and relapse of mood disorders postpartum, when accompanied by rapid hormonal fluctuation as well as other factors such as sleep deprivation and the psychological adjustment to parenthood.

Sleep regulation. The psychobiological pathways involved in sleep may contribute to the development of perinatal mood and anxiety disorders. Women experience dramatic changes to their sleep pattern and sleep quality beginning in late pregnancy and extending well into the postpartum period, including frequent awakenings, fewer hours of total sleep, reduced sleep efficiency and shorter rapid eye movement (REM) sleep latency (Karacan, Williams et al. 1969; Coble, Reynolds et al. 1994). A systematic review on the topic reported women at risk of postpartum depression demonstrated reduced REM latency, increased total sleep time during pregnancy and decreased total sleep time in the postpartum period (Ross, et al. 2005). Lending support to this finding, a recent prospective study found that mothers who slept less than four hours between midnight and 6 a.m., and mothers who napped for less than one hour during the day were at higher risk of postpartum depression three months after delivery than women who got more sleep (Goyal, et al. 2009).

Reduced sleep has always been considered a major risk factor (or harbinger) of postpartum psychotic episodes. There is some support for this hypothesis, although sample sizes have been small (Sharma, et al. 2004) and complicated by clinical management affecting sleep (Bilszta, et al. 2010). Regardless of these study limitations, because of the known relationship between reduced sleep and the onset of bipolar mood episodes outside the perinatal period, sleep protection is considered an important part of preventive management for women with mood disorders in the perinatal period.

Consequences of untreated perinatal mental illness

Depression is a leading cause of disability worldwide, and causes impairment of function in many spheres. It can affect interpersonal relationships, occupational function and has been linked with a significantly increased risk of adverse child outcomes. In its most severe form, it can lead to suicide, and has been identified as one of the leading causes of maternal mortality in developed countries (Oates 2003; Austin, et al. 2007; Palladino, et al. 2011). Anxiety disorders can also be associated with significant morbidity that interferes with function, concentration, sleep and parenting ability. Depression and anxiety in pregnancy are strong risk factors for the persistence of depression, anxiety and stress in the postpartum period, where the links between these illnesses and adverse child outcomes have been well-established.

Impact of depression and anxiety on the developing fetus

Perinatal depression, anxiety and stress are clearly associated with adverse effects on the developing fetus (Dipietro 2012). The mechanism for the associations between mental distress during pregnancy and adverse outcomes in the offspring is not fully understood, but dysregulation of the maternal-placental-fetal axis as a result of neuroendocrine changes related to depression has been suggested (Wadhwa, et al. 2001). In addition, the importance of environmental factors associated with depression and anxiety such as maternal smoking, drug/alcohol use, poor nutrition and a low socioeconomic status may also play a role. In particular, exposure to maternal depression, anxiety and stress in pregnancy has been shown in multiple studies to be associated with an increased rate of preterm deliveries, lower APGAR scores, lower birth weights and smaller head circumference (Davalos, et al. 2012). Depression in late pregnancy is also associated with an increased risk for operative deliveries and admission to a neonatal intensive care unit (Chung, et al. 2001). While the magnitude of risk does not appear to be large in population-based studies, these outcomes have clinical significance for long-term trajectories of the developing child.

A number of studies have examined cognitive and emotional outcomes of infants of mothers who were depressed or anxious in pregnancy. Newborns of depressed mothers consistently show behavioral differences and developmental problems when compared to infants born to nondepressed mothers (Jones, et al. 1998; Weinberg & Tronick 1998; Martins & Gaffan 2000; Grace, et al. 2003). Prenatal depression has been associated with lower levels of attachment (Goecke, et al. 2012), and infants of depressed and anxious mothers may be less likely to identify their mother's voice in the early weeks (Pacheco & Figueiredo 2012). Studies have also linked perinatal symptoms of anxiety with behavioral problems in early childhood (O'Connor, et al. 2002; Glasheen, et al. 2010), and suggest that physiological changes related to anxiety could affect fetal brain development. In fact, fetal changes, including increased activity and growth delays, as well as low neurotransmitter concentrations and changes in EEG activity in the newborns, have been noted in children of women with high levels of anxiety, depression and anger in the second trimester of pregnancy (Field, et al. 2003). There has also been a report of increased risk for criminality in the offspring of women who reported symptoms of depression during pregnancy (Maki, et al. 2003).

Children exposed to maternal depression and anxiety

The ill effects of maternal depression and anxiety on the offspring are well documented. Infants tend to be withdrawn, exhibit behavioral difficulties and have a higher rate of insecure or avoidant attachments (Murray & Copper 1997; Glasheen, et al. 2010). Children of depressed mothers exhibit ineffective emotional regulation, poor social skills, delays in cognitive development and are more likely to experience emotional instability later in life (Murray & Cooper 1997; Weinberg & Tronick 1998; Newport, et al. 2002). Few studies report longer-term follow-up beyond childhood and findings are less consistent. Those mothers who have childhood abuse and neglect histories as risk factors for depression are particularly likely to have problematic behaviors and attachment (Muzik, et al. 2013). Importantly, treatment of maternal psychiatric illness can change and improve the trajectory of a child's development. In the Sequenced Treatment Algorithm for Depression (STAR-D) treatment trial, remission of depressive symptoms had a positive effect on both mothers and children, with children of mothers who remained depressed demonstrating an increased incidence of both externalizing and internalizing disorders (Weissman, Pilowsky et al. 2006).

Case identification

Case identification is an important part of the management of depression during pregnancy and postpartum. There is strong evidence that mood and anxiety disorders are underidentified and undertreated in the perinatal period – particularly when formal case identification programs are not in place (Byatt, et al. 2012). This may in part be due to lack of knowledge on the part of women and their providers about what is a "normal" reaction to pregnancy-induced physiological and psychological changes as well as to the adjustment to parenthood. Stigma around mental disorders, particularly as they relate to women's ability to parent, may also play a role. In addition, providers have reported that discomfort about how to manage perinatal mental health issues as well as lack of specialist referral pathways can also be barriers to case identification and care (Buist, et al. 2005).

In response to these issues, clinical practice guidelines focused on management of perinatal mental health have begun to make recommendations about when and how to screen for perinatal mental disorders, as well as when to send for specialist referral (Austin, et al. 2011). These guidelines recommend that efforts to identify mood disorders be integrated into routine antenatal care as early as possible in the pregnancy – and that appropriate treatment pathways should be available for women who are identified. There is some controversy regarding whether *all* women should be screened (hence potentially increasing the rate of false positive screenings) or whether in-depth screening should focus only on women at high-risk (increasing the specificity, but potentially excluding women who do require care, but were not identified as part of a high-risk category). It is generally agreed that in-depth assessment should be offered to women with a personal history of a psychiatric disorder, a family history of psychiatric disorder and/or major psychosocial risk factors for perinatal mental health issues such as poor social support, intimate partner violence and/or other major life stressors.

Psychosocial risk assessment in and of itself is not adequate for the prediction and/or detection of perinatal mood and anxiety disorders (Austin, et al. 2011). Many systems have implemented routine screening of perinatal mental health issues, including jurisdictions in Canada, the United States, the UK, Israel and Australia.

The goal of a screening program for perinatal mental health is to identify women who require in-depth mental health assessment and may require treatment. Case identification can take several forms, and the case finding tool that is used may be dependent on the setting. For example, the UK's National Institute for Health and Care Excellence (NICE) clinical guidelines recommend that *all* women are asked two questions at the first visit in pregnancy, as well as at postpartum follow-up to identify the possible presence of depression: 1) "During the past month, have you often been bothered by feeling down, depressed, or hopeless?" and 2) "During the past month, have you often been bothered by having little interest or pleasure in doing things?" (National Collaborating Centre for Mental Health 2007). In the case of a positive response, then the following question is asked as well: "Is this something you feel you need or want help with?" In addition, there are some structured self-report tools that are used to screen for perinatal depression and anxiety. Of these, the Edinburgh Postnatal Depression Scale (EPDS) (Cox, et al. 1987) is the most widely accepted. It has been used in a number of countries, and has been translated into more than 30 languages (Cox & Holden 2003). The EPDS is brief (10 questions), inexpensive to use, and has a high sensitivity and validity for detection of current depression. A total score of 12 or more represents women at high risk of having major depression in the postpartum period (with scores of 14 or higher having better specificity during pregnancy) (Murray & Cox 1990). The EPDS also contains three questions that screen for anxiety, a common presentation for women with major depression in the perinatal period (Matthey 2008). Australia's "Beyond Blue" Clinical Practice Guidelines for depression and related disorders in the perinatal period recommend specifically that the EPDS be used to screen for perinatal depression and anxiety (Austin, et al. 2011).

For conditions other than depression, no perinatal specific screening tools have been well-studied. However, there is evidence that the Spielberg State-Trait Anxiety Inventory (STAI), although not a perinatal-specific tool, has utility in detecting clinical significant anxiety in a manner that is stable across the early postpartum period (Meades & Ayers 2011; Dennis, et al. 2013). We have recently piloted the use of the Generalized Anxiety Disorder 7-item (GAD-7) scale (Spitzer, et al. 2006) as a screening tool in a perinatal population. Results indicated that the GAD-7 yielded a sensitivity of 69.3% and specificity of 67.3% at an optimal cutoff score of 12. However, compared to the EPDS and the EPDS-3A anxiety subscale, the GAD-7 displayed greater specificity over a greater range of cut-off scores and could more accurately identify GAD in patients with comorbid MDD. Therefore, we suggest that at a higher cut-off score of ≥ 14, the GAD-7 represents a clinically useful scale for the

detection of GAD in perinatal psychiatric populations (Glazer, et al. 2013).

There are no perinatal-specific screening questionnaires for bipolar disorder. The Mood Disorder Questionnaire (MDQ) covers a wide breadth of manic and hypomanic symptoms, is brief and has been validated for use in a perinatal population (Frey, et al. 2012). As such, it has been recommended for use in perinatal settings. However, it suffers from the limitations of a self-report measure in that it requires that the individual have insight into manic and hypomanic symptoms to be identified (Zimmerman & Galione 2011). Also, it should be used in conjunction with a depression assessment tool such as the EDPS because it does not screen for depressive symptoms.

Regardless of the method used to identify women with perinatal mental illness, it is important to emphasize that case identification must be linked to an appropriate care pathway.

Prevention

Prevention is considered to be the first line of treatment for perinatal depression and other perinatal mental illnesses. To prevent relapse for women with preexisting disorders, it is recommended that informed and collaborative prenatal planning take place, preferably before pregnancy, to discuss issues related to birth control and planning pregnancy, the potential risks and benefits of psychotropic medication use and to outline plans in the case of relapse.

For women with a history of mood disorders (and particularly those with previous mood episodes in the perinatal period), who are currently pregnant or planning pregnancy, individualized and collaborative prenatal planning is indicated. Depending on the woman's particular situation, this will likely involve planning to reduce psychosocial risk factors and decisions regarding psychotropic medication treatment during pregnancy. Reduction or discontinuation of psychotropic medication in pregnancy can be a risk factor for relapse, particularly in women with severe depression and bipolar disorder. It should be noted, however, that the prophylactic use of medication in euthymic women with a history of unipolar depression (but not taking medication at baseline) has not been demonstrated to be an effective prevention strategy (Dennis 2004). Decisions about prophylactic use of pharmacotherapy for women with previous episodes must be made on a case-by-case basis.

Severity of illness is a key factor to consider, as are the preferences of the woman and her partner, if she has one. These aspects are addressed further in Chapters 19, 20 and 21 of this book.

Women with subsyndromal mood and/or anxiety symptoms are also important to target for intervention because these symptoms may increase the risk for full disorder with accompanying functional impairment, particularly in the postpartum period. In such cases, optimization of any current psychiatric or psychological treatment as well as consideration of the addition of psychological interventions to achieve symptoms remission are likely indicated. A Cochrane Review of 28 trials on psychosocial interventions to prevent postpartum depression concluded that: "Overall, psychosocial and psychological interventions significantly reduce the number of women who develop postpartum depression. Promising interventions include the provision of intensive, professionally-based postpartum home visits, telephone-based peer support and interpersonal psychotherapy" (Dennis & Dowswell 2013). Other general factors include minimizing stress and promoting family support, reduction (or cessation) of smoking, alcohol and illicit drug use; promoting health sleep, dietary and exercise habits; and close monitoring with aggressive treatment if early signs of depression are detected.

There is limited evidence for the prevention of postpartum depression and postpartum psychosis with exogenous administration of estrogen shortly after childbirth, as well as some evidence for the use of estrogen to treat postpartum depression (Ahokas, et al. 2000; Ahokas, et al. 2001).

High-dose oral estrogen was used as a prophylactic strategy in seven women with history of severe postpartum affective disorder (including both postpartum depression and postpartum affective psychosis); six of the seven remained well throughout the first postpartum year (Sichel, et al. 1995), but the high dose administered in this study is unlikely to be routinely given as a result of potential safety concerns.

Issues for treatment

Decision making about treatment of perinatal mood and anxiety disorders can be complex. Treatment decisions should take into account patient preference, seriousness of psychiatric illness, risk of relapse, as well as treatment risks and benefits. Clinical practice guidelines recommend a stepped treatment approach where women with mild symptoms are treated with supportive and psychological interventions within public health and/or primary care settings (National Collaborating Centre for Mental Health 2007). With increasing severity, pharmacological strategies are considered with the input of specialist consultation. Recent systematic reviews and meta-analyses have addressed the risk-benefit assessment of exposure to antidepressant medication during pregnancy (Grigoriadis, et al. 2013a; Grigoriadis, et al. 2013b; Ross, et al. 2013). In more extreme cases, psychiatric care, inpatient hospitalization and the consideration of somatic therapies such as electroconvulsive therapy may be required.

Treatment options
Psychological

Supportive therapies. It is not uncommon for first-time mothers to experience difficulty with the transition to motherhood. Supportive counseling can be adequate to help most new mothers deal with issues of unmet expectations and feelings of inadequacy (Murray, et al. 2003). Social support is also a key factor in recovery. Specifically, the involvement of the partner in treatment for postpartum depression results in improved outcomes (Misri, et al. 2000; Dennis & Ross 2006). With decreasing birth rates in many countries and more women joining the work force, the traditional social supports such as an extended family and a network of friends are often absent. Thus, maternal and child health nurses and postnatal depression support groups play a valuable role in helping mothers to recover. In addition, differing expectations of parenthood frequently increase stress on relationships. Marital difficulties predating the birth are often accentuated, and these further deplete the support base available to both parties. Relationship counseling is an important part of stress management in this context. Failure to address these issues between couples can result in ongoing marital difficulties and can contribute to parenting difficulties and later marital breakups. Fathers may also develop depression in the postpartum period and might require specific care.

Structured psychotherapies. Structured psychotherapies, such as cognitive behavior therapy (CBT) and interpersonal psychotherapy (IPT), have the strongest evidence for the treatment of mood disorders outside of the perinatal period. CBT is also considered a very effective treatment for many anxiety disorders (Hofmann, et al. 2012; Barth, et al. 2013). There have been some studies assessing these treatments specifically in the perinatal period. In a Cochrane database systematic review of randomized controlled trials for psychological and psychosocial interventions for *antenatal* mood disorders, only one trial (of IPT) met criteria. This study showed a reduction in depressive symptoms, but the authors concluded that the trial was too small, and with a nongeneralizable sample, to make specific recommendations on psychological/psychosocial treatment (Dennis, et al. 2007). However, a Cochrane systematic review of psychological therapies to treat *postpartum* depression included ten trials, and provided support for their efficacy (Dennis & Hodnett 2007). Using broader inclusion criteria for their review, another group conducted a meta-analysis to evaluate various psychological and psychosocial treatments for depression in pregnancy and postpartum. The largest effect size was found for CBT in combination with medication, but CBT alone also demonstrated significant effects. The review also supported the efficacy of IPT, with intervention effects postpartum greater than for treatment during pregnancy. Other interventions with significant beneficial effects included group therapy with cognitive behavioral, educational and transactional analysis components; psychodynamic therapy; counseling; and telephone-based and internet-based therapies (Bledsoe & Grote 2006). Simple educational interventions have not been shown to be effective in treating depression during pregnancy or postpartum.

It is important, however, to consider some potential disadvantages to psychotherapeutic and psychosocial interventions for depression and anxiety during pregnancy and postpartum. For example, treatment of mood and anxiety disorders using psychotherapeutic options may require more time (and effort) than pharmacological therapies – potentially increasing the amount of time that a developing fetus or young child is exposed to maternal depression and/or anxiety. Further, women with severe depression or anxiety may be less likely to respond to psychotherapy alone. This may be less of a problem with CBT where the treatment can focus on behavioral activation, but women with severe functional and cognitive impairment from depression may have difficulty with the cognitive and interpersonal interaction requirements

of IPT. Other potential limits to the application of psychotherapy are more practical, in that it requires access to trained psychotherapists (not readily available in some areas), and may represent a large time investment (difficulty for mothers with young children) as well as a large financial investment in some jurisdictions. More recently, telephone-based and internet-based therapies are increasingly being developed and evaluated in an attempt to overcome some of these access barriers (Dennis & Kingston 2008).

Biological

Psychopharmacological interventions. The guidelines that inform pharmacological treatments for perinatal psychiatric disorders are generally the same as those used for treatment of the disorders in women at other times in their lives (Altshuler, et al. 2001; Yonkers, et al. 2011). However, safety of the therapy for the fetus or breastfeeding infant is an important consideration in clinical decision-making. These are covered in detail in Chapters 9, 11, 19 and 21 of this book.

Hormonal interventions. Because of the dramatic reduction in sex hormones (estrogen and progesterone) postpartum, hormonal treatments have been considered for the prevention and treatment of postpartum mood disorders. Ahokas and colleagues reported that women with severe postpartum depression or postpartum psychosis responded rapidly to sublingual estrogen treatment (Ahokas, et al. 2001; Ahokas, et al. 2000). However, all patients in these trials were hypo-estrogenic at the time therapy was initiated and hypo-estrogenic states have not been consistently reported across patients with postpartum depression. The only published placebo-controlled trial of estrogen in postpartum depression involved administration of 200µg/day transdermal 17β-estradiol or placebo to 61 women with severe postpartum depression (Gregoire, et al. 1996). While the estrogen-treated participants appeared to improve more rapidly and to a greater extent than controls, differences between the groups were small in magnitude, and confounded by concomitant use of traditional antidepressant medication. Because of the potential adverse effects of exogenous hormonal administration coupled with the dearth of supporting literature, these data have not translated into recommendations for clinical practice.

Electroconvulsive therapy (ECT). ECT has been long considered to have a role in the more severe perinatal depressions and psychosis (Anderson & Reti 2009). Because of issues of stigma, and a high rate of relapse, ECT is used in only severe cases where there is poor nutritional intake, a strong risk of suicide or a high level of tormenting thoughts. A recent systematic review examined the literature from 1941 to 2007 to try to evaluate the safety of ECT during pregnancy. This review found a total of 339 cases, with at least partial remission reported in 78% of treated women. Fetal and neonatal complications possibly related to ECT were reported in 11 cases (3.2%), with maternal complications reported in 18 cases (5.3%). There were no comparisons made to women with untreated severe mental illnesses, so the level of morbidity attributable to ECT is uncertain, but the risk of serious complications from ECT during pregnancy is likely to be low (Anderson & Reti 2009).

Other interventions. Other interventions that have been evaluated for treatment of perinatal mood disorders include bright light therapy, massage therapy, exercise/yoga, acupuncture, sleep deprivation and omega-3 fatty acid supplementation; however, there is limited randomized controlled trial evidence to support their use (Richards & Payne 2013). Most research suggests that these treatments would be more helpful for women with subsyndromal or mild depression. For women who are not responsive to antidepressant medications or who do not want to use psychotropic medication, alternative brain stimulation treatments for depression such as repetitive transcranial magnetic stimulation (rTMS) are also being evaluated (Zhang, et al. 2010; Kim, et al. 2011).

Treatment settings

While most women with mood and anxiety problems can be treated in the community, hospitalization may be required for the acute management of psychosis, suicidal and/or infanticidal intent or severe psychiatric symptomatology impairing a woman's functional ability. However, admitting women without their babies can have negative consequences for the mother as it can enhance her guilt for abandoning her child. This separation may have consequences for the children in addition to any consequences of the maternal mental illness. As mother-infant attachment is often a central element in the woman's depression, mother-baby admission allows for parenting and attachment to be addressed as part of the treatment plan, while ensuring a safe environment for mother and baby (Milgrom, et al. 1998).

Mother-baby units originated in the United Kingdom and have now been implemented worldwide, including Australia, France, Germany and the United States. Reports of these mother-baby units have been limited to reviews of inpatient admissions because a randomized control trial is ethically and practically difficult to implement (Joy & Saylan 2007). A report on a large cohort of women admitted to mother-baby units in the UK over six years found that in a majority of the 848 cases (78%), outcomes were positive with respect to clinical improvement and capacity to care for the child (Salmon, et al. 2003). A smaller review of the admissions to four inpatient units in Melbourne, Australia, found similar results. Predictors of poor outcomes (separation from child, involvement of protective services) included low socioeconomic class, poor or no relationship to partner and a diagnosis of schizophrenia (Buist, et al. 2004). A recent French study involving 869 women jointly admitted with their infants to 13 mother-baby units found that two-thirds of women were significantly improved at discharge, with good prognostic factors being diagnosis of a mood disorder (vs. schizophrenia) and poor prognostic factors being comorbid personality disorder and poor social integration (Glangeaud-Freudenthal, et al. 2011). Despite their political popularity, no randomized controlled trial evidence is yet available of mother-baby units' clinical and cost effectiveness. This is important given their cost and the relative scarcity of mother-baby unit beds. A major new UK study comparing outcomes of mothers and children with alternative acute care pathways is currently underway.

Special populations

Certain populations have been identified as being at increased risk for mood and anxiety disorders in the perinatal period, likely because of a high prevalence of major psychosocial risk factors. These vulnerable populations are important to highlight because of their unique management needs (Clare & Yeh 2012). Adolescent and/or single mothers have been identified as having increased risk of postpartum depression, potentially related to the unique developmental and psychosocial challenges of being an adolescent or a single parent (Yozwiak 2010). Recent immigrant pregnant women and mothers may also be at increased risk in some contexts (Miszkurka, et al. 2010; Collins, et al. 2011).

Fathers. In recent years there has been increasing interest in the experience of fathers postpartum. Although recent meta-analysis reported that 10.4% of fathers experience depression in the first postpartum year, a significantly higher rate than that would be observed in the general population (Paulson & Bazemore 2010). Munk-Olsen's recent high-quality population study in Denmark reported that although the risk of postpartum mental disorders among primiparous mothers is increased for several months after childbirth, among fathers there is no excess of severe mental disorders necessitating admission or outpatient contacts (Munk-Olsen, et al. 2006). This is important considering that paternal mental health has been associated with child internalizing and externalizing behaviors (Kane & Garber 2004). Studies suggest that men in Western societies are grappling with changes in societal expectations, which result in conflicts between the traditional breadwinner role and that of equal sharing of childcare responsibilities (Morse, et al. 2000). The area of paternal depression remains under-researched; it is essential for further work to be done. In particular the impact of dual parental depression on the child is a key area requiring further investigation.

Same-sex couples. Although most research on perinatal depression has included samples of predominantly or exclusively heterosexual women, increasing numbers of lesbian and bisexual women are choosing to become parents (Patterson & Friel 2000). Lesbian mothers of toddlers and school-age children have been found to have equivalent levels of depressive symptoms relative to either published normal scores (Patterson 2001) or to heterosexual control groups (Chan, et al. 1998; Golombok, et al. 2003; Borneskog, et al. 2013). However, in the early postpartum period, there is some evidence that lesbian mothers may have higher depression scores (Ross, et al. 2007). While many of the fundamental aspects of the transition to parenthood are likely experienced similarly in lesbian and heterosexual mothers, lesbian mothers may differ from heterosexual parents on a number of variables that have been previously associated with parental mental health. For example, the potential lack of family and societal support for lesbian mothers, together with stress associated with homophobia and heterosexism, could make the transition to parenthood difficult for these women, and, in particular, for nonbiological lesbian parents. However, some characteristics of lesbian families may also protect against perinatal mental illness; for example, their preparedness for pregnancy and their relatively equal division of child-care labor (Ross 2005). There has been almost no research focused on male same-sex couples.

Adoptive parents. Mothers who adopt children are subject to the same psychological and social stressors that can affect all new parents, including sleep deprivation and issues related to social support and other life stressors. Studies without comparison groups of nonadoptive mothers demonstrate that adoptive mothers do experience depression, with prior depression a major predictive factor (Senecky, et al. 2009). A study comparing 147 adoptive mothers to a set of 147 postpartum women found that the groups experienced similar levels of depressive symptoms, although adoptive mothers did report less anxiety symptoms and better overall well-being (Mott, et al. 2011).

Conclusions

Perinatal psychiatric disorders present a particular challenge to clinicians and families alike. They are common, yet can readily be missed because of overlap with pregnancy and postnatal symptoms and the social pressures to attain an ideal of motherhood. These disorders confer risks to the whole family, but can present an ideal opportunity for early identification and prevention. Research and clinical interests are imperative to provide a path toward improved treatment outcomes and a clearer understanding of these disorders.

References

Ahokas, A., M. Aito, et al. (2000). "Positive treatment effect of estradiol in postpartum psychosis: a pilot study." *J Clin Psychiatry* 61(3): 166–169.

Ahokas, A., J. Kaukoranta, et al. (2001). "Estrogen deficiency in severe postpartum depression: successful treatment with sublingual physiologic 17beta-estradiol: a preliminary study." *J Clin Psychiatry* 62(5): 332–336.

Akincigil, A., S. Munch, et al. (2010). "Predictors of maternal depression in the first year postpartum: marital status and mediating role of relationship quality." *Soc Work Health Care* 49(3): 227–244.

Alcorn, K. L., A. O'Donovan, et al. (2010). "A prospective longitudinal study of the prevalence of post-traumatic stress disorder resulting from childbirth events." *Psychol Med* 40(11): 1849–1859.

Altemus, M., C. C. Neeb, et al. (2012). "Phenotypic differences between pregnancy-onset and postpartum-onset major depressive disorder." *J Clin Psychiatry* 73(12): e1485–1491.

Altshuler, L. L., L. S. Cohen, et al. (2001). "The Expert Consensus Guideline Series. Treatment of depression in women." *Postgrad Med*(Spec No): 1–107.

American Psychiatric Association. (2013). *Diagnostic and Statistical Manual of Mental Disorders, 5th Edition (DSM-5)*. Washington, DC: American Psychiatric Association.

Anderson, E. L. and I. M. Reti (2009). "ECT in pregnancy: a review of the literature from 1941 to 2007." *Psychosom Med* 71(2): 235–242.

Appleby, L., P. B. Mortensen, et al. (1998). "Suicide and other causes of mortality after post-partum psychiatric admission." *Br J Psychiatry* 173: 209–211.

Austin, M. P. (2010). "Classification of mental health disorders in the perinatal period: future directions for DSM-V and ICD-11." *Arch Womens Ment Health* 13(1): 41–44.

Austin, M.-P., N. Highet, et al. (2011). "Clinical practice guidelines for depression and related disorders – anxiety, bipolar disorder and puerperal psychosis – in the perinatal period." *A guideline for primary care health professionals*. Melbourne: beyondblue: the national depression initiative.

Austin, M. P., S. Kildea, et al. (2007). "Maternal mortality and psychiatric morbidity in the perinatal period: challenges and opportunities for prevention in the Australian setting." *Med J Aust* 186(7): 364–367.

Banti, S., M. Mauri, et al. (2011). "From the third month of pregnancy to 1 year postpartum. Prevalence, incidence, recurrence, and new onset of depression. Results from the perinatal depression-research & screening unit study." *Compr Psychiatry* 52(4): 343–351.

Barth, J., T. Munder, et al. (2013). "Comparative efficacy of seven psychotherapeutic interventions for patients with depression: a network meta-analysis." *PLoS Med* 10(5): e1001454.

Beck, C. T. (1998). "The effects of postpartum depression on child development: a meta-analysis." *Arch Psychiatr Nurs* 12(1): 12–20.

Beck, C. T. (2002). "Postpartum depression: a metasynthesis." *Qual Health Res* 12(4): 453–472.

Beck, C. T., R. K. Gable, et al. (2011). "Posttraumatic stress disorder in new mothers: results from a two-stage U.S. national survey." *Birth* 38(3): 216–227.

Beck, C. T. and S. Watson (2010). "Subsequent childbirth after a previous traumatic birth." *Nurs Res* 59(4): 241–249.

Belmaker, R. H. and G. Agam (2008). "Major depressive disorder." *N Engl J Med* 358(1): 55–68.

Bennett, H. A., A. Einarson, et al. (2004). "Prevalence of depression during pregnancy: systematic review." *Obstet Gynecol* 103(4): 698–709.

Bergink, V., S. A. Kushner, et al. (2011). "Prevalence of autoimmune thyroid dysfunction in postpartum psychosis." *Br J Psychiatry* 198(4): 264–268.

Beydoun, H. A., M. A. Beydoun, et al. (2012). "Intimate partner violence against adult women and its association with major depressive disorder, depressive symptoms and postpartum depression: a systematic review and meta-analysis." *Soc Sci Med* 75(6): 959–975.

Bilszta, J. L., D. Meyer, et al. (2010). "Bipolar affective disorder in the postnatal period: investigating the role of sleep." *Bipolar Disord* 12(5): 568–578.

Blackmore, E. R., D. R. Rubinow, et al. (2013). "Reproductive outcomes and risk of subsequent illness in women diagnosed with postpartum psychosis." *Bipolar Disord* 15(4): 394–404.

Bledsoe, S. E. and N. K. Grote (2006). "Treating depression during pregnancy and the postpartum: a preliminary meta-analysis." *Research on Social Work Practice* 16(2): 109–120.

Bodnar, L. M. and K. L. Wisner (2005). "Nutrition and depression: implications for improving mental health among childbearing-aged women." *Biol Psychiatry* 58(9): 679–685.

Boorman, R. J., G. J. Devilly, et al. (2013). "Childbirth and criteria for traumatic events." *Midwifery* 30(2): 255–261.

Borneskog, C., G. Sydsjo, et al. (2013). "Symptoms of anxiety and depression in lesbian couples treated with donated sperm: a descriptive study." *BJOG* 120(7): 839–846.

Buist, A., J. Bilszta, B. Barnett, J. Milgrom, J. Condon, and B. Hayes (2005). "Recognition and management of perinatal depression in general practice: results of an Australian National Survey." *Australian Family Physician* 34(9): 787–790.

Buist, A., N. Gotman, et al. (2011). "Generalized anxiety disorder: course and risk factors in pregnancy." *J Affect Disord* 131(1–3): 277–283.

Buist, A., B. Minto, et al. (2004). "Mother-baby psychiatric units in Australia-the Victorian experience." *Arch Womens Ment Health* 7(1): 81–87.

Bunevicius, R., L. Kusminskas, et al. (2009a). "Psychosocial risk factors for depression during pregnancy." *Acta Obstet Gynecol Scand* 88(5): 599–605.

Bunevicius, R., L. Kusminskas, et al. (2009b). "Depressive disorder and thyroid axis functioning during pregnancy." *World J Biol Psychiatry* 10(4): 324–329.

Byatt, N., T. A. Simas, et al. (2012). "Strategies for improving perinatal depression treatment in North American outpatient obstetric settings." *J Psychosom Obstet Gynaecol* 33(4): 143–161.

Chan, R. W., B. Raboy, et al. (1998). "Psychosocial adjustment among children conceived via donor insemination by lesbian and heterosexual mothers." *Child Dev* 69(2): 443–457.

Chaudron, L. H. and R. W. Pies (2003). "The relationship between postpartum psychosis and bipolar disorder: a review." *J Clin Psychiatry* 64(11): 1284–1292.

Chung, T. K., T. K. Lau, et al. (2001). "Antepartum depressive symptomatology is associated with adverse obstetric and neonatal outcomes." *Psychosom Med* 63(5): 830–834.

Clare, C. A. and J. Yeh (2012). "Postpartum depression in special populations: a review." *Obstet Gynecol Surv* 67(5): 313–323.

Coble, P. A., C. F. Reynolds, 3rd, et al. (1994). "Childbearing in women with and without a history of affective disorder. II. Electroencephalographic sleep." *Compr Psychiatry* 35(3): 215–224.

Cohen, L. S., L. L. Altshuler, et al. (2006). "Relapse of major depression during pregnancy in women who maintain or discontinue antidepressant treatment." *JAMA* 295(5): 499–507.

Collins, C. H., C. Zimmerman, et al. (2011). "Refugee, asylum seeker, immigrant women and postnatal depression: rates and risk factors." *Arch Womens Ment Health* 14(1): 3–11.

Cox, J. and J. Holden (2003). *Perinatal Mental Health: A Guide to the Edinburgh Postnatal Depression Scale*. London: RCPsych Publications.

Cox, J. L., J. M. Holden, et al. (1987). "Detection of postnatal depression. Development of the 10-item Edinburgh Postnatal Depression Scale." *Br J Psychiatry* 150: 782–786.

Dannon, P. N., I. Iancu, et al. (2006). "Recurrence of panic disorder during pregnancy: a 7-year naturalistic follow-up study." *Clin Neuropharmacol* 29(3): 132–137.

Davalos, D. B., C. A. Yadon, et al. (2012). "Untreated prenatal maternal depression and the potential risks to offspring: a review." *Arch Womens Ment Health* 15(1): 1–14.

de Rosnay, M., P. J. Cooper, et al. (2006). "Transmission of social anxiety from mother to infant: an experimental study using a social referencing paradigm." *Behav Res Ther* 44(8): 1165–1175.

Dennis, C. L. (2004). "Preventing postpartum depression part I: a review of biological interventions." *Can J Psychiatry* 49(7): 467–475.

Dennis, C. L., M. Coghlan, et al. (2013). "Can we identify mothers at-risk for postpartum anxiety in the immediate postpartum period using the State-Trait Anxiety Inventory?" *J Affect Disord* 150(3): 1217–1220.

Dennis, C. L. and T. Dowswell (2013). "Psychosocial and psychological interventions for preventing postpartum depression." *Cochrane Database Syst Rev* 2: CD001134.

Dennis, C. L. and E. Hodnett (2007). "Psychosocial and psychological interventions for treating postpartum depression." *Cochrane Database Syst Rev*(4): CD006116.

Dennis, C. L. and D. Kingston (2008). "A systematic review of telephone support for women during pregnancy and the early postpartum period." *J Obstet Gynecol Neonatal Nurs* 37(3): 301–314.

Dennis, C. L. and L. Ross (2006). "Women's perceptions of partner support and conflict in the development of postpartum depressive symptoms." *J Adv Nurs* 56(6): 588–599.

Dennis, C. L., L. E. Ross, et al. (2007). "Psychosocial and psychological interventions for treating antenatal depression." *Cochrane Database Syst Rev*(3): CD006309.

Di Florio, A., L. Forty, et al. (2013). "Perinatal episodes across the mood disorder spectrum." *JAMA Psychiatry* 70(2): 168–175.

Dietz, P. M., S. B. Williams, et al. (2007). "Clinically identified maternal depression before, during, and after pregnancies ending in live births." *Am J Psychiatry* 164(10): 1515–1520.

Dipietro, J. A. (2012). "Maternal stress in pregnancy: considerations for fetal development." *J Adolesc Health* 51(2 Suppl): S3–8.

Doornbos, B., D. A. Dijck-Brouwer, et al. (2009). "The development of peripartum depressive symptoms is associated with gene polymorphisms of MAOA, 5-HTT and COMT." *Prog Neuropsychopharmacol Biol Psychiatry* 33(7): 1250–1254.

Doornbos, B., D. Fekkes, et al. (2008). "Sequential serotonin and noradrenalin associated processes involved in postpartum blues." *Prog Neuropsychopharmacol Biol Psychiatry* 32(5): 1320–1325.

Doucet, S., N. Letourneau, et al. (2012). "Support needs of mothers who experience postpartum psychosis and their partners." *J Obstet Gynecol Neonatal Nurs* 41(2): 236–245.

Edge, D. (2007). "Ethnicity, psychosocial risk, and perinatal depression – a comparative study among inner city women in the UK." *Journal of Psychosomatic Research*, 63(3), 291–295. eScholarID:1d27626, doi:10.1016/j.jpsychores.2007.02.013.

Edhborg, M. (2008). "Comparisons of different instruments to measure blues and to predict depressive symptoms 2 months postpartum: a study of new mothers and fathers." *Scand J Caring Sci* 22(2): 186–195.

Engineer, N., L. Darwin, et al. (2013). "Association of glucocorticoid and type 1 corticotropin-releasing hormone receptors gene variants and risk for depression during pregnancy and post-partum." *J Psychiatr Res* 47(9): 1166–1173.

Engqvist, I. and K. Nilsson (2013). "Experiences of the first days of postpartum psychosis: an interview study with women and next of kin in Sweden." *Issues Ment Health Nurs* 34(2): 82–89.

Fernandez, J. W., J. A. Grizzell, et al. (2013). "The role of estrogen receptor beta and nicotinic cholinergic receptors in postpartum depression." *Prog Neuropsychopharmacol Biol Psychiatry* 40: 199–206.

Field, T., M. Diego, et al. (2003). "Pregnancy anxiety and comorbid depression and anger: effects on the fetus and neonate." *Depress Anxiety* 17(3): 140–151.

Figueiredo, B. and A. Conde (2011). "Anxiety and depression in women and men from early pregnancy to 3-months postpartum." *Arch Womens Ment Health* 14(3): 247–255.

Forray, A., M. Focseneanu, et al. (2010). "Onset and exacerbation of obsessive-compulsive disorder in pregnancy and the postpartum period." *J Clin Psychiatry* 71(8): 1061–1068.

Forty, L., L. Jones, et al. (2006). "Familiality of postpartum depression in unipolar disorder: results of a family study." *Am J Psychiatry* 163(9): 1549–1553.

Frey, B. N., W. Simpson, et al. (2012). "Sensitivity and specificity of the Mood Disorder Questionnaire as a screening tool for bipolar disorder during pregnancy and the postpartum period." *J Clin Psychiatry* 73(11): 1456–1461.

Ganjekar, S., G. Desai, et al. (2013). "A comparative study of psychopathology, symptom severity, and short-term outcome of postpartum and nonpostpartum mania." *Bipolar Disord* 15(6): 713–718.

Gavin, N. I., B. N. Gaynes, et al. (2005). "Perinatal depression: a systematic review of prevalence and incidence." *Obstet Gynecol* 106(5 Pt 1): 1071–1083.

Gaynes, B. N., N. Gavin, et al. (2005). "Perinatal depression: prevalence, screening accuracy, and screening outcomes." *Evid Rep Technol Assess (Summ)*(119): 1–8.

Glangeaud-Freudenthal, N. M., A. L. Sutter, et al. (2011). "Inpatient mother-and-child postpartum psychiatric care: factors associated with improvement in maternal mental health." *Eur Psychiatry* 26(4): 215–223.

Glasheen, C., G. A. Richardson, et al. (2010). "A systematic review of the effects of postnatal maternal anxiety on children." *Arch Womens Ment Health* 13(1): 61–74.

Glazer, M., W. Simpson, et al. (2013). *The use of the GAD-7 as a screening tool for Generalized Anxiety Disorder in pregnant and postpartum women.* San Francisco, CA: 166th Annual Meeting of the American Psychiatric Association.

Glover, V., T. G. O'Connor, et al. (2010). "Prenatal stress and the programming of the HPA axis." *Neurosci Biobehav Rev* 35(1): 17–22.

Goecke, T. W., F. Voigt, et al. (2012). "The association of prenatal attachment and perinatal factors with pre- and postpartum depression in first-time mothers." *Arch Gynecol Obstet* 286(2): 309–316.

Golombok, S., B. Perry, et al. (2003). "Children with lesbian parents: a community study." *Dev Psychol* 39(1): 20–33.

Gonzalez, A., J. M. Jenkins, et al. (2012). "Maternal early life experiences and parenting: the mediating role of cortisol and executive function." *J Am Acad Child Adolesc Psychiatry* 51(7): 673–682.

Gorman, L. L., M. W. O'Hara, et al. (2004). "Adaptation of the structured clinical interview for DSM-IV disorders for assessing depression in women during pregnancy and post-partum across countries and cultures." *Br J Psychiatry Suppl* 46: s17–23.

Goyal, D., C. Gay, et al. (2009). "Fragmented maternal sleep is more strongly correlated with depressive symptoms than infant temperament at three months postpartum." *Arch Womens Ment Health* 12(4): 229–237.

Grace, S. L., A. Evindar, et al. (2003). "The effect of postpartum depression on child cognitive development and behavior: a review and critical analysis of the literature." *Arch Womens Ment Health* 6(4): 263–274.

Gregoire, A. J., R. Kumar, et al. (1996). "Transdermal oestrogen for treatment of severe postnatal depression." *Lancet* 347(9006): 930–933.

Grigoriadis, S., D. de Camps Meschino, et al. (2011). "Mood and anxiety disorders in a sample of Canadian perinatal women referred for psychiatric care." *Arch Womens Ment Health* 14(4): 325–333.

Grigoriadis, S., E. H. VonderPorten, et al. (2013a). "The effect of prenatal antidepressant exposure on neonatal adaptation: a systematic review and meta-analysis." *J Clin Psychiatry* 74(4): e309–320.

Grigoriadis, S., E. H. VonderPorten, et al. (2013b). "Antidepressant exposure during pregnancy and congenital malformations: is there an association? A systematic review and meta-analysis of the best evidence." *J Clin Psychiatry* 74(4): e293–308.

Grigoriadis, S., E. H. VonderPorten, et al. (2013c). "The impact of maternal depression during pregnancy on perinatal outcomes: a systematic review and meta-analysis." *J Clin Psychiatry* 74(4): e321–341.

Guler, O., G. N. Koken, et al. (2008). "Course of panic disorder during the early postpartum period: a prospective analysis." *Compr Psychiatry* 49(1): 30–34.

Guler, O., F. K. Sahin, et al. (2008). "The prevalence of panic disorder in pregnant women during the third trimester of pregnancy." *Compr Psychiatry* 49(2): 154–158.

Halbreich, U. and S. Karkun (2006). "Cross-cultural and social diversity of prevalence of postpartum depression and depressive symptoms." *J Affect Disord* 91(2–3): 97–111.

Hall, E. and M. Steiner (2013). "Serotonin and female psychopathology." *Womens Health (Lond Engl)* 9(1): 85–97.

Healey, C., R. Morriss, et al. (2013). "Self-harm in postpartum depression and referrals to a perinatal mental health team: an audit study." *Arch Womens Ment Health* 16(3): 237–245.

Heron, J., N. Gilbert, et al. (2012). "Information and support needs during recovery from postpartum psychosis." *Arch Womens Ment Health* 15(3): 155–165.

Heron, J., M. McGuinness, et al. (2008). "Early postpartum symptoms in puerperal psychosis." *BJOG* 115(3): 348–353.

Hofmann, S. G., A. Asnaani, et al. (2012). "The efficacy of cognitive behavioral therapy: a review of meta-analyses." *Cognit Ther Res* 36(5): 427–440.

Howard, L. M., S. Oram, et al. (2013). "Domestic violence and perinatal mental disorders: a systematic review and meta-analysis." *PLoS Med* 10(5): e1001452.

Jones, I. and R. Cantwell (2010). "The classification of perinatal mood disorders—suggestions for DSMV and ICD11." *Arch Womens Ment Health* 13(1): 33–36.

Jones, N. A., T. Field, et al. (1998). "Newborns of mothers with depressive symptoms are physiologically less developed." *Infant Behav Dev* 21(3): 537–541.

Joy, C. B. and M. Saylan (2007). "Mother and baby units for schizophrenia." *Cochrane Database Syst Rev*(1): CD006333.

Kane, P. and J. Garber (2004). "The relations among depression in fathers, children's psychopathology, and father-child conflict: a meta-analysis." *Clin Psychol Rev* 24(3): 339–360.

Kaplan, B. J., G. F. Giesbrecht, et al. (2012). "The Alberta Pregnancy Outcomes and Nutrition (APrON) cohort study: rationale and methods." *Matern Child Nutr* [Epub ahead of print].

Karacan, I., R. L. Williams, et al. (1969). "Some implications of the sleep patterns of pregnancy for postpartum emotional disturbances." *Br J Psychiatry* 115(525): 929–935.

Khalafallah, A. A. and A. E. Dennis (2012). "Iron deficiency anaemia in pregnancy and postpartum: pathophysiology and effect of oral versus intravenous iron therapy." *J Pregnancy* 2012: 630519.

Kim, D. R., N. Epperson, et al. (2011). "An open label pilot study of transcranial magnetic stimulation for pregnant women with major depressive disorder." *J Womens Health (Larchmt)* 20(2): 255–261.

Kitamura, T., K. Yoshida, et al. (2006). "Multicentre prospective study of perinatal depression in Japan: incidence and correlates of antenatal and postnatal depression." *Arch Womens Ment Health* 9(3): 121–130.

Le Strat, Y., C. Dubertret, et al. (2011). "Prevalence and correlates of major depressive episode in pregnant and postpartum women in the United States." *J Affect Disord* 135(1–3): 128–138.

Leung, B. M. and B. J. Kaplan (2009). "Perinatal depression: prevalence, risks, and the nutrition link—a review of the literature." *J Am Diet Assoc* 109(9): 1566–1575.

Leung, B. M., B. J. Kaplan, et al. (2013). "Prenatal micronutrient supplementation and postpartum depressive symptoms in a pregnancy cohort." *BMC Pregnancy Childbirth* 13: 2.

Lilliecreutz, C., G. Sydsjo, et al. (2011). "Obstetric and perinatal outcomes among women with blood- and injection phobia during pregnancy." *J Affect Disord* 129(1–3): 289–295.

Maki, P., H. Hakko, et al. (2003). "Parental separation at birth and criminal behaviour in adulthood—a long-term follow-up of the Finnish Christmas Seal Home children." *Soc Psychiatry Psychiatr Epidemiol* 38(7): 354–359.

Martins, C. and E. A. Gaffan (2000). "Effects of early maternal depression on patterns of infant-mother attachment: a meta-analytic investigation." *J Child Psychol Psychiatry* 41(6): 737–746.

Matthey, S. (2008). "Using the Edinburgh Postnatal Depression Scale to screen for anxiety disorders." *Depress Anxiety* 25(11): 926–931.

Matthey, S., B. Barnett, et al. (2003). "Diagnosing postpartum depression in mothers and fathers: whatever happened to anxiety?" *J Affect Disord* 74(2): 139–147.

Meades, R. and S. Ayers (2011). "Anxiety measures validated in perinatal populations: a systematic review." *J Affect Disord* 133(1–2): 1–15.

Meltzer-Brody, S., A. Stuebe, et al. (2011). "Elevated corticotropin releasing hormone (CRH) during pregnancy and risk of postpartum depression (PPD)." *Journal of Clinical Endocrinology & Metabolism* 96(1): E40–47.

Meng, X. and C. D'Arcy (2012). "Common and unique risk factors and comorbidity for 12-month mood and anxiety disorders among Canadians." *Can J Psychiatry* 57(8): 479–487.

Metz, A., K. Stump, et al. (1983). "Changes in platelet alpha 2-adrenoceptor binding post partum: possible relation to maternity blues." *Lancet* 1(8323): 495–498.

Mileva-Seitz, V., A. S. Fleming, et al. (2012). "Dopamine receptors D1 and D2 are related to observed maternal behavior." *Genes Brain Behav* 11(6): 684–694.

Mileva-Seitz, V., J. Kennedy, et al. (2011). "Serotonin transporter allelic variation in mothers predicts maternal sensitivity, behavior and attitudes toward 6-month-old infants." *Genes Brain Behav* 10(3): 325–333.

Mileva-Seitz, V., M. Steiner, et al. (2013). "Interaction between Oxytocin Genotypes and Early Experience Predicts Quality of Mothering and Postpartum Mood." *PLoS One* 8(4): e61443.

Milgrom, J., G. D. Burrows, et al. (1998). "Psychiatric illness in women: a review of the function of a specialist mother-baby unit." *Aust N Z J Psychiatry* 32(5): 680–686.

Misri, S., X. Kostaras, et al. (2000). "The impact of partner support in the treatment of postpartum depression." *Can J Psychiatry* 45(6): 554–558.

Miszkurka, M., L. Goulet, et al. (2010). "Contributions of immigration to depressive symptoms among pregnant women in Canada." *Can J Public Health* 101(5): 358–364.

Morse, C. A., A. Buist, et al. (2000). "First-time parenthood: influences on pre- and postnatal adjustment in fathers and mothers." *J Psychosom Obstet Gynaecol* 21(2): 109–120.

Mota, N., B. J. Cox, et al. (2008). "The relationship between mental disorders, quality of life, and pregnancy: findings from a nationally representative sample." *J Affect Disord* 109(3): 300–304.

Mott, S. L., C. E. Schiller, et al. (2011). "Depression and anxiety among postpartum and adoptive mothers." *Arch Womens Ment Health* 14(4): 335–343.

Munk-Olsen, T., T. M. Laursen, et al. (2006). "New parents and mental disorders: a population-based register study." *JAMA* 296(21): 2582–2589. doi:10.1001/jama.296.21.2582.

Murgatroyd, C. A. and B. C. Nephew (2013). "Effects of early life social stress on maternal behavior and neuroendocrinology." *Psychoneuroendocrinology* 38(2): 219–228.

Murphy-Eberenz, K., P. P. Zandi, et al. (2006). "Is perinatal depression familial?" *J Affect Disord* 90(1): 49–55.

Murray, D. and J. L. Cox (1990). "Screening for depression during pregnancy with the Edinburgh Depression Scale (EPDS)." *Journal of Reproductive and Infant Psychology* 8: 99–107.

Murray, L., P. Cooper, et al. (2007). "The effects of maternal social phobia on mother-infant interactions and infant social responsiveness." *J Child Psychol Psychiatry* 48(1): 45–52.

Murray, L. and P. Cooper (1997). "Effects of postnatal depression on infant development." *Arch Dis Child* 77(2): 99–101.

Murray, L. and P. J. Copper, Eds. (1997). *Postpartum depression and child development.* New York: The Guilford Press.

Murray, L., M. Woolgar, et al. (2003). "Self-exclusion from health care in women at high risk for postpartum depression." *J Public Health Med* 25(2): 131–137.

Muzik, M., E. L. Bocknek, et al. (2013). "Mother-infant bonding impairment across the first 6 months postpartum: the primacy of psychopathology in women with childhood abuse and neglect histories." *Arch Womens Ment Health* 16(1): 29–38.

Nager, A., R. Szulkin, et al. (2013). "High lifelong relapse rate of psychiatric disorders among women with postpartum psychosis." *Nord J Psychiatry* 67(1): 53–58.

National Collaborating Centre for Mental Health (2007). *Antenatal and Postnatal Mental Health: The NICE Guideline on Clinical Management and Service Guidance.* Leicester (UK), British Psychological Society.

Navarro, P., L. Garcia-Esteve, et al. (2008). "Non-psychotic psychiatric disorders after childbirth: prevalence and comorbidity in a community sample." *J Affect Disord* 109(1–2): 171–176.

Newport, D. J., Z. N. Stowe, et al. (2002). "Parental depression: animal models of an adverse life event." *Am J Psychiatry* 159(8): 1265–1283.

O'Connor, T. G., J. Heron, et al. (2002). "Antenatal anxiety predicts child behavioral/emotional problems independently of postnatal depression." *J Am Acad Child Adolesc Psychiatry* 41(12): 1470–1477.

O'Hara, M. W. and J. E. McCabe (2013). "Postpartum depression: current status and future directions." *Annu Rev Clin Psychol* 9: 379–407.

O'Hara, M. W. and A. M. Swain (1996). "Rates and risk of postpartum depression-A meta-analysis." *International Review of Psychiatry* 8(1): 37–54.

O'Keane, V., S. Lightman, et al. (2011). "Changes in the maternal hypothalamic-pituitary-adrenal axis during the early puerperium may be related to the postpartum 'blues'." *Journal of Neuroendocrinology* 23(11): 1149–1155.

Oates, M. (2003). "Perinatal psychiatric disorders: a leading cause of maternal morbidity and mortality." *Br Med Bull* 67: 219–229.

Olde, E., O. van der Hart, et al. (2006). "Posttraumatic stress following childbirth: a review." *Clin Psychol Rev* 26(1): 1–16.

Pacheco, A. and B. Figueiredo (2012). "Mother's depression at childbirth does not contribute to the effects of antenatal depression on neonate's behavioral development." *Infant Behav Dev* 35(3): 513–522.

Palladino, C. L., V. Singh, et al. (2011). "Homicide and suicide during the perinatal period: findings from the National Violent Death Reporting System." *Obstet Gynecol* 118(5): 1056–1063.

Patterson, C. J. (2001). "Families of the lesbian baby boom: Maternal mental health and child adjustment." *Journal of Gay & Lesbian Psychotherapy* 4(3–4): 91–107.

Patterson, C. J. and L. V. Friel (2000). Sexual orientation and fertility. In *Infertility in the modern world: Biosocial perspectives*. G. Bentley and N. Mascie-Taylor (eds). Cambridge, Cambridge University Press: 238–260.

Paulson, J. F. and S. D. Bazemore (2010). "Prenatal and postpartum depression in fathers and its association with maternal depression: a meta-analysis." *JAMA* 303(19): 1961–1969.

Pedersen, C. A., J. L. Johnson, et al. (2007). "Antenatal thyroid correlates of postpartum depression." *Psychoneuroendocrinology* 32(3): 235–245.

Pinsonneault, J. K., D. Sullivan, et al. (2013). "Association study of the estrogen receptor gene ESR1 with post-partum depression – a pilot study." *Arch Womens Ment Health* [Epub ahead of print].

Reck, C., E. Stehle, et al. (2009). "Maternity blues as a predictor of DSM-IV depression and anxiety disorders in the first three months postpartum." *J Affect Disord* 113(1–2): 77–87.

Richards, E. M. and J. L. Payne (2013). "The management of mood disorders in pregnancy: alternatives to antidepressants." *CNS Spectr*: 1–11.

Robertson, E., S. Grace, et al. (2004). "Antenatal risk factors for postpartum depression: a synthesis of recent literature." *Gen Hosp Psychiatry* 26(4): 289–295.

Robertson, E., I. Jones, et al. (2005). "Risk of puerperal and non-puerperal recurrence of illness following bipolar affective puerperal (post-partum) psychosis." *Br J Psychiatry* 186: 258–259.

Ross, L. E. (2005). "Perinatal mental health in lesbian mothers: a review of potential risk and protective factors." *Women Health* 41(3): 113–128.

Ross, L. E., S. Grigoriadis, et al. (2013). "Selected pregnancy and delivery outcomes after exposure to antidepressant medication: a systematic review and meta-analysis." *JAMA Psychiatry* 70(4): 436–443.

Ross, L. E. and L. M. McLean (2006). "Anxiety disorders during pregnancy and the postpartum period: A systematic review." *J Clin Psychiatry* 67(8): 1285–1298.

Ross, L. E., B. J. Murray, et al. (2005). "Sleep and perinatal mood disorders: a critical review." *J Psychiatry Neurosci* 30(4): 247–256.

Ross, L. E., E. M. Sellers, et al. (2004). "Mood changes during pregnancy and the postpartum period: development of a biopsychosocial model." *Acta Psychiatr Scand* 109(6): 457–466.

Ross, L. E., L. Steele, et al. (2007). "Perinatal depressive symptomatology among lesbian and bisexual women." *Arch Womens Ment Health* 10(2): 53–59.

Rubertsson, C., U. Waldenström, et al. (2003). "Depressive mood in early pregnancy: Prevalence and women at risk in a national Swedish sample" *Journal of Reproductive and Infant Psychology* 21(2): 113–123.

Russell, E. J., J. M. Fawcett, et al. (2013). "Risk of obsessive-compulsive disorder in pregnant and postpartum women: a meta-analysis." *J Clin Psychiatry* 74(4): 377–385.

Russell, J. A., A. J. Douglas, et al. (2001). "Brain preparations for maternity—adaptive changes in behavioral and neuroendocrine systems during pregnancy and lactation. An overview." *Prog Brain Res* 133: 1–38.

Sacher, J., A. A. Wilson, et al. (2010). "Elevated brain monoamine oxidase A binding in the early postpartum period." *Arch Gen Psychiatry* 67(5): 468–474.

Salmon, M., K. Abel, et al. (2003). "Clinical and parenting skills outcomes following joint mother-baby psychiatric admission." *Aust N Z J Psychiatry* 37(5): 556–562.

Sanjuan, J., R. Martin-Santos, et al. (2008). "Mood changes after delivery: role of the serotonin transporter gene." *Br J Psychiatry* 193(5): 383–388.

Sasson, Y., J. Zohar, et al. (1997). "Epidemiology of obsessive-compulsive disorder: a world view." *J Clin Psychiatry* 58 Suppl 12: 7–10.

Schiller, C. E., M. W. O'Hara, et al. (2013). "Estradiol modulates anhedonia and behavioral despair in rats and negative affect in a subgroup of women at high risk for postpartum depression." *Physiology & Behavior* 119: 137–144.

Schmied, V., M. Johnson, et al. (2013). "Maternal mental health in Australia and New Zealand: A review of longitudinal studies." *Women Birth* 26(3): 167–178.

Senecky, Y., H. Agassi, et al. (2009). "Post-adoption depression among adoptive mothers." *J Affect Disord* 115(1–2): 62–68.

Sharma, V. and D. Mazmanian (2003). "Sleep loss and postpartum psychosis." *Bipolar Disord* 5(2): 98–105.

Sharma, V., A. Smith, et al. (2004). "The relationship between duration of labour, time of delivery, and puerperal psychosis." *J Affect Disord* 83(2–3): 215–220.

Sichel, D. A., L. S. Cohen, et al. (1995). "Prophylactic estrogen in recurrent postpartum affective disorder." *Biol Psychiatry* 38(12): 814–818.

Skrundz, M., M. Bolten, et al. (2011). "Plasma oxytocin concentration during pregnancy is associated with development of postpartum depression." *Neuropsychopharmacology* 36(9): 1886–1893.

Soderquist, J., B. Wijma, et al. (2009). "Risk factors in pregnancy for post-traumatic stress and depression after childbirth." *BJOG* 116(5): 672–680.

Speisman, B. B., E. A. Storch, et al. (2011). "Postpartum obsessive-compulsive disorder." *J Obstet Gynecol Neonatal Nurs* 40(6): 680–690.

Spinelli, M. G. (2004). "Maternal infanticide associated with mental illness: prevention and the promise of saved lives." *Am J Psychiatry* 161(9): 1548–1557.

Spitzer, R. L., K. Kroenke, et al. (2006). "A brief measure for assessing generalized anxiety disorder: the GAD-7." *Arch Intern Med* 166(10): 1092–1097.

Steiner, M., E. Dunn, et al. (2003). "Hormones and mood: from menarche to menopause and beyond." *J Affect Disord* 74(1): 67–83.

Stuebe, A. M., K. Grewen, et al. (2013). "Association between maternal mood and oxytocin response to breastfeeding." *J Womens Health (Larchmt)* 22(4): 352–361.

Treloar, S. A., N. G. Martin, et al. (1999). "Genetic influences on post-natal depressive symptoms: findings from an Australian twin sample." *Psychol Med* 29(3): 645–654.

Uguz, F., C. Akman, et al. (2007). "Postpartum-onset obsessive-compulsive disorder: incidence, clinical features, and related factors." *J Clin Psychiatry* 68(1): 132–138.

Uguz, F., K. Gezginc, et al. (2007). "Obsessive-compulsive disorder in pregnant women during the third trimester of pregnancy." *Compr Psychiatry* 48(5): 441–445.

Vesga-Lopez, O., C. Blanco, et al. (2008). "Psychiatric disorders in pregnant and postpartum women in the United States." *Arch Gen Psychiatry* 65(7): 805–815.

Vigod, S. N., L. Villegas, et al. (2010). "Prevalence and risk factors for postpartum depression among women with preterm and low-birth-weight infants: a systematic review." *BJOG* 117(5): 540–550.

Viguera, A. C., L. Tondo, et al. (2011). "Episodes of mood disorders in 2,252 pregnancies and postpartum periods." *Am J Psychiatry* 168(11): 1179–1185.

Viguera, A. C., T. Whitfield, et al. (2007). "Risk of recurrence in women with bipolar disorder during pregnancy: prospective study of mood stabilizer discontinuation." *Am J Psychiatry* 164(12): 1817–1824; quiz 1923.

Vythilingum, B. (2010). "Should childbirth be considered a stressor sufficient to meet the criteria for PTSD?" *Arch Womens Ment Health* 13(1): 49–50.

Wadhwa, P. D., C. A. Sandman, et al. (2001). "The neurobiology of stress in human pregnancy: implications for prematurity and development of the fetal central nervous system." *Prog Brain Res* 133: 131–142.

Watanabe, M., K. Wada, et al. (2008). "Maternity blues as predictor of postpartum depression: a prospective cohort study among Japanese women." *J Psychosom Obstet Gynaecol* 29(3): 206–212.

Weinberg, M. K. and E. Z. Tronick (1998). "The impact of maternal psychiatric illness on infant development." *J Clin Psychiatry* 59(Suppl 2): 53–61.

Weisberg, R. B. and J. A. Paquette (2002). "Screening and treatment of anxiety disorders in pregnant and lactating women." *Womens Health Issues* 12(1): 32–36.

Weissman, M. M., D. J. Pilowsky, et al. (2006). "Remissions in maternal depression and child psychopathology: a STAR*D-child report." *JAMA* 295(12): 1389–1398.

Wisner, K. L., E. L. Moses-Kolko, et al. (2010). "Postpartum depression: a disorder in search of a definition." *Arch Womens Ment Health* 13(1): 37–40.

Wisner, K. L., D. K. Sit, et al. (2013). "Onset timing, thoughts of self-harm, and diagnoses in postpartum women with screen-positive depression findings." *JAMA Psychiatry* 70(5): 490–498.

Yawn, B. P., A. L. Olson, et al. (2012). "Postpartum depression: screening, diagnosis, and management programs 2000 through 2010." *Depress Res Treat* 2012: 363964.

Yonkers, K. A., S. Vigod, et al. (2011). "Diagnosis, pathophysiology, and management of mood disorders in pregnant and postpartum women." *Obstet Gynecol* 117(4): 961–977.

Yozwiak, J. A. (2010). "Postpartum depression and adolescent mothers: a review of assessment and treatment approaches." *J Pediatr Adolesc Gynecol* 23(3): 172–178.

Zambaldi, C. F., A. Cantilino, et al. (2009). "Postpartum obsessive-compulsive disorder: prevalence and clinical characteristics." *Compr Psychiatry* 50(6): 503–509.

Zhang, X., K. Liu, et al. (2010). "Safety and feasibility of repetitive transcranial magnetic stimulation (rTMS) as a treatment for major depression during pregnancy." *Arch Womens Ment Health* 13(4): 369–370.

Zimmerman, M. and J. N. Galione (2011). "Screening for bipolar disorder with the Mood Disorders Questionnaire: a review." *Harv Rev Psychiatry* 19(5): 219–228.

Pharmacological treatment of mental health problems in pregnancy and lactation

Angelika Wieck and Margareta Reis

Introduction

At least one in ten women is affected by mental ill health during pregnancy or the postpartum period (see Chapter 10). In most mild to moderate cases, nonpharmacological interventions will be appropriate. In women with more severe illness, however, psychotropic medication is often the mainstay of management. The focus of this chapter is the reproductive safety of the main psychotropic medications used in psychiatric disorders and how this can be applied to the management of women across childbearing.

A drug may harm a fetus early on in organogenesis, when major structural anomalies could occur, or later in pregnancy, when functional problems or suboptimal obstetric outcomes can result. Although advances have recently been made in this area, most evidence is very limited. Rigorous enquiry cannot include randomized controlled trials in pregnant or lactating women as they are not considered ethical. The next best approach is prospective cohort studies that include control groups and data collection before the studied outcome occurs. This reduces selection and recall bias, but cannot avoid "confounding by indication." A confounder is a factor that is associated independently with both the exposure (to the medication) and the outcome (e.g., malformation). Confounding by indication implies that because women treated with antipsychotic medication are unwell, any adverse effects in their children may be associated with the illness for which the medication is prescribed rather than the medication itself.

Pregnancy registers with a prospective design have been established, particularly for antiepileptic drugs, and have begun to publish results. However, there are problems with the small size of these datasets and the bias in their sampling. If a study is set up to test whether an agent taken in the first trimester of pregnancy increases the risk of major congenital malformations two-fold above a similarly sized control group where the expected incidence is, say, 2%, then approximately 900 cases need to be included in both groups (Dellicour et al., 2008). More relevant for clinical practice is whether the risk of specific congenital malformations that have a major impact on the survival or functioning of the child is increased. If the background rate of such a condition is very small, 0.1%, for example, as it is for persistent pulmonary hypertension, and a study aims to test a clinically meaningful five-fold increase, then the required sample size is about 2,300 in each group (Dellicour et al., 2008). Existing pregnancy registers are beginning to approach such numbers, but usually only for groups of drugs, rather than individual agents, which may well differ in their potential for reproductive toxicity. Larger sample sizes can be achieved by epidemiological cohort and case-control studies, but the advantages of these may be offset in some population cohorts by uncertainty about timing and duration of exposure to the offending agent, as well as the accuracy of diagnosis and clinical significance of malformations. One example of a large pregnancy register prospectively collecting data about drug use in early pregnancy is the Swedish Medical Birth Register. The register has been covering around 98% of all pregnancies since 1995, including 1,764,458 deliveries to date. At the first antenatal care appointment the woman is questioned about any drug use since she became pregnant, hence recall bias is avoided.

Other challenges in this research are confounding factors for infant and pregnancy outcomes. Although suboptimal pregnancy and developmental outcomes in offspring of mothers with mental illness have been

Comprehensive Women's Mental Health, ed. David J. Castle and Kathryn M. Abel. Published by Cambridge University Press. © Cambridge University Press 2016.

reported, it is not yet clear how much of this effect can be attributed to psychiatric disorders themselves, that is, confounding by indication. A host of other parameters can also act as confounders, including psychiatric comorbidities, physical illnesses, concomitant medication, smoking, maternal age, maternal obesity and low socioeconomic status. In women with mental illness, several of these characteristics are often present.

In this chapter, we discuss the challenges of the research in this complex area and consider classes of psychotropic drugs and individual agents to which mothers and their offspring are exposed. We not only review the literature on safety and potential adverse effects but also discuss implications for clinical practice.

Pharmacokinetics in pregnancy

Pharmacokinetics is the science describing what "the body does with the drug," that is, how the drug is absorbed, distributed and eliminated from the body. Pharmacokinetic data from studies in men or non-pregnant women cannot necessarily be extrapolated to pregnant women. The continuous physiological changes throughout pregnancy, particularly during the second and third trimester, alter pharmacokinetic properties for many drugs. Some examples of pregnancy-induced changes are slowed gastric emptying, increased volume of distribution, changes in hepatic clearance and decreases in $\alpha1$-glycoprotein, which results in a higher proportion of the unbound, biologically active fraction of a drug. Furthermore, the activity of hepatic drug metabolizing enzymes changes during pregnancy. For example, the activity of cytochrome P4502D6 is increased and of P4502C19 decreased (see review by Hodge and Tracy, 2007). The renal elimination of drugs also changes across childbearing with rises from early pregnancy to a peak by the end of the second trimester up to 150% above baseline. In some women, decreases begin to occur in the third trimester and others only in the first few weeks postpartum. Little is as yet known about the net effect of these changes on the concentration of free and total parent compounds and their biologically active metabolites in human pregnancy.

Transfer of drugs to the fetus occurs mainly via diffusion across the placenta, favoring movement of smaller, lipophilic agents, such as psychotropic drugs. The rate-limiting step of this process is placental blood flow. Both the fetal liver and the placenta can metabolize drugs: Immature phase I and II metabolism can occur

in the fetus at 8 weeks post conception. Metabolic enzyme activity, however, is low and 50% of the fetal circulation from the umbilical vein bypasses the fetal liver to the cardiac and cerebral circulation. Elimination from the fetus is by diffusion back to the maternal compartment. As most drug metabolites are polar, this favors accumulation of metabolites in the fetus.

Psychotropic drugs and breastfeeding

The amount of maternal drug present in the blood circulation of a breastfed infant is the result of complex interactions that could be regarded among the most challenging in pharmacology. Factors involved include maternal pharmacokinetics, the molecular size, lipophilicity and protein binding of the drug; the fat content of the milk; volume and frequency of feeding; the fate of the drug in the infant's gut; the absorption rate; the maturity of the infant's liver; and the infants volume of distribution. The concentration of psychotropic drugs and their metabolites in infants' serum has seldom been measured, but where it is has, it has often fallen below the limit of detection of the estimation method used.

Overall, available studies of drug transfer into milk suggest that, compared with pregnancy, much smaller amounts of most psychotropic drugs are ingested by the offspring during breastfeeding although there are significant differences between drugs. One standardized measure of exposure that is frequently used in pediatric practice is the relative infant dose. This is defined as the daily amount of drug ingested by the infant during exclusive breastfeeding per kg bodyweight divided by the maternal daily dose per kg body weight. A value of more than 10% is regarded as indicating a higher probability of side effects in the infant (Bennett, 1996). Research into the potential behavioral and physical effects of psychotropic drugs to which infants are exposed to during breastfeeding is scarce and suffers from perhaps the most methodological problems in the field of reproductive psychopharmacology. Observations of infants involve isolated cases or case series and have not usually used standardized assessment tools or timing relative to drug exposure or control groups. Long-term effects have not been investigated.

Antidepressant drugs

Antidepressant drugs (ADs) are prescribed not only for unipolar depression, but also for a number of other psychiatric conditions, such as anxiety disorders, post-traumatic stress disorders, obsessive-compulsive disorder and bipolar depression. It has been estimated that up to 3% of women in Europe and 13% of women in the United States use antidepressant drugs during pregnancy. The choice of antidepressant is similar to that in other psychiatric patients; selective serotonin re-uptake inhibitors (SSRIs) are the most commonly prescribed. In a recent UK study, prescription rates decreased from 4.7% in the 3 months to conception to 2.8%, 1.3% and 1.3% in the first, second and third trimester and increased again to 5.5% in the first 3 months postpartum (Margulis et al., 2014). A large proportion of women (79.6%) discontinued ADs at some stage in pregnancy whereas only 0.4% of those who had not taken them before pregnancy commenced them in the third trimester.

Pharmacokinetics of antidepressants in pregnancy

The net result of pregnancy-induced pharmacokinetic changes on the pharmacokinetics of AD varies greatly among pregnant women, with some but not all experiencing faster AD metabolism in late pregnancy (for review see Deligiannidis et al., 2014). The lack of systematic studies of the relationship between drug levels and clinical response in pregnancy does not allow for any firm conclusions to be drawn for clinical practice.

All antidepressants readily cross the placenta, but to differing degrees. Existing studies of maternal serum and umbilical cord serum concentrations of SSRIs and their metabolites consist of descriptions of cases or case series with a tendency of fetal:maternal ratios at delivery being the lowest for sertraline and at the higher end for citalopram. Little is known about differences among tricyclic (TCAs) and other drugs.

The reproductive safety of antidepressant drugs in early pregnancy

An abundance of literature exists on the use of antidepressants during pregnancy, notably of SSRIs as the most commonly used drugs. A review of the literature on the association between antidepressant use and any infant congenital malformations and neonatal morbidity was recently published (Källén et al., 2013). The recently published analysis by Grigoriadis et al.

(2013) found no association between exposure to SRRIs and other antidepressants and overall congenital anomalies or major congenital anomalies, but a small increase in the risk of cardiovascular malformations with an odds ratio of 1.40 (CI 1.10-1.77). A small effect was found specifically for paroxetine (RR = 1.43; CI 1.08-1.88). The meta-analysis of Myles et al. (2013) looked at four SSRIs individually. Fluoxetine and paroxetine were associated with an increased risk of major malformations (ORs of 1.14, CI 1.01-1.30 and 1.29, CI 1.11-1.49) and paroxetine was associated with a small excess of cardiovascular anomalies (1.44, CI 1.12-1.86). In contrast, sertraline and citalopram were not linked with any teratogenic potential.

Although TCAs were introduced in the 1950s, comparatively little has been published on these agents and sample sizes have been too small to test reliably for an increase in congenital malformation rate above the general population rate. One notable signal, however, comes from two large Swedish epidemiological studies which have linked clomipramine use with a small increase in the risk for cardiovascular defects (Källén and Otterblad Olausson, 2006; Reis and Källén, 2010).

The use of antidepressants in late pregnancy

Many studies have shown an increased risk for infant morbidity after antidepressant exposure during the latter part of pregnancy. Delivery results in a neonatal antidepressant withdrawal syndrome that is fairly common, occurring in about 30% of exposed neonates compared to only about 10% of nonexposed children (Kieviet et al., 2013) which represents a three-fold increase over unexposed newborns (Moses-Kolko et al., 2005). The syndrome includes feeding difficulties, irritability, abnormal crying, jitteriness and cerebral excitation. Respiratory distress and tremors are also more common (Grigoriadis et al., 2013). In general, the neonatal effects are transient; most symptoms develop within 48 hours after birth and last for 2–6 days (Kieviet et al., 2013).

An increased risk for low Apgar score, hypoglycemia, prematurity and low birth weight (but not small for gestational age) has been reported (e.g., Källén et al., 2013). In a recent meta-analysis of published studies on the effects of antidepressant use in pregnancy on the preterm birth rate, Huybrechts et al. (2014) found an increased odds ratio (adjusted OR 1.53, CI 1.40 – 1.66), which was still significant when a diagnosis of depression was taken into account. The effect was significant if the exposure occurred in the second and third trimester but not in the first. Huang et al. (2014) confirmed in their meta-analysis an effect on preterm birth but also found evidence for lower birth weight.

Persistent hypertension of the newborn (PPHN) is a rare but potentially fatal complication, with a population incidence of 1–2 cases per 1000 live births (Walsh-Sukys et al., 2000). Several studies have suggested an increased risk for PPHN after maternal use of SSRIs late in pregnancy. Grigoriadis et al. (2014) conducted a meta-analysis and confirmed an effect of late pregnancy exposure, which was still significant after moderator variables were taken into account. Although the odds ratio was 2.50 (CI 1.32 to 4.73), the risk is still small for any given pregnancy considering the base rate. So far TCAs and other antidepressants have not been related to PPHN.

Some other pregnancy complications and maternal delivery diagnoses have been reported to occur more frequently after treatment with SSRIs, TCAs and other antidepressants. Examples are an increased risk for preeclampsia, hyperemesis and intrapartum bleeding, which was seen in a large Swedish sample (Reis and Källén, 2010). Palmsten et al. (2013) found a significant risk increase of postpartum hemorrhage. Moreover, an association between the use of SSRI and an increased risk of gestational hypertension and preeclampsia has been described (Toh et al., 2009). In women using antidepressants, however, factors that predispose to these conditions, such as higher maternal age, smoking, higher body mass index and the use of other drugs (Reis and Källén, 2010) are also more commonly present, suggesting that further research on these outcomes is required.

Neurodevelopment in children with intrauterine exposure to antidepressants

Nulman et al. (2012) conducted a small prospective study of children between 1.5 and 6 years old who were exposed to TCAs, SSRIs, venlafaxine or untreated maternal depression during fetal development. An unexposed control group of children with healthy mothers was included. An effect of antidepressant drug exposure on the children's cognitive development or behavior was not found. Rather, the authors emphasized that untreated depression during pregnancy was associated with a high risk for postpartum depression.

Further, fetal and childhood exposure to maternal depression was a predictor of child behavioral problems and long-term child psychopathology.

A concern was recently raised about the effects of intrauterine SSRI exposure on the social development of offspring. Of five epidemiological and case control studies, three found a significantly increased rate of autism spectrum disorder or autistic traits with odds ratios ranging between 1.9 and 3.3 (Croen et al., 2011; Rai et al., 2013; El Marroun et al., 2014). However, two studies did not find an association when the maternal mood disorder was controlled for (Sørensen et al., 2013; Clements et al., 2014). Interestingly, in one of these studies (Clements et al., 2014) exposed children had the same rate as their unexposed siblings, suggesting that there is a genetic link between maternal depression and autism spectrum disorders and that antidepressant therapy is not causally related. Further family genetic studies are needed to clarify this important question.

Antidepressants and breastfeeding

Most antidepressants are excreted in low concentrations in breast milk (Hale, 2012). Paroxetine and sertraline produce low relative infant doses in the 0.5 to 3% range, while fluoxetine, venlafaxine, and citalopram produce milk levels closer to, and sometimes even above, the 10% limit (Chad et al., 2013). In a pooled analysis of 57 studies, Weissman et al. (2004) found usually undetectable plasma levels for nortriptyline, paroxetine and sertraline during lactation in more than 200 infants tested, whereas fluoxetine, citalopram and the metabolite of venlafaxine, O-desmethylvenlafaxine, produced measurable but low levels in some infants.

Case reports and case series have reported some adverse events in infants who ingested antidepressants via breastmilk. These studies observed nonspecific symptoms such as irritability, decreased feeding and sleep problems, which were more often reported during exposure to citalopram and fluoxetine (see review by Weissman et al., 2004). However, the observations were uncontrolled and unstandardized and definitive conclusions about differences between drugs and how they affect breastfed children cannot be drawn.

Antipsychotic drugs

Consistent with pharmacoepidemiological studies in other psychiatric patient groups, two studies from the

United States and UK have shown an increase in recent years in the prescribing of atypical antipsychotics to pregnant women, whilst the use of typical antipsychotics has remained the same or decreased (Toh et al., 2013; Petersen et al., 2014). The rate of prescribing was 8/1000 any time during pregnancy in the United States, and 3/1000 any time from 6 weeks post conception in the UK (Toh et al., 2013; Petersen et al., 2014). In the UK study, prescriptions for antipsychotic medications were often discontinued or no longer claimed by pregnant patients. Only 38% of atypical and 19% of typical antipsychotics were still prescribed in the third trimester (Petersen et al., 2014).

Pharmacokinetics of antipsychotics in pregnancy

In a first study of serial plasma level estimations of antipsychotics, Windhager et al. (2014) found large decreases in three women taking aripiprazole during pregnancy, followed by an increase in levels in the early postpartum period. Clear deteriorations in mental state were not seen. No other systematic data are available on how antipsychotic drug levels may change during pregnancy and whether this would affect the course of illness.

When measuring the transplacental passage of several antipsychotic drugs at birth, Newport et al. (2007) found the highest fetal-to-maternal serum concentration ratio for olanzapine, followed by haloperidol, risperidone and quetiapine. Whether differences in placental transfer translate into differences in infant outcome is currently unknown.

Congenital anomalies associated with first trimester exposure to antipsychotics

When considering potential teratogenicity, the challenges in existing datasets outlined earlier mean that most antipsychotic drugs have not been studied as individual agents but within groups. In a meta-analysis of (predominantly) prospective cohort studies, first-trimester use of phenothiazines was associated with a small but significant excess of congenital anomalies in infants exposed to phenothiazines as a group (odds ratio: 1.21, 95% CI 1.01–1.45), but there was no association with a specific anomaly or a specific agent (Altshuler et al., 1996). In the population study by Reis and Källen (2008), there was a nonsignificant trend

for an association of antipsychotic drugs (mostly first generation, but second generation agents were included as well) with an excess of anomalies (odds ratio 1.45, CI 0.99-1.41). The authors noted that the excess seemed to be due to cardiovascular anomalies, and in particular ventricular and atrial septum defects. In a prospective cohort study of women contacting a teratology information service (Habermann et al., 2013) only second generation antipsychotics were associated with an increased risk of congenital malformations (OR 3.21, CI 1.34-7.67) and again there seemed to be an excess of septal defects which mostly occurred as isolated anomalies. In these three studies, limited adjustments were made for confounding factors, which are known to be associated independently with cardiovascular anomalies and which are more prevalent in women who suffer from psychosis. No conclusions can be drawn in respect of individual antipsychotic agents as data are too limited (Barnes et al., 2011).

The literature indicates therefore that antipsychotic therapy is associated with a small increase in the risk of cardiovascular (mainly septal) defects. However, it is at present uncertain whether this is a causal relationship and how clinically significant these findings are, or whether there are differences among antipsychotics.

Other pregnancy outcomes

Obesity and diabetes mellitus are two side effects of antipsychotic medication that are particularly important in the context of childbearing since they are independently associated with adverse pregnancy and infant outcomes (Aberg et al., 2001; Sebire et al., 2001; Owens et al., 2010). There are differences among antipsychotic drugs in their propensity to cause weight gain and increases in blood glucose levels, with olanzapine and clozapine having the greatest impact (Rummel-Kluge et al., 2010).

The rate of diabetes increases from the second trimester onwards and antipsychotic medication may amplify this effect. In two population studies from Sweden (Reis and Källen, 2008; Bodén et al., 2012a), antipsychotic therapy was indeed associated with a significant, almost two-fold, increase of gestational diabetes. Bodén et al. (2012a) also controlled for confounding factors, and when they took early pregnancy BMI into account, the odds ratios for gestational diabetes were slightly attenuated and no longer significant. Gestational exposure was based on pharmacy claims data in this study and the duration and precise timing in pregnancy was not reported. Despite this, it is noteworthy that the two epidemiological studies found similar odds ratios.

There is evidence that antipsychotic therapy is associated with an increased rate of preterm birth (Reis and Källén, 2008) with more support for an effect of first-generation agents than second-generation agents (Diav-Citrin et al., 2005; Bodén et al., 2012a; Lin et al., 2010; Newham et al., 2008). Whether severe mental illness itself contributes to early delivery is unclear (Bodén et al. 2012a; Lin et al., 2010). Studies of the effect of antipsychotic drugs on infant birth weight, length and head circumference have resulted in conflicting findings. Although most of these studies controlled for other factors that influence birth weight, the inconsistent results may be due to differences in their relative balance, the diagnostic profile and other population characteristics. In two epidemiological studies, there was no increased risk of stillbirth following the use of antipsychotics in pregnancy (Reis and Källén, 2008; Bodén et al., 2012b).

Neonatal effects

Motor or withdrawal symptoms have been described in neonates following late pregnancy exposure to antipsychotic medication in case reports, retrospective case series and small prospective observational studies (American College of Obstetricians and Gynecologists, 2008; Gentile, 2010; Gilad et al., 2011). In a search of their spontaneous Adverse Event Reporting System Database the US Food and Drug Administration (2011) reported that, up to 2008, 69 cases of neonatal extrapyramidal or withdrawal symptoms after late pregnancy antipsychotic exposure had been identified. Some neonates recovered within hours or days without specific treatment, while others required intensive care unit support and prolonged hospitalization. In the majority of cases, there were confounding factors, including concomitant use of other drugs known to be associated with withdrawal symptoms, prematurity, congenital malformations and obstetric and perinatal complications. However, there were some cases where these symptoms were associated with antipsychotic medication alone. Habermann et al. (2013) found an increased risk of discontinuation symptoms in their prospectively followed

cohort of exposed and control children, but whether the result remained significant after accounting for concomitant medication was not reported.

Because of these concerns, the Federal Drug Administration in the United States added information about neonatal effects to the pregnancy risk labeling for all antipsychotic drugs in 2011. In the UK, the Medicines and Health Care Products Regulatory Agency (2011) also issued advice to healthcare professionals to examine neonates for discontinuation symptoms.

Neurodevelopmental effects

Data on neurodevelopmental effects of antipsychotics are sparse. In a prospective study of 2,141 children exposed to phenothiazines in the first 4 lunar months of pregnancy and 26,217 unexposed children, there were no differences in IQ in children with heavy, intermediate and no intrauterine exposure (Slone et al., 1977). Many of these mothers were mentally well and took phenothiazines for nausea. A different result was found in a recent prospective study. Johnson et al. (2012) examined the effects of psychotropic exposure in pregnancy on neuromotor performance in 6-month-old infants. All mothers had a psychiatric history with predominantly affective disorders but they differed in medication status in pregnancy. Infants prenatally exposed to first or second generation antipsychotic drugs demonstrated significantly lower scores compared with both antidepressant-exposed infants and infants with no psychotropic exposure. Results were also significantly associated with variables relating to maternal psychiatric history, including depression, psychosis and overall severity or chronicity. However, the study sample was very small and the majority of women taking antipsychotics during pregnancy were also co-prescribed antidepressants, anxiolytics or hypnotics. In a well-designed, prospective study of 76 infants whose mothers had taken first or second generation antipsychotics in pregnancy and 76 unexposed children of mothers without severe mental illness, the Bayley's neurodevelopment scores indicated delay in several domains in the early postnatal months in the exposed children (Peng et al., 2013). However, these differences resolved by the end of the first year, indicating that any potential adverse effects were only temporary.

These studies suggest that there are no long-term neurodevelopmental disadvantages arising from antipsychotic exposure in pregnancy. However, the database remains small and further prospective investigations of monotherapy exposure with larger samples, longer follow up and measures of potential confounders (e.g., maternal physical and mental health, socioeconomic status, social environment) are needed.

Antipsychotic drugs and breastfeeding

Based on the best available published evidence, Hale (2012) summarized relative infant doses for several frequently used antipsychotics. The small case numbers to date suggest relative infant doses of much less than 10% except for amisulpride, haloperidol, sulpiride and risperidone, where doses can approach or exceed 10% (Hale, 2012; Teoh et al., 2011). In published clinical observations of breastfed infants, relatively few adverse effects have been reported (Gentile, 2008; Dayan et al., 2011) although definite conclusions cannot be drawn because of the small numbers of infants observed and a lack of standardized assessments. Dev and Krupp (1995) reported agranulocytosis in one breastfed infant whose mother took clozapine.

Antiepileptic mood stabilizers

The antiepileptic mood stabilizers valproate, carbamazepine and lamotrigine are used for the treatment of bipolar disorder in acute phases of illness and in maintenance therapy. Over the last two decades, there has been a large decline in the UK in the use of carbamazepine and sodium valproate in pregnant women; lamotrigine is now the most commonly prescribed antiepileptic in this patient group with 0.25% of pregnancies affected (Man et al., 2012). Similar trends have been reported for other countries (Man et al., 2012). Little data exist about prescribing of antiepileptic mood stabilizers specifically to pregnant women with psychiatric disorders, but it is of concern that a nationally representative survey in the United States recently reported no decline in the recent prescribing of valproate to women of childbearing age with nonepileptic conditions (Adedinsewo et al., 2013).

Pharmacokinetics of antiepileptic medication in pregnancy

As pregnancy progress, the serum concentrations of total and free lamotrigine decline markedly. This may be because of pregnancy-induced alterations in the activity of glucuronosyl transferases or renal function. The extent is highly variable with values of 248% being reported (Pennell et al., 2008; Tomson et al., 2013). The return to the nonpregnant baseline occurs within the first month postpartum. In a prospective study of pregnant women with epilepsy on lamotrigine monotherapy, seizure control significantly decreased when serum lamotrigine concentrations had fallen by more than 35% from their optimal serum concentration before pregnancy (Pennell et al., 2008). In a case series of bipolar patients, Clark et al. (2013) found that several women required dose increases of lamotrigine in pregnancy. However, the threshold at which deterioration in mental state becomes likely has not been explored.

The changes in total and unbound carbamazepine levels seem to be small in pregnancy (Tomson et al., 2013). Little reliable data are as yet available in respect of the pharmacokinetics of valproate that could inform clinical practice (Tomson et al., 2013).

The extent to which total valproate is transferred from the maternal to the fetal circulation is high, whereas the concentration of biologically active free fraction is lower in the fetal than the maternal circulation with a ratios between 0.5 and 0.8 (see review by Wieck, 2011). A reverse relationship exists for carbamazepine where the ratio for the free fraction is higher and ranges between 1.0 and 1.4 (for review see Wieck, 2011). About 90% of total lamotrigine is transferred to the fetus (for review see Wieck, 2011).

Major congenital anomalies after pregnancy exposure to antiepileptic drugs

It has been known for several decades that maternal use of valproate is associated with congenital anomalies. In their systematic review and meta-analysis of cohort and pregnancy register studies, Meador et al. (2008) found an anomaly rate for monotherapy with valproate in the first trimester of 10.7% which was much higher than among the offspring of healthy control mothers (3.3%). Among specific anomalies, significant differences were found for spina bifida with a particularly high odds ratio (12.7), atrial septal defects, cleft palate, hypospadias, polydactyly and craniosynostosis (Jentink et al., 2010a). A relationship of the teratogenic effect with daily dose has been widely described although the critical threshold has varied between daily doses of 600–1500 mg (Tomson and Battino, 2012).

Carbamazepine and lamotrigine have consistently been shown to be less teratogenic than valproate, and in the study by Meador et al. (2008) they were associated with congenital malformation rates similar to those of children of healthy mothers. However, carbamazepine has been implicated in an increased risk of spina bifida (Matalon et al., 2002; Jentink et al., 2010b) with an odds ratio of 2.6 compared to no antiepileptic exposure (Jentink et al., 2010b). An earlier finding of an increased rate of oral clefts following pregnancy exposure to lamotrigine has not been substantiated by subsequent studies (Tomson and Battino, 2012).

The general population incidence of neural tube defects and several other congenital anomalies can be markedly reduced by folic acid use from preconception to early pregnancy. However, clinical guidelines are misleading if they recommend high-dose folic acid (4–5 mg daily) to women taking antiepileptic drugs since there is little evidence that this will prevent their teratogenic effect (Wlodarczyk et al., 2012).

Other pregnancy outcomes

In a population-based cohort study, Bech et al. (2014) found an increased risk of spontaneous abortion in women filling prescriptions for high, but not low doses of antiepileptic drugs irrespective of diagnosis and even after adjusting for measured confounders. In a Swedish population study, valproate exposure was associated with preterm birth and increased neonatal morbidity in the form of respiratory problems, hypoglycemia and central nervous system symptoms (Källén et al., 2013).

Neurodevelopmental effects

Meador et al. (2013) followed children who were exposed to valproate in pregnancy until age 6 and found that their cognitive abilities were reduced across a range of domains in a dose-dependent fashion. They also found that these children were at a greater risk of being diagnosed with attention deficit hyperactivity disorder (Cohen et al., 2013).

Furthermore, a recent population study from Denmark (Christensen et al., 2013) added to earlier findings that valproate can also cause deficits in social development. Children with fetal exposure to valproate were at greater risk of autism spectrum disorder

(absolute risk 4.42%; adjusted hazard ratio: 2.9; CI 1.7-4.9) and childhood autism (absolute risk 2.50%, adjusted hazard ratio: 5.2; CI 2.7-10.0).

Like congenital malformations, the adverse effects of valproic acid on cognitive development have been related to dose, with an increased risk being documented only with doses above 800–1000 mg/day (Adab et al., 2004; Meador et al., 2013).

Because of mounting evidence for widespread harm to offspring, the European Medicines Agency (2014) has recently recommended that valproate is not used to treat epilepsy, bipolar disorder or migraine in girls and women who are pregnant or who can become pregnant unless other treatments are ineffective or not tolerated. Should valproate be the only option, the woman should use effective contraception and a physician experienced in treating these conditions should commence and supervise treatment (European Medicines Agency, 2014). The guidelines of the National Institute of Health and Care Excellence on antenatal and postnatal mental health (NICE, 2014) for England and Wales go even further. They state that no woman of childbearing potential with a mood disorder should be treated with valproate, irrespective of their contraceptive status. This recommendation has arisen from clinical audit data from several perinatal services in the UK, that prescribers of valproate have, despite earlier warnings by NICE (2007), given little consideration to the issue of childbearing in their patients.

Breastfeeding and antiepileptic drugs

The ratios of breastmilk:maternal serum concentrations are low for valproate, and measured plasma levels in infants ingesting this drug via breast milk have been reported to be less than 2.3% of maternal serum levels (reviewed by Wieck, 2011). No adverse effects have been reported in any reported breastfed infants except for one case of thrombocytopenic purpura and anemia. However, women with childbearing potential (and that includes breastfeeding women) should not be offered valproate (NICE, 2014), unless there are exceptional circumstances as discussed earlier.

The concentration of carbamazepine in breast milk compared to maternal serum is higher than for valproate, ranging between 10 and 30% of the maternal serum concentration (see Wieck, 2011 for review). Pharmacological concentrations of carbamazepine are sometimes found in breastfed infants (Tomson, 2005). Exposure during pregnancy and breastfeeding was associated with cholestatic hepatitis in three infants (Frey et al., 2002), consistent with the occurrence of this side effect in adults.

Newport et al. (2008) also reported high total lamotrigine serum levels in infants exposed via breast-milk with an average of 18.3% of the maternal value whereas the infant/maternal ratio for the free fraction was as high as 30.9%. Similar mean values (concentration fraction in neonatal versus maternal plasma of 0.23–0.50) were found in a smaller study of mother-infant pairs in the early postnatal period (Ohman et al., 2000). Despite this, in neither study did infants show adverse events (Ohman et al., 2000; Newport et al., 2008) except for mild and asymptomatic thrombocytosis (Newport et al., 2008).

Lithium
Pharmacokinetics in pregnancy

The increased glomerular filtration rate in pregnancy means that lithium serum levels tend to become lower as pregnancy progresses (Schou et al., 1973) and dosing requires adjustments. During, or soon after delivery, the glomerular filtration rate decreases and lithium levels become difficult to predict. Particular caution needs to be exercised during this period and in particular if there is a risk of sodium depletion since this can lead to intoxication of the mother and neonate (Schou et al., 1973). Lithium readily equilibrates across the placenta with similar concentrations being reported in fetal and maternal serum at birth (Newport et al., 2005). Whether more than once daily dosing offers greater protection to the fetus is currently unknown.

Reproductive safety of lithium

Concerns about the teratogenic effects of lithium arose from the "lithium baby register" that was established in Denmark, Canada and the United States following reports of reproductive toxicity in preclinical studies. Its report on 225 infants exposed to lithium in utero suggested a high risk of cardiovascular anomalies (18/225, 8%) compared to the general population incidence of less than 1%. In particular, the severe Ebstein anomaly that occurs rarely in the general population (about 1:20,000) was extraordinarily overrepresented with 6 of the 225 cases affected

(2.3%). Selection bias was a major problem in this study and subsequent cohort and case-control studies have shown that the magnitude of the risks was over-estimated in the lithium register (McKnight et al., 2012; Diav-Citrin et al., 2014). Current evidence suggests that there is a small increase in the risk of cardiac malformations after first trimester exposure (Diav-Citrin et al., 2014; NICE, 2014), but sample numbers are still small and further studies are needed. McKnight et al. (2012) did not specifically find an increased risk of the Ebstein anomaly in their meta-analysis but point out that the finding is unstable because of the low number of events.

There have been no systematic studies of the physical health in neonates exposed in pregnancy to lithium but cases have been reported who suffered from a variety of problems (including cardiac arrhythmias, hypoglycemia, diabetes insipidus, polyhydramnios, thyroid dysfunction, goiter, floppiness, lethargy, hepatic anomalies and respiratory difficulties; American College of Obstetricians and Gynecologists, 2008). There is one five-year prospective study of 60 children who showed no excess of physical or mental anomalies compared to their siblings (Schou et al., 1976).

Breastfeeding and lithium

Lithium easily enters breast milk and case reports have indicated that the amount of lithium an infant is ingesting via breast milk results in lithium serum levels that are between 10 and 56% of the maternal value (Lact med, 2014). Several instances of infant health problems were described in these reports, including suspected lithium intoxication, abnormal thyroid function tests, slow weight gain and delay in motor development (Lact med, 2014). In some cases, it was difficult to establish whether these problems were the result of the lithium in breast milk.

Anxiolytic and hypnotic drugs

Countries vary in how commonly anxiolytic and hypnotic drugs are prescribed in pregnancy, ranging from very few cases in the United States to a rate of 3% in France (Bellantuono et al., 2013). This may reflect both concerns about the dependency potential for mother and child but also the increased risk of orofacial clefts that was reported in case control studies of first trimester exposure to benzodiazepines (BZDs) in the 1970s. However, this has not been confirmed in a recent meta-analysis (Enato et al., 2011) or a UK population-based cohort study (Ban et al., 2014), which found no evidence for teratogenicity.

Hypnotic benzodiazepine receptor agonists, which include zopiclone, zaleplon and zolpidem, have been studied less extensively. In a Swedish population study by Wikner and Källén (2011), there was no evidence for overall teratogencity. A statistically significant increased risk for intestinal malformations other than atresias/stenosis was based on only four infants. Ban et al. (2014) found in their recent meta-analysis no evidence for teratogenicity after first trimester exposure to zopiclone.

The second generation antiepileptic drug, pregabalin, is increasingly used in psychiatry for the treatment of generalized anxiety disorder. There are no studies of its reproductive safety aspects in humans as yet. Teratogenic effects in mice at suprapharmacological doses have been reported in one study (Etemad et al, 2013). The use of this drug is therefore not recommended during pregnancy or during breastfeeding pending further studies.

Maternal use of benzodiazepines during late pregnancy has been associated with neonatal morbidity, including withdrawal symptoms and the so-called "floppy baby" syndrome. An increased risk for preterm birth and low birth weight was found in singleton infants exposed to benzodiazepines or HBRA during late pregnancy and also an increased rate of infants with a low Apgar score, also among term infants. An increased risk for respiratory problems was also seen (for review see Källén et al., 2013). Furthermore, an increased risk for neonatal morbidity with the combination of SSRIs and all types of sedatives/hypnotics has been shown but this may reflect a confounding by indication (Källén and Reis, 2012).

Anxiolytic and hypnotic drugs during breastfeeding

There is evidence that benzodiazepines are excreted into breast milk with a maternal weight adjusted dose above 10% (Hale, 2012). Hence, there is a risk for an accumulation of drug in the suckling infant if the ingestion by the mother is on a continuous basis. On the other hand, occasional use of therapeutic doses is unlikely to affect the baby. Hypnotic benzodiazepine receptor agonists are excreted to a much lower degree than benzodiazepines (Hale, 2012) at

< 3% of the maternal weight adjusted dose and breastfeeding is not contraindicated.

Conclusions

Weighing up the benefits and risks of continuing or stopping medication in pregnancy and the choice of medications poses difficult challenges. Since half of all pregnancies are unplanned, clinicians should discuss family planning and the fetal effects of psychotropic medication, but also the effect of childbearing on mental illness in women with recurrent or chronic mental illnesses. It is essential that the woman is involved in making decisions as an equal partner and that she and her carer/partner are given correct and adequate information. The first step in making this decision is to establish whether medication can be stopped or whether the likelihood of a recurrence in pregnancy and the postpartum period is too high and has serious consequences for the mother and her family. This requires a careful analysis of the woman's past course of illness, her personal history and social circumstances and what level of risk is acceptable to her and others around her. A high degree of clinical skill and expertise, but also sufficient consultation time is needed and, if available, a referral to a specialist in perinatal psychiatry should be considered.

If it is decided to continue medication in pregnancy, the choice of drug should be guided by the principle of avoiding drugs with higher risks of teratogenicity. Because of its widespread fetal toxicity, valproate should not be prescribed to women with psychiatric disorders who could become pregnant. On account of the potential severity of neural tube defects and the relative lack of evidence for its efficacy in bipolar disorder, carbamazepine should also not be offered to women who could conceive or are pregnant. If mood stabilizing medication is needed, mood stabilizing antipsychotics can be considered as an alternative. Lithium should also not be offered to women who are planning a pregnancy or are pregnant, unless no other medication is likely to be effective (NICE, 2014).

Differences in reproductive safety profiles among antidepressant and antipsychotic drugs are often uncertain and small in size and should not be the only consideration in selecting medication. At least equally important is how effective a medication is for the particular woman's mental illness, how she has responded to other medications in the past and what her experience of side effects has been. Often this process narrows the choice of medication to a few agents that can be further considered.

Pregnancy-induced changes of the pharmacokinetics of lithium require close monitoring in pregnancy, in particular the last month of gestation and intrapartum to avoid underdosing, but also maternal and infant toxicity. Detailed guidelines are provided by NICE (2014). Research is needed for all other psychotropic drugs, which may identify individuals at particular genetic risk of low serum concentrations and lack of efficacy in pregnancy. In clinical practice, practitioners often reduce the dose of medication on learning of pregnancy in the belief that this may reduce harm to the fetus. This approach may lower drug levels further and is likely to lead to loss of efficacy and at the same time expose the fetus unnecessarily. When lamotrigine is prescribed to a pregnant woman, her mental state should be monitored closely combined with lamotrigine serum estimations in each trimester. Thus, potential loss of efficacy due to falling serum concentrations can be avoided. Our understanding of psychotropic metabolism across childbearing is in its infancy and future research may show that other agents also require therapeutic drug monitoring (Hiemke et al., 2011).

The benefits of breastfeeding are well documented. Women are strongly encouraged to breastfeed exclusively for the first six months after childbirth (World Health Organization, 2003; American Academy of Pediatrics, 2012). With a few exceptions, which include clozapine, lithium and carbamazepine, women taking psychotropic medication in therapeutic doses should be allowed to breastfeed but asked to monitor their babies for sedation or other side effects that may occur in adults. Little is as yet known about the safety of breastfeeding when the mother takes several psychotropic drugs and decisions have to be made on an individual basis. When discussing psychotropic medication with women who are breastfeeding, they should be informed that the exposure to the child is much smaller than during pregnancy, but that there are still uncertainties about potential adverse effects.

A large number of new compounds are currently in development in an attempt to improve our treatment of severe mental illness. These include, for example, new compounds of existing drug classes with a dopamine and/or 5HT receptor profile but also representatives of new drug classes, such as oxytocin, glutamate, glycine and phosphodiesterase-10 for the treatment of schizophrenia and ketamine as an adjunct treatment in the context of severe resistant for depression (Aids Profile Summary, 2014). Research of the reproductive safety of new psychotropic compounds has been haphazard and undirected up to date, usually following the pattern of initial case reports, then case series and finally, in the best case scenario, the establishment of pregnancy registers or large pharmaco-epidemiological studies. It has taken two decades for a more consistent picture to emerge about the reproductive safety of some SSRI antidepressants, and antipsychotic pregnancy registers have only recently been set up. To the benefit of the patient and clinician, it is important that in future, as soon as a drug is licensed, an independent prospective pregnancy register is set up that records the outcome of pregnancies that were inadvertently exposed. This may require health regulatory policy.

In the treatment of a woman of childbearing potential or in pregnancy who has a severe or enduring mental illness, clinicians and women should be aware that one treatment does not necessarily fit all women with the same diagnosis, nor are there any risk-free options. A good treatment plan is one that has been arrived at jointly by the patient and her mental health team and takes into account – apart from the reproductive safety of considered medications – the woman's individual illness history, perceptions and experiences, and optimizes pharmacological, psychological, physical and social interventions in a holistic approach.

References

Aberg, A., Westbom, L., Källén, B. (2001). Congenital malformations among infants whose mothers had gestational diabetes or preexisting diabetes. *Early Human Development*, 61, 85–95.

Adab, N., Kini, U., Vinten, J., et al. (2004). The longer term outcome of children born to mothers with epilepsy. *J Neurol Neurosurg Psychiatry*, 75, 1575–1583.

Adedinsewo, D. A., Thurman, D. J., Luo, Y. H., et al. (2013). Valproate prescriptions for nonepilepsy disorders in reproductive-age women. *Birth Defects Research Part A: Clinical and Molecular Teratology*, 97, 403–408.

Aids Profile Summary. (2014). *Pharm Med*, 28, 265–271.

Altshuler, L. L., Cohen, L., Szuba, M. P., et al. (1996). Pharmacologic management of psychiatric illness during pregnancy: dilemmas and guidelines. *American Journal of Psychiatry*, 153, 592–606.

American Academy of Pediatrics (2012). Breastfeeding and the use of human milk. *Pediatrics*, 129, e827–e841.

American College of Obstetricians and Gynecologists. (2008). ACOG Practice Bulletin: clinical management guidelines for obstetrician-gynecologists number 92, April 2008. Use of psychiatric medications during pregnancy and lactation. *Obstetetrics and Gynecology*, 111, 1001–1020.

Ban, L., West, J., Gibson, J. E., et al. (2014). First trimester exposure to anxiolytic and hypnotic drugs and the risks of major congenital anomalies: a United Kingdom population-based cohort study. *PLoS One*, 9(6), e100996. doi: 10.1371/journal.pone.0100996. eCollection 2014.

Barnes, T. R. (2011). Schizophrenia Consensus Group of British Association for Psychopharmacology. Evidence-based guidelines for the pharmacological treatment of schizophrenia: recommendations from the British Association for Psychopharmacology. *J Psychopharmacol*, 25, 567–620.

Bech, B. H., Kjaersgaard, M. I., Pedersen, H. S., et al. (2014). Use of antiepileptic drugs during pregnancy and risk of spontaneous abortion and stillbirth: population based cohort study. *BMJ*, 349, g5159. doi: 10.1136/bmj.g5159.

Bennett, P. N. (1996). Use of monographs in drugs. In: Bennett, P. N. (Ed.), *Drugs and Human Lactation* (pp. 67–74). Amsterdam: Elsevier Science Publishers.

Bodén, R., Lundgren, M., Brandt, L., et al. (2012a). Risks of adverse pregnancy and birth outcomes in women treated or not treated with mood stabilisers for bipolar disorder: population based cohort study. *BMJ*, 345, e7085. doi: 10.1136/bmj.e7085.

Bodén, R., Lundgren, M., Brandt, L., et al. (2012b). Antipsychotics during pregnancy: relation to fetal and maternal metabolic effects. *Arch Gen Psychiatry*, 69: 715–721.

Bellantuono, C., Tofani, S., Di Sciascio, G., Santone, G. (2013). Benzodiazepine exposure in pregnancy and risk of major malformations: a critical overview. *Gen Hosp Psychiatry*, 35, 3–8.

Chad, L., Pupco, A., Bozzo, P., Koren, G. (2013). Update on antidepressant use during breastfeeding. *Can Fam Physician*, 59, 633–634.

Clark, E. C., Klein, A. M., Perel, J. M., et al. (2013). Lamotrigine dosing for pregnant patients with bipolar disorder. *Am J Psychiatry*, 170, 1240–1247.

Christensen, J., Grønborg, T. K., Sørensen, M. J., et al. (2013). Prenatal valproate exposure and risk of autism spectrum disorders and childhood autism. *JAMA*, 309, 1696–1703.

Clements, C. C., Castro, V. M., Blumenthal, S. R., et al. (2014). Prenatal antidepressant exposure is associated with risk for attention-deficit hyperactivity disorder but not autism spectrum disorder in a large health system. *Mol Psychiatry*, Aug 26, doi: 10.1038/mp.2014.90. [Epub ahead of print]

Cohen, M. J., Meador, K. J., Browning, N., et al. (2013). Fetal antiepileptic drug exposure: Adaptive and emotional/behavioral functioning at age 6 years. *Epilepsy Behav*, 29, 308–315.

Croen, L. A., Grether, J. K., Yoshida, C. K., et al. (2011). Antidepressant use during pregnancy and childhood autism spectrum disorders. *Arch Gen Psychiatry*, 68, 1104–1112.

Dayan, J., Graignic-Philippe, R., Seligmann, C., Andro, G. (2011). Use of antipsychotics and breastfeeding. *Current Women's Health Reviews*, 7, 37–45.

Deligiannidis, K. M., Byatt, N., Freeman, M. P. (2014). Pharmacotherapy for mood disorders in pregnancy: a review of pharmacokinetic changes and clinical recommendations for therapeutic drug monitoring. *J Clin Psychopharmacol*, 34, 244–255.

Dellicour, S., ter Kuile, F. O., Stergachis, A.(2008). Pregnancy exposure registries for assessing antimalarial drug safety in pregnancy in malaria-endemic countries. *PLoS Med*, 5(9):e187. doi: 10.1371/journal.pmed.0050187. Epub Sep 2008.

Dev, V. J., Krupp, P. (1995) Adverse event profile and safety of clozapine. *Rev Contemp Pharmacother*, 6, 197–208.

Diav-Citrin, O., Shechtman, S., Ornoy, S., et al. (2005). Safety of haloperidol and penfluridol in pregnancy: a multicenter, prospective, controlled study. *J Clin Psychiatry*, 66, 317–322.

Diav-Citrin, O., Shechtman, S., Tahover, E., et al. (2014). Pregnancy outcome following in utero exposure to lithium: a prospective, comparative, observational study. *Am J Psychiatry*, 171, 785–794.

El Marroun, H., White, T. J., van der Knaap, N. J., et al. (2014). Prenatal exposure to selective serotonin reuptake inhibitors and social responsiveness symptoms of autism: population-based study of young children. *Br J Psychiatry*, 205, 95–102.

Enato, E., Moretti, M., Koren, G. (2011). The fetal safety of benzodiazepines: an updated meta-analysis. *J Obstet Gynaecol Can*, 33, 46–48.

Etemad, L., Mohammad, A., Mohammadpour, A. H. et al. (2013) Teratogenic effects of pregabalin in mice. *Iran J Basic Med Sci*, 16, 1065–1070.

European Medicines Agency, Pharmacovigilance and Risk

Assessment Committee (2014). PRAC recommends strengthening the restrictions on the use of valproate in women and girls. www.ema.europa.eu/ema/index.jsp?curl=pages/news_and_events/news/2014/10/news_detail_002186.jsp&mid=WC0b01ac058004d5c1

Frey, B., Braegger, C. P., Ghelfi, D. (2002).Neonatal cholestatic hepatitis from carbamazepine exposure during pregnancy and breast feeding. *Ann Pharmacother*, 36, 644–647.

Gentile, S. (2008). Infant safety with antipsychotic therapy in breast-feeding: a systematic review. *J Clin Psychiatry*, 69, 666–673.

Gentile, S. (2010). Antipsychotic therapy during early and late pregnancy. A systematic review. *Schizophr Bull*, 36, 518–544.

Gilad, O., Merlob, P., Stahl, B., Klinger, G. (2011). Outcome of infants exposed to olanzapine during breastfeeding. *Breastfeed Med*, 6, 55–58.

Grigoriadis, S., VonderPorten, E. H., Mamisashvili, L., et al. (2013). Antidepressant exposure during pregnancy and congenital malformations: is there an association? A systematic review and meta-analysis of the best evidence. *J Clin Psychiatry*, 74(4), e293-308. doi: 10.4088/JCP.12r07966.

Grigoriadis, S., Vonderporten, E. H., Mamisashvili, L., et al. (2014). Prenatal exposure to antidepressants and persistent pulmonary hypertension of the newborn: systematic review and meta-analysis. *BMJ*, 348, f6932. doi: 10.1136/bmj.f6932.

Habermann, F., Fritzsche, J., Fuhlbrück, F., et al. (2013). Atypical antipsychotic drugs and pregnancy outcome: a prospective, cohort study. *J Clin Psychopharmacol*, 33, 453–462.

Hale, T. (2012). *Medications and mother's milk*. Amarillo: Hale Publishing.

Hiemke, C., Baumann, P., Bergemann, N. et al. (2011). AGNP Consensus Guidelines for Therapeutic Drug Monitoring in Psychiatry: Update 2011.

Hodge, L. S. and Tracy, T. S. (2007). Alterations in drug disposition during pregnancy: implications for drug therapy. *Expert Opin Drug Metab Toxicol*, 2007, 3, 557–571.

Huang, H., Coleman, S., Bridge, J. A., et al. (2014). A meta-analysis of the relationship between antidepressant use in pregnancy and the risk of preterm birth and low birth weight. *Gen Hosp Psychiatry*, 36, 13–8.

Huybrechts, K. F., Sanghani, R. S., Avorn, J., Urato, A. C.(2014). Preterm birth and antidepressant medication use during pregnancy: a systematic review and meta-analysis. *PLoS One*, 9(3):e92778. doi: 10.1371/journal.pone.0092778. eCollection 2014.

Jentink, J., Loane, M. A., Dolk, H., et al. (2010a). Valproic acid monotherapy in pregnancy and major congenital malformations. *N Engl J Med*, 362, 2185–2193.

Jentink, J., Dolk, H., Loane, M. A., et al. (2010b). Intrauterine exposure to carbamazepine and specific congenital malformations: systematic review and case-control study. *BMJ*, 341:c6581. doi: 10.1136/bmj.c6581.

Johnson, K. C., LaPrairie, J. L., Brennan, P. A., et al. (2012). Prenatal antipsychotic exposure and neuromotor performance during infancy. *Arch Gen Psychiatry*, 69, 787–794.

Källén, B., Borg, N. and Reis, M. (2013). The use of central nervous system active drugs during pregnancy. *Pharmaceuticals (Basel)*, 6, 1221–1286.

Källén, B. and Otterblad Olausson, P. (2006). Antidepressant drugs during pregnancy and infant congenital heart defect. *Reprod Toxicol*, 21, 221–222.

Källén, B. and Reis, M. (2012). Neonatal complications after

maternal concomitant use of SSRI and other central nervous system active drugs during the second or third trimester of pregnancy. *J Clin Psychopharmacol*, 32, 608–614.

Kieviet, N., Dolman, K. M., and Honig, A. (2013). The use of psychotropic medication during pregnancy: how about the newborn? *Neuropsychiatr Dis Treat*, 9, 1257–1266.

Lact med, accessed October 19, 2014; http://toxnet.nlm.nih.gov/cgi-bin/sis/search2

Lin, H. C., Chen, I. J., Chen, Y. H., et al. (2010). Maternal schizophrenia and pregnancy outcome: does the use of antipsychotics make a difference? *Schizophr Res*, 116, 55–60.

Man, S. L., Petersen, I., Thompson, M., Nazareth, I. (2012). Antiepileptic drugs during pregnancy in primary care: a UK population based study. *PLoS One*, 7(12):e52339. doi: 10.1371/journal.pone.0052339. Epub Dec 18, 2012.

Margulis, A. V., Kang, E. M., Hammad, T. A. (2014). Patterns of prescription of antidepressants and antipsychotics across and within pregnancies in a population-based UK cohort. *Matern Child Health J*, 18, 1742–1752.

Matalon, S., Schechtman, S., Goldzweig, G., Ornoy, A. (2002). The teratogenic effect of carbamazepine: a meta-analysis of 1255 exposures. *Reprod Toxicol*, 16, 9–17.

McKnight, R. F., Adida, M., Budge, K., et al. (2012). Lithium toxicity profile: a systematic review and meta-analysis. *Lancet*, 379, 721–728.

Meador, K., Reynolds, M. W., Crean, S., et al. (2008). Pregnancy outcomes in women with epilepsy: a systematic review and meta-analysis of published pregnancy registries and cohorts. *Epilepsy*, 81, 1–13.

Meador, K. J., Baker, G. A., Browning, N., et al. (2013). Fetal antiepileptic drug exposure and cognitive outcomes at age 6 years (NEAD study): a prospective observational study. *Lancet Neurol*, 12, 244–252.

Medicines and Health Care Products Regulatory Agency. (2011). Drug Safety Update, Sept 2011, vol. 5, issue 2: A2. www.mhra.gov.uk/home/groups/dsu/documents/publication/con129002.pdf

Moses-Kolko, E. L., Bogen, D., Perel, J., et al. (2005). Neonatal signs after late in utero exposure to serotonin reuptake inhibitors: literature review and implications for clinical applications. *JAMA*, 293, 2372–2383.

Myles, N., Newall, H., Ward, H., Large, M. (2013). Systematic meta-analysis of individual selective serotonin reuptake inhibitor medications and congenital malformations. *Aust NZ J Psychiatry*, 47, 1002–1012.

National Institute for Care and Health Excellence (2014). Antenatal and postnatal mental health – Clinical management and service guidance. Full guideline. NICE clinical guideline 192.

Newham. J. J., Thomas, S. H., MacRitchie, K., et al. (2008). Birth weight of infants after maternal exposure to typical and atypical antipsychotics: prospective comparison study. *Br J Psychiatry*, 192, 333–337.

Newport, D. J., Calamaras, M. R., DeVane, C. L., et al. (2007). Atypical antipsychotic administration during late pregnancy: placental passage and obstetrical outcomes. *Am J Psychiatry*, 164, 1214–1220.

Newport, D. J., Viguera, A. C., Beach, A. J., et al. (2005). Lithium placental passage and obstetrical outcome: implications for clinical management during late pregnancy. *Am J Psychiatry*, 162, 2162–2170.

Newport, D. J., Pennell, P. B., Calamaras, B. S., et al (2008). Lamotrigine in breast milk and nursing infants: determination of exposure. *Pediatrics*, 122, e223–e231.

Nulman, I., Koren, G., Rovet, J., et al. (2012). Neurodevelopment of children following prenatal exposure to venlafaxine, selective serotonin reuptake inhibitors, or untreated maternal depression. *Am J Psychiatry*, 169, 1165–1174.

Ohman, I., Vitols, S., Tomson, T. (2000). Lamotrigine in pregnancy: pharmacokinetics during delivery, in the neonate, and during lactation. *Epilepsia*, 41, 709–713.

Owens, L. A., O'Sullivan, E. P., Kirwan, B., et al. (2010). ATLANTIC DIP: the impact of obesity on pregnancy outcome in glucose-tolerant women. *Diabetes Care*, 33, 577–579.

Palmsten, K., Hernández-Díaz, S., Huybrechts, K. F., et al. (2013). Use of antidepressants near delivery and risk of postpartum hemorrhage: cohort study of low income women in the United States. *BMJ*, 347, f4877. doi: 10.1136/bmj.f4877.

Peng, M., Gao, K., Ding, Y., et al. (2013). Effects of prenatal exposure to atypical antipsychotics on postnatal development and growth of infants: a case-controlled, prospective study. *Psychopharmacology (Berl)*, 228, 577–584.

Pennell, P. B., Peng, L., Newport, D. J., et al. (2008). Lamotrigine in pregnancy: clearance, therapeutic drug monitoring, and seizure frequency. *Neurology*, 70, 2130–2136.

Perucca, E., Battino, D., Tomson, T. (2014). Gender issues in antiepileptic drug treatment. *Neurobiol Dis*, 72 Pt B, 217–223.

Petersen, I., McCrea, R. L., Osborn, D. J., et al. (2014). Discontinuation of antipsychotic medication in pregnancy: A cohort study. *Schizophr Res*, 159, 218–225.

Rai, D., Lee, B. K., Dalman, C., et al. (2013). Parental depression, maternal antidepressant use during pregnancy, and risk of autism spectrum disorders: population based case-control study. *BMJ*, 346, f2059. doi: 10.1136/bmj.f2059.

Reis, M. and Källén, B. (2008). Maternal use of antipsychotics in early pregnancy and delivery outcome. *J Clin Psychopharmacol*, 28, 279–288.

Reis, M. and Källén, B. (2010). Delivery outcome after maternal use of antidepressant drugs in pregnancy: an update using Swedish data. *Psychol Med*, 40, 1723–1733.

Rummel-Kluge, C., Komossa, K., Schwarz, S., et al. (2010). Head-to-head comparisons of metabolic side effects of second generation antipsychotics in the treatment of schizophrenia: a systematic review and meta-analysis. *Schizophr Res*, 123, 225–233.

Schou, M. (1976). What happened later to the lithium babies? A follow-up study of children born without malformations. *Acta Psychiatr Scand*, 54, 193–197.

Schou, M., Amdisen, A., Steenstrup, O. R. (1973). Lithium and pregnancy. II. Hazards to women given lithium during pregnancy and delivery. *Br Med J*, 2(5859), 137–138.

Sebire, N. J., Jolly, M., Harris, J. P., et al. (2001). Maternal obesity and pregnancy outcome: a study of 287,213 pregnancies in London. *Int J Obes Relat Metab Disord*, 25, 1175–1182.

Slone, D., Siskind, V., Heinonen, O. P., et al. (1977). Antenatal exposure to the phenothiazines in relation to congenital malformations, perinatal mortality rate, birth weight, and intelligence quotient score. *Am J Obstet Gynecol*, 128, 486–488.

Sørensen, M. J., Grønborg, T. K., Christensen, J., et al. (2013). Antidepressant exposure in pregnancy and risk of autism spectrum disorders. *Clin Epidemiol*, 5, 449–459.

Teoh, S., Ilett, K. F., Hackett, L. P., Kohan, R.(2011). Estimation of rac-amisulpride transfer into milk and of infant dose via milk during its use in a lactating woman with bipolar disorder and schizophrenia. *Breastfeed Med*, 6, 85–88.

Toh, S., Li, Q., Cheetham, T. C., et al. (2013). Prevalence and trends in the use of antipsychotic medications during pregnancy in the U.S., 2001–2007: a population-based study of 585,615 deliveries. *Arch Womens Ment Health*, 16, 149–157.

Toh, S., Mitchell, A. A., Louik, C., et al. (2009). Selective serotonin reuptake inhibitor use and risk of gestational hypertension. *Am J Psychiatry*, 166, 320–328.

Tomson, T. (2005). Gender aspects of pharmacokinetics of new and old AEDs: pregnancy and breastfeeding. *Ther Drug Monit*, 27, 718–721.

Tomson, T., Battino, D. (2012). Teratogenic effects of antiepileptic drugs. *Lancet Neurol*, 11, 803–813.

Tomson, T., Landmark, C. J., Battino, D. (2013). Antiepileptic treatment in pregnancy: changes in drug disposition and their clinical implications. *Epilepsia*, 54, 405–414.

US Food and Drug Administration. (2011). FDA Drug Safety Communication: Antipsychotic drug labels updated on use during pregnancy and risk of abnormal muscle movements and withdrawal symptoms in newborns. www.fda .gov/drugs/drugsafety/ucm243903 .htm.

Walsh-Sukys, M. C., Tyson, J. E., Wright, L. L., et al. (2000). Persistent pulmonary hypertension of the newborn in the era before nitric oxide: practice variation and outcomes. *Pediatrics*, 105(1 Pt 1), 14–20.

Weissman, A. M., Levy, B. T., Hartz, A. J., et al (2004). Pooled analysis of antidepressant levels in lactating mothers, breast milk, and nursing infants. *Am J Psychiatry*, 161, 1066–1078.

Wieck, A. (2011). The use of anti-epileptic medication in women with affective disorders in early and late pregnancy and during breastfeeding. *Current Women's Health Reviews*, 7, 50–57.

Wikner, B. N., Källén, B. (2011). Are hypnotic benzodiazepine receptor agonists teratogenic in humans? *J Clin Psychopharmacol*, 31, 356–359.

Windhager, E., Kim, S. W., Saria, A., et al. (2014). Perinatal use of aripiprazole: plasma levels, placental transfer, and child outcome in 3 new cases. *J Clin Psychopharmacol*, 34, 637–641.

Wlodarczyk, B. J., Palacios, A. M., George, T. M., et al. (2012). Antiepileptic drugs and pregnancy outcomes. *Am J Med Genet A*, 158A(8): 2071–2090.

World Health Organization. (2013). Global Strategy for Infant and Young Child Feeding. ISBN 92 4 156221 8. Accessible at: www.who .int/nutrition/publications/ infantfeeding/9241562218/en/.

Borderline personality disorder

12 Sex differences

Andrew M. Chanen and Katherine Thompson

Borderline personality disorder (BPD) is a severe mental disorder characterized by a pervasive pattern of impulsivity, emotional instability, interpersonal dysfunction and disturbed self-image (American Psychiatric Association, 2013: refer to Table 12.1). The recently published DSM-5 rejected a proposed dimensional model of personality disorder (PD); the reasons for this decision are beyond the scope of this chapter. Consequently, DSM-5 retained the nine DSM-IV polythetic diagnostic criteria for BPD and these are reproduced in Table 12.1. A diagnosis is made when any five of these criteria are met. Despite retaining a categorical personality disorder (PD) diagnostic system in the DSM-5, there is substantial evidence that BPD is a dimensional construct (Trull, Distel, & Carpenter, 2011; Zimmerman, Chelminski, Young, Dalrymple, & Martinez, 2012), existing along a continuum of severity.

BPD is common in clinical practice (Zimmerman, Chelminski, & Young, 2008) and is associated with severe distress and persistent functional disability, which is at least as severe as that associated with major depression (Gunderson et al., 2011). There is also high family and carer burden (Goodman et al., 2011; Hoffman, Buteau, Hooley, Fruzzetti, & Bruce, 2003) and high rates of continuing resource utilization (Horz, Zanarini, Frankenburg, Reich, & Fitzmaurice, 2010). Despite persistent help seeking, 8–10% of adults with BPD will die by suicide (Paris & Zweig-Frank, 2001; Pompili, Girardi, Ruberto, & Tatarelli, 2005).

The long-term outcomes for adults presenting with BPD have been well characterized, mostly in samples from the United States. "Remission" of the categorical diagnosis (i.e., no longer meeting five or more DSM-IV BPD criteria) and attenuation of the specific diagnostic features of BPD is common and tends to be stable (Gunderson et al., 2011; Zanarini, Frankenburg, Reich, & Fitzmaurice, 2010), but *recovery* is more elusive. When recovery is defined as 2 years of both remission of BPD diagnostic features and good social and vocational functioning (Zanarini et al., 2010), only half of adult BPD patients will recover by 10 years. One-third of those recovered will later "relapse."

Table 12.1 DSM-5 Borderline Personality Disorder Criteria

A pervasive pattern of instability of interpersonal relationships, self-image, and affects, and marked impulsivity, beginning by early adulthood and present in a variety of contexts, as indicated by five (or more) of the following:

1. Frantic efforts to avoid real or imagined abandonment.
2. A pattern of unstable and intense interpersonal relationships characterized by alternating between extremes of idealization and devaluation.
3. Identity disturbance: markedly and persistently unstable self-image or sense of self.
4. Impulsivity in at least two areas that are potentially self-damaging (e.g., spending, sex, substance use, reckless driving, binge eating).
5. Recurrent suicidal behavior, gestures, or threats, or self-mutilating behavior.
6. Affective instability due to a marked reactivity of mood (e.g., intense episodic dysphoria, irritability, or anxiety usually lasting a few hours and only rarely more than a few days).
7. Chronic feelings of emptiness.
8. Inappropriate, intense anger or difficulty controlling anger (e.g., frequent displays of temper, constant anger, recurrent physical fights).
9. Transient, stress-related paranoid ideation or severe dissociative symptoms.

(American Psychiatric Association, 2013)

Comprehensive Women's Mental Health, ed. David J. Castle and Kathryn M. Abel. Published by Cambridge University Press.
© Cambridge University Press 2016.

BPD is moderately heritable and appears to arise from the interaction of biological and environmental risk and protective factors, but the developmental pathways remain unclear (Chanen & Kaess, 2012). A variety of genetic, neurobiological, psychopathological and environmental risk factors have been suggested for BPD (Chanen & Kaess, 2012), but these risk factors are common to other mental disorders and are generally not specific for BPD (Chanen & McCutcheon, 2013).

BPD is of particular relevance to this volume because, according to DSM-5, it is diagnosed predominantly in women (75%) (American Psychiatric Association, 2013). While this appears to be true in many clinical settings, recent evidence suggests that these differences are less marked in the community (Lenzenweger, Lane, Loranger, & Kessler, 2007). This chapter provides an overview of sex differences in BPD, covering clinical presentation, longitudinal course, etiological factors and neurobiological underpinnings. Given the recency of DSM-5's publication, this chapter reports data relating to the DSM-IV-TR personality disorders and their predecessors.

Possible sources of sex differences in BPD rates

There has been debate about whether reported sex differences in personality disorders (PDs) in clinical samples, including BPD, reflect true biological, psychological or social differences between females and males or whether they are an artifact of sampling or diagnostic biases (Skodol, 2003). Borderline, histrionic and dependent PDs are diagnosed more frequently in women, whereas schizoid, schizotypal, paranoid, antisocial, narcissistic and obsessive-compulsive PDs are more often diagnosed in males. The largest sex difference in the prevalence of PDs has been reported to be between antisocial PD (ASPD) and BPD, with ASPD believed to be up to 5 times more common in men than women. In the past, it was believed that the reverse was true for BPD, with greater prevalence in women. Taken together with the evidence that ASPD and BPD share the traits of antagonism (hostility) and disinhibition (impulsivity and risk taking), together with many of the psychosocial risk factors of family dysfunction and exposure to trauma, abuse and neglect (Paris, Chenard-Poirier, & Biskin, 2013), this caused Paris (1997) to question whether these disorders might be two aspects of the same psychopathology.

However, recent high-quality, community-based, epidemiological studies (see following) have found either equal prevalence among women and men for BPD or only a slightly elevated prevalence in females (Paris et al., 2013). Based upon this and other literature published in the past 15 years on prevalence, prognosis and treatment outcome for BPD, Paris and colleagues (Paris et al., 2013) revised their original (Paris, 1997) hypothesis. They concluded that BPD and ASPD are in fact different disorders and that the influence of sex upon symptoms is not an artifact. Rather, the differences between these disorders are embedded in trait dimensions that are shaped by sex and sex is a factor that partly determines the specific psychopathological profile.

The higher prevalence of BPD among women has been a long-standing clinical assumption, but whether this really is the case, and what the potential sources for this difference might be requires further scrutiny. We have considered the most recent epidemiological data, along with potential sources of this bias, including a biased application of diagnostic criteria, sex bias in the DSM-5 criteria, and social and cultural factors.

Prevalence of BPD in population samples

The DSM-IV-TR and previous versions of this manual stated that there is a 3:1 female to male sex ratio for BPD, perpetuating the belief that this disorder is much more prevalent among females (Sansone & Sansone, 2011). Numerous high-quality epidemiological studies of the population prevalence of DSM-IV PDs have now been published. Among these, the National Comorbidity Survey Replication (Lenzenweger et al., 2007), based upon a representative sample of 9,282 adults from the United States, reported the prevalence of BPD to be 1.4%, with no sex difference. Torgensen and colleagues' (Torgersen, Kringlen, Cramer, 2001) study of a representative community sample of 2,053 adult residents of Oslo, Norway and found the prevalence of BPD to be 0.7%, with no sex differences. The British National Survey of Psychiatric Morbidity (Coid et al., 2006) studied a representative sample of 8,886 16- to 74-year-olds reported the prevalence of BPD to be 0.7%, with no sex differences. Finally, Wave 2 of the National Epidemiological Survey on Alcohol and Related Conditions (NESARC; Grant et al., 2008) studied a representative sample of 34,653 American adults. The lifetime prevalence of BPD was 5.9%, with no sex differences. The NESARC has been criticized for its measurement of PD and a conservative re-analysis of the data by Trull and colleagues (2010) reported the overall prevalence of BPD to be 2.7%, with a statistically significant but slight preponderance of BPD among females (3.02% *vs.* 2.44% among males).

The only study to report reliably on sex differences among young people with BPD (Zanarini et al., 2011), assessed a community sample of 6,330 11-year-olds from Bristol, England and found the prevalence of BPD to be 3.2%, with no statistically significant sex difference.

Taken together, the results from these population studies do not support the assumption that BPD is much more prevalent among females. In fact, the rate of BPD is either equal or only slightly higher in females.

Biased sampling in research studies

Contrary to the aforementioned studies, clinical epidemiological studies do reveal sex differences, with a preponderance of females (around 75–80%) in clinical services. It has been suggested that this might be the reason why clinicians perceive more females have BPD (Skodol, 2003). This might be due to sampling biases associated with the clinical presentation of BPD. For example, it has been argued that males with BPD are more likely to present to drug and alcohol treatment services and are less likely to utilize pharmacotherapy and psychotherapy (Sansone & Sansone, 2011), thereby accounting for the greater proportion of women with BPD in clinical services. This is supported by data from the Collaborative Longitudinal Personality Disorders Study (CLPS), which investigated differences among their sample of 175 females and 65 males with BPD (Johnson et al., 2003). Males with BPD were more likely to present with substance use disorders, and with schizotypal, narcissistic and antisocial PDs, while females with BPD were more likely to present with post traumatic stress disorder (PTSD), eating disorders and the BPD criterion of identity disturbance.

Biased application of diagnostic criteria

Another reason for a possible disparity between the actual prevalence of BPD among females and the assumed prevalence might be biased (unequal) application of diagnostic criteria (Widiger, 1998). Anderson, Sankis, and Widiger (2001) asked 720 members of the American Psychological Association to judge the frequency of DSM-IV personality pathology in female and male patients. They cross-validated these results in a second sample of 900 additional members of the American Psychological Association. The findings of this study indicated that when clinicians applied the DSM-IV PD criteria, they rated BPD symptoms to be as infrequent in males, and as pathological in males, as they were in females. There was no significant statistical difference between sexes. This suggests that the application of diagnostic criteria might be neutral.

Sex bias in the DSM criteria

Few studies have investigated the DSM-IV criteria for sex bias. The most robust and largest study conducted used factor analytic strategies to investigate the measurement invariance for these criteria using the Norwegian Twin database (Aggen, Neale, Roysamb, Reichborn-Kjennerud, & Kendler, 2009). A total of 2,794 twins were interviewed, 1772 females and 1022 males, and the SCID-II interview was administered for DSM-IV PDs. The results of the statistical analyses confirmed the coherence of the nine criteria in a general population sample. This BPD factor differed according to sex and age in relation to affective instability and impulsivity. Females reported more affective instability and less impulsivity than males. In younger females, impulsivity was more prominent and this changed over time.

Social constructivism

The tendency to diagnose BPD more often in women than men might be partly due to sociocultural factors and the cultural history of BPD (Bjorklund, 2006). The basis of this hypothesis has been informed by cross-cultural studies where, for example, in Ethiopia and India only 1–3% of psychiatric outpatients were diagnosed with PDs compared with a rate as high as 32% in the United Kingdom. This variation might be due to different diagnostic practices and the way people seek help in these societies. Other factors might include economic status, optimism, religion, psychological awareness and medical orientation of the society. Cultural factors also influence the way mental illness manifests in relation to sex. Expectations exist concerning women's tendency to be more emotional and relational and relationship-dependent than men (see Chapter 1). Therefore, it is possible for diagnostic constructs to be gender-biased. Sexist characterizations of women's health and illness are affected by political, economic and cultural factors along with biomedical ones. Sex differences exist in normal behavior (Simmons, 1992).

For example, excessive anger, argumentativeness and sexual promiscuity are described as pathological behaviors that might lead to BPD diagnosis. However, if displayed by men, these behaviors might be seen as acceptable, expected or even admirable. It might be rare for a man to be diagnosed as having BPD based upon these behaviors. He would be more likely to be diagnosed as having ASPD, if at all. More research is clearly needed in this area.

Sex differences in clinical presentation

Having established that the population prevalence of BPD is more equal than first assumed, it is relevant to investigate whether those who come to the attention of mental health services actually do show sex differences in clinical presentation and/or symptom profile.

When sex differences in clinical variables are considered, females presenting with BPD have been reported to be younger than males and these males presented clinically at a later age (McCormick et al., 2007). They were also less likely to seek mental health treatment. Women rated themselves as having worse mental health functioning and social role functioning, and tended to be more self-critical than men.

Sex differences in BPD symptom criteria

Studies have investigated the prevalence of individual diagnostic criteria for BPD in females and males and found a sex difference in the type of psychopathology associated with this diagnostic label. A study of 11-year-old children with BPD found that girls were significantly more likely to fulfill DSM-IV criteria for mood reactivity, frantic efforts to avoid abandonment and unstable relationships, compared with boys who were more likely to evidence impulsivity and physically self-destructive acts (Zanarini et al., 2011). The Collaborative Longitudinal Personality Disorders Study (CLPS) found females were significantly more likely to rate higher than males for affective instability and identity disturbance (Johnson et al., 2003). Whereas other studies have reported that males more commonly endorsed the item "intensive anger" (and to some degree "impulsivity"), and that females more commonly endorsed "affective instability" (Tadic et al., 2009). By contrast, some researchers have reported no sex differences in BPD criteria, except for dissociation, which is more prevalent among females (McCormick et al., 2007). Therefore, while there were few differences among the majority of

BPD criteria, there was evidence of some difference in terms of affective instability, anger and impulsivity.

Sex differences in the traits and behaviors underlying BPD

Widiger (1998) suggests that trait-based models of personality disorder, in particular the five-factor model (Wiggins, 1996), might provide some assistance in resolving the sex bias controversy by providing a theoretical basis for sex prevalence rates. He hypothesizes that, if personality disorders are extreme maladaptive variants of normal personality traits, the prevalence of personality disorders would be expected to mirror any differential sex prevalence of the factors and facets of the five-factor model. In fact, in the literature on normal personality, consistent sex differences have been obtained for most of the domains and facets of the five-factor model (Widiger, 1998) and for some other trait measures (Jang, McCrae, Angleitner, Riemann, & Livesley, 1998). Furthermore, there are also significant sex differences in the magnitude of heritability of those traits and some evidence of sex-specific genetic effects (Jang et al., 1998).

A study of maladaptive personality among 681 volunteer twin pairs from the general population showed that most maladaptive traits are heritable in both sexes (Jang et al., 1998). Cognitive dysregulation, suspiciousness and self-harm were the only traits that did not have a significant heritable component in females and likewise for submissiveness in males. Sex-specific genetic effects were detected for all traits, except insecure attachment. There was no evidence to support sex-specific, non-shared environmental influences for any traits underlying BPD. It is also noteworthy that callousness and conduct problems, along with their higher order *dissocial* factor were not significantly heritable for females.

The DSM-5 BPD diagnostic criteria comprise a mixture of more stable traits (e.g., chronic anger, intolerance of aloneness) and unstable symptomatic behaviors (e.g., self-mutilation) (Gunderson et al., 2011; Zanarini et al., 2007). Several studies have examined sex differences among the traits that underlie BPD, using measures of normal and pathological personality. In a community sample of 263 children aged between 9 and 13 years (Gratz et al., 2009), affective dysfunction and disinhibition significantly predicted borderline personality symptoms in both girls and boys, and that there were no sex differences in the level of BPD symptoms. Among girls, affective dysfunction and sensation seeking accounted for a significant amount of additional variance in BPD symptoms, whereas among boys, only affective dysfunction accounted for a significant amount of unique variance. Likewise, a study of undergraduate university students found that women rated significantly higher on affective instability, abandonment and relationships; and men on impulsiveness (Fonseca-Pedrero et al., 2011). However, these findings are limited by their reliance on a self-report borderline personality disorder scale, not a formal DSM-IV diagnostic interview.

In a study comparing male and female adolescents with BPD (measured by the SWAP-200, which uses a Q-sort methodology), girls showed more internalizing psychopathology and were more emotionally dramatic, whereas boys were more behaviorally disinhibited, externalizing and angry (Bradley, Zittel Conklin, & Westen, 2005). The young women in this study were described as more likely to be drawn into relationships where they could be emotionally or physically abused, choose inappropriate romantic partners, be overly sexually seductive or provocative, make suicidal threats or gestures, have uncontrolled eating binges, and be preoccupied by food-related issues. In contrast, the young men were described as more likely to bully others, feel self-important, show reckless disregard for the rights of others, prefer to operate as if emotions were irrelevant, take advantage of others, have trouble making decisions, seek to dominate others, show no remorse, not need contact with other people, and promise to change but then revert to their previous maladaptive behavior.

There is also some evidence to suggest there are sex differences in behavioral symptoms in BPD. In a sample of internal medicine patients screened (but not formally assessed) for BPD, women were more likely to be engaged in a sexually abusive relationship, whereas men were significantly more likely to bang their head or to lose a job on purpose (Sansone, Lam, & Wiederman, 2010). In a sample of low socio-economic status middle- and high-school students, males were significantly more likely to burn or punch themselves (Gratz et al., 2012). Another study compared female and male offenders and found that, in females, the combination of interpersonal-affective traits and impulsive-antisocial traits combined to increase the risk of self-directed violence, whereas in males, interpersonal-affective traits were associated

with reduced symptoms of BPD, which in turn reduced the risk of self-directed violence (Verona, Sprague, & Javdani, 2012).

Sex differences in co-occurring disorders

Aside from differences in how the BPD criteria are manifest, it is possible that sex differences occur in regard to co-occurring mental state (*aka* axis I) and trait (*aka* axis II) pathology.

The Methods to Improve Diagnostic Assessment and Services (MIDAS) study used semi-structured DSM-IV diagnostic interviews to investigate the pattern of comorbidity among 130 outpatients (71 women, 30 men) with BPD (Zlotnick, Rothschild, & Zimmerman, 2002). They found that there were sex differences in the pattern of lifetime impulse-related disorders. Women were more likely to have a history of eating disorder, but in contrast it was more common to find substance abuse disorders, intermittent explosive disorder and ASPD histories among males. There were no differences in rates of comorbid PTSD.

A study of comorbidity among 484 consecutively admitted outpatients with a diagnosis of BPD, where most participants were female (83%), found 74% met criteria for at least one co-occurring DSM-IV PD, 33.5% had two or three PDs, and 7.6% had between four and eight PDs (Barrachina et al., 2011). Women tended to have more disorders than men. In women, the most frequent co-occurring disorders (from highest to lowest) were depressive, paranoid, passive-aggressive, dependent, avoidant and obsessive-compulsive PDs. In contrast, among men the most frequent (from highest to lowest) were paranoid, antisocial, passive-aggressive, depressive and avoidant PDs. Of particular relevance were the significantly higher rates of dependent PD in women, supporting their tendency to internalize symptoms and among males with BPD the significantly higher prevalence of antisocial PD, which gives further support to the suggestion that males manifest impulsivity through externalising behaviors.

Another study investigated DSM-IV axis I and axis II comorbidity among patients with BPD (Tadic et al., 2009). Of the 110 women and 49 men studied using a standardized diagnostic interview, they found women were significantly more likely to have a co-occurring eating disorder and affective instability. Males were significantly more likely to have a co-occurring substance use disorder, disorder of social behavior, antisocial PD and intensive anger. Their findings further support the hypothesis that women and men have more similarities than differences in the number of comorbid axis I disorders, axis II disorders and BPD criteria. However, women tend to have more internalizing psychopathology and men more externalizing psychopathology associated with BPD. With regard to mental state disorders, females have higher rates of anxiety, affective and eating disorders, whereas males have higher rates of substance use disorders. With regard to personality disorder, compared to males, females show significantly lower rates of behavioral problems in childhood and adolescence and ASPD.

When standard personality tests and structured clinical interviews were used to investigate sex differences among 114 female and 57 male patients with BPD (Banzhaf et al., 2012), they found that women with BPD were significantly more likely to meet criteria for PTSD, panic disorder with agoraphobia and bulimia nervosa. Men with BPD were more likely to meet criteria for binge eating disorder, a disorder of social behavior in childhood, and antisocial and narcissistic PDs. These findings are comparable with those reported by other studies, except for the absence of substance use disorders among males with BPD.

Another study investigated comorbidity in BPD and found no differences in the frequency of axis I disorders, except that women were significantly less likely to have alcohol use disorders (Barnow et al., 2007). Patients with BPD had, on average, three additional PDs. Women were more likely to have an avoidant PD, whereas men had significantly higher rates of antisocial personality disorder.

These studies suggest that there are sex differences in clinical presentation of patients with BPD in terms of criteria, patterns of co-occurring PD and mental state pathology. In all these aspects of presentation, females tend to have more internalizing symptoms and males tend to have more externalizing symptoms (Eaton et al., 2011). Most striking, however, is that females and males with BPD generally display more similarities than differences, a fact that often seems to be overlooked in clinical practice and which might contribute to the misdiagnosis of BPD among males (Johnson et al., 2003). Where differences occur, the studies above indicate that females with BPD tend to have greater affective instability and to engage in a variety of methods of self-harm and may place themselves in situations where they are vulnerable to being mistreated by others. In contrast, males with BPD pathology tend to be more impulsive and to physically harm themselves using greater self-directed violence.

Clinical studies indicate there are sex differences in the way BPD presents, with females having more affective instability and males being more impulsive. This in turn is reflected in sex differences in co-occurring disorders, functioning and traits. Women with BPD tend to have greater rates of internalizing psychopathology, whereas males have a greater number of externalizing behaviors.

Sex differences in temporal stability, longitudinal course and functioning

BPD is increasingly seen as a lifespan developmental disorder that exists on a dimensional continuum of severity (Chanen & McCutcheon, 2013). There is a normative rise in BPD pathology at puberty, which peaks in the teens and emerging adulthood and then wanes across the lifespan (Bernstein et al., 1993; Crawford, Cohen, & Brook, 2001; Gunderson et al., 2011; Johnson, Cohen, Kasen, Skodol, Hamagami, & Brook, 2000; Zanarini, Frankenburg, Reich, & Fitzmaurice, 2012). However, data on sex differences in stability of BPD over time are scant. Chanen and colleagues (2004) examined the 2-year stability of categorical and dimensional PD in 101 psychiatric outpatients 15–18 years old. Of those with any categorical PD diagnosis at baseline, 74% still met criteria for a PD at follow-up, with marked sex differences (83% of females and 56% of males). The small sample size prevented analysis of sex differences among specific PDs.

Only limited cross-sectional data are available on functioning. Findings from Wave 2 of the NESARC study (Grant et al., 2008) indicate that respondents with BPD were more likely to have low income, lower educational attainment and to be separated/divorced/widowed. Generally, individuals with BPD had greater physical and mental disability than those who did not have BPD, and this disability was greater among women with BPD, which might be another contributor to their presentation at treatment services. However, these findings are not supported by data from the CLPS study (Johnson et al., 2003), which found no significant sex differences in functioning.

In short, published studies of the longitudinal course and functional outcomes for BPD do not address the issue of sex differences adequately. This is likely to be because most studies have been conducted in clinical settings, where males with BPD are comparatively rare. The instability of categorical diagnoses of BPD is striking. Most individuals with BPD tend to "lose" their diagnosis over time by falling below definitions of "caseness" for the disorder. The data of Chanen and colleagues (2004) suggest that, for PD in general, this might be more likely for males than females in older adolescents. However, it is noteworthy that large-scale community-based studies of the traits underlying PD have not found any significant sex differences in mean level or rank order stability over lengthy follow-up periods (Caspi, Roberts, & Shiner, 2005). Further research is required, notably to explore what particular features of particular PDs might change differentially with time in females and males. In the absence of comprehensive data, we turn to a consideration of etiological parameters in BPD, with a view to whether there are clues to sex divergence in the disorder.

Sex differences in heritability and risk factors for BPD

Heritability estimates for BPD (or dimensional representations of BPD) in large scale twin studies range from 0.3 to 0.5 (Bornovalova, Hicks, Iacono, & McGue, 2009; Distel et al., 2008), with no sex differences reported. More recently, Torgersen and colleagues (2012) used a more rigorous diagnostic methodology in the 2,800 twins from the Norwegian Institute of Public Health Twin Panel and found the heritability for BPD to be 0.69. They did not report on sex differences.

Sex differences in risk factors for BPD have been infrequently reported. Childhood adversity (including childhood abuse and neglect, adverse family environment and familial psychopathology) (Chanen & Kaess, 2012) is common in BPD (Zanarini, 2000; Zanarini et al., 2002) and is thought to be an important etiological factor for the disorder, although it is neither necessary nor sufficient for development of BPD (Johnson, Cohen, Brown, Smailes, & Bernstein, 1999; Paris, 1998; Zanarini, 2000). In epidemiological studies of community samples, childhood sexual abuse is more common among women (Fergusson, Lynskey, & Horwood, 1996), although not uncommon among

men (Johnson et al., 2003). This appears to be the case in BPD (Paris, Zweig-Frank, & Guzder, 1994) and might contribute to sex differences in the prevalence of BPD.

Overall, the etiological underpinnings of sex differences in PD in general and BPD, in particular, involve complex and dynamic genetic and environmental interactions throughout development (Chanen & Kaess, 2012). However, sex differences have rarely been investigated among genetic and environmental risk factors. Individuals with a "sensitive" genotype have been found to be at greater risk of BPD in the presence of a predisposing environment, supporting a stress-diathesis model. Furthermore, the genes that influence BPD features also increase the likelihood of comorbidity, and of being exposed to certain adverse life events. Finally, a range of childhood and parental demographic characteristics, adverse childhood experiences, early relational difficulties and forms of maladaptive parenting have been identified as risk factors for BPD.

Sex differences in the neurobiology of BPD

The vast majority of neurobiological studies of BPD have been conducted with female participants. As discussed, this reflects the relative scarcity of potential male research participants in clinical services where such research is carried out. Studies implicate a neurobiological circuit involving abnormalities in fronto-limbic networks including regions involved in emotion processing (e.g., the amygdala and insula) and frontal brain regions implicated in regulatory control processes (e.g., anterior cingulate cortex, medial frontal cortex, orbitofrontal cortex, and dorsolateral prefrontal cortex) (Krause-Utz, Winter, Niedtfeld, & Schmahl, 2014; Tebartz van Elst, 2003). Studies of young people early in the course of BPD suggest that some structural changes (e.g., amygdala and hippocampal volume reduction) might be a consequence of living with the disorder (Chanen & Kaess, 2012). There is also some evidence that patients with BPD show hyperconnectivity between brain regions involved in emotion processing (e.g., the amygdala, insula, occipito-frontal cortex and putamen) and this might reflect the affective hyperarousal and intense emotional reactions observed in BPD (Krause-Utz et al., 2014). Studies focusing on emotional processing and emotional regulation similarly show hyperactivity of limbic brain areas in response to negative emotional stimuli followed by a slower return of the amygdala to baseline (Krause-Utz et al., 2014). However, the effect of sex on either vulnerability to, or expression of these pathologies remains unclear.

Altered function has been reported in serotonergic, glutamatergic and GABAergic systems in patients with BPD but sex differences have not been systematically examined in all these systems, but sex differences have been reported in serotonergic functioning in BPD (Leyton et al., 2001; Soloff, Kelly, Strotmeyer, Malone, & Mann, 2003). Leyton and colleagues (2001) studied 13 medication-free patients with BPD (8 females) using a PET scanning technique that indexes serotonin synthesis capacity, and compared them to 11 healthy controls (5 female). Males with BPD had significantly lower serotonin synthesis in corticostriatal sites, including the medial frontal gyrus, anterior cingulate gyrus, superior temporal gyrus and corpus striatum. In females with BPD, these changes were seen in fewer regions.

In a study specifically looking for sex differences in central serotonergic function in BPD (Soloff et al., 2003), a fenfluramine challenge test was conducted in 64 BPD participants (44 female) and 57 control participants (21 female). Male BPD participants had significantly diminished prolactin responses compared with healthy controls, but female BPD participants did not. Measures of impulsivity and aggression were inversely related to prolactin responses among male but not female subjects. The authors concluded that sex differences in central serotonergic function might contribute to variations in impulsivity in BPD.

A more recent study (Perez-Rodriguez et al., 2012) investigated striatal function in 38 BPD patients with intermittent explosive disorder (BPD-IED; 22 male) and 36 healthy controls (18 male) using an aggression-provocation task in PET scanning. Male BPD-IED patients had significantly lower striatal relative glucose metabolism compared with controls during the behavioral aggression task under the provoking and nonprovoking conditions, although female and male BPD-IED patients did not differ in clinical or behavioral measures. This suggests differential involvement of frontal-striatal circuits in men with BPD-IED.

Thus, the neurobiology of BPD is beginning to inform our understanding of sex differences in the disorder, most notably with respect to serotonergic systems and striatal functioning. However, most studies have not been designed to investigate potential sex differences in BPD or the specificity of these findings to BPD, and much more work is required in this area.

Conclusions

There has been debate about whether reported sex differences in BPD reflect true biological, psychological or social differences between females and males or whether they are an artifact of sampling, diagnostic or other biases. While approximately 75% of patients presenting to clinical services with BPD are female, recent evidence suggests that sex differences in the prevalence of BPD are much less marked in the community. There is evidence to support sampling biases as a source of these differences associated with the clinical presentation of BPD, along with sex differences in affective instability and impulsivity, in the prevalence of individual diagnostic criteria for BPD, and in the prevalence of co-occurring syndromes. Moreover, sex differences in BPD are likely also to reflect sex differences in the personality traits that underlie personality disorder. The evidence does not support biased application of the diagnostic criteria for BPD. Finally, although the vast majority of neurobiological studies of BPD have been conducted with women, studies do suggest some sex differences. Men have been reported to have lower serotonin synthesis in corticostriatal areas of brain and diminished prolactin response to a fenfluramine challenge test. One study also reported differential involvement of frontal-striatal circuits in men with BPD plus intermittent explosive disorder.

The evidence is unclear regarding the sources of sociocultural biases in BPD or any sex differences in the temporal stability of BPD. More research is needed in these areas, along with studies of sex differences in the risk factors for BPD.

References

Aggen, S. H., Neale, M. C., Roysamb, E., Reichborn-Kjennerud, T., & Kendler, K. S. (2009).

A psychometric evaluation of the DSM-IV borderline personality disorder criteria: age and sex moderation of criterion functioning. *Psychol Med*, 39(12), 1967–1978.

American Psychiatric Association. (2013). *Diagnostic and Statistical Manual of Mental Disorders.* Retrieved from dsm. psychiatryonline.org

Anderson, K. G., Sankis, L. M., & Widiger, T. A. (2001). Pathology versus statistical infrequency: potential sources of gender bias in personality disorder criteria. *J Nerv Ment Dis*, 189(10), 661–668.

Banzhaf, A., Ritter, K., Merkl, A., Schulte-Herbruggen, O., Lammers, C. H., & Roepke, S. (2012). Gender differences in a clinical sample of patients with borderline personality disorder. *J Pers Disord*, 26(3), 368–380.

Barnow, S., Herpertz, S. C., Spitzer, C., Stopsack, M., Preuss, U. W., Grabe, H. J., ... Freyberger, H. J. (2007). Temperament and character in patients with borderline personality disorder taking gender and comorbidity into account. *Psychopathology*, 40(6), 369–378.

Barrachina, J., Pascual, J. C., Ferrer, M., Soler, J., Rufat, M. J., Andion, O., ... Perez, V. (2011). Axis II comorbidity in borderline personality disorder is influenced by sex, age, and clinical severity. *Compr Psychiatry*, 52(6), 725–730.

Bernstein, D. P., Cohen, P., Velez, C. N., Schwab-Stone, M., Siever, L. J., & Shinsato, L. (1993). Prevalence and stability of the DSM-III-R personality disorders in a community-based survey of adolescents. *Am J Psychiatry*, 150(8), 1237–1243.

Bjorklund, P. (2006). No man's land: gender bias and social contructivism in the diagnosis of borderline personality disorder. *Issues in Mental Health Nursing*, 27, 3–23.

Bornovalova, M. A., Hicks, B. M., Iacono, W. G., & McGue, M. (2009). Stability, change, and heritability of borderline personality disorder traits from adolescence to adulthood: a longitudinal twin study. *Dev Psychopathol*, 21(4), 1335–1353.

Bradley, R., Zittel Conklin, C., & Westen, D. (2005). The borderline personality diagnosis in adolescents: gender differences and subtypes. *J Child Psychol Psychiatry*, 46(9), 1006–1019.

Caspi, A., Roberts, B. W., & Shiner, R. L. (2005). Personality development: stability and change. *Annual Review of Psychology*, 56, 453–484.

Chanen, A. M., Jackson, H. J., McGorry, P. D., Allot, K., Clarkson, V., Yuen, H. P. (2004). Two-year stability of personality disorder in older adolescent outpatients. *J Pers Disord*, 18(6), 526–541.

Chanen, A. M., & Kaess, M. (2012). Developmental pathways to borderline personality disorder. *Curr Psychiatry Rep*, 14(1), 45–53.

Chanen, A. M., & McCutcheon, L. (2013). Prevention and early intervention for borderline personality disorder: current status and recent evidence. *British Journal of Psychiatry*, 202, s24–s29.

Coid, J., Yang, M., Roberts, A., Ullrich, S., Moran, P., Bebbington, P., ... Singleton, N. (2006). Violence and psychiatric morbidity in a national household population – a report from the British Household Survey. *Am J Epidemiol*, 164(12), 1199–1208.

Crawford, T. N., Cohen, P., & Brook, J. S. (2001). Dramatic-erratic personality disorder symptoms: I. Continuity from early adolescence into adulthood. *J Pers Disord*, 15(4), 319–335.

Distel, M. A., Trull, T. J., Derom, C. A., Thiery, E. W., Grimmer, M. A., Martin, N. G., ... Boomsma, D. I. (2008). Heritability of borderline personality disorder features is similar across three countries. *Psychol Med*, 38(9), 1219–1229.

Eaton, N. R., Krueger, R. F., Keyes, K. M., Skodol, A. E., Markon, K. E., Grant, B. F., & Hasin, D. S. (2011). Borderline personality disorder co-morbidity: relationship to the internalizing-externalizing structure of common mental disorders. *Psychol Med*, 41(5), 1041–1050.

Fergusson, D. M., Lynskey, M. T., & Horwood, L. J. (1996). Childhood sexual abuse and psychiatric disorder in young adulthood: I. Prevalence of sexual abuse and factors associated with sexual abuse. *J Am Acad Child Adolesc Psychiatry*, 35(10), 1355–1364.

Fonseca-Pedrero, E., Paino, M., Lemos-Giraldez, S., Sierra-Baigrie, S., Gonzalez, M. P., Bobes, J., & Muniz, J. (2011). Borderline personality traits in nonclinical young adults. *J Pers Disord*, 25(4), 542–556.

Goodman, M., Patil, U., Triebwasser, J., Hoffman, P., Weinstein, Z. A., & New, A. (2011). Parental burden associated with borderline personality disorder in female offspring. *J Pers Disord*, 25(1), 59–74.

Grant, B. F., Chou, S. P., Goldstein, R. B., Huang, B., Stinson, F. S., Saha, T. D., ... Ruan, W. J. (2008). Prevalence, correlates, disability, and comorbidity of DSM-IV borderline personality disorder: results from the Wave 2 National Epidemiologic Survey on Alcohol and Related Conditions. *J Clin Psychiatry*, 69(4), 533–545.

Gratz, K. L., Latzman, R. D., Young, J., Heiden, L. J., Damon, J., Hight, T., Tull, M.T. (2012). Deliberate self-harm among underserved adolescents: the moderating roles of gender, race, and school-level and association with borderline personality features. *Personality Disorders: Theory, Research, and Treatment*, 3(1), 39–54.

Gratz, K. L., Tull, M. T., Reynolds, E. K., Bagge, C. L., Latzman, R. D., Daughters, S. B., & Lejuez, C. W. (2009). Extending extant models of the pathogenesis of borderline personality disorder to childhood borderline personality symptoms: the roles of affective dysfunction, disinhibition, and self- and emotion-regulation deficits. *Dev Psychopathol*, 21(4), 1263–1291.

Gunderson, J. G., Stout, R. L., McGlashan, T. H., Shea, M. T., Morey, L. C., Grilo, C. M., ... Skodol, A. E. (2011). Ten-year course of borderline personality disorder: psychopathology and function from the Collaborative

Longitudinal Personality Disorders study. *Arch Gen Psychiatry*, 68(8), 827–837.

Hoffman, P. D., Buteau, E., Hooley, J. M., Fruzzetti, A. E., & Bruce, M. L. (2003). Family members' knowledge about borderline personality disorder: correspondence with their levels of depression, burden, distress, and expressed emotion. *Fam Process*, 42(4), 469–478.

Horz, S., Zanarini, M. C., Frankenburg, F. R., Reich, D. B., & Fitzmaurice, G. (2010). Ten-year use of mental health services by patients with borderline personality disorder and with other axis II disorders. *Psychiatr Serv*, 61(6), 612–616.

Jang, K. L., McCrae, R. R., Angleitner, A., Riemann, R., & Livesley, W. J. (1998). Heritability of facet-level traits in a cross-cultural twin sample: support for a hierarchical model of personality. *J Pers Soc Psychol*, 74(6), 1556–1565.

Johnson, J. G., Cohen, P., Brown, J., Smailes, E. M., & Bernstein, D. P. (1999). Childhood maltreatment increases risk for personality disorders during early adulthood. *Arch Gen Psychiatry*, 56(7), 600–606.

Johnson, J. G., Cohen, P., Kasen, S., Skodol, A.E., Hamagami, F., Brook, J.S. (2000). Age-related change in personality disorder trait levels between early adolescence and adulthood: a community-based longitudinal investigation. *Acta Psychiatrica Scandinavica*, 102, 265–275.

Johnson, D. M., Shea, M. T., Yen, S., Battle, C. L., Zlotnick, C., Sanislow, C. A., ... Zanarini, M. C. (2003). Gender differences in borderline personality disorder: findings from the Collaborative Longitudinal Personality Disorders Study. *Compr Psychiatry*, 44(4), 284–292.

Krause-Utz, A., Winter, D., Niedtfeld, I., & Schmahl, C. (2014). The latest neuroimaging findings in borderline personality disorder. *Curr Psychiatry Rep*, 16(3), 438.

Lenzenweger, M. F., Lane, M. C., Loranger, A. W., & Kessler, R. C. (2007). DSM-IV personality disorders in the National Comorbidity Survey Replication. *Biol Psychiatry*, 62(6), 553–564.

Leyton, M., Okazawa, H., Diksic, M., Paris, J., Rosa, P., Mzengeza, S., ... Benkelfat, C. (2001). Brain Regional alpha-[11C]methyl-L-tryptophan trapping in impulsive subjects with borderline personality disorder. *Am J Psychiatry*, 158(5), 775–782.

McCormick, B., Blum, N., Hansel, R., Franklin, J. A., St John, D., Pfohl, B., ... Black, D. W. (2007). Relationship of sex to symptom severity, psychiatric comorbidity, and health care utilization in 163 subjects with borderline personality disorder. *Compr Psychiatry*, 48(5), 406–412.

Paris, J. (1997). Antisocial and borderline personality disorders: two separate diagnoses or two aspects of the same psychopathology? *Compr Psychiatry*, 38(4), 237–242.

Paris, J. (1998). Does childhood trauma cause personality disorders in adults? *Can J Psychiatry*, 43(2), 148–153.

Paris, J., Chenard-Poirier, M. P., & Biskin, R. (2013). Antisocial and borderline personality disorders revisited. *Compr Psychiatry*, 54(4), 321–325.

Paris, J., & Zweig-Frank, H. (2001). A 27-year follow-up of patients with borderline personality disorder. *Compr Psychiatry*, 42(6), 482–487.

Paris, J., Zweig-Frank, H., & Guzder, J. (1994). Risk factors for borderline personality in male outpatients. *J Nerv Ment Dis*, 182(7), 375–380.

Perez-Rodriguez, M. M., Hazlett, E. A., Rich, E. L., Ripoll, L. H., Weiner, D. M., Spence, N., ... New, A. S. (2012). Striatal activity in borderline personality disorder with comorbid intermittent explosive disorder: sex differences. *J Psychiatr Res*, 46(6), 797–804.

Pompili, M., Girardi, P., Ruberto, A., & Tatarelli, R. (2005). Suicide in borderline personality disorder: a meta-analysis. *Nord J Psychiatry*, 59(5), 319–324.

Sansone, R. A., Lam, C., & Wiederman, M. W. (2010). Self-harm behaviors in borderline personality: an analysis by gender. *J Nerv Ment Dis*, 198(12), 914–915.

Sansone, R. A., & Sansone, L. A. (2011). Gender patterns in borderline personality disorder. *Innov Clin Neurosci*, 8(5), 16–20.

Simmons, D. (1992). Gender issues and borderline personality disorder: why do females dominate the diagnosis? *Arch Psychiatr Nurs*, 6(4), 219–223.

Skodol, A. E., & Bender, D. S. (2003). Why are women diagnosed borderline more than men? *Psychiatric Quarterly*, 74(4), 349–360.

Soloff, P. H., Kelly, T. M., Strotmeyer, S. J., Malone, K. M., & Mann, J. J. (2003). Impulsivity, gender, and response to fenfluramine challenge in borderline personality disorder. *Psychiatry Res*, 119(1–2), 11–24.

Tadic, A., Wagner, S., Hoch, J., Baskaya, O., von Cube, R., Skaletz, C., ... Dahmen, N. (2009). Gender differences in axis I and axis II comorbidity in patients with borderline personality disorder. *Psychopathology*, 42(4), 257–263.

Tebartz van Elst, L., Hesslinger, B., Thiel, T., Geiger, E., Haegele, K., Lemieux, L., Lieb, K., Bohus, M., Hennig, J., Ebert, D. (2003). Frontolimbic brain abnormalities in patients with borderline personality disorder: a volumetric magnetic resonance imaging study. *Biological Psychiatry*, 54(2), 163–171.

Torgersen, S., Kringlen, E., & Cramer, V. (2001). The prevalence of personality disorders in a community sample. *Archives of General Psychiatry*, 58, 590–596.

Torgersen, S., Myers, J., Reichborn-Kjennerud, T., Roysamb, E., Kubarych, T. S., & Kendler, K. S. (2012). The heritability of Cluster

B personality disorders assessed both by personal interview and questionnaire. *J Pers Disord*, 26(6), 848–866.

Trull, T. J., Distel, M. A., & Carpenter, R. W. (2011). DSM-5 Borderline personality disorder: at the border between a dimensional and a categorical view. *Curr Psychiatry Rep*, 13(1), 43–49.

Trull, T. J., Jahng, S., Tomko, R. L., Wood, P. K., & Sher, K. J. (2010). Revised NESARC personality disorder diagnoses: gender, prevalence, and comorbidity with substance dependence disorders. *J Pers Disord*, 24(4), 412–426.

Verona, E., Sprague, J., & Javdani, S. (2012). Gender and factor-level interactions in psychopathy: implications for self-directed violence risk and borderline personality disorder symptoms. *Personal Disord*, 3(3), 247–262.

Widiger, T. A. (1998). Four out of five ain't bad. *Archives of General Psychiatry*, 55(10), 865–866.

Wiggins, C. (1996). Counting gender: does gender count? *J Health Adm Educ*, 14(3), 379–388.

Zanarini, M. C. (2000). Childhood experiences associated with the development of borderline personality disorder. *Psychiatr Clin North Am*, 23(1), 89–101.

Zanarini, M. C., Frankenburg, F. R., Reich, D. B., & Fitzmaurice, G. (2010). Time to attainment of recovery from borderline personality disorder and stability of recovery: a 10-year prospective follow-up study. *Am J Psychiatry*, 167(6), 663–667.

Zanarini, M. C., Frankenburg, F. R., Reich, D. B., & Fitzmaurice, G. (2012). Attainment and stability of sustained symptomatic remission and recovery among patients with borderline personality disorder and axis II comparison subjects: a 16-year prospective follow-up study. *Am J Psychiatry*, 169(5), 476–483.

Zanarini, M. C., Frankenburg, F. R., Reich, D. B., Silk, K. R., Hudson, J. I., & McSweeney, L. B. (2007). The subsyndromal phenomenology of borderline personality disorder: a 10-year follow-up study. *Am J Psychiatry*, 164(6), 929–935.

Zanarini, M. C., Horwood, J., Wolke, D., Waylen, A., Fitzmaurice, G., & Grant, B. F. (2011). Prevalence of DSM-IV borderline personality disorder in two community samples: 6,330 English 11-year-olds and 34,653 American adults. *J Pers Disord*, 25(5), 607–619.

Zanarini, M. C., Yong, L., Frankenburg, F. R., Hennen, J., Reich, D. B., Marino, M. F., & Vujanovic, A. A. (2002). Severity of reported childhood sexual abuse and its relationship to severity of borderline psychopathology and psychosocial impairment among borderline inpatients. *J Nerv Ment Dis*, 190(6), 381–387.

Zimmerman, M., Chelminski, I., & Young, D. (2008). The frequency of personality disorders in psychiatric patients. *Psychiatr Clin North Am*, 31(3), 405–420.

Zimmerman, M., Chelminski, I., Young, D., Dalrymple, K., & Martinez, J. (2012). Does the presence of one feature of borderline personality disorder have clinical significance? Implications for dimensional ratings of personality disorders. *J Clin Psychiatry*, 73(1), 8–12.

Zlotnick, C., Rothschild, L., & Zimmerman, M. (2002). The role of gender in the clinical presentation of patients with borderline personality disorder. *J Pers Disord*, 16(3), 277–282.

Chapter

13

Women offenders and mental health

Sandra Flynn, Naomi Humber, Annie Bartlett and Jenny Shaw

Which women offend?

Women constitute half the population but only a small number break the law (Kong and AuCoin, 2008; Ministry of Justice, 2012a; Sipes, 2012). Women account for 5% of the prison population in England and Wales. In March 2013, 3,860 of 3,869 (99%) women in prison were aged over 18 (Ministry of Justice, 2013a) and 23% were from Black and Minority Ethnic groups, a significant overrepresentation compared to the general population. Before entering prison custody, 28% of women were living with a partner (HM Chief Inspector of Prisons for England and Wales, 2011).

What are the rates of offending among women?

In many countries worldwide the women's prison population rate is increasing faster than for men (Walmsley, 2012). In England and Wales the number of women in prison increased by 85% between 1996 and 2011 (Ministry of Justice, 2012b) and in the United States between 1990 and 2009 the number increased by 153% (Glaze, 2009). Worldwide, women constitute between 2% and 9% of the prison population (Walmsley, 2012), 5% in England and Wales in 2012. A greater number were serving short sentences of 12 months or less (21% women compared with 10% of men). In 2011 a greater proportion of women than men who were sentenced for an indictable offense had no previous cautions or convictions (15% compared to 9%).

The nature and seriousness of criminal offenses by women have remained relatively stable over time (Medlicott, 2007). The Ministry of Justice (2012a) reported figures for women in the criminal justice system between 2006 and 2011. Women consistently accounted for between 13% and 18% of adult arrests.

In each year, the most common offense group, in approximately a third of arrestees, was violence against the person (most of which were minor assaults) followed by theft and handling stolen goods (29%) (Ministry of Justice, 2012a).

In 2011, women comprised 24% of court disposals and criminal court proceedings, a rise of 3% from 2007. Of the 14,200 women tried at Crown Court in 2011, 20% received a custodial sentence and 10% a community sentence (Table 13.1). Men were more likely to re-offend at 1-year follow up (29% versus 19%). After leaving prison, 51% of women were reconvicted within 1 year and for those serving sentences of less than 12 months this increased to 62% (Ministry of Justice, 2011a).

What distinguishes women offenders from men?

There are several criminogenic factors common to both men and women including antisocial attitudes, weak social ties and identification with criminal/antisocial models, dependency on alcohol and drugs, social and economic adversity such as unemployment or family breakdown, and poor cognitive skills and abilities (Bonta et al., 1995; Gelsthorpe and Morris, 2002). However, it has been suggested that there are significant differences between men and women in terms of the types of offenses, the context in which the offenses occurred and the women's past history and experiences (Hannah-Moffat, 1999). It is widely recognized that compared to male offenders, women often have different personal pathways and histories to men (Bloom, Owen and Covington, 2005; Hooper, 2003; McIvor, 2004; Ministry of Justice, 2009; Ministry of Justice, 2012c; Rumgay, 2004). Women offenders have commonly experienced stressful life events including

Comprehensive Women's Mental Health, ed. David J. Castle and Kathryn M. Abel. Published by Cambridge University Press.
© Cambridge University Press 2016.

Table 13.1 Key statistics of women prisoners

Characteristics	%
Women in the prison population	5%
Demographic characteristics of women prisoners	
Age group[1]:	
15–17 years	<1%
18–20 years	5%
21+ years	95%
Black and minority ethnic group	23%
Living with partner prior to prison[2]	28%
Dependent children <18 years[7]	66%
Dependent children between 5 and 10 years[7]	40%
Dependent children <5 years[7]	34%
Clinical characteristics of women prisoners	
Lifetime history of attempted suicide[4]	37%
Psychiatric diagnoses:	
Severe and enduring mental illness[3]	51%
Major depressive disorder[3]	47%
Psychosis[3]	6%
Schizophrenia[3]	3%
Offense type of women prisoners:[6]	
Violence against the person	27%
Theft and handling	13%
Drug offenses	21%
Sexual offenses	2%
Prison sentence length for women:[5]	
≤ 6 months	61%
> 6 months and < 12 months	10%
12 months to < 4 years	22%
4 years or more (excluding indeterminate)	4%
Fine defaulter	2%
Indeterminate	<1%
Women prisoners: no previous convictions[5]	28%
Court outcomes for women offenders:[6]	
Women tried at Crown Court in 2011 (N=14,200):	
Received a custodial sentence	20%
Received a community sentence	10%
Received a suspended sentence	8%
Received a fine	5%

[1]Ministry of Justice (2013a) Offender Management Statistics Quarterly. March 31, 2013. www.gov.uk/government/publications/offender-management-statistics-quarterly-2
[2]HM Chief Inspector of Prisons for England and Wales (2011). Annual Report 2010/2011. London: The Stationary Office.
[3]The Offender Health Research Network (2009) A National Evaluation of Prison In-Reach Services: a report to the National Institute of Health Research. Manchester: The University of Manchester. www.ohrn.nhs.uk/resource/Research/Inreach.pdf.

[4]Home Office (2007) The Corston Report: a report by Baroness Jean Corston of a review of women with particular vulnerabilities in the criminal justice system. March 2007. London: Home Office.
[5]Ministry of Justice (2010) Table 2.1c Offender Management Caseload Statistics 2010. London: Ministry of Justice.
[6]Ministry of Justice (2012a) Statistics on Women and the Criminal Justice System: A Ministry of Justice publication under Section 95 of the Criminal Justice Act 1991, November 2012. London: Ministry of Justice.
[7]Home Office Research Study 208, cited in Prison Reform Trust (2007) Bromley Briefings Prison Factfile December 2007. London: Prison Reform Trust.

childhood abuse (Home Office, 2007). They have high rates of substance abuse, traumatic histories of victimization, damaged social networks, detached family relationships and parenting problems (Alexander, 1996; Borrill et al. 2003; McDaniels-Wilson and Belknap, 2008; Teplin et al., 1996). The causal pathways between these factors and offending are unclear.

Vulnerable background

In 2007, the Corston review of vulnerable women in the criminal justice system commissioned by the Home Secretary reported three categories of vulnerabilities for women:

- domestic circumstances and problems, such as domestic violence, childcare and being a single parent;
- personal circumstances such as mental illness, low self-esteem, eating disorders and substance misuse;
- socioeconomic factors such as unemployment, poverty and isolation (Home Office, 2007).

In the UK, 53% of women and 27% of male prisoners reported experiencing emotional, physical or sexual abuse as a child (Ministry of Justice, 2012c). Over half the women in prison custody reported having experienced domestic violence (Howard League for Penal Reform, 2006; Social Exclusion Unit, 2002). Compared to nearly a quarter of male prisoners nearly one-third of women prisoners report to having been in local authority care as a child (Ministry of Justice, 2012c). In the prison population, 89% of men and 84% of women left school at or before the age of 16 years (Singleton et al, 1998).

History of mental illness

Compared to women in the general population, women in prison custody are five times more likely to have mental health problems with 78% demonstrating psychological disturbance on reception into prison (Plugge et al., 2006). They have higher rates of mental health problems than men. Thus, 30% of women have been a psychiatric in-patient prior to prison compared to 10% of men (Department of Health, 2007), and 25% having been treated/counseled for a mental health or emotional problem in the year prior to custody, compared to 16% of men (Cabinet Office Social Exclusion Task Force, 2009). Regarding diagnosis, 50% had a personality disorder, 66% neurotic disorder and 14% functional psychosis (Singleton et al., 1998). There is also a high prevalence of comorbidity, with 83% of women remand prisoners and 70% of women sentenced prisoners having two or more mental disorders (ONS, 1997). The Cabinet Office Social Exclusion Task Force (2009) reported that 51% of women sent to prison have severe and enduring mental illness.

History of substance dependence/misuse

In the year prior to prison, 44% of women prisoners reported drug dependence, and 34% hazardous drinking (ONS, 1997). Compared to men, women prisoners were more likely to be dependent on opiates (ONS, 1997). Whilst in prison, 27% had used heroin and 9% crack cocaine. Light, Grant and Hopkins (2013) in a sample comprising 1,303 male and 132 women sentenced prisoners found that women prisoners reported more Class A drug use in the 4 weeks prior to custody than male prisoners and were more likely to report that their offending was supporting both theirs and someone else's drug use.

Self-harm and suicide

In 2011, the Ministry of Justice (2011b) reported a total of 24,648 incidents of self-harm in prisons with 6,854 prisoners recorded as having self-harmed. The self-harm rate in women was 10 times higher than for men. The rate was 2,104 incidents per 1,000 women prisoners and 194 per 1,000 male prisoners. Women account for approximately 47% of all incidents of self-harm despite representing only 5% of the total prisoner population. Repeated self-harm impacts on this comparison as women who self-harmed in 2011 did so more often than men with an average of 7.1 compared with 2.8 incidents per person (Ministry of Justice, 2013b). Across the 5-year period studied by the Ministry of Justice between 2007 and 2011, there were 329

self-inflicted deaths with 15 (5%) involving women, reflecting the representation of women in the general prison population. Compared to the general population, women recently released from prison are 36 times more likely to take their own life, compared to men who are 8 times more likely (Pratt et al. 2006).

Domestic circumstances and needs

Two-thirds of women in prison have dependent children less than 18 years old and of those women, a third have children under 5 (Home Office, 2003). At least one-third of mothers are lone parents prior to imprisonment (Social Exclusion Unit, 2002). It is estimated that more than 17,700 children each year are separated from their mother by imprisonment (Home Office, 2003). Women are more likely than men to say that getting support from their family would help to stop their recidivism (51% versus 39% respectively) (Ministry of Justice, 2012c).

Women and violence

In 2009, a third of all women arrested were detained for violence against the person (34%), similar to the proportion for men (31%) (Ministry of Justice, 2010). The same proportion of girls (<17 years) are recorded as having an act of violence as their first offense, and violence was the most common offense group among juvenile females. However, in terms of actual numbers, compared to men, women rarely commit violent crime (United Nations, 2000). The gender gap is greatest for serious crime such as homicide, with women comprising 11% of homicide perpetrators (ONS, 2013).

There has been increased interest in "violent women" in recent years, with the majority of studies focused on homicide committed by women in a domestic setting, more specifically in the context of intimate partner violence or child abuse and maltreatment. Few studies have been undertaken on nationally representative samples. Consequently, robust generalizable data on the circumstances and risk factors for serious violence by women is limited. Notable exceptions to this were studies by Eronen (1995) and Putkonen et al. (1998), which analyzed national register data in Finland; and a recent study by Flynn et al. (2011) reporting data from a national population of homicide offenders in England and Wales. Factors associated with violent behavior have been identified as self-defense, retaliatory violence, alcohol and drug misuse (Table 13.2), a history of violent behavior, delinquency and criminality,

Table 13.2 Substance use prior to homicide in women offenders

Study	Sample of women who commit homicide	Substance use
Flynn et al., 2011	England and Wales N=446	45% history of alcohol misuse 37% history of drug misuse
Goetting, 1988	Detroit, Michigan N=136	35.3% of women offenders had been drinking before the homicide
Mann, 1996	6 cities in the USA N=296	36.2% of women had been drinking before the offense
Sprunt et al., 1996	New York, USA N=215	70% history of drug misuse, a third were intoxicated at the time of the offense

and antisocial personality disorder (Dasguta, 1999; Moffitt et al, 2001; Graham-Kevan and Archer, 2005; Weizmann-Henelius et al. 2003).

Who are the victims?

The relationship between violent women offenders and their victims follows a different pattern to men. Violence by women is commonly characterized by interpersonal conflicts. The evidence suggests that the victims of homicide perpetrated by women are more likely to be close family members (Cooper and Smith, 2011; Flynn et al., 2011; Hakkanen-Nyholm et al., 2009). Findings from Flynn et al. (2011) for England and Wales have shown that the victims of women convicted of homicide were overwhelmingly immediate family members, either a spouse/partner/ex-spouse partner (36%) or a son or daughter (19%).

Intimate partners

There is a large body of research examining intimate partner homicide. The evidence suggests a substantial proportion of women who killed a partner had previously been subjected to intimate partner violence (Websdale, 1999). "Battered person syndrome" was first used as a legal defense for an act of homicide in the 1970s. It is now a recognized diagnosis in both the *International Classification of Disease 10th Revision* (code 995.81; WHO, 1993) and the *Diagnostic and Statistical Manual of Mental Disorders, 4th Edition* (DSM-IV; APA, 1994) as a form of post-traumatic stress. The association between gender-based violence and mental illness was recently shown by Rees et al. (2011).

Children

The definition of filicide is the killing of one's own son or daughter and includes infanticide (the killing of an infant within 12 months of birth) and neonaticide (the killing of a newborn less than 24 hours old). Contributions to our knowledge and understanding of filicide come from two main fields of inquiry: (1) perpetrator-centered research focusing on situational factors, motivation and parental mental illness and; (2) victim-focused research on the ecology of the family, child abuse and maltreatment and child protection issues (Chistoffel, 1984; Wilcznski, 1997). The findings from previous research on filicide have been remarkably consistent internationally. Flynn et al. (2013), in a study of 297 filicides in England and Wales, reported that men more commonly killed their own child (ratio of 2:1). Over half of the victims were infants (51%). Mental illness was found to be a common feature of maternal filicide and infant homicide (Flynn et al., 2007); 40% of the women who killed their child had a longstanding history of mental health problems, 53% had symptoms of mental illness at the time of offense. Depression was noted as the most common diagnosis.

Mental illness in women who commit homicide

The association between violence and mental illness has been the focus of much academic and clinical research. In a recent study of serious violence in England and Wales over a 12-month period, Flynn et al. (2013) found 8% of serious violent offenses in the general population were committed by women and 10% of these women had been recently under the care of mental health services. That study was based on a national sample, but other research has been undertaken in specific populations. For example, findings of Monahan et al. (2001) from the MacArthur Risk Assessment Study on violence by patients following discharge from psychiatric hospitals found no overall significant difference in offending by gender. However, when specific diagnoses were examined, Fazel and Grann (2006) revealed that compared to men, women with psychosis had a greater attributable risk of violence in all age groups. Serious mental illness has been shown to be an important feature in homicides by women. Flynn et al. (2011) showed 28% of women compared with 20% of men had symptoms of mental illness at the time of offense and half had a prior history of mental disorder compared to less than a third of men (50% vs. 30%).

It has been argued that research relying on pretrial forensic evaluations of the perpetrator as the main measure of mental illness can be subject to bias and potentially overestimate mental illness in female offenders (Eronen, 1995; Nielssen, 2007; Schanda et al., 2004). Consequently, there is evidence to suggest a leniency towards women. Although there is evidence to support potential bias, particularly in sentencing (Hoyt and Scherer, 1998; Flynn et al., 2011), it is difficult to prove due to numerous confounders that may influence the judicial outcomes. The clinical differences between men and women with mental illness committing violent acts may be moderate but this does warrant further research to ensure women are receiving services that are appropriate to their needs.

Systems of care for women offenders

The system of care for women offenders is constantly changing. Sexual segregation was introduced into prisons by the middle of the nineteenth century doing much to reduce prison pregnancy and the exploitation of vulnerable women incarcerated alongside men (Zedner, 1998). This was echoed in the first provision of secure hospital care for women in the UK in 1860. The current, interconnected system of care, treatment, supervision and punishment is designed to ensure that women who offend are correctly placed in terms of the gravity of their actions, the presence of treatable mental disorders and the need for supervision, in order to protect the public and to prevent re-offending. The particular roles of health, social care and criminal justice agencies are both specific and different (Bartlett and Kesteven, 2009), but in practice much more similar than many practitioners might wish to admit.

Currently there are only about 50 women in high secure hospital care and 1,314 in enhanced medium, medium and low secure care in the UK (Bartlett et al., 2014b). These units undertake assessments and treatment of women with and without criminal convictions who are thought to require secure hospital environments. A small proportion of women remanded to prison are transferred to hospital care under the 1983 Mental Health Act (revised 2007). Both the National Health Service (NHS) and the Independent Sector health care providers have secure hospital beds and undertake prison health care, now commissioned by NHS England, in line with the changes in the Health and Social Care Act (2012). Third-sector providers also have roles in liaison and diversion schemes whose intention is both to avoid unnecessary remands in custody, particularly of women with major mental illness, and also to foster rehabilitation and prevent family disruption.

Ways of understanding the needs of women offenders

There is no single agreed way to conceptualize the needs of women offenders. There are a number of cogent frameworks evident in clinical work, research, policy initiatives and in funding for service innovation. These include:

- Epidemiological studies based on diagnostic categories
- Trauma-informed formulations
- Personality disorder (diagnosed or inferred)
- Complex needs

None of the frameworks considered here are exclusive but there is considerable work to be done to establish a shared understanding across and within agencies with responsibility for women offenders.

Epidemiological studies (e.g., Coid et al., 2000; O'Brien et al., 2003) have tended to rely on psychiatric diagnostic systems based on standardized assessments and, where possible, large-scale projects. These have generated a comprehensive account of the psychiatric problems of women in prison and to some extent in secure hospital care, but are limited by using gender-blind approaches. Studies on self-harm in women and suicide in both prisons and hospitals (Marzano et al., 2010; Shaw et al., 2004) have been revealing, and environments and practice have changed in women's prisons in response to concerns about preventable deaths (NOMS, 2013).

Trauma-informed formulation both of individual women and of the environments in which they live have influenced policy in this area and led to specific interventions (Covington, 1998; Najavits et al., 1998). This discourse highlights the impact in adult life of earlier sexual and physical abuse and creates a narrative for individual women to understand adult problems, particularly repetitive self-harm and pseudo-hallucinatory voices. It allows practitioners in both custodial and clinical environments to grasp that systems of care and supervision (e.g., male staff, restraint) can echo, inadvertently, unwanted earlier experiences of disempowerment and coercion, especially by men (Heney and Kristiansen, 1997; Henderson et al., 1998, Aitken and Logan, 2004; Benda et al., 2005). The fact that many women offenders have involvement in sex work and are further abused as adults (see US prison literature on this especially) reinforces the relevance of this approach.

There has been a range of policy and practice initiatives in the field of Personality Disorder (PD) since 1999. The impetus behind the Dangerous and Severe Personality Disorder (DSPD) programme (Eastman, 1999) was the management of mainly male violence and the only tangible outcome for women was the creation of the Low Newton 12 bedded DSPD unit. Changes in the direction of policy and the funding of initiatives by government have meant that there is now an offender PD strategy for women (Department of Health/NOMS, 2011). The epidemiology established that patterns of PD in male and women offenders are different and that Emotionally Unstable Personality Disorder (Singleton et al., 1998), for which the evidence base for treatment is slightly stronger, is more common in women. The direction of policy is not to deliver treatment per se, but to promote interventions and practical support and enhanced understanding within the Criminal Justice System (rather than in the health sector) for those likely to have a PD. National Offender Management Service (NOMS) commissions a range of providers to undertake this work including, but far from exclusively, health providers. "PD: no longer a diagnosis of exclusion" (Department of Health, 2003) does not seem to have led to comprehensive PD services in the community and a range of nonhealth providers are responding with innovative provision of services (e.g., Women in Prison).

There is no accepted definition of the term "complex needs." In practice, it appears to have become shorthand for multiple health and social care, gender-specific needs (children and separation, the avoidance of cycles of deprivation and the management of disrupted attachments) in women offenders. A formulation of complete needs incorporates social roles as well as psychological issues and has a practical focus on accommodation, training and educational opportunities.

In the UK, there is a large gap in conceptual frameworks around drug and alcohol problems. Both are very common in women offenders, in hospital and prison populations, often in combination with other difficulties (Bland et al., 1999; Coid et al., 2000; Singleton et al., 1998; O'Brien et al., 2003; Abram et al., 2003). The separate commissioning structure in substance misuse services, including in prison, could be argued to have impaired a comprehensive, gendered understanding of women's use of legal and illegal substances in the UK. Detoxification services and psychosocial programs focus on the addiction itself, rather than the person with the addiction and have protocol driven approaches. Within prisons, until recently, psychosocial programs neglected alcohol in favor of street drugs. Therefore, the reasons why women use alcohol and drugs, their patterns of use and the links with trauma and mental health problems can be poorly operationalized in clinical practice, despite a robust evidence base in the United States (Peugh and Belenko 1999; McCellan et al. 1997). This undermines a coherent understanding of the reasons for abuse/dependence and also the consequences in terms of well-being (Chapter 15).

These competing but overlapping frameworks may provide a degree of flexibility in terms of models of care but risk leaving frontline practitioners at sea and talking past each other. Multiple reviews of women offenders have made recommendations for treatment (Henderson, 1998; Baletka and Shearer, 2001; Nicholls et al., 2001). However, treatment based on these concepts has been poorly anchored by evidence of efficacy per se or of cost effectiveness; this is curious given the size of the populations and the cost of institutional rather than community care and supervision.

Evidence that treatment and interventions work?

There is, therefore, a sense of despondency in some writing about women offenders. Authors note repeatedly the absence of interventions in situ (Covington, 1998; Ford et al., 2013) as well as the lack of an evidence base for efficacy (Bartlett, 2001, 2007; Nee and Farman, 2007; Drapalski et al., 2009).

Possible frameworks of evaluation would include: mental health outcome measures, length of stay required for change, quality of life, re-offending rates and community survival. Where possible these would use similar tools of measurement to maximize useful cross-referencing. This would inform commissioners about cost-effective care and improve the chances of sustainable effective services being provided. Patient generated measures have been strikingly absent from the evaluations that do exist but would warrant a place in contemporary research (Bartlett et al., 2014c).

Bartlett (2001) reviewed the evidence base for treatment studies in secure settings and found sparse information on women leaving secure hospital care and those women who had received care and treatment in medium and high secure care had contested its value at the same time as it being far from clear what was delivered to them. The exception to the general statement about poor evaluation was in the US prison system where treatment initiatives directed at trauma symptoms and substance misuse were showing promising findings.

These observations remained largely true 6 years later (Bartlett, 2007) compounded in the UK by a recognition that even the size of the secure hospital population of women in the UK was unknown at that time and needed mapping. Currently, the psychiatric epidemiology of the women prison population is seriously out of date as the last major study was over 15 years ago. This creates real difficulty in designing services and evaluating interventions.

Interventions in secure hospitals

Existing descriptions of the women secure population indicate diagnostic heterogeneity (Coid et al. 2000; Bartlett et al., 2007) with high proportions of the women having multiple diagnoses (Bartlett et al., 2014b).

Long is conspicuous in the UK in articulating a model of gender sensitive care (Long et al., 2008) and delineating and assessing hospital interventions in a modest-sized cohort (Long et al., 2010, 2011a, 2011b, 2012, 2013). Hitherto the treatment offered has been poorly described and change, whilst discharge and

community survival had not been attributable to specified interventions. Evidence from this cohort suggests that group interventions within secure services reduce symptoms of anxiety and suicidality, that treatment engagement reduces risk and that short length of stay is associated with treatment completion. Noncompletion of interventions is common and has economic as well as individual health implications.

Nee and Farman (2007) reviewed dialectic behavioral therapy (DBT) in hospital settings noting encouraging results in terms of reductions in self-harm and psychiatric symptoms in low and high secure inpatient and outpatient settings. Barr et al. (2013) examined the usefulness of high support housing after discharge for women in secure hospital care, finding it to be linked to improvements in psychological health, without increased risk.

These recent findings are important given that traditionally women have had longer lengths of stay than men in high secure care (Butwell et al., 2000) and have been more likely to be readmitted to medium secure hospital care (Coid et al., 2000). Maden et al. (2004, 2006) followed up women from secure hospital care (who were markedly different from men also discharged) and found they had a reconviction rate of 9% at 1 year, less than the rate for men (16%).

Interventions in prison

The paucity of robust empirical research on the expensive secure hospital population of women sits in some contrast to the larger, although still inconclusive body of work conducted in prison. Almost without exception, this work is conducted outside of the UK and so its importance for the UK is debatable. Much is pilot or small-scale research. Programs that ostensibly target one problem can also be seen to have more widespread benefits. Key outcome measures include recidivism but are not restricted to this.

Substance misuse programmes show an impact on re-offending (Dowden and Blanchette, 2002) better compliance if women remained in contact with their children (Nishimoto and Roberts, 2001) and desistance if women were moved away from their home area (Strauss and Falkin, 2001). Drapalski et al. (2009) noted greater help seeking in women in prison, not least because they sought help with traumatic sequelae. Staton-Tindall et al. (2009) noted that some gender-specific aspects of previous community treatment have potential implications for treatment success in prison.

Trauma programs, which can include substance misuse work, resulted in fewer symptoms of post-traumatic stress disorder (Valentine, 2000; Valentine and Smith, 2001; Zlotnick et al., 2003) in some early studies but negative findings have also been reported (e.g., Bradley and Follingstad, 2003). Messina et al. (2010) took a trauma-informed approach to intervention with substance misuse women in prison. In a randomized trial comparing the gender-responsive treatment (GRT) to a therapeutic community, GRT produced better integration into aftercare, less re-incarceration and greater reduction in drug use. Ford et al. (2013), reviewing this body of work, argued that it was hard to specify what was responsible for the mixed results. Nee and Farnam (2005) evaluated DBT with 30 prisoners. Despite a high attrition rate completers did better than noncompleters and controls. In a pilot study in a UK women's prison, Gee and Reed (2013) found modified DBT to be helpful in producing fewer incidents warranting adjudication, less use of self-harm management processes in prison and improved mental health. Gussak (2009) evaluated art therapy with male and women prison inmates and found reductions in depression and improved locus of control after a period of group treatment.

Interventions in the community

The population statistics would suggest this is a key area of intervention. However, by comparison with both prisons and secure hospitals, the evidence base for work with women offenders in the community is even more limited. Jolliffe et al. (2011) reviewed the impact of women's centers and found equivocal support for this new area of investment which is currently subject to transformation and further scrutiny (NOMS, 2013a). Unknown numbers of women in the UK are under the care of community forensic health provision. Van den Bosch (2012) notes the relevance of mainstream treatments for this group.

In sum, there is a need to capitalize on programs of intervention and scale up studies to provide an evidence base that would allow for specification in national services and for individuals to have some degree of personal choice in what would help them.

Future developments

Recent interest in women offenders has improved understanding of both their criminality and associated health and social care needs. It is clear that women are less likely than men to have contact with the criminal justice system and that they will rarely be involved in serious violent offending. However, their involvement is routinely complicated by profound health and social care difficulties, which demand a response from relevant criminal justice and other agencies that includes a gender dimension. In the UK and elsewhere a range of agencies has been developed to meet these needs but until recently there was little evidence to support one intervention rather than another. In the UK, hospital or prison-based services have routinely lacked a theoretically driven approach to care. Encouraging findings for trauma-informed interventions, work on substance misuse and more detailed articulation of some secure hospital programs all need pursuing. A conspicuous gap, which stands out in terms of population statistics, is work with women offenders in the community, where most reside, most of the time.

References

Abram, K. M., Teplin, L.A. and McClelland, G. M. 2003. Co-morbidity of severe psychiatric disorders and substance use disorders among women in jail, *American Journal of Psychiatry* 160(5): 1007–1010.

Aitken, G. and Logan, C. 2004. Dangerous women? A UK response, *Feminism & Psychology* 14(2): 262–267.

Alexander, M. J. 1996. Women with co-occurring addictive and mental disorders: An emerging profile of vulnerability, *American Journal of Orthopsychiatry*, 66(1): 61–70.

American Psychiatric Association 1994. *Diagnostic and Statistical Manual of Mental Disorder, Fourth Edition*. Washington, DC: American Psychiatric Association.

Baletka, D. M. and Shearer, R. A. 2001. Counselling female offenders who abuse substances, *TCA Journal* 29(2): 140–148.

Barr, W., Brown, A., Quinn, B., Mcfarlane, J., Mccabe, R. and Whittington, R. 2013. How effective is high-support community-based step-down housing for women in secure mental health care? A quasi-experimental pilot study, *Journal of Psychiatric & Mental Health Nursing* 20:41–49.

Bartlett, A. 2001. *NHS Expert Paper: Women. National Programme on Forensic Mental Health Research and Development*, University of Liverpool.

Bartlett, A. 2007. *Expert Paper. Social Difference and Division: Women NHS National Programme on Forensic Mental Health Research and Development*. www.nfmhp.org.uk/expert paper.htm.

Bartlett, A., Johns, A., Jhawar, H. and Fiander, M. 2007. *Report of the London Forensic Units Benchmarking Project*.

Bartlett, A. and Kesteven, S. 2009. 'Organisational and Conceptual Frameworks and the Mentally Disordered Offender', in Bartlett and McGauley (eds.), pp. 327–338, *Forensic Mental Health: Concepts, Systems and Practice*. Oxford: Oxford University Press.

Bartlett, A., Abel, K. M. Walker, T. and Harty, M. 2014a. Health & social care services for women offenders: Current provision and a future model of care, *The Journal of Forensic Psychiatry & Psychology*, doi:10.1080/14789949.2014.944202.

Bartlett, A., Somers, N., Fiander, M. and Harty, M. 2014b Pathways of care for women in secure hospital: Which women go where and why?, *British Journal of Psychiatry* 205:298–306. doi: 10.1192/bjp.bp.113.137547.

Bartlett, A., Walker, T., Harty, M. A. & Abel, K. M. 2014c. Health and social care services for women offenders: current provision and a future model of care, *The Journal of Forensic Psychiatry & Psychology*, doi: 10.1080/14789949.2014.944202.

Benda, B. B, Harm, N. J. and Toombs, N. J. 2005. 'Survival Analysis of Male and Female Boot Camp Graduates Using Life Course Theory', in Benda and Pallone (eds.) *Rehabilitation Issues, Problems, and Prospects in Boot Camp*. New York, NY: Haworth Press.

Bland, J., Mezey, G. & Dolan, B. 1999. Special women, special needs:

a descriptive study of female special hospital patients, *The Journal of Forensic Psychiatry* 10(1), 34–45.

Bloom, B., Owen, B. and Covington, S. 2005. *A Summary of Research, Practice, and Guiding Principles for Women Offenders. The Gender-Responsive Strategies Project: Approach and Findings*. Washington, DC: National Institute of Corrections.

Bonta, J., Pang, B. and Wallace-Capretta, S. (1995). Predictors of recidivism among incarcerated female offenders, *The Prison Journal* 75(3): 277–295.

Borrill, J., Maden, A., Martin, A., Weaver, T., Stimson, G., Farrell, M. and Barnes, T. 2003. *Differential substance misuse treatment needs of women, ethnic minorities and young offenders in prison: prevalence of substance misuse and treatment needs (Home Office Online Report 33/03)*. London: Home Office Research, Development and Statistics Directorate.

Bradley, R. G. and Follingstad, D. R. 2003. Group therapy for incarcerated women who experienced interpersonal violence: A pilot study, *Journal of Traumatic Stress*, 16(4): 337–340.

Butwell, M., Jamieson, E., Leese, M. and Taylor, P. J. 2000. Trends in special (high-security) hospitals: 2: Residency and discharge episodes, 1986-1995, *British Journal of Psychiatry* 176:260–265.

Cabinet Office Social Exclusion Task Force 2009. *Social Exclusion Task Force. Short Study on Women Offenders*. May 2009. London: Cabinet Office.

Cooper, A. and Smith, E. L. 2011. *US Department of Justice Bureau of Justice Statistics 2011. Homicide Trends in the United States, 1980–2008. Annual Rates for 2009 and 2010*.

Christoffell, K. K. 1984. Homicide in childhood: a public health problem in need of attention, *American Journal of Public Health* 74: 68–70.

Coid, J., Kahtan, N., Gault, S. and Jarman, B. 2000. Women admitted to secure psychiatric facilities: comparison of men and women, *Journal of Forensic Psychiatry* 11(2): 275–295.

Covington, S. S. 1998. Women in prison: approaches in the treatment of our most invisible population, *Women & Therapy* 21(1): 141–155.

Dasguta, S. D. 1999 'Just Like Men? A Critical View of Violence by Women', in Shepard and Pearce (eds.), pp. 195–222, *Coordinating Community Responses to Domestic Violence*. Thousand Oaks, CA: Sage.

Department of Health. 2003. *Personality disorder: no longer a diagnosis of exclusion-policy implementation guidance for the development of services for people with personality disorder*, webarchive.nationalarchives.gov.uk/+/www.dh.gov.uk/en/Publicationsandstatistics/Publications/PublicationsPolicyAndGuidance/DH_4009546 (Accessed 10.03.14).

Department of Health. 2007. *Conference Report, Sharing Good Practice in Prison Health, 4/5 June 2007*. London: Department of Health.

Department of Health /NOMS. 2011. *Offender personality disorder strategy for women*, www.womensbreakout.org.uk/wp-content/uploads/downloads/2012/07/Offender-Personality-Disorder-Strategy-Summary.pdf (Accessed 07.03.14).

Dolan, M. and Vollm, B. 2009. Anti-social personality disorder and psychopathy in women: A literature review on the reliability and validity of assessment instruments, *International Journal of Law and Psychiatry* 32: 2–9.

Dowden, C. and Blanchette, K. 2002. An evaluation of the effectiveness of substance abuse programming for female offenders, *International Journal of Offender Therapy and*

Comparative Criminology 46(2): 220–230.

Drapalski, A. L., Youman, K., Stuewig, J. and Tangney, J. 2009. Gender differences in jail inmates' symptoms of mental illness, treatment history and treatment seeking, *Criminal Behaviour and Mental Health* 19: 193–2006.

Eastman, N. 1999. Public health psychiatry or crime prevention?, *British Medical Journal* 318: 549–551.

Eronen, M. 1995. Mental disorders and homicidal behavior in female subjects, *The American Journal of Psychiatry* 152: 1216–1218.

Fazel, S. and Grann, M. 2006. The population impact of severe mental illness on violent crime, *The American Journal of Psychiatry* 163: 1397–1403.

Flynn, S., Abel, K. M., While, D., Mehta, H. and Shaw, J. 2011. Mental illness, gender and homicide: a population-based descriptive study, *Psychiatric Research* 185:368–375.

Flynn, S., Rodway, C., Appleby, L. and Shaw, J. 2013. Serious violence by people with mental illness: national clinical survey, *Journal of Interpersonal Violence*. doi: 10.1177/ 0886260513507133.

Flynn, S. M., Shaw, J. J. and Abel K. M. 2007. Homicide of infants: a cross-sectional study, *Journal of Clinical Psychiatry* 68: 1501–1509.

Flynn, S. M. , Shaw J. J., and Abel, K. M. 2013. Filicide: mental illness in those who kill their children, *PLoS ONE* 8(4): e58981. doi:10.1371/ journal.pone.0058981.

Ford, J. D., Chang, R., Levine, J. and Zhang, W. 2013. Randomized clinical trial comparing affect regulation and supportive group therapies for victimization-related PTSD with incarcerated women, *Behavior Therapy* 44: 262–276.

Gee, J. and Reed, S. 2013. The HoST programme: A pilot evaluation of modified dialectical behaviour therapy with female offenders diagnosed with borderline personality disorder, *European Journal of Psychotherapy & Counselling*, 1–19.

Gelsthorpe L. and Morris A. 2002. Women's imprisonment in England and Wales: A penal paradox, *Criminal Justice*, 2(3): 277–301.

Glaze, L. E. 2009. *Correctional populations in the United States 2009*, Washington DC: Bureau of Justice Statistics US Department of Justice.

Goetting, A. 1988. Patterns of homicide among women, *Journal of Interpersonal Violence* 3(1): 3–19.

Graham-Kevan, N. and Archer, J. 2005. Investigating three explanations of women's relationship aggression, *Psychology of Women Quarterly* 29(3): 270–277.

Gussak, D. 2009. The effects of art therapy on male and female inmates: Advancing the research base, *Arts in Psychotherapy* 36: 5–12.

Hakkanen-Nyholm, H., Putkonen, H., Lindberg, N., Holi, M., Rovamo, T. and Weizmann-Henelius, G. 2009. Gender differences in Finnish homicide offence characteristics, *Forensic Science International* 186: 75–80.

Hannah-Moffit, K. 1999. Moral agent or actuarial subject: Risk and Canadian women's imprisonment, *Theoretical Criminology* 3:71–94.

Health and Social Care Information Centre. 2012. Inpatients formally detained in hospitals under the Mental Health Act, 1983 and patients subject to supervised community treatment, Annual figures, England, 2011/12, November 2012. www.hscic.gov.uk/ catalogue/PUB08085.

Henderson, D., Schaeffer, J. and Brown, L. 1998. Gender-appropriate mental health services for incarcerated women: Issues and challenges, *Family & Community Health* 21(3): 42–53.

Heney, J. and Kristiansen, C. M. 1997. An analysis of the impact of prison on women survivors of childhood sexual abuse, *Women & Therapy* 20(4): 29–44.

HM Chief Inspector of Prisons for England and Wales. 2011. *Annual Report 2010/2011*. London: The Stationary Office.

Home Office. 2003. Research, Development and Statistics Directorate. *Offending Surveys and Research, National Centre for Social Research and BMRB. Social Research, Offending, Crime and Justice Survey, 2003. 3rd Edition*. Colchester Essex: Home Office.

Home Office. 2007. *The Corston Report: a report by Baroness Jean Corston of a review of women with particular vulnerabilities in the criminal justice system*. March 2007. London: Home Office.

Hooper, C. A. 2003. *Abuse, Interventions and Women in Prison: A Literature Review*. London: Home Office/HM Prison Service.

Howard League for Penal Reform. 2006. *Prison Information Bulletin 2. Women and girls in the penal system*. London: Howard League for Penal Reform.

Hoyt, S. and Scherer, D. G. 1998. Female juvenile delinquency: misunderstood by the juvenile justice system, neglected by social science, *Law and Human Behavior*, 22.81.

Jolliffe, D., Hedderman, C., Palmer, E. and Hollins, C. 2011. Re-offending analysis of women offenders referred to Together Women and the scope to divert from custody. Ministry of Justice Research Series 11/11, www.gov.uk/government/ uploads/system/uploads/ attachment_data/file/217364/ women-offenders-referred-together-women.pdf (Accessed 09.21.15).

Kong, R. and K. AuCoin. 2008. Female offenders in Canada, *Juristat*, 28(1). Statistics Canada Catalogue no. 85-002-X. Ottawa.

Light, M., Grant, E. and Hopkins, K. 2013. *Gender differences in substance misuse and mental health amongst prisoners*. London: Ministry of Justice.

Long, C. G., Dickens, G., Sugarman, P., Craig, L., Mochty, U. and Hollin, C. 2010a. Tracking risk profiles and outcome in a medium secure service for women: Use of the HoNOS-Secure, *International Journal of Forensic Mental Health* 9: 215–225.

Long, C. G., Dolley, O., Barron, R. and Hollin, C. R. 2012. Women transferred from prison to medium-secure psychiatric care: The therapeutic challenge, *Journal of Forensic Psychiatry and Psychology* 23: 261–273.

Long, C. R., Dolley, O. and Hollin, C. 2013. Engagement in psychosocial treatment: its relationship to outcome and care pathway progress for women in medium secure settings, *Criminal Behaviour and Mental Health*, 22:336–349.

Long, C. G., Fulton, B., Fitzgerald, K. A. and Hollin, C. R. 2010b. Group substance abuse treatment for women in secure services, *Mental Health and Substance Use: Dual Diagnosis* 3: 227–237.

Long, C. G., Fulton, B. and Hollin, C. R. 2008. The development of a "Best practice" service for women in a medium secure psychiatric setting: treatment components and evaluation, *Clinical Psychology and Psychotherapy* 15:304–319.

Long, C., Hall, L., Craig, L., Mochty, U. and Hollin, C. R. 2011. Women referred for medium secure inpatient care: a population study over a six-year period, *Journal of Psychiatric Intensive Care* 7: 17–26.

Maden, A., Scott, F., Burnett, R., Lewis, G. L. and Skapinakis, P. 2004. Offending in psychiatric patients after discharge from medium secure units: Prospective National Cohort Study, *British Medical Journal* 328:1534.

Maden, A., Skapinakis, P., Lewis, G., Scott, F. and Jamieson, E. 2006.

Gender differences in reoffending after discharge from medium-secure units. National cohort study in England and Wales, *British Journal of Psychiatry* 189, 168–72.

Mann, C. R. 1996. *When Women Kill*. New York, State University of New York Press.

Marzano, L., Fazel, S., Rivlin, A. and Hawton, K. 2010. Psychiatric disorders in women prisoners who have engaged in near-lethal self-harm: case–control study, *British Journal of Psychiatry* 197: 219–226.

McCellan D. S., Farabee, D. and Crouch, B. M. 1997. Early victimisation, drug use and criminality: a comparison of male and female prisoners, *Criminal Justice and Behaviour* 24(4): 455–476.

McDaniels-Wilson, C. and Belknap, J. 2008. The extensive sexual violation and sexual abuse histories of incarcerated women. *Violence Against Women* 14: 1090–1127.

McIvor, G. 2004. 'Service with a Smile? Women and Community Punishment', in McIvor (ed.) *Women who Offend*, pp. 126–41. London: Jessica Kingsley.

Medlicott, D. 2007. 'Women in prison' in Jewkes (ed.), *Handbook on Prisons*. Devon: Willan Publishing, 245–267.

Mental Health Act (MHA) (1983 as amended 2007). Accessed October 23, 2013 from www.legislation.gov .uk/ukpga/1983/20/contents.

Messina, N., Grella, C. E., Cartier, J. and Torres, S. 2010. A randomized experimental study of gender-responsive substance abuse treatment for women in prison, *Journal of substance abuse treatment* 38(2):97–107.

Ministry of Justice. 2009. *Offender Management Caseload Statistics 2009: an overview of the main findings*. London: Ministry of Justice Statistics Bulletin.

Ministry of Justice. 2010. *Table 2.1c Offender Management Caseload*

Statistics 2010, London: Ministry of Justice.

Ministry of Justice. 2011a *Proven Reoffending Statistics Quarterly Bulletin January to December 2009, England and Wales*. London: Ministry of Justice.

Ministry of Justice. 2011b. *Safety in Custody 2010 England and Wales. Statistics Bulletin July 2010*. London: Ministry of Justice.

Ministry of Justice. 2012a. *Statistics on Women and the Criminal Justice System: A Ministry of Justice publication under Section 95 of the Criminal Justice Act 1991, November 2012*. London: Ministry of Justice.

Ministry of Justice. 2012b. *Annual tables – Offender management caseload statistics 2011 tables. Prison Population Tables*. London: Ministry of Justice.

Ministry of Justice. 2012c. *Prisoners' childhood and family backgrounds. Ministry of Justice Research Series 4/ 12 March 2012*. London: Ministry of Justice.

Ministry of Justice. 2013a. *Offender Management Statistics Quarterly*. March 31, 2013. https://www.gov .uk/government/publications/ offender-management-statistics- quarterly–2.

Ministry of Justice. 2013b. *Safety in Custody Statistics England and Wales update to December 2012. Ministry of Justice Statistics Bulletin. April 25, 2013*. London: Ministry of Justice.

Moffitt, T. E., Caspi, A., Rutter, M. and Silva, P. A. 2001. *Sex differences in antisocial behaviour: Conduct disorder, delinquency and violence in the Dunedin longitudinal study*, New York: Cambridge University Press.

Monahan, J., Steadman, H. J., Silver, E., Applebaum, P., Robbins, P., Mulvey, E., Roth L., Grisso, T. and Banks, S. 2001. *Rethinking risk assessment: The MacArthur Study of Mental Disorder and Violence*. New York: Oxford University Press.

Najavits, L. M., Weiss, R. D., Shaw, S. R. and Muenz, L. 1998. "Seeking Safety" outcome of a new cognitive behavioural psychotherapy for women with post traumatic stress disorder and substance dependence, *Journal of Traumatic Stress* 11: 437–456.

Nee, C. and Farman, S. 2005. Female prisoners with borderline personality disorder: some promising treatment developments, *Criminal Behaviour and Mental Health* 15(1): 2–16.

Nee, C. and Farman, S. 2007. Dialectical behaviour therapy as a treatment for borderline personality disorder in prisons: three illustrative case studies. *Journal of Forensic Psychiatry and Psychology* 18:160–180.

Nicholls, T. L., Hemphill, J. F., Boer, D. P., Kropp, P., Randall, Z. and Patricia, A. 2001. 'The Assessment and Treatment of Offenders and Inmates: Specific Populations', in Schuller and Ogloff (eds.) pp. 248–262, *Introduction to Psychology and Law: Canadian Perspectives*. Toronto: University of Toronto Press.

Nielsson, O. B., Westmore, B. D. Large, M.M.B. and Hayes, R. A. 2007. Homicide during psychotic illness in New South Wales between 1993 and 2002, *Med J Aust*, 186(6):301–304.

Nishimoto, R. H., and Roberts, A. C. 2001. Coercion and drug treatment for postpartum women. *The American Journal of Drug and Alcohol Abuse* 27.1: 161–181.

NOMS. 2013. Management of prisoners at risk of harm to self, to others and from others (Safer Custody) PSI 64/2011 Ministry of Justice. www.justice.gov.uk/downloads/offenders/psipso/psi-2011/psi-64-2011-safer-custody.doc (Accessed 07.03.14).

NOMS. 2013a. Stocktake of Women's Services for Offenders in the Community www.justice.gov.uk (Accessed 05.03.14).

O'Brien, M., Mortimer, L., Singleton, N., Meltzer, H., and Goodman, R. 2003. Psychiatric morbidity among women prisoners in England and Wales, *International Review of Psychiatry* 15(1–2): 153–157.

Office for National Statistics (ONS). 1997. Singleton, N., Meltzer, H., and Gatward, R. *Psychiatric Morbidity among Prisoners in England and Wales*. London: Stationery Office.

Office for National Statistics (ONS). 2013. *Focus on: Violent Crime and Sexual Offences, 2011/12*. www.ons.gov.uk/ons/rel/crime-stats/crime-statistics/focus-on-violent-crime/stb-focus-on–violent-crime-and-sexual-offences-2011-12.ht.

Peugh, J. and Belenko, S. 1999. Substance-involved women inmates: Challenges to providing effective treatment, *Prison Journal*, 79(1):23–44.

Plugge, E., Douglas, N. and Fitzpatrick, R. 2006. *The Health of Women in Prison Study Findings*. Department for Public Health, University of Oxford.

Pratt, D., Piper, M., Appleby, L., Webb, R. and Shaw, J. 2006. Suicide in recently released prisoners: a population-based cohort study, *The Lancet*, 368(9530): 119–123.

Prison Reform Trust. 2007. *Bromley Briefings Prison Factfile December 2007*. London: Prison Reform Trust.

Putkonen, H., Collander, J., Honkasalo, M. L.. and Lonnqvist, J. 1998. Finnish female homicide offenders 1982-92, *The Journal of Forensic Psychiatry* 9(3): 672–684.

Rees, S., Silove, D., Chey, T., Ivancic, L., Steel, Z., Creamer, M., Teeson, M., Bryant, R., McFarlane, A. C., Mills, K. L., Slade, T., Carragher, N., O'Donnell, M. and Forbes, D. 2011. Lifetime prevalence of gender-based violence in women and the relationship with mental disorders and psychosocial function, *JAMA* 306(5): 513–521.

Rumgay, J. 2004. *When victims become offenders: In search of coherence in policy and Practice*. London School of Economics, London: Fawcett Society.

Schanda H., Knect G. and Schreinzer D. 2004. Homicide and major mental disorders: a 25-year study, *Acta Psychiatrica Scandinavica*, 110(2): 98–107.

Shaw, J., Baker, D., Hunt, I. M., Moloney, A. and Appleby, L. 2004. Suicide by prisoners: National Clinical Survey, *British Journal of Psychiatry* 184:263–267.

Singleton. N., Meltzer. H., Gatward. R. et al. 1998. *Psychiatric morbidity among prisoners in England and Wales. Office of National Statistics*. London: Stationery Office.

Sipes, L. A. 2012. Statistics on Women Offenders. Senior Public Affairs Specialist/Social Media Manager Court Services and Offender Supervision Agency.

Social Exclusion Unit. 2002. *Reducing Reoffending by Ex-Prisoners*. London: Social Exclusion Unit.

Sprunt, B., Brownstein, H. H., Crimmins, S. M. and Langley, S. 1996. Drugs and homicide by women, *Substance Use and Misuse* 31(7):825–845.

Staton-Tindall, M., Havens, J. R., Oser, C. B., Prendergast, M. and Leukefeld, C. 2009. Gender-specific factors associated with community substance abuse treatment utilization among incarcerated substance users, *Int Journal of Offender Ther Comp Criminol*, 53:401–419.

Strauss, S. M. and Falkin, G.P. 2001. The first week after drug treatment: the influence of treatment on drug use among women offenders. *American Journal of Drug and Alcohol Abuse* 27(2):241–264.

Taylor, P. J. and Bragado-Jimenez, M.D. 2009. Women psychosis and violence, *International Journal of Law and Psychiatry* 32.1: 56–64.

Teplin, L. A., Abram, K. M. and McClelland, G. M. 1996. Prevalence of psychiatric disorders among incarcerated women. *Archives of General Psychiatry*, 53: 505–512.

The Offender Health Research Network. 2009. A National Evaluation of Prison In-Reach Services: a report to the National Institute of Health Research. Manchester: The University of Manchester. www .ohrn.nhs.uk/resource/Research/ Inreach.pdf

United Nations. 2000. *Women and Men in Europe and North America*. Geneva: United Nations.

Valentine, P. V. 2000. Traumatic incident reduction I: traumatized women inmates: particulars of practice and research, *Journal of Offender Rehabilitation* 31(3–4):1–15.

Valentine, P. V. and Smith, T. E. 2001. Evaluating traumatic incident

reduction therapy with female inmates: a randomized controlled clinical trial, *Research on Social Work Practice* 11(1): 40–52.

Van den Bosch L.M.C., Hysaj, M. and Jacobs, P. 2012. DBT in an outpatient forensic setting, *International Journal of Law and Psychiatry* 35:311–316.

Walmsley, P. 2012. World Female Imprisonment List (Women and girls in penal institutions, including pre-trial detainees/remand prisoners). International Centre for Prison Studies.

Websdale, N. 1999. *Understanding Domestic Violence*. Boston, MA: Northeastern University Press.

Weizmann-Henelius, G., Viemero, V. and Eronen, M. 2003. 'The violent female perpetrator and her victim', *Forensic Science International* 133(3):197–203.

Wilczynski, A. 1997. *Child Homicide*. London: Greenwich Medical Media.

World Health Organization. 1993. *The ICD-10 classification of mental and behavioural disorders: diagnostic criteria for research*. Geneva: World Health Organization.

Zedner, L. 1998. 'Wayward Sisters: The Prison for Women', in Morris and Rothman (eds.), pp. 295–324, *The Oxford History of the Prison: the Practice of Punishment in Western Society*, Oxford: Oxford University Press.

Zlotnick, C., Najavits, L. M., Rohsenow, D. J. and Johnson, D. M. 2003. A cognitive-behavioral treatment for incarcerated women with substance abuse disorder and posttraumatic stress disorder: findings from a pilot study, *Journal of Substance Abuse Treatment* 25: 99–105.

Chapter

14

Domestic violence and women's mental health

Roxane Agnew-Davies

A public health problem

This chapter considers domestic violence to be a major public health problem that causes acute and long-term psychological distress as well as physical injury and chronic illness (Roberts, et al., 2006). Domestic violence does not respect geographical, cultural or (to the surprise of many) socioeconomic boundaries and is recognized by the World Health Organization as a global issue that urgently requires the attention of all health and mental health professionals (Garcia-Moreno et al., 2006; Krug et al., 2002). This chapter outlines the impacts of domestic violence on the mental health of women and offers best practice guidelines for identifying victims, responding to their disclosures appropriately as well as simple strategies to promote their recovery.

The British Crime Survey (2010–2011), a face-to-face survey of around 51,000 individuals aged between 16 and 59 and living across England and Wales, reported that 27% of women experience intimate partner abuse at some point in their lives, with 7% reporting abuse in the preceding year. These findings are consistent with treating domestic violence as a major public health problem. Although men are also victims of domestic violence (14% lifetime prevalence) women are more likely to be injured, more likely to need medical attention, more likely to be afraid and more likely to be raped (Howarth & Feder, 2013); 89% of incidents of intimate partner violence are perpetrated by men against women (Walby & Allen, 2004). Indeed, the most reliable defining characteristic of a victim of domestic violence is that she is a woman (e.g., Jonas et al., 2014). Younger women (under 34 years old), women who are deprived (Pickett & Wilkinson 2009) and women with disabilities (Khalifeh, 2013) may experience higher rates of domestic violence,

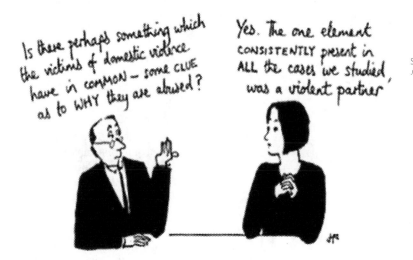

Source: C. Jacky Fleming. www.jackyfleming.co.uk. Printed with permission.

---

although these women may also be more likely to depend on and come to the attention of statutory services.

The prevalence of domestic violence is much higher for people accessing health, maternity and psychiatric services than in the general population, partly because they seek medical attention after abuse (Feder, et al., 2009.; Howard, et al., 2009). In a global systematic review of 134 prevalence studies, the highest rates were in psychiatric and gynecology clinics and in accident and emergency departments (Alhabib, et al., 2010). Studies are not always explicit about the relationship between victim and offender but people with mental disorders are between 4 and 11 times more likely to have experienced recent violence than people in the general population (Trevillion, et al., 2013). A systematic review of studies in mental health settings, albeit most based on small numbers (Oram, et al., 2013), found a median lifetime prevalence of intimate partner violence of 32% among female in-patients and 33% among female in-patients.

The higher prevalence of domestic violence for women accessing psychiatric services extends across different diagnoses and may be bidirectional. The median prevalence of lifetime intimate partner violence (IPV) amongst women was reported as 61% of those with post-traumatic stress disorder (PTSD), 46% of those with depressive disorder and 28% of those with anxiety disorders (Trevillion, et al., 2012). The review found that women with PTSD were seven times more likely [odds ratio (OR)= 7.34], women with anxiety disorders four times more likely [OR=4.08] and women with depressive disorders three times more likely [OR=2.77] to have experienced IPV than women without mental disorders. The few studies to date have been based on small sample sizes but the prevalence of IPV among women with schizophrenia and non-affective psychosis ranged between 42% and 83% (Trevillion, et al., 2013). In UK community mental health services, one study detected 60% of female service users had experienced IPV, 15% reporting abuse in the previous year (Morgan, et al., 2010).

Understanding the nature of domestic violence

Understanding what is meant by domestic violence will not only influence what health-care professionals look for (that is, help or hinder their detection of patients at risk) but will affect the nature of their enquiries and

responses to disclosures. For example, it is not confined to abuse by a partner, which to date has constrained much of the research focused on intimate partner violence (IPV). This constraint is not matched by reality; for instance, over 2010/2011 22% of all homicides in London were domestic related, with the murder of a parent by a son being most prevalent (Metropolitan Police, 2011). Moreover, the term IPV itself can mislead a mental health professional to focus on the relationship, in a way they would not for another trauma, such as a road traffic accident or mugging.

It is critical to understand that domestic violence is a multifaceted problem, not simply concerned with inflicting physical pain. Psychological abuse often precedes, accompanies and follows physical abuse and may also be experienced by women whose partners are never physically abusive (Rivas, Kelly & Feder, 2013). It is almost always underpinned by psychological control and often characterized by sexual abuse or coercion (Stark, 2007). As such, the Home Office (2013) revised their definitions in 2013 to acknowledge the centrality of coercive control and to highlight the risks to 16- to 18-year-olds, as follows:

[Domestic violence is characterized by] Any incident or pattern of incidents of controlling, coercive or threatening behaviour, violence or abuse between those aged 16 or over who are or have been intimate partners or family members regardless of gender or sexuality.

Controlling behaviour is a range of acts designed to make a person subordinate and/or dependent by isolating them from sources of support, exploiting their resources and capacities for personal gain, depriving them of the means needed for independence, resistance and escape and regulating their everyday behaviour.

Coercive behaviour is an act or a pattern of acts of assault, threats, humiliation and intimidation or other abuse that is used to harm, punish, or frighten their victim.

Evan Stark (2007) has expanded Johnson's (2006) categories of "situational" or "common couple violence," when equal force might be used in response to situationally specific stressors, and "intimate terrorism," more akin to a pattern of torture. Terms like "coercive control" draw out the inequality within a relationship whereby one adult misuses their power to frighten and control what another thinks, feels or does. Most victims are afraid, comply with and can describe their abuser's controlling behaviors or "rules." There is empirical support (Agnew-Davies, 2006; Stark, 2007; Rivas et al., 2013) that women can be effectively held hostage (a useful metaphor) or become isolated at home through powerful dynamics such as:

- Violence – to establish dominance, prevent escape, repress resistance;
- Sexual abuse – through invading bodily integrity, inspections, accusations, coercion;
- Intimidation – active threats (including to kill or hurt others), stalking (so he appears omnipresent) or passive threats (e.g., sulking); withholding money, food, medication;
- Emotional abuse – public and private insults, swearing, criticism, degradation;
- Shaming – marking ownership, enforcing behaviors against her values or standards;
- Social isolation, deprivation of movement to hinder escape and induce dependency;
- Control or micromanagement of the basic necessities of daily living and money.

There are specific, additional dynamics of domestic violence in some cultures that can overlap with child abuse including traditional practices such as pressures to maintain the so-called honor of the family (EACH, 2009), forced marriage (FCO, 2007), female genital mutilation and trafficking for exploitation (Zimmerman, et al., 2006).

The impacts of domestic violence on health

Domestic violence is life-threatening. Across England and Wales, about two women are killed every week by a partner or ex-partner (Povey, 2004), nearly always preceded by a history of abuse and coercive control (Richards, et al., 2008; Stark, 2007). The State of Victoria in Australia has identified intimate partner violence as the leading contributor to death, disability and illness in women aged 15 to 44, accounting for a higher proportion of the disease burden than diabetes, high blood pressure, smoking and obesity (Vos, et al., 2006). Mortality statistics related to domestic violence include deaths by suicide and the deaths of children, including by miscarriage and forced abortion.

Physical assaults often result in injury, ranging from minor abrasions to more serious trauma, typically to the head, face and neck (Wu, et al., 2010). Facial injuries range from zygomatic complex fractures and perforated tympanic membranes to dental damage. Common musculoskeletal injuries include sprains, fractures, dislocations and blunt-force

trauma to the forearms, a product of trying to block being struck (Howarth & Feder, 2013).

Violence often increases in frequency and severity over time. The cumulative effect of frequent but relatively minor assaults can be just as damaging to an individual's physical and emotional health as a more severe but one-off violent act (Hegarty, 2006). Living in fear day to day in the context of repeated, prolonged abuse is associated with a number of chronic physical health conditions. Reviews show that women experiencing domestic violence are at increased risk of gastrointestinal, neurological, musculoskeletal and cardiovascular symptoms (Ramsay, 2009). Women who experienced violence from a partner are two to four times more likely to report disability preventing them from work, chronic neck or back pain, arthritis, hearing loss, angina, bladder and kidney infections, sexually transmitted infections, chronic pelvic pain or irritable bowel syndrome (Coker, et al., 2002). A review of nursing studies has shown that women who are physically or sexually assaulted by partners suffer from significantly more gynecological problems, sexually transmitted infections, sexual difficulties and gynecological pain (Campbell, 2002).

Research shows that psychological abuse can have severe consequences, even after controlling for the effects of physical abuse (Arias & Pape, 1999; Marshall, 1996). Many victims of IPV rate the impact of emotional abuse on their lives and health as more profound than that of the physical abuse (Coker, et al., 2000; Follingstad, et al., 1990; Murphy & Hoover, 1999; O'Leary, 1999). For example, women exposed to psychological abuse were not significantly different from women exposed to physical and psychological abuse with regards to the severity and incidence of symptoms of depression, anxiety and PTSD, whilst both groups reported a higher incidence and severity than the control sample (Pico-Alfonso, et al., 2006).

Systematic reviews suggest that there is a causal association between domestic violence and mental disorder. People with mental disorders are also at increased risk of violence victimization (Trevillion & Howard, 2013). Golding (1999) found large associations between domestic violence and PTSD, depression, suicidality and problematic substance use. (PTSD avoidance behaviors can be exhibited in problematic substance use, with suicidal ideation at the extreme end of that spectrum.) The more severe and prolonged the violence, the greater the risk of mental disorder. There is also a temporal effect in that the violence typically precedes rather than postdates the mental illness and if the violence stops, mental health can recover. Women who are revictimized or who experience more than one form of abuse are at increased risk of mental illness and comorbidity (Jones, et al., 2001; Golding, 1999).

Depression and PTSD are prevalent and often comorbid conditions in victims of domestic violence and sexual violence (Warburton and Abel, 2006; Mechanic, 2004; Zimmerman, et al., 2006; Campbell, 2002). Systematic reviews have identified a 2-to-3-fold increase in the odds of depression in women who experienced partner violence, including for postnatal depression and domestic abuse during pregnancy, as well as increased odds of having experienced domestic violence among women with high levels of depressive, anxiety, and PTSD symptoms in both antenatal and postnatal periods (Howard, et al., 2013; Devries, et al., 2013).

More research is required on the associations between domestic violence and other mental health conditions, but there are indications that eating disorders are associated with a high prevalence and increased odds of lifetime IPV (Bundock, et al., 2013).

Judith Herman (1992) purports that violence against women involving repeated trauma, is followed by a *complex* form of PTSD, the symptoms of which include:

- Difficulties regulating affect (emotion), including anger and mood;
- Altered consciousness including amnesia, dissociation;
- Altered self-perception, including a sense of helplessness, shame, guilt;
- Altered perception of the perpetrator, including preoccupation with the relationship, unrealistic attribution of total power to the perpetrator, acceptance of their belief system;
- Altered relationships, for example, mistrust, failures of self-protection, search for a rescuer;
- Altered belief system, including altered faith, hopelessness, despair.

Along similar lines, in recognition of the wider impacts of trauma, the diagnostic criteria of PTSD within the revised DSM-5 now includes a symptom cluster of "negative cognitions and mood," both highly likely to be affected by exposure to domestic violence (Chapter 17).

Understanding the causes of domestic violence

There have been many competing theories to account for domestic violence, often based on examining the associations between specific variables and the characteristics of abusers (e.g. Barnish, 2004). Although a number of factors have been correlated with abuse, no single theory can explain it or the variance (Howarth & Feder, 2013; Krug, et al., 2002). For example, most perpetrators do not have a personality disorder and have not been diagnosed with a serious mental illness. Most individuals exposed to violence as children do not go on to commit violence as adults, not all abusers have violent upbringings and witnessing domestic violence in childhood does not distinguish between perpetrators or victims as adults. There are likely multiple causes for its occurrence, some of which is captured in an integrative multidimensional approach or social ecology model (Heise, 1998).

Figure 14.1 illustrates the need for multi-level interventions to tackle and prevent domestic violence including through domestic violence advocacy, social work and education. It is a salutary lesson to medical professionals of the danger of focusing on personal history or characteristics, particularly of a victim. Discussions about abuse should hold an abuser accountable whilst acknowledging contributory factors and asking what is needed.

Questioning victims about "reasons" or what they have done to invite or trigger the abuse is akin to holding a rape victim responsible for contributory negligence and can verge on victim-blaming. The medical professional has an important role in asserting that no violence is justified and that every individual is responsible for his or her actions. Focusing on the behavior of the perpetrator rather than the victim can reattribute the problem to the abuse and can help reveal that a "loss of control" by the abuser (for instance, when intoxicated) is in fact a pattern of selective targeting of the victim to which other people (such as the bar manager or boss) are not subjected.

"Why doesn't she leave?"

That domestic violence, harassment and stalking often continue after separation can be masked by questions as to why the victim does not leave, as if separation necessarily improves safety. In fact, data have shown that women are at greatest risk of violence from their

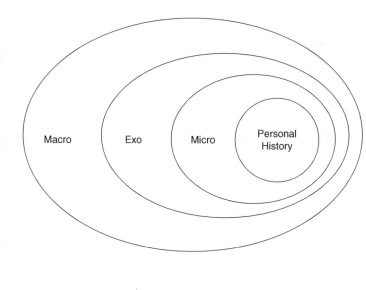

Personal history
○ Witnessing marital violence as a child
○ Being abused oneself as a child
○ Absent or rejecting father

Microsystem
○ Male dominance in the family
○ Male control of wealth in the family
○ Use of alcohol
○ Marital/verbal conflict

Exosystem
○ Low socioeconomic status/unemployment
○ Isolation of woman and family
○ Delinquent peer associations

Macrosystem
○ Male entitlement/ownership of women
○ Masculinity linked to aggression and dominance
○ Rigid gender roles
○ Acceptance of interpersonal violence
○ Acceptance of physical chastisement

Figure 14.1 Social ecology model reproduced with permission (Heise,1998)

partners when or just after they attempt to leave. In other words, advising victims to leave could put them at greater risk of serious injury or homicide. Practitioners should also understand that victims who do not leave their home are often deploying various strategies to minimize the risk of further abuse (Rivas, et al., 2013). These include legal action, help-seeking behaviors, escape strategies, appeals to the abuser, compliance with his rules, resistance and efforts to protect the children (Agnew-Davies, 2013b).

The role of health and mental health professionals

Domestic violence is a common problem that underlies victims seeking primary health care, especially to cope with the medical effects but sometimes in the hope of emotional support (Rivas, et al., 2013). Yet most victims do not identify or disclose their abuse as the causative agent, especially in the absence of direct questions, whilst health professionals frequently fail to ask about or recognize domestic violence as the primary etiological factor in their patient's poor health

and mental health (Hegarty, et al., 2006). Many clinicians report a variety of barriers that impede their identification of victims and feel that they lack training regarding how to ask victims appropriate questions about domestic violence or how to refer them appropriately for help (Warburton & Abel, 2006). In a sample of UK primary care clinicians, 80% said that their knowledge about local domestic violence services was inadequate (Ramsay, et al., 2012). Mental health-care professionals also do not ask routinely about domestic violence (Howard, et al., 2009).

Good practice guidelines for mental health professionals have been burgeoning over the last decade within the UK (e.g., Howard, et al., 2013) and globally (WHO, 2013). Women who experience domestic violence can have very different needs, depending on their circumstances and the severity of the violence and its consequences. Furthermore, women may need different types of support over time. Nevertheless, the WHO recommends a minimum set of actions to guide health-care responses. Thus, women who disclose any form of domestic violence should be offered immediate support. This includes:

- ensuring consultation is conducted in private;
- ensuring confidentiality (while being clear about the limits of confidentiality);
- being non-judgmental and supportive and validating what the woman is saying;
- providing practical care and support in response to the woman's concerns;
- asking about her history of violence;
- listening carefully, without pressuring her to talk;
- helping access to information about resources, including legal and specialist services;
- assisting the victim to increase safety for herself and her children, where needed;
- providing or mobilizing social support.

Improving practice is underpinned by better partnership work between mental health services and domestic violence services. For instance, even 4-hour training programs in domestic violence can improve the identification and referral practices of clinicians in mental health teams (Trevillion, et al., 2013).

Setting the scene

In the first instance, asking for materials such as posters or leaflets from local or national domestic violence services that are then made available in departments can increase the rate of self-referral to specialist services (Feder, et al., 2011).

Recognizing victims of domestic violence

An earlier section in this chapter reviewed the impacts of domestic violence on health and mental health. These effects can be harnessed to guide recognizing or identifying signs of abuse, as outlined in Table 14.1. Selective enquiry when these signs are evident is recommended (WHO, 2013).

Selective enquiry about domestic violence

Questions to help practitioners enquire about physical abuse, sexual abuse and psychological control have been suggested elsewhere (Agnew-Davies, 2013a). Questions about abuse should always be asked in private to ensure the safety of the victim. An e-learning facility for mental health professionals

Table 14.1 Recognizing signs of domestic abuse

1. Acute physical injuries following assault

- Bruising and injuries, e.g., bi-lateral bruising, burns, bite marks; genital trauma; injuries to face, head, neck, chest
- Breaks and fractures, e.g., broken bones, orbital fractures, lost teeth
- Miscarriage, fetal trauma, abdominal trauma
- Injuries or bruises in various stages of healing
- Injury inconsistent with explanation offered

2. Chronic health problems

- Gynecological problems, e.g., pelvic pain, vaginal bleeding, STIs
- HIV
- Heart and circulatory conditions
- Complaints of aches and pains, e.g., headaches, back pain
- Gastrointestinal disorders, e.g., irritable bowel syndrome
- Stress-related symptoms, e.g., dizziness, chronic headache

3. Psychological indicators

- Post-traumatic stress (PTSD)
- Depression including suicide attempts and self-harming behaviors
- Problematic substance use (including prescribed drugs and alcohol)
- Anxiety disorders
- Sleep problems
- Exacerbation of psychotic symptoms

4. Indicators in the behavior of the victim

- Covering the body to hide marks (long sleeves, trousers or scarves)
- Attending late or often missing appointments
- Frequent visits with vague complaints or different symptoms
- Seeming anxious, fearful or passive (particularly in presence of others)
- Giving inconsistent explanations for injuries or is evasive or embarrassed
- Not wanting letters, visits or contact at home

5. Possible indicators in the behavior of partner/another person

- Cancellation of appointments on patient's behalf
- Always attends, talking on behalf of patient or appearing overly protective

Table 14.1 (cont.)

- Bullying or aggressive; critical, judgmental or insulting about patient
- Evasive or conversely, adamant about the cause of injury
- Overvehement denial of violence or minimizes its severity
- Does not consult patient about their wishes, needs or feelings

Trevillion, Howard & Agnew-Davies (2010) with permission

to help develop confidence in asking service users questions and responding appropriately to promote their sexual and reproductive health as well as their recovery from abuse can be found on www.scie .org.uk/assets/elearning/sexualhealth/Web/Object3/ main.html.

Questions to help tease out the dynamics of the abuse might explore whether the patient is frightened of anyone or what they might do. The patient may have been scared of, or hurt by, more than one person and the abuse is likely to have happened more than once. Some women face abuse from wider family and community networks so questions should not focus just on intimate partners. An alternative to explore the pattern of domestic violence is to ask someone who discloses about the first incident, the worst and the most recent.

The Power and Control Wheel (see Figure 14.2) is a useful tool for exploring psychological abuse. Simply providing a copy to the patient and asking whether they recognize any of these behaviors can help open up further discussion.

The Power and Control Wheel is a conceptual tool to represent the tactics typically used by perpetrators of domestic violence. It was developed in 1982 in Duluth, Minnesota (Pence & Paymar, 1986), but has been translated into forty languages and is used across the world. The tactics do not in and of themselves constitute domestic violence. Abuse involves the patterned and intentional use of these tactics to control the victim's autonomy and instil fear and compliance. The wheel can help victims to see patterns in behavior and their unconscious significance. Simply showing them the wheel and asking if anyone treats or has treated them in any of these ways can be very powerful and helpful. Thinking about the wheel can help a patient to

understand the multiple aspects of abuse, to identify behaviors as domestic violence and to counteract feelings of being alone or to blame.

Responding to disclosures of domestic violence

Victims of domestic violence often hope for emotional support from their health-care practitioners, and appreciate it when it is offered (Malpass, et al., 2014). The immediate response can be in the form of a key message to raise awareness, validate the patient's reaction and name the problem (Agnew-Davies, 2013b). Box 14.1 outlines some examples of key messages in response to a disclosure of domestic violence.

Assessing risk

Assessing risk is important not only to safeguard vulnerable adults and children but can be a step towards safety planning. Independent Domestic Violence Advisors (IDVAs) offer emotional and practical support to victims and conduct risk assessments prior to referring those at high risk to MARACs (Multiple Agency Risk Assessment Conferences). MARACs are staffed by representatives from police, social care, housing, health, substance use and specialist domestic violence services amongst others and aim to share information about high-risk cases and build and implement a shared safety plan to reduce the risk of further harm (Richards, et al., 2008).

Using a police data base of over 2,000 incidents of domestic abuse across the UK, Laura Richards (2008) developed a comprehensive risk assessment model; an adapted risk assessment checklist with explanatory notes can be downloaded from the Coordinated Action Against Domestic Abuse (CAADA) website (www.caada.org.uk/marac/RIC_with_guidance.pdf).

Referring to domestic violence specialists

Referring victims at risk to a specialist domestic violence service can be a critical part of treatment planning and promoting their safety, as well as a means to meet their needs more effectively, enhance their social inclusion and safeguard children (e.g., Howarth, et al., 2009; Trevillion, et al., 2013; Coy & Kelly, 2011).

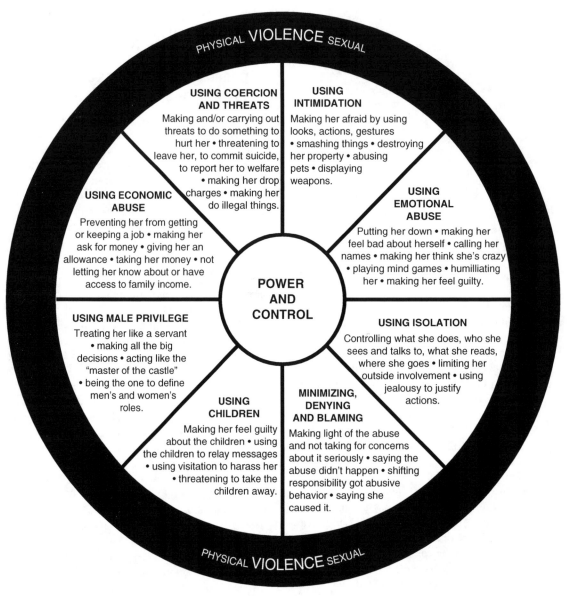

Figure 14.2 Power and Control Wheel

Ongoing support

Victims have repeatedly stated that they most value ongoing support from their health-care provider and that abuse is recognized as the cause of their difficulties. They prefer talking treatment to medication, joined-up services (e.g., mental health and substance use) and need information about their choices, without undue pressure to act (e.g., Stella Project, 2012). Principles underlying practice are outlined in Table 14.2.

The effectiveness of advocacy and mental health interventions

Evidence has accumulated that routine enquiry into domestic violence is not in itself sufficient to effect change. However, if enquiry is followed by referral to specialist domestic violence advocacy services, the outlook for the victim is likely to be improved. Domestic violence advocacy typically offers victims practical and emotional support, such as help with their welfare, housing and legal rights as well as their safety planning and access to other services. Tailored advocacy support in the UK has led to reductions in the severity and frequency of domestic violence, as well as improvements in coping behaviors and social support networks (Howarth, et al., 2009).

A systematic review in 2009 (Ramsay, et al., 2009) concluded after analyzing 10 trials involving 1,527 participants who received a wide range of brief advocacy interventions (of less than 12 hours duration)

seemed to increase the use of safety behaviors for over 2 years. Longer-term advocacy (12 hours or more) helped reduce physical abuse for victims leaving refuges between 1 and 2 years later and may improve their quality of life at up to 12 months follow-up, but it did not significantly alleviate their symptoms of depression or psychological distress. The authors concluded that the evidence was equivocal whether or not intensive advocacy for women recruited in refuges has a beneficial effect on their physical and psychosocial well-being, and that it was not known whether less intensive interventions in health-care settings are effective for women who still live with abusive partners.

In summary, mental health professionals can improve their practice by developing partnerships with local domestic violence services including by designing referral pathways. More research is required, especially with regards to supporting victims in the community.

Regarding psychological interventions, there is as yet limited evidence of their effectiveness for victims of domestic violence, especially for those with mental

---

Box 14.1: Examples of immediate responses to disclosures

- Domestic violence can negatively affect mental health.
- Service users with mental health problems have the right to be safe.
- The victim is not alone and it is not her fault.
- There is help available.
- People have the right to talk about it in privacy.

Table 14.2 Helpful and unhelpful responses to domestic violence disclosures

Helpful	Unhelpful	Your Role
help to name domestic violence and hold perpetrator accountable	failing to recognize the abuse; blaming the victim; focusing on the relationship not the abuse	be aware of the signs, ask questions about abuse; identify the abuse as the problem; make it safe to talk about experiences
give attention to risk and focus on safety of victim and children	reacting with disbelief or skepticism, telling her what to do; suggesting family therapy or couple counseling involving the perpetrator	be knowledgeable about key risks; record evidence; do not talk to victim in presence of abuser about abuse; explore how victim can put a plan in place to increase safety
respond to special needs	focusing simply on medication or substance use without recognizing the complexity of partner violence; working in isolation	be prepared to work in partnership with other agencies; have information available in different formats; acknowledge the complexities and long-term nature of abuse
help recovery from experiences of abuse	making the abuser invisible by focusing only on the victim's mental health	be nonjudgmental; set the symptoms in the context of trauma; hold the abuser not the victim accountable; acknowledge her range of survival strategies
offer support for children	focusing on failure to protect children rather than the source of abuse	give information and refer to relevant agencies with consent; promote children's well-being by support for the nonabusive parent
recognize stages of change	withholding treatment because the victim is living in an abusive situation	adapt intervention to suit client's needs and the stage the victim has reached; risk assess and safety plan, or refer to someone who can

Adapted from Howard, Feder & Agnew-Davies (2013) with permission of the Royal College of Psychiatry

illness (Trevillion & Agnew-Davies, 2013). However, it is well understood that standard therapies for victims of domestic violence suffering from mental illnesses may not be effective if the domestic violence is not addressed. In addition, a failure to acknowledge the abuse, assess risk or assist with safety planning may not only fail to safeguard a vulnerable adult and her children but there is an implicit risk that the intervention medicalizes and pathologizes the individual without addressing the etiology of their problems.

Although many studies are based on small sample sizes or have methodological limitations, a range of psychological interventions, usually based on cognitive behavioral therapy (CBT) principles with modules to empower women (e.g., through self-advocacy, assertion and skills training) have reduced depressive and PTSD symptoms and improved the self-esteem of victims of domestic violence, especially victims of historic rather than current abuse (Feder, et al., 2009). For example, Kubany and colleagues in Hawaii have designed a package called Cognitive Trauma Therapy to include i) exploring the history of abuse, ii) psycho-education on PTSD, iii) imaginal and invivo exposure to alleviate PTSD symptoms, iv) psycho-education on maladaptive self-talk, v) stress management and relaxation training, vi) cognitive therapy for trauma-related guilt, vii) assertiveness training, viii) safety planning, ix) strategies to avoid revictimization and x) positive strategies to increase self-empowerment (Kubany & Watson, 2002). These researchers have reported reductions in depression, guilt and remittance of PTSD in 87% of women completers, maintained at 6-month follow-up, along with significant improvements in self-esteem (Kubany, et al., 2004). Another manualized treatment, Psychological Advocacy Towards Healing (PATH) comprising ten sessions of psychological support alongside advocacy and delivered by trained Special Psychological Advocates (SPAs) is being subjected to a randomized controlled trial in the UK (Brierley, et al., 2013).

El-Mohandes et al. (2008) developed a CBT program for depression and smoking cessation in 913 pregnant African-American women, with an individualized program to raise awareness about domestic violence, conduct simple risk assessments and develop safety planning. The program was delivered over at least four sessions prenatally and up to two sessions postpartum. Reductions in depression (from 83% to 55%) and partner violence (from 51% to 28%) were reported by the intervention group but failed to reach statistical significance.

Mueser et al. (2008) designed a 21-week, gender-neutral, trauma-focused group therapy program for patients with schizophrenia or major mood disorders and comorbid PTSD, although the traumas were not confined to domestic violence. Of the 80 patients who attended 11 or more sessions, 59% reported significant improvements in symptoms of PTSD, depression and trauma-related cognitions post-treatment although longer-term outcomes including revictimization were not assessed.

Further research on the effectiveness of psychological interventions for victims of domestic violence, particularly within the statutory sector, is urgently required.

A note for health service commissioners

Population attributable fractions (PAFs) have been used to quantify the public health implications of domestic violence. For instance, domestic violence-related PAFs have been estimated in an Australian study at 21% for major depression and 17% for anxiety (Vos, et al., 2006). Tackling domestic violence could therefore reduce the disease burden of mental health disorder and lower health service costs.

Training health and mental health professionals in domestic violence can significantly improve their knowledge, attitudes and behaviors including their rates of detection, enquiry and referrals to domestic violence advocacy services (Feder, et al., 2011; Trevillion, et al., 2013) and is likely to be cost-effective (Norman, et al., 2010).

Conclusions

Domestic violence is a common feature in the histories of at least a third of female psychiatric patients and a significant proportion of these are at current risk. However, the detection of abuse by health-care professionals has been inadequate and as such is likely to contribute to the ineffectiveness of treatment. To improve practice, mental health services need to access training to increase their confidence to ask questions about domestic violence and refer high-risk victims to local domestic violence services. Interagency partnership work with domestic violence services and substance use teams can improve safeguarding and mental health care. Trauma-focused specialist therapies can help victims recover from their psychological distress once their safety has improved.

References

Agnew-Davies, R. (2013a). Identifying domestic violence experienced by service users. In L. M. Howard, G. Feder & R. Agnew-Davies (eds.), *Domestic Violence & Mental Health*, ch. 3. London: Royal College of Psychiatry.

Agnew-Davies, R. (2013b). Responding to disclosures of domestic violence. In L. M. Howard, G. Feder & R. Agnew-Davies (eds.), Op. cit, ch. 4.

Agnew-Davies, R. (2006). *Experience of Abuse Questionnaire. Presentation in a Panel Domestic Violence and Mental Health*. June, Edinburgh: Society for Psychotherapy Research.

Alhabib, S., Nur, U., Jones, R. (2010). Domestic violence against women: systematic review of prevalence studies. *Journal of Family Violence*, 25, 369–382.

Arias, I., & Pape, K. T. (1999). Psychological abuse: Implications for adjustment and commitment to leave violent partners. *Violence and Victims*, 14(1), 55–67.

Barnish, M. (2004). *Domestic Violence: A Literature Review*. London: HM Inspectorate of Probation. http://webarchive.nationalarchives.gov.uk/+/http:/www.justice.gov.uk/inspectorates/hmi-probation/docs/thematic-dv-literaturereview-rps.pdf.

Brierley, G., Agnew-Davies, R., Bailey, J., Evans, M., Fackrell, M., Ferrari, G., Hollinhurst, S., Howard, L., Howarth, E., Malpass, A., Metters, C., Peters, T. L., Saeed, F., Sardhina, L,. Sharp, D. & Feder, G. (2013). Psychological advocay towards healing (PATH): study protocol for a randomized contrelled trial. *Trials*, 14, 221.

Bundock, L., Howard, L. M., Trevillion, K., Malcolm, E., Feder, G. & Oram, S. (2013). Prevalence and risk of experiences of intimate partner violence among people with eating disorders: a systematic review. *J. Psychiatr. Res.*, 47(9), 1134–1142.

Campbell, J. (2002). Health consequences of intimate partner violence. *Lancet*, 359, 1131–1136.

Coker, A. L., Davis, K. E., Arias, I., Desai, S., Sanderson, M., Brandt, H. M. & Smith, P. H. (2002). Physical and mental health effects of intimate partner violence for men and women. *American Journal of Preventative Medicine*, 23, 260–268.

Coy, M. & Kelly, L. (2011). *Islands in the Stream: An Evaluation of Four London Independent Domestic Violence Advocacy Services*. London: Henry Smith Charity.

Devries, K. M., Mak, J. Y., Bacchus, L. J., Child, J. C., Falder, G., Petzold, M., Astbury, J. & Watts, C. H. (2013). Intimate partner violence and incident depressive symptoms and suicide attempts: a systematic review of longitudinal studies. *PLoS Med* 10(5), e1001439.

EACH. (2009). *Asian Women, Domestic Violence and Mental Health: A Toolkit for Health Professionals*, pp. 1–60. London: EACH.

El-Mohandes, A. A. E, Kiely, M., Joseph, J. G. et al. (2008). An intervention to improve postpartum outcomes in African-American mothers: a randomised controlled ctrial. *Obstetrics & Gynecology*, 112, 611–620.

Feder, G., Agnew-Davies, R., Baird, K., Dunne, D., Eldridge, S., Griffiths, C., Gregory, A., Howell, A., Johnson, M., Ramsay, J., Rutterford, C. & Sharp, D. (2011). Identification and Referral to Improve Safety (IRIS) of women experiencing domesitc violence with a primary care training and support programme: a cluster randomised controlled trial. *Lancet*, 11, 1–8.

Feder, G., Ramsay, J., Dunne, D. et al. (2009). How far does screening women for domestic (partner) violence in different health-care settings meet criteria for a screening programme? Systematic reviews of nine UK National Screening

Committee criteria. *Health Technology Assessment*, 13, iii–xiii.

Follingstad, D. R., Rutledge, L. L., Berg, B. J., Hause, E. S., & Polek, D. S. (1990). The role of emotional abuse in physically abusive relationships. *Journal of Family Violence*, 5(2), 107–120.

Foreign & Commonwealth Office (2007). *Dealing with Cases of Forced Marriage: Practice Guidance for Health Professionals* (1st edn). London: FCO Services: Publishing.

Garcia-Moreno, C., Jansen, H. A., Ellsberg, M., Heise, L., & Watts, C. H. (2006). Prevalence of intimate partner violence: findings from the WHO multi-country study on women's health and domestic violence. *The Lancet*, 368, 1260–1269.

Golding, M. J. (1999). Intimate partner violence as a risk factor for mental disorders: a meta-analysis. *Journal of Family Violence*, 14, 99–132.

Hegarty, K. (2006). What is intimate partner abuse and how common is it? In G. Roberts, K. Hegarty, & G. Feder (eds.), *Intimate Partner Abuse and Health Professionals: New Approaches to Domestic Violence*, pp. 19–40. Edinburgh: Elsevier.

Hegarty, K., Feder, G. & Ramsay, J. (2006). Identification of intimate partner abuse in health care settings: should health professionals be screening? In G. Roberts, K. Hegarty, & G. Feder (eds.), *Intimate Partner Abuse and Health Professionals: New Approaches to Domestic Violence*, pp. 81–92. Edinburgh: Elsevier.

Heise, L. L. (1998). Violence against women an integrated, ecological framework. *Violence Against Women*, 4(3), 262–290.

Herman, J. L. (1992). *Trauma and Recovery: From Domestic Abuse to Political Terror*. London: Pandora.

Home Office. (2013). Home Office Circular 003/2013. Broad Subject: Crime and Disorder Issue. www.gov.uk/government/publications/

new-government-domestic-violence-and-abuse-definition.

Howard, L. M., Feder, G. & Agnew-Davies, R. (eds). *Domestic Violence & Mental Health*. London: Royal College of Psychiatry.

Howard, L. M., Oram, S., Galley, H., Trevillion, K. & Feder, G. (2013). Domestic Violence and perinatal disorders: a systematic review and meta-analysis. *PLoS Med.*, 10(5): e1001452. doi: 10.1371.

Howard, L. M., Trevillion, K. & Agnew-Davies, R. (2010). Domestic violence and mental health. *International Review of Psychiatry*, 22(5), 525–534.

Howard, L. M., Trevillion, K., Khalifeh, H., Woodall, A., Agnew-Davies, R. & Feder, G. (2009). Domestic violence and severe psychiatric disorders: prevalence and interventions. *Psychological Medicine*, 40, 881–893.

Howarth, E. & Feder, G. (2013) Prevalence and physical impact of domestic violence. In L.M. Howard, G. Feder & R. Agnew-Davies (eds)., *Domestic Violence & Mental Health*, ch. 1. London: Royal College of Psychiatry.

Howarth, E., Stimpson, L., Barron, D. & Robinson, A. (2009). *Safety in Numbers: A Multi-Site Evaluation of Independent Domestic Violence Advisor Services*. The Henry Smith Charity.

Johnson, M. P. (2006). Conflict and control. *Violence Against Women*, 12, 1003–1018.

Jonas, S., Khalifeh, H., Bebbington, P. E., McManus, S., Brugha, T., Meltzer, H., & Howard, L. M. (2014). Gender differences in intimate partner violence and psychiatric disorders in England: results from the 2007 adult psychiatric morbidity survey. *Epidemiology and Psychiatric Sciences*, 23(2), 189–199.

Jones, L, Hughes, M. & Unterstaller, U. (2001). Post traumatic stress disorder (PTSD) in victims of domestic violence: a review of the research. *Trauma, Violence & Abuse*, 2, 99–119.

Khalifeh, H., Howard, L. M., Osborn, D., Moran, P. & Johnson, S. (2013). Violence against people with disability in England and Wales: findings from a National Cross-Sectional Survey. *PLoS ONE*, 8(2), e55952. doi:10.1371/journal. pone.0055952.

Krug, E. G., Mercy, J. A., Dahlberg, L. L. & Zwi, A. B. (2002). The world report on violence and health. *Lancet*, 360, 1083–1088.

Kubany, E. S., Hill, E. E., Owens, J. A., Iannce-Spencer, C., McCaig, M. A, Tremayne, K. J. & Williams, P. L. (2004). Cognitive trauma therapy for battered women with PTSD (CTT-BW). *Journal of Consulting & Clinical Psychology*, 72(1), 1–17.

Kubany, E. S., & Watson, S. B. (2002). Cognitive trauma therapy for formerly battered women with PTSD: Conceptual bases and treatment outlines. *Cognitive and Behavioral Practice*, 9(2), 111–127.

Malpass, A., Sales, K., Johnson, M., Howell, A., Agnew-Davies, R., & Feder, G. (2014). Women's experiences of referral to a domestic violence advocate in UK primary care settings: a service-user collaborative study. *British Journal of General Practice*, 64(620), e151–e158.

Marshall, L. L. (1996). Psychological abuse of women: Six distinct clusters. *Journal of Family Violence*, 11(4), 379–409.

Mechanic, M. B. (2004). Beyond PTSD: Mental health consequences of violence against women. A response to Briere and Jordan. *Journal of Interpersonal Violence*, 19(11), 1283–1289.

Metropolitan Police. (2011). Domestic and Sexual Violence Board Final Report 2006-2011. London: Metropolitan Police Authority.

Morgan, J. F., Zolese, G., McNulty, J. et al. (2010). Domestic violence among female psychiatric out-patients: cross-sectional survey. *Psychiatrist*, 34, 461–464.

Mueser, K. T., Rosenberg, S. D., Xie, H., et al. (2008). A randomised controlled trial of cognitive-behavioral treatment for post traumatic stress disorder in severe mental illness. *Journal of Consulting and Clinical Psychology*, 76, 259–271.

Murphy, C. M., & Hoover, S. A. (1999). Measuring emotional abuse in dating relationships as a multifactorial construct. *Violence and Victims*, 14(1), 39–53.

Norman, R., Spence, A., Eldridge, S. & Feder, G. (2010). Cost-effectiveness of a programme to detect and provide better care for female victims of intimate partner violence. *J. Health Service Research Policy*, doi: 10.1258/jhsrp.2009.009032.

O'Leary, K. D. (1999). Psychological abuse: A variable deserving critical attention in domestic violence. *Violence and Victims*, 14(1), 3–23.

Oram, S., Trevillion, K., Feder, G. et al. (2013). Prevalence of experiences of domestic violence among psychiatric patients: systematic review. *British Journal of Psychiatry*, 202, 94–99.

Pence, E. & Paymar, M. (1986). *Power and Control: Tactics of Men who Batter*. Duluth, MN: Minnesota Program Development, Inc. Revised, 1990.

Pickett, K., & Wilkinson, R. (2009). *The Spirit Level: Why Equality is Better for Everyone*. London: Allen Lane.

Pico-Alfonso, M. A., Garcia-Linares, M., Celda-Navarro, N., et al. (2006). The impact of physical, psychological, and sexual intimate male partner violence on women's mental health: depressive symptoms, posttraumatic stress disorder, state anxiety and suicide. *Journal of Women's Health*, 15, 599–611.

Povey, D. (2004). *Crime in England and Wales 2002/3: Supplementary*

Volume 1-Homicide and Gun Crime. London: Home Office.

Ramsay, J., Carter, Y., Davidson, L., Dunne, D., Eldridge, S., Feder, G., Hegarty, K., Rivas, C., Taft, A. & Warburton, A. (2009). Advocacy interventions to reduce or eliminate violence and promote the physical and psychosocial well-being of women who experience intimate partner abuse. *Cochrane Database of Systematic Reviews*, 3, CD005043.

Ramsay, J., Rutterford, C., Gregory, A., Dunne, D., Eldridge, S., Sharp, D. & Feder, G. (2012). Domestic violence: knowledge, attitudes and clinical practice of selected UK primary health care clinicians. *British Journal of General Practice*, September, 647–655.

Richards, L., Letchford, S. & Stratton, S. (2008). *Policing Domestic Violence*. Oxford: Oxford University Press.

Rivas, C., Kelly, M. & Feder, G. (2013). Drawing the line: how African, Caribbean and White British women live out psychologically abusive experiences. *Violence Against Women*, 19(9), 1104–1132.

Roberts, G., Hegarty, K. & Feder, G. (eds.). (2006). *Intimate Partner Abuse and Health Professionals: New Approaches to Domestic Violence*. Edinburgh: Churchill Livingstone Elsevier.

Smith, K., Coleman, K, Eder, S., et al. (2011). *Homicides, Firearm Offences and Intimate Violence 2009/2010* (Supplementary to Volume 2 to Crime in England & Wales 2009/10 2nd Edition). Home Office Statistical Bulletin.

Stark, E. (2007). *Coercive Control: How Men Entrap Women in Personal Life*. Oxford: Oxford University Press.

Stella Project (2012). *"Treat me like a human being, like someone who matters": Findings of the Stella Project Mental Health Initiative Survivor Consultation*. London: AVA. www.avaproject.org.uk/our-projects/stella-project/stella-project-mental-health-initiative.aspx.

Trevillion, K. & Agnew-Davies, R. (2013). Interventions for mental health service users who experience domestic violence. In L. M. Howard, G. Feder & R. Agnew-Davies (eds), *Domestic Violence & Mental Health*, ch. 5. London: Royal College of Psychiatry.

Trevillion, K., Agnew-Davies, R. & Howard, L. M. (2011). Domestic violence: responding to the needs of patients. *Nursing Standard*, 25(26), 48–56.

Trevillion, K., Byford, S., Cary, M., Rose, D., Oram, S., Feder, G., Agnew-Davies, R. & Howards, L. M. (2013). Linking abuse and recovery through advocacy: an observational study. *Epidemiol Psychiatr Sci.*, 30, 1–15.

Trevillion, K., Oram, S., Feder, G., & Howard, L. M. (2012). Experiences of domestic violence and mental disorders: a systematic review and meta-analysis. *PLoS One*, 7(12), e51740.

Trevillion, K., Oram, S. & Howard, L. M. (2013). Domestic violence and mental health. In L. M. Howard, G. Feder & R. Agnew-Davies (eds.),

Domestic Violence & Mental Health, ch. 2. London: Royal College of Psychiatry.

Walby, S. & Allen, J. (2004). *Domestic Violence, Sexual Assault & Stalking: Findings from the British Crime Survey*. Home Office Research Study 276. London: Home Office.

Warburton, A. L. & Abel, K. M. (2006). Domestic violence and its impact on mood disorder in women: implications for mental health workers. In D. Castle, J. Kulkarni, & K.M. Abel (eds.), *Mood and Anxiety Disorders in Women*, ch. 6. Cambridge University Press.

World Health Organisation (2013). *Responding to intimate partner violence and sexual violence against women: WHO clinical and policy guidelines*. Geneva: WHO.

Wu, V., Huff, H., & Bhandari, M. (2010). Pattern of physical injury associated with intimate partner violence in women presenting to the emergency department: A systematic review and meta analysis. *Trauma, Violence and Abuse*, 11, 71–82.

Vos, T., Astbury, J., Piers, L. S. et al. (2006). Measuring the impact of intimate partner violence on the health of women in Victoria, Australia. *Bulletin of World Health Organisation*, 84, 739–744.

Zimmerman, C., Hossain, M., Yun, K. et al. (2006) *Stolen Smiles. The physical and psychological health consequences of women and adolescents trafficked in Europe*. London School of Hygiene & Tropical Medicine.

Chapter 15

Women and addiction

Sally Marlow and Emily Finch

Introduction

Addiction is as old as civilization itself, with the deliberate brewing of beer first recorded in the Bronze Ages. Opium is known to have been used for medicinal reasons around 6,000 years ago, and cannabis and cocaine also have long histories. Tobacco is a relatively new arrival in Europe, in the fifteenth century, but elsewhere has been part of daily life for centuries more. From the beginning, the ability of drugs to alter mood and their addictive properties had important implications for women. Initially this was vicariously, as women experienced the fallout from male use of drugs, but more recently, increasingly as users in their own right. As women have achieved the vote and marriage property rights, stepped into the workplace and gained financial independence, their hard-won freedoms have included the right and the ability to take mood-altering substances, just as men have for centuries before them. Unfortunately, alongside that right have come harms, from addiction itself as well as from related physical, psychological and social damage.

Over the past few decades women's problematic use of substances has increased, yet being a woman is still a protective factor for addiction, with rates of addiction in women being lower than in men. However, the picture is complicated. Despite less use, women suffer greater harms from alcohol, tobacco and drugs, and in a shorter space of time than men. Rates of alcohol use in young women overall have been falling in Western societies over the last five years, but those who do drink consume more alcohol than ever. While younger women drink less, some countries are reporting increases in alcohol-related mortality in middle-aged women. The confusion is not helped by the fact that, even in the twenty-first century, addiction in women remains stigmatized and shrouded in secrecy, viewed as deviant behavior, a perception fuelled by media images of women out of control whilst intoxicated. All of this makes understanding what addiction is and what it means in relation to women particularly difficult.

Defining and diagnosing addictions

Definitions

The term "addiction" has been adopted into everyday language, where it is used to describe a range of experiences. Sometimes these experiences fall within what would be clinically recognized as being addiction, but more often the word addiction in common parlance is used as a shortcut to describe wanting or liking: "She's addicted to shoes"; "I'm a chocolate addict." The addiction described in this chapter denotes something more than wanting and liking. Addiction is considered here in its clinical sense to capture the spectrum of addictive disorders and behaviors described in both the *International Classification of Diseases, 10th Edition* (ICD-10) and the *Diagnostic and Statistical Manual of Mental Disorders, 5th Edition* (DSM-5). ICD-10 describes addiction within its category F10–F19: "Mental and behavioural disorders due to psychoactive substances" (World Health Organisation [WHO] 1993), whereas DSM-5 describes "Substance-Related and Addictive Disorders" (American Psychiatric Association [APA] Task Force, 2013).

Under the previous version of the DSM, DSM-IV (APA 1994), the differences between how addiction was classified in DSM and ICD nosologies were arguably minimal. Both made a distinction between "dependence," a more severe form of addiction, and "harmful use" (WHO 1993) or "abuse" (APA 1994) of

---

Comprehensive Women's Mental Health, ed. David J. Castle and Kathryn M. Abel. Published by Cambridge University Press.
© Cambridge University Press 2016.

substances. In dependence, both highlighted the two physiological criteria of withdrawal and tolerance alongside a range of psychological criteria, which include compulsions, lack of control, preoccupation with substance use and persisting despite knowledge of harm to self and others. In harmful use/abuse, both focused on the harms caused by the substance. However, DSM-5 does not separate the diagnoses of substance abuse and dependence, plus it has added a new criterion, that of craving. The number of criteria necessary for diagnosis has also been changed. It is not currently known whether these changes will have particular implications for how women with addiction problems are identified and diagnosed.

Although categories of addiction may be necessary for diagnostic and research purposes, these are based on convenient cutoff points, determined by statistical techniques and expert opinion. Categories may not always be the best way to understand addiction, which clearly exists on a continuum, and is affected by several dimensions: consumption levels, addiction-related problems and pattern of use.

What is addictive is also subject to some debate, with both substances and behaviors coming under scrutiny. Often addictions are all lumped together under one "substance misuse" heading. The legal drugs alcohol, tobacco and caffeine are recognized to have addictive properties. The main illicit drugs of addiction identified by the WHO are cannabis, stimulants (ecstasy-type drugs and amphetamine-type stimulants such as methamphetamine), cocaine and opioids/opiates. There is also an identified problem with addiction to certain prescription medications, in particular opiate-based painkillers and sedatives/tranquilizers. Alongside these substances, it has also been argued that some behaviors can be addictive. DSM-5 has included gambling amongst the addictive disorders. Gambling is included in ICD-10, but not under the same heading as substances: F63.0, "Pathological gambling" is categorized as a habit and impulse disorder rather than an addictive disorder.

Other behaviors may also be addictive. Neuroscientific findings suggest that sugar, fat and other types of food are not in themselves addictive, but that the act of eating may be, and addictive eating may be behavioral rather than substance related (Hebebrand et al. 2014). Other candidates for addictive behaviors include sex, excessive exercise and internet use. However, research into whether these can truly be described as addictive is inconclusive.

Box 15.1 Emerging trends

Online access to drugs

Availability of drugs has been enhanced by the development of the internet; in particular, the so-called dark net, a network where users remain anonymous by using encryption techniques and IP addresses stay hidden, hosts many sites where drugs of all types can be purchased. These are often not accessible by traditional search engines. The most well-known is Silk Road, which was closed down by the FBI recently, although in its place others have sprung up, and at the time of writing these include Black Markey Reloaded, The Armoury, and The General Store. Payment is often also anonymous, made in Bitcoins, an anonymous virtual currency. There is very little data about the use of these sites and the quantities of drugs purchased through them, and women-specific data are not available.

Club drugs and legal highs

The terms "club drugs" and "legal highs" are used to refer to synthetic compounds that may be taken in a nightclub, but are also often taken recreationally at home. Some are legal, but others are not. At the time of writing, the most common of these drugs are gamma hydroxybutrate (GHB) and gamma butyrolactone (GBL), along with ketamine and mephedrone (M-Cat, meow-meow, drone), but there are many more and different variations of compounds go in and out of fashion. Club drugs are a phenomenon of youth, with only 2% of those in treatment over the age of 18 being treated for club drugs, compared to 10% of the under 18s. Of all those in treatment for club drugs, 87% are aged between 15 and 17. Club drugs are still a relatively small problem, and whether usage will increase remains to be seen. However, there are some significant problems that accompany club drug use in some people, including psychosis and mood disturbance. Severe dependence and withdrawal have been noted with GHB. Research in this area is difficult – compounds change from week to week, and it is difficult to know exactly what people are taking and in what dosage. There is currently no research specifically into women's usage of club drugs.

Electronic cigarettes

Electronic cigarettes (also known as e-cigs and e-cigarettes) are a relatively newly developed method of delivering nicotine, via a battery-powered device that vaporizes the nicotine from a liquid in order to allow its inhalation, rather than using the

Box 15.1 *(cont.)*

combustion method as in regular cigarettes. This is argued to result in a much less harmful form of nicotine delivery. However, opinion is divided on the evidence for harm. The WHO reviewed the evidence (Grana et al. 2013), and released a series of conclusions that have been disputed by scientists, many of them in the public health arena, as "creating an impression of alarming possibilities" (McNeill et al. 2014). In particular, scientists took issue with WHO statements implying that electronic cigarettes encourage young people to smoke; that they are not beneficial for helping people to quit smoking; and that the differences in toxin levels, harms and risk of passive harms between conventional and electronic cigarettes are not large. To date, gender differences in e-cigarettes have not been examined.

In this chapter, therefore, the relationships of women with the main drugs of addiction are considered: alcohol, cannabis, stimulants, cocaine, opioids/opiates (including illicit opioids/opiates and painkillers), along with prescription sedatives/tranquilizers. We also summarize what is known about women and nicotine – smoking is most often considered under the public health umbrella, but nicotine is the most addictive of all known substances and responsible for more deaths in women than any of the other drugs under consideration (WHO 2011). Novel psychoactive compounds are also briefly discussed. In terms of behaviors, we include some data on gambling, although research in this area specifically into women is sparse.

Identification and diagnosis

Different methods of identification may be appropriate for different points on the continuum of addiction, and for different substances/behaviors. Risky substance use, which although not classified as an addictive disorder can certainly be argued to be on a continuum, is generally identified using biomarkers and self-report screening tools. These not only differ from drug to drug, but also differ in terms of their sensitivity and specificity. Particular problems may exist with some of these biomarkers, as women metabolize most psychoactive substances differently to men. In particular, it is known that carbohydrate deficient transferrin (CDT) levels vary between women and men, with women showing lower elevations of CDT after drinking alcohol than men (Golka & Weise 2004).

Problems also exist with the use of self-report methods for women. Differing levels and effects of consumption in women compared to men could have implications for key screening tools containing consumption measures, such as the Alcohol Use Disorders Identification Test (AUDIT, Saunders et al. 1993), which is used to screen for hazardous and harmful drinking, and the Severity of Alcohol Dependence Questionnaire (Stockwell et al. 1983), which is used to determine severity of alcohol dependence. Lower cutoff points may be appropriate for women to take these consumption differences into account (Bradley et al., 1998). Also, women may be less likely to report substance misuse than men because of stigma and fear of social service scrutiny of parenting capacity (Wilsnack & Wilsnack 2002), and identification may be further complicated by the fact that women may be less likely to be screened for alcohol misuse than men in primary care (Kaner et al., 2001). Chang et al. (2002) report that screening and subsequent brief interventions for women are not consistently helpful, and that more research is needed.

Clinical assessments are used by a variety of health care professionals and service providers to identify and diagnose more severe addiction problems. These may be more or less structured, depending on the experience and preference of the clinician or service provider. Diagnostic criteria for ICD-10 and DSM-IV and 5 have been operationalized into a range of structured diagnostic interviews, validated in populations of women for use with different types of addiction (e.g., Gibbon et al. 1997).

Epidemiology
Consumption

If identification, diagnosis and measurement are complex, then so too are estimates of prevalence. Different countries and organizations have different measures, some to inform health and treatment policies, some to inform crime policies. On a global level, data are collected on production, trafficking and consumption of drugs (United Nations Office on Drugs and Crime [UNODC] 2014). Estimates of consumption levels can help illuminate the prevalence of addiction and addiction disorders, and on a country-by-country basis many Western countries collect consumption data using general population surveys, sometimes in combination with examinations of health care and crime data. Methodologies and analyses vary widely from study to study, and this may contribute to variations in estimates. Regardless of how the data are collected, it is consistently shown that despite a narrowing of the gender gap over the last few decades, women still consume less than men, and engage in risky use of substances less than men (with the exception of some studies examining prescription medicines, in particular, sedatives or tranquilizers). Also, fewer women than men are arrested for possession of illicit substances (UNODC 2014).

There is also enormous variation between countries in terms of what is consumed and how much. For example, in countries where there are religious and/or cultural reasons for not drinking, particularly women not drinking, rates of alcohol use and misuse are generally much lower than in Western countries. Average global consumption to 2005 was 6.13 liters pure alcohol per capita, whereas in Europe it was more than double that amount, 13.37 liters per capita (WHO 2014). Not surprisingly, therefore, there are wide variations in alcohol misuse from country to country for women (Kerr-Corrêa et al., 2007). There are also country-to-country variations in illicit drugs, with South American countries showing relatively high prevalence of cocaine and low prevalence of heroin, whereas in Asia and Europe heroin prevalence is relatively high, and in Africa rates of cannabis use are relatively high, with little cocaine and heroin use (UNODC 2014).

All estimates, however, should be treated with caution. Underreporting of use is ubiquitous in all areas of addiction. For legal drugs, for example, a recent study (Boniface & Shelton, 2013) found that when the general population self-reports drinking more than the UK weekly guidelines it underestimates by 11% for women (15% for men). In drinking above the daily limit, there is a mismatch of 26% in women (19% in men) between what is reported and what is actually consumed; in binge drinking the mismatch is 28% in women (20% in men), assuming people underreport equally across consumption levels. This suggests women underreport single episodes of drinking more than men, and although it is not known why, lack of knowledge of alcohol units could provide a partial explanation, as could reasons of social desirability. It is well known that women who misuse alcohol experience more stigma than men (Nolen-Hoeksema 2004). For illegal drugs, their very illegality may mean that estimates based on self-report are even more problematic.

Table 15.1 summarizes consumption estimates for alcohol, tobacco and the main illicit drugs.

Addiction disorders

As is the case for consumption, recent decades have seen rates of problematic use and addiction in women and men converge, but women are still less likely than men to have an addiction problem, and this finding is consistent across substances and behaviors (with the exception of addiction to prescription medications such as tranquilizers, sedatives and opiate/opioid painkillers, where women take more of these types of drugs, and show higher rates of problematic use). It is widely agreed that addiction problems in women are more hidden than in men, and this may be due in part to the stigma women experience, along with concerns about childcare, child protection issues, and negative attitudes from health professionals (Gilchrist et al. 2011).

Not every woman who uses alcohol or drugs will become addicted, and addiction disorders may take some time to develop. Table 15.2 summarizes the rates of various addiction disorders.

Course and consequences

Addiction disorders develop over time, and those who become addicted start from the same place as those who do not, with initial use or experimentation with alcohol and drugs.

How addiction develops does not lend itself to a single parsimonious theory, and many explanations have been proposed. It is beyond the scope of this chapter to discuss each of these in detail, but a summary of the predominant theories is given in Table 15.3, grouped into headings/categories suggested by West and Hardy (2006), and three of these theories are described in detail in Box 15.2.

For the majority of people, and for alcohol and for the majority of illicit drugs, levels of initial consumption do not progress to addiction. However, sizeable minorities who try a substance will go on to develop a problem with that substance, and this is not something that happens overnight, it is something that takes time.

Age of onset, adolescence and young adulthood

Women tend to start using alcohol and drugs slightly later in life than men, and there are often gender differences for motivation to start using. However,

177

Table 15.1 Prevalence estimates for consumption of addictive substances and behaviors

Addiction	Source	Country	Measure	Estimate: Women	Estimate: men
Alcohol	WHO 2014	Global	Current drinkers age 15+	28.9%	47.7%
			Annual alcohol per capita	8.9 liters	21.2 liters
			Prevalence of heavy episodic drinking (HED)	5.7%	21.5%
	(i) SAMHSA 2013b	USA	Young people "Binge drinking" aged 12–20 yrs	14%	16.5%
	HSCIC 2014	UK	Drinking > weekly guidelines	18%	24%
			Drinking > 2x daily guidelines	24%	31%
			High risk: W35,M50 units/week	4%	5%
			Children aged 15 who have drunk	74%	74%
Any drug	UNODC 2014	Global	Use of any illicit drug	2–3x less likely	2–3x more likely
	British Crime Survey 2013	UK	% using illicit drug in the last year	5.4%	11.0%
Any Class A drug	British Crime Survey 2013	UK	% using Class A drug in the last year	1.5%	3.7%
Cannabis	British Crime Survey 2013	UK	% using cannabis in last year	4.1%	8.6%
Cocaine	British Crime Survey 2013	UK	% using powder cocaine in last year	1.1%	2.7%
Gambling	McManus et al. 2009	UK	Any gambling	61.3%	70.8%
Heroin	McManus et al. 2009	UK	Lifetime use	0.2%	1.1%
Amphetamine	British Crime Survey 2013	UK	% ecstasy use in last year	0.7%	1.9%
Opium and/or crack	Hay et al. 2010	UK	Estimated number users	70,040	235,110
			Estimated % overall users	23.2%	76.8%
Nicotine	Hammond 2009	China	Current smoker	2%	57%
	Hammond 2009	Developed countries	Current smoker	24%	42%
Prescription painkillers	Back et al. 2010	USA	Lifetime nonmedical use	11%	16%
			Past year nonmedical use	4%	6%

to many adolescents, female and male, experimentation with mood-altering substances is attractive and behavior of peers can contribute to this. For girls and young women whose onset of drug and alcohol use is the teenage years, there are particular risks: brains and bodies are still developing and susceptible to damage and some hormones that are thought to play a role in metabolism and in developing and maintaining addiction problems may be in a state of flux. Further, young women receive confusing messages about the acceptability of alcohol and drug use. Alcohol use is more acceptable now in young women, but when women do drink, particularly younger women, there is greater censure than for men when they drink excessively, and this censure comes from both women and men (de Visser et al., 2012).

Table 15.2 Prevalence of addiction disorders

Addiction	Source	Country	Problematic use described	Estimates for women	Estimates for men
Alcohol	WHO 2014	Southeast Asia	Heavy episodic drinking	10.9x less likely	10.9x more likely
	SAMSHA 2013	USA	Binge drinking 18–25 yrs old	33.2%	45.8%
			Binge drinking 26+ yrs	14.7%	30.7%
	McManus et al. 2009	UK	Hazardous drinking	15.7%	33.2%
			Dependent on alcohol	3.3%	8.7%
All drugs	National Treatment Agency (NTA) 2010	UK	Numbers entering treatment	21,038	63,488
Cannabis	Degenhardt et al. 2013	Global	Cannabis dependence	0.14%	0.23%
	McManus et al. 2009	UK	Signs of dependence	1.7%	3.7%
	EMCDDA 2014	Europe	% of total number in treatment	17%	83%
Cocaine	McManus et al. 2009	UK	Signs of dependence	0.2%	0.7%
	EMCDDA 2014	Europe	% of total number in treatment	16%	84%
Tranquilizers	McManus et al. 2009	UK	Signs of dependence	0.3%	0.3%
Gambling	McManus et al. 2009	UK	Problem gambling	0.2%	1.2%
Amphetamines	EMCDDA 2014	Europe	% total number in treatment	21%	79%
Heroin	EMCDDA 2014	Europe	% total number in treatment	21%	79%
	McManus et al. 2009	UK	Signs of dependence	0.0%	0.3%
All prescription drugs	Culberson & Ziska 2008	USA	Abuse in elderly females	11%	–
Prescription opiates	Back et al. 2010	USA	Prescription opiate abuse or dependence	0.58%	0.74%

A particular harm in young people who use alcohol and drugs is risk-taking, which may manifest itself in behaviors such as driving whilst intoxicated, or result in outcomes such as accidental injury. Women are less likely to engage in risk-taking behaviors, but such behaviors do still occur (e.g., Lex et al. 1994).

Girls are more likely to smoke for reasons of appetite reduction and weight control than boys and men, and, compared to boys who smoke, tend to have stronger peer attachments; to have parents and friends who smoke; to be less committed to school; and to have less knowledge about nicotine, addiction and prevalence of smoking (US Department of Health and Human Services 2001). Escalating rates of smoking in young girls have recently been noted in Southeast Asia – whereas smoking rates for women in general are one-tenth of those for men; for 13–15 year olds, boys are only 2.5x more likely to smoke than girls (Hammond 2009).

Transition to problematic use

Although fewer women than men use drugs, alcohol and nicotine, those who do tend to have a more rapid acceleration of use than men, and this appears across drugs such as alcohol, cannabis, cocaine and opiates/opioids (Brady 1999, Hernandez-Avila 2004). The transition in women from use to hazardous use to harmful

Table 15.3 Major theories of addiction

Type of theory	Examples	Refs
Addiction as rational choice	Rational Informed Stable Choice models The Theory of Rational Addiction Self-Medication model Opponent Process Theory	e.g., Davies 1992 Becker & Murphy 1988 Khantzian 1997 Solomon 1980
Addiction as irrational choice	Expectancy Theories Skog's (conflicted) Choice Theory Slovic's Affect Heuristic Cognitive bias theories Behavioral Economic Theory Gateway Drug Theory The Transtheoretical Model of Behavior Change Identity Shift Theory	e.g., Christiansen & Goldman 1983 Skog 2000 Slovic et al. 2002 Field et al. 2004; Franken et al. 2003 Bickel et al. 1995 Kandell et al. 1992 Prochaska & DiClemente 1985 Kearney & O'Sullivan 2003
Addiction as a disorder of impulse and/or self-control: a combination of conscious, automatic and semi-automatic brain processes are responsible for addiction	Disease Model of Addiction Addictive personality types Self-efficacy Theory The Abstinence Violation Effect Inhibition Dysregulation Theory Self-regulation theory Cognitive model of drug urges	Jellinek 1960 Cloninger 1987 Bandura 1977 Marlatt 1979 Lubman et al. 2004 Baumeister et al. 1994 Tiffany and Conklin 2000
Addiction as a learning disorder	Classical conditioning Operant conditioning/Instrumental learning theories Social learning theory Dopamine reward theory and other theories arising from the functional neurotoxicity of drugs Multiple Memory System Theory of Addiction Incentive Sensitisation Theory Theory of differential drug effects	e.g., Drummond 1990 e.g., O'Brien et al. 1992 Bandura et al. 1971 e.g., Weiss & Koob 2001 White 1996 Robinson & Berridge 1993, Balfour 2004
Comprehensive theories of addiction	Addiction as Excessive Appetite PRIME theory	Section 1.02 Orford 2001 West & Hardy 2006

Adapted from West & Hardy 2006

use to dependence is less clear. Late 20s is often a time when women cut back on use, and both marriage and pregnancy seem to have a protective effect in reducing substance use (Leonard & Eiden 2007). Child-rearing is often accompanied by less money and less time, along with the increased responsibilities of motherhood, and these all may contribute to how mothers modify their drinking and drug-taking behavior.

Women transition to problematic alcohol use more quickly than men (Zilberman et al. 2003). The reproductive years also carry increased risks of harm for women who misuse alcohol. Alcohol misuse can disrupt the menstrual cycle and reproductive function and has been implicated in infertility and spontaneous abortion (Jones et al., 2008). Women who binge drink are more likely to engage in risky sexual behaviors, with increased risk of both sexually transmitted diseases (Thomas et al. 2001) and unplanned pregnancy (Naimi et al. 2003). There is also some evidence in young women that alcohol use by both perpetrator and victim is a risk factor for sexual assault (Abbey 2002; Mohler-Kuo 2004).

Box 15.2 Three theories of addiction

The Opponent Process Theory of Addiction (Solomon 1980)

The transition to addiction has been described as a model of opponent processes. In this model, initial drug taking is accompanied by high levels of pleasure and low levels of withdrawal, but over time the physiological process of tolerance reduces the levels of pleasure as more and more of the drug is needed to obtain the same effect, and at the same time withdrawal symptoms increase, leading to increasing discomfort. Drug taking becomes necessary to relieve withdrawal, with little pleasure attached.

The Transtheoretical Model of Behavior Change (Prochaska & DiClemente 1985)

This theory (commonly also known as the Stages of Change Model) has been operationalized into a treatment model widely found in addiction services. Several stages of change are proposed, from pre-contemplation of making a change through contemplation of that change; preparation for it; action, that is, making the change; then maintenance of the new behavior. Processes of change are often represented as a circle, with individuals progressing through the stages, sometimes with backwards movements, before reaching maintenance.

Addiction as Excessive Appetite (Orford 2001)

The conceptualization of addiction as being disordered appetite allows for a consideration of several primary and secondary psychological processes, including restraint, control, cues and complex memory schemata processes. The model can incorporate other theories, such as neuroadaptation, the abstinence violation effect and conflict. Importantly, this theory was the first to propose that it is possible to be addicted not just to substances, but also to behaviors, for example, sex and gambling.

There is clear evidence of a quicker transition in cocaine use too: women begin taking cocaine earlier, then progress from initial use to dependence more rapidly than men and enter treatment earlier. They also report higher levels of craving in response to cues, and if they relapse, have longer periods of use than men (Becker & Hu 2008). These findings are supported by animal studies, where sex differences are

Box 15.3 Special population: pregnant women and mothers

Addiction problems are particularly concerning in women who are pregnant, as harms may be caused not only to the expectant mother, but also to the child in utero. In 2010, in the USA, 4% of women entering drug and/or alcohol treatment were pregnant (SAMSHA 2010). Specialist treatment services for pregnant women should be working together with other agencies in order to address the pregnancy, safeguarding and housing.

Fetal Alcohol Spectrum Disorders (FASD) occur when alcohol, ingested during pregnancy by the mother, adversely affects the cells and organs of the unborn child in several ways, as alcohol passes through the placenta into the blood of the developing fetus. Effects can be mild or severe. They occur because of the neurotoxic and teratogenic effects of alcohol, exacerbated by the fact that the liver of the fetus is not sufficiently developed to metabolize the alcohol it receives from the mother through the placenta (Howell et al. 2006, Plant 1985, Plant & Plant 1988). In FASD, alcohol ingested by the fetus in utero results in neuropsychological deficits and behavioral features (for a full review see Mattson et al. 2011) as well as physiological impairments (Russell et al. 1991) in the child. Birth abnormalities occur most often in the children of women who drink heavily, but small amounts of alcohol might also be harmful, and in the United States advice is given that "no amount of alcohol is safe for pregnant women to drink" (National Institute on Alcohol Abuse and Alcoholism 2015). In the UK, advice remains confusing and contradictory, between total abstinence during pregnancy and small amounts. In a large part because of public health education programs, pregnant women are much less likely to drink alcohol than nonpregnant women, for example around 1 in 10 in the UK drinking in the last week, compared to 5 in 10 non-pregnant women (HSCIC 2014). In 2010, a survey indicated that 48% of women stopped drinking completely during pregnancy, and a further 47% reduced how much they drank (HSCIC 2010). However, in pregnant women who drink excessively FASD is a major of concern, and the prevalence of FASD in the United States has been estimated to be between 0.5 and 3 per 1,000 (Stratton, Howe et al. 1996), although a more recent study estimated it could be as high as 20–50 per 1,000 (May, Gossage et al. 2009).

Pregnant women who use illicit substances are also of concern to agencies and those who are receiving opiate substitution treatment have an increased risk of their baby being born with neonatal

Box 15.3 *(cont.)*

abstinence syndrome, (that is, exhibiting signs of opiate withdrawal). Women who are pregnant or who have children are often pressurized to come off methadone or buprenorphine and services can be perceived to be very judgmental. In family drug and alcohol courts (FDACs), abstinence is very highly correlated with family reunification (Harwin et al. 2014), and although no one would argue that abstinence alone necessarily equates to good parenting, it is often a prerequisite of the Court if a woman is to keep care of her children. The FDAC model has been far more successful at achieving sustained abstinence for substance-addicted parents than previous models and is currently being considered for longer-term funding and evaluation of cost-effectiveness (Advisory Council for the Misuse of Drugs 2003). Other psychosocial factors accompanying misuse also contribute and disentangling the contributions of each to those outcomes is difficult (e.g., Cleaver et al. 2011).

Smoking during pregnancy is known to contribute to poorer outcomes for offspring in a range of areas, and has been described as the most important environmental risk to an unborn child. The adverse outcomes it contributes could also be avoided with smoking cessation (Mund et al. 2013).

consistently found in the area of cocaine self-administration (Roth et al. 2004).

Women who have transitioned into cannabis misuse show increased analgesia, depression, anxiety and catalepsy compared to men. Further, they show increased sexual behavior, whereas in men the opposite is the case (Fattore & Fratta 2010).

In opiates, findings differ, although some studies do suggest that women escalate more rapidly to problematic use than men and experience addiction in a shorter period (Anglin et al. 1987, Hser et al. 1987, Greenfield et al. 2007). However, women are somewhat less likely to have injected than men, although if they do inject, they are more likely to share needles than men (24% vs. 17%) (NTA 2010), leading to increased risk for blood-borne viruses such as Hepatitis A, B and C, and HIV. Menstrual disorders have also been associated with opiate use (Busch et al. 1986) and are thought to be caused by disruption to the hypothalamic pituitary axis (HPA) (Vuong et al. 2010).

Nicotine is highly addictive and the transition to dependence can take as little as 3 months (WHO 2011). There is also evidence that nicotine has specific effects on sexual and reproductive health and smoking has been implicated in infertility problems, ectopic pregnancies and preterm problems including preterm delivery, stillbirth, neonatal deaths, Sudden Infant Death Syndrome and lower birth weight (US Department of Health and Human Services 2001).

Addiction in middle age

Middle age is when many of the physical and psychological consequences of long-term substance misuse begin to take their toll. The contribution of alcohol to mortality and morbidity increases (Jones et al. 2008). The health risks of smoking are well documented and also begin to manifest themselves in middle age. In women, smoking is a major cause of mortality and morbidity from various cancers, coronary heart disease, stroke and chronic obstructive pulmonary disease (US Department of Health and Human Services 2001), and women have a 1.5-to-2-fold higher risk for lung cancer than men at the same level of tar exposure (Harris et al. 1993).

Further problems for women can occur when children grow into adults and leave the family home, and some women may question their social roles (Nolen-Hoeksema 2004). Rates of divorce and separation are higher in middle age and these are risk factors for women for alcohol misuse (Leonard & Eiden 2007).

Reproductive problems may continue in middle age. The onset of menopause is earlier in women who misuse alcohol than in women who do not (Eagon 2010) and women smokers are also at increased risk of early menopause (US Department of Health and Human Services 2001).

Addiction in the elderly

For many women, numerous challenges accompany old age: bereavement, failing physical health, depression, isolation, loneliness and poverty. Those who have developed addiction problems over the lifespan may be particularly difficult to identify in old age. Shame and stigma are particularly prevalent in this group and symptoms of, for example, alcohol dependence might be mistaken for symptoms of dementia, and vice versa (NIAAA 1998). Further, for those who take medications, there may be harmful interactive effects between those medications and alcohol. Elderly women appear to be particularly vulnerable to addiction to opioid-based painkillers, and at time of writing the CODEMISUSED project at http://codemisused.org is investigating this group in the UK, Ireland and South Africa.

For elderly women who smoke, there are increased risks of osteoporosis. Postmenopausal smoking women have lower bone density and increased risks of hip fractures than do nonsmoking women (WHO 2010).

Consequences over the life span

Although on a population level women suffer fewer harms from addiction than men, there is good evidence that women are suffering increasing addiction-related harms over the life span (e.g., Jones et al. 2008, Jones et al. 2011). This has been exacerbated by the increase in women's use of alcohol and drugs over the past few decades, within a context of economic development and changing gender roles. A well-recognized phenomenon is that of the "telescoping effect," when women transition to dependence more rapidly than men, and suffer greater harms more quickly and with less consumption/use than men. This phenomenon has been found in a range of addictive drugs and behaviors, including alcohol (e.g., Diehl et al. 2007) and gambling (Slutske et al. 2014).

The WHO estimates that alcohol contributes to 4% of deaths in women, compared to 7.6% in men, but women appear to be more vulnerable to alcohol-related harm than men: while intoxicated, they have higher Blood Alcohol Content (BAC) after consuming the same amount of alcohol (Nolen-Hoeksema 2004). Women also suffer memory blackouts while drinking much lower levels of alcohol than men (White et al. 2002). With longer-term, chronic alcohol misuse, women develop alcohol liver injury and cirrhosis having consumed less alcohol than men and for a shorter time, and it is suggested that, as well as body mass and composition of fat versus water, sex hormones play a part in this (Eagon 2010).

There is enormous variation from country to country. In the United States, alcohol-related deaths averaged 26,000 for women and 62,000 for men between 2006 and 2010. Rates of harms are strongly correlated with rates of consumption: in the Russian Federation, consumption is high and 6% of deaths among women are attributable to alcohol misuse (Kerr-Correâ et al. 2007). In England, alcohol contributes to 2.0% of deaths in women, compared to 4.4% in men. There are differences in causes of alcohol-attributable deaths across the life course: under the age of 25, the leading cause is intentional self-harm; between the ages of 25 and 34 spontaneous abortion; between the ages of 35–54 mental and behavioral disorders; post 55 hypertensive diseases; and over 75 cardiac arrhythmias (Jones et al., 2008).

In drug-taking populations, women may also have poorer health outcomes: Neale (2004) reports women drug takers scoring significantly lower on six out of eight health dimensions than men.

Alcohol and drugs are also significant contributors to a range of health harms; Table 15.4 lists the key harms associated with use of addictive substances.

Risk factors

Given that women as a whole consume less alcohol and overall have fewer alcohol-related harms than men, being a woman in itself could be considered a protective factor. Certain women are more vulnerable than others to addiction problems and the reasons for this can be viewed within a biopsychosocial model (Mueller et al. 2009, Knibbe et al. 2006).

Biological

Biological risk factors for women are considered in four main areas: metabolism, genes, sex hormones and neuroscience.

Women have differences in biological mechanisms relating to the metabolism of alcohol and to body water content, compared to men. This means that women are more likely to experience harm related to drinking at the same level of alcohol consumption, even controlling for body mass (Zakhari 2006). Levels of alcohol dehydrogenase tend to be lower in women, resulting in less efficient metabolism of alcohol and higher levels remaining in the bloodstream (Frezza et al. 1990). In smoking, women have greater sensitivity to the effects of nicotine at lower levels, and do not take in as much nicotine as men (Benowitz 1998). However, in pregnant women and in women taking oral contraceptives, metabolism of nicotine is much higher than in women who are not (Dempsey et al. 2002, Matta et al. 2007). Metabolic differences have also been noted in cannabis users, with women taking longer to clear tetrahydrocannabinol (THC) than men, which is thought to be related to the lipophyllic properties of THC and the greater proportion of fat in women's bodies. In benzodiazepines, gender differences have been observed in

Table 15.4 Addiction-related harms

Addictive substance	Harms	Specific harms for women
Alcohol	Various forms of liver disease Increased risk of cancer Alcoholic cardiomyopathy Cognitive impairment Dementia Brain damage Stroke Reproductive problems Poor nutrition and low weight	More harm, sooner and at lower levels More harm, sooner and at lower levels More harm, sooner and at lower levels More harm, sooner and at lower levels More harm, acute and chronic drinking Fertility problems, early menopause
Cannabis	Poor nutrition and low weight Psychosis and schizophrenia	Fewer women than men
Cocaine and crack cocaine	Burns to fingers, lips and mouth Blood-borne viruses: Hep A, B & C, and HIV Risky environment	Women more likely to share needles Women particularly vulnerable
Heroin	Overdose Blood-borne viruses: Hep A,B & C, and HIV Dental problems Reproductive problems Poor nutrition and low weight Risky environments	Fewer women than men overdose Women more likely to share needles Amenorrhea Women particularly vulnerable
Nicotine	Various cancers including lung, esophagus, throat Emphysema Coronary heart disease, stroke Chronic obstructive pulmonary disease	
Prescription painkillers and tranquilizers	Overdose	More women than men

both directions, with some linked to faster metabolism, and some linked to lower (Howell et al. 2001).

Sex hormones are also thought to contribute to risk factors for the harms associated with alcohol misuse in women (Eagon 2010). Gonadal hormones are thought to contribute to neurobiological sex differences in cannabinoid action (Fattore & Fratta 2010). In animal models, estrogen has been found to facilitate drug-seeking behavior, whereas progesterone has been found to reduce drug seeking, contributing to an increased vulnerability in females. There may also be different responses to substances at different stages in the menstrual cycle: in human studies, increased responsivity to stimulants has been observed during the follicular phase, but lower responsivity during the luteal phase (Sofuoglu et al. 1999). Other candidates for sex differences, particularly in treatment

responses, are the hypothalamic pituitary axis (HPA), dopamine (DA) and gamma-hydroxy-butyric acid (GABA) (Carroll & Anker 2010). Oral contraceptive pills have been noted to affect clearance rates, in both directions, of different types of benzodiazepine (Howell et al. 2001)

Recent research has started to find different associations between neurobiological processes underlying motivations for drug and alcohol use in women and men. Becker et al. (2012) propose that sex differences in brain function may contribute to different pathways to addiction for women and men. They hypothesize that more men than women begin taking drugs for sensation-seeking reasons, receiving positive reinforcement of drug taking initially in the form of euphoria (related to dopamine, norepinephrine, endogenous opioids and acetylcholine), which over time becomes negative reinforcement, leading to dysphoria and eventually to drug dependence. Women, they argue, are less likely to initiate drug use for the positive euphoriant effects. (See also Bobzean et al. 2014.)

Most studies in genetics suggest that genes play a role in alcohol misuse in both women and men, with heritability estimates in both groups clustering at around 50%. Early genetic studies suggested that alcohol misuse might be more heritable in men than in women, although more recent reviews suggest this is not the case (Plomin et al. 2008, Agrawal & Lynskey 2008). Genetic factors are thought to contribute to smoking initiation, where women have higher rates of heritability than men (66% vs. 49%) (Hamdani et al. 2006).

Box 15.4   Special population: lesbian women

As with heterosexual women, there is tremendous diversity amongst lesbians. There is no single pattern of drink or drug taking amongst lesbians, although higher rates of problem drinking are often reported in lesbian women than in heterosexual women. Research into lesbians and substance misuse is lacking, and often findings for gay males have been misguidedly generalized across to lesbians (SAMSHA 2001). Heterogeneity amongst lesbians means that some may be comfortable with and public about their sexuality, for others it may be hidden. Structural heterosexism may contribute to drug and alcohol problems, reinforcing feelings of alienation and shame and individual experiences of homophobia may also contribute to these.

Particular risk factors include a high reliance on lesbian bars as a source of social support; feelings of alienation from family and friends as a result of sexuality and/or of coming out; and interactions between sexism, stress and trauma with substance misuse. Lesbians also have increased rates of sexual abuse, both as children and as adults (SAMSHA 2001).

Female-only treatment programs are more attractive to lesbians (Copeland et al. 1993) and some lesbians are unwilling to join Alcoholics Anonymous or Narcotics Anonymous programs as they view these as being male organizations (SAMSHA 2001).

Psychological

Psychological comorbidity with use of alcohol and drugs is common and clinically important. However, there is often a lack of clarity on the direction of causation and investigating psychological factors can be further complicated by different patterns of use, with women's use being more stigmatized and therefore more hidden (Bradly & Randall 1999).

Studies have shown the tendency for women to self-medicate with alcohol (Smith et al. 2012), and some with cocaine (Waldrop et al. 2007). The same may also be the case for opiates: rates of psychiatric comorbidity have been reported to be twice as high in women opiate users when compared to men (Brooner et al. 1997), although the problems of establishing causation remain. Smoking is thought to be used as a means of self-medication (US Department of Health and Human Services 2001) and this may be more the case in women than in men.

Depression is diagnosed more often in women than in men (Hammen 1997) and is a major comorbidity in women with addiction problems (e.g., Brady et al. 1993). Depression and anxiety are particularly prevalent in women who misuse alcohol (Nolen-Hoeksema 2004, Dawson et al. 2010), and more often a primary diagnosis than in men (Zilberman et al. 2003). Depression in young women has also been identified as a risk factor for alcohol misuse in later life (Fillmore et al. 1979). Women who have been diagnosed with alcohol use disorders and depression have been shown to have improved outcomes if treatment has a depression focus rather than a primary alcohol focus (Baker et al. 2010), underlining the strong relationship between alcohol and depression in women. Substance misuse should therefore be a consideration for clinicians examining women presenting with depression and anxiety. In cocaine users, however, women have shown the same rates of depression as men (Rounsaville et al. 1991) or lower (Griffin et al. 1989). In opiate users, the pattern appears to be similar to alcohol, with women opiate users reporting more depression than men (Brooner et al. 1997). Women who smoke tobacco are also more likely to report depression than men (US Department of Health and Human Services 2001, Perkins 1996).

Alcohol is also associated with suicide in women and men (Kaplan et al. 2013); however, consumption has been found to be a predictor in suicide rates in women aged 29 and under, but not in men of that age (Innamorati et al. 2010). Young women with alcohol use disorders have been found to be more likely to have suicidal ideation, whilst rates of adverse life events and mental health problems are associated with alcohol use disorders and suicidal ideation in young women (Agrawal et al. 2013). Suicides involving prescription painkillers in the United States are increasing at an alarming rate (McCarthy 2013), more than five-fold over 10 years.

Women with Generalized Anxiety Disorder (GAD) have higher rates of alcohol use than women without GAD and moderate anxiety increases the risk for alcohol abuse in women (Howell et al. 2001). Also, alcohol withdrawal symptoms may be difficult to differentiate from symptoms of anxiety disorders such as GAD and panic disorder.

Substance misuse in women, including alcohol misuse, is more often accompanied by eating disorders such as anorexia nervosa and bulimia nervosa, either in parallel, or sequentially, than it is in men. For a full review see National Center on Addiction and Substance Abuse at Columbia University (2003).

Rates of various personality disorders have also been found to be higher in women who misuse alcohol than women in the general population (Grant et al. 2004). Borderline personality disorder is more common in women who misuse alcohol than in men who misuse alcohol (Sinha & Rounsaville, 2002), but this is also the case in the general population (McManus et al. 2009). Rates of personality disorders such as anti-social personality disorder and conduct disorder have been noted to be higher in drug using women than in the general population (Lex 1994). As with other comorbidities, the direction of causation is unclear.

Although post-traumatic stress disorder (PTSD) has historically been studied in men, women who have been subjected to partner violence have increased rates of PTSD and increased rates of alcohol misuse (Sinha & Rounsaville, 2002). There is also evidence that for some women who experience childbirth as traumatic, childbirth could be considered a stressor sufficient to meet the criteria for PTSD (Alcorn et al. 2010). Studies have found that trauma exposure and PTSD in women is more strongly associated with binge drinking when compared to men (Kachadourian et al. 2014).

Other psychological findings include that women who misuse alcohol are less likely to do so for sensation-seeking or impulsive reasons than men (Dawson et al. 2010) and that there may be neuropsychological reasons for this (Becker et al. 2012). Women also report that smoking tobacco gives them greater subjective pleasurable effects than men report (Perkins et al. 1999).

Social

Women experiencing adverse life events or family problems are known to be more vulnerable to substance misuse than men (Copeland & Hall 1992). Divorce and separation are risk factors for alcohol misuse (Leonard & Eiden 2007). It is also known that childhood sexual abuse plays a role in later substance misuse. Almost two-thirds of US women drug users in treatment reporting physical, sexual or emotional abuse in childhood (National Institute for Drug Abuse [NIDA] 1998). In Scotland nearly two-thirds of women in treatment report physical abuse and one-third report sexual abuse (McKeganey et al. 2005).

Rates of domestic violence are particularly high in women with addiction problems and often run alongside comorbid psychiatric problems, so much so that practitioners refer to addiction, domestic violence and mental health problems as a "toxic triangle" in women. Alcohol is particularly implicated in domestic violence and a myriad of studies across low- and middle-income countries consistently demonstrate a strong association between alcohol use in men and experiencing domestic violence in women. A large portion of partner violence occurs after drinking and the risks are particularly high during heavy episodic drinking (for an in-depth review see Heise 2011). See also Chapter 14.

> **Box 15.5 Special population: sex workers**
>
> Women with addiction problems may turn to prostitution to finance their addictions, with up to two-thirds of opiate users in one study funding their drug use in this way (Gossop et al. 1994). Sex work carries with it high risks, particularly from unsafe sex and assault, and women using cocaine have been found to be particularly likely to be exposed to violence and criminal activities (Goldstein et al. 1991). Sex workers are less likely than other women to access health services (Clements 1996), leading to poorer health outcomes. Opiate substitution treatment has shown to lead to a reduction in exchanges of sex for drugs and/or money (Gowing et al. 2006).

There is mixed evidence in women for the role of socioeconomic status and social roles in increased alcohol consumption and related problems (Nolen-Hoeksema, 2004). Traditionally, feminine traits such as nurturance appear to be protective factors against alcohol misuse, although this is the case in both sexes. Women, however, perceive greater social censure than men (Nolen-Hoeksema 2004) and, for women drug takers, stigma is known to be a particularly pertinent issue (Brown 2011). Recent decades have seen increased targeting of alcohol and nicotine advertising and branding specifically at women, from sugary alcohol drinks in pink packaging marketed as low calorie, to "light" cigarettes, smoked by two-thirds of women compared to one-half of men (Shifman et al. 2001).

Treatment

Brickman et al. (1982) described four approaches to treatment of substance use disorders. First, what they termed the "moral model," which emphasizes punishment and incarceration; second, the "disease model," which does not include elements of blame or coercion, but rather considers the role of genetics and biological vulnerabilities; third, the "spiritual model," which is a recognition of the treatment power of 12-step programs and similar; and lastly the "compensatory model," which posits that biopsychosocial risk factors vary between individuals and that treatment should also vary, based on the goals of the individual. The debate in recent years about how best to approach treatment has become less nuanced and more polarized, with discussion focusing on concepts of harm reduction, where a pragmatic approach is taken to addiction and ways in which the harms can be minimized are explored (examples include opioid substitution treatment, overdose prevention, needle exchanges, nicotine replacement therapy and controlled drinking), and on abstinence-base recovery ideas, where the end goal is no drug use. This harm reduction versus abstinence-based recovery debate has specific implications for pregnant women and women with children (see Box 15.3). There is huge heterogeneity in addiction treatment services from country to country, and even within countries, not only in their philosophical approaches to harm reduction and abstinence, but also in their service delivery.

A stepped approach to care is sometimes proposed, with the aim first of stabilizing those whose drug use is volatile, and once stabilized, offering psychotherapeutic treatments (Wanigaratne 2006). Treatment is further complicated by the high rate of comorbid psychiatric disorders found in those misusing drugs and alcohol and whether those disorders are primary or secondary to any addiction disorder – this may have particular implications for women. Furthermore, addiction is a chronic disorder with high rates of relapse, and this is reflected in the terminology often used to refer to treatment as "relapse prevention."

In the United States in 2010, around 30% of those who enter state funded drug and/or alcohol treatment programs were women (28% in treatment for alcohol, 33% for heroin, 32–46% for cocaine, 27% for cannabis, 49–55% for tranquilizers and sedatives and 46% for opiates other than heroin) (SAMSHA 2010). Women in England come to treatment at a younger age than men (30 years, compared to 32 for men) and, on average, at an early stage in their drug-taking career (7 years, compared to 9 for men).

Much of the treatment provision for women has historically been based on research into what is effective for men (Greenfield et al. 2007, Greenfield et al. 2009). For example, in detoxification programs for alcohol, benzodiazepines are routinely prescribed to prevent seizures, yet it is not known whether there are gender differences in terms of the efficacy of these drugs (Amato et al. 2010). Women may have particular treatment needs and services are rarely designed with those in mind (Marsh et al. 2000). Increasingly, there is a realization that women may need specialist services and some service providers do indeed offer those, but these are in the minority. In particular, all-women treatment services are the exception rather than the norm and mother-and-baby treatment units are very scarce. The lack of specialist services for women may be reducing the rates of successful outcomes. Recently, more women-only treatment services have emerged, but few randomized controlled trials have been conducted, and with small sample sizes it is not possible to say with any certainty whether they are superior (Greenfield et al. 2010).

It may also be important in women to take a multi-agency approach, particularly for those women with children, coordinating support from social services, help with housing and benefits and access to mental health services as well as drug/alcohol treatment services.

Women who do come into treatment tend to be younger than men, to have had an earlier onset of drug use, to be more likely to be married and less likely to be employed (Acharyya et al. 2003). They also have more physical and psychological problems at entry than do men (Chatham et al. 1999)

Retention in treatment

The longer a person with addiction problems remains in treatment, the more likely a successful outcome, so much so that retention in treatment is measured as a treatment outcome in its own right in some countries (Marsden et al. 2008). However, treatment drop-out rates are concerningly high for both women and men, as those who leave treatment are less likely to address their addiction problems. Despite best efforts, researchers have been unable to identify clear reasons why people drop out of treatment. Although there do not appear to be gender differences in treatment retention, gender-specific factors have been identified that improve treatment retention in women, including social support, psychological functioning, personal stability, low levels of anger, belief in treatment efficacy and referral source. These run alongside factors that improve outcomes for both women and men: fewer mental health problems, less severe addiction problems and access to greater financial resources (Greenfield et al. 2010).

Treatment outcomes

Data on treatment outcomes are patchy and there is much heterogeneity in findings. Treatment programs vary widely, so it is not surprising that treatment outcomes also vary. However, it has been reported that women who are dependent on alcohol can have higher relapse rates than men (Breese et al. 2005). Research also seems to suggest that women find it more difficult to quit smoking than men (Perkins 2001, Mackay & Amos 2003) and that nicotine replacement therapy is less successful in women than in men (Perkins & Scott 2008).

Treatment outcomes for opiates have been found to be about the same for women and men when measured by abstinence (around 34%) and when measured by reduction of use (NTA 2010). There is little research in this area, although at the time of writing Bawor et al. (2014) have published a protocol to review gender differences in opiate substitution treatment. What is known is that women in drug treatment are less likely than men to achieve abstinence from crack cocaine (49% vs. 42%) (NTA 2010). It is also thought that certain factors that may contribute to positive outcomes are more prevalent in women: these include stronger family and social relationships, better money management and more access to informal support, including housing and material assistance (Neale et al. 2013).

Barriers to treatment

Barriers to addiction treatment specific to women include stigma, lack of childcare, child custody issues, psychiatric comorbidity and victimization (Brady & Randall 1999). Other problems specific to women that may also be a barrier to treatment include maternity, physical and sexual abuse, prostitution, sexual and mental health (NTA 2010). In England, around 60% of women entering treatment are mothers, but there is a perception amongst service users that entering treatment will increase the likelihood of their children being taken into care (NTA 2010). For those women who have children, parenthood can be a barrier to treatment, but for some it can be a key motivator for engaging with and staying with treatment.

Shand et al. (2003a, 2003b) strongly recommended in order to improve treatment outcomes for women, that issues particular to women should be treated with greater sensitivity in clinical settings; that the therapeutic environment should be safe, with provision for the tackling issues such as mental health and physical and sexual abuse; and that treatment services should have strong relationships with and easy access to other specialist services. They further recommended that women should be able to choose the gender of their therapist, that a range of services should be offered, and that awareness of services and working to decrease fear of service involvement should be addressed.

Treatment of women in relationships with another alcohol/drug user

Being in a relationship with another alcohol or drug user is a risk factor for addiction problems in women, may prove a barrier to treatment and may increase the chances of relapse. Women with addiction problems are thought to select intimate partners who have similar addiction problems, a phenomenon known as "assortative mating" (Leonard & Eiden 2007). Rates of domestic violence in such couples are high (Heise 2011). Behavioral couples' treatment, where couples are treated together, has shown improved outcomes in substance use, but also in partner violence, marital satisfaction and outcomes for children, when compared to individual treatment (Greenfield et al. 2010).

Opiate substitution treatment

The predominant treatment for opiate users in most countries is opiate substitution treatment in the form of methadone and/or buprenorphine and this has been shown to improve a range of outcomes from physical, social and psychological functioning, to reduction in criminal activity and illicit drug use. For women, there may be particular side effects of treatment, including weight gain and, if amenorrhea has occurred during drug use, the return of menstruation. This may require a woman to reevaluate her need for contraception.

Mutual aid organizations

Mutual aid organizations can be a very effective method of treatment, providing a potent combination of structured contact in the form of regular group meetings and individual peer support, and almost exclusively work towards total abstinence rather than harm reduction. The most well-known are the 12-step recovery-based programs, the original of which was Alcoholics Anonymous (www.aa.org), a model which has been developed to include other substances (e.g., Narcotics Anonymous) and behavioral addictions (e.g., Gamblers Anonymous). Women have been involved in these 12-step programs since they began, with Marty Mann playing a key role in the 1950s, promoting their treatment approach and tackling stigma around alcohol addiction, and writing a chapter in the second edition of the key Alcoholics Anonymous text, *The Big Book*, entitled "Women Suffer Too" (Alcoholics Anonymous 1955). The 12-step programs have a spiritual element in them and require the invoking of a "Higher Power," which has drawn some criticism. In 1994, SMART Recovery was established, a less spiritually based organization with a four-point program dealing with motivations, urges, feelings and behaviors, with an emphasis on living a balanced life (www.smartrecovery.org). Although these organizations do have women-only meetings, some women have found them to be too male-focused. Women for Sobriety was set up in 1976 in response to a need for an organization exclusively for women (www.women forsobriety.org).

Conclusions

Most research into addictions of all types has taken place in men. Yet the clear gender differences in prevalence, risk factors, course, consequences and treatment mean there remains a large gap in the information needed to plan effective services for women. Addiction in women, whilst less prevalent than in men, develops quicker with less use and brings with it more harms. Those harms may affect others in particular ways, especially in women who are pregnant and/or who have children. There is a need to develop the evidence base by examining women as a separate group and by examining subgroups of women. Policy makers and treatment services should give more consideration to gender-sensitive treatment, whilst bearing in mind that there is much heterogeneity in women and that what is appropriate for one will not necessarily be appropriate for another. Women who are addicted represent a complex and challenging group both for researchers and for treatment services because of concurrent problems with comorbidity, stigma and family and other carer responsibilities.

Suggested reading

Becker, J. B., Perry, A. N. & Westenbroek, C. (2012). Sex differences in the neural mechanisms mediating addiction: a new synthesis and hypotheseis. *Biology of Sex Differences*, 3: 14.

Dawson, D. A., Goldstein, R. B., Moss, H. B., Li, T. K. & Grant, B. F. (2010) Gender differences in the relationship of internalizing and externalizing psychopathology to alcohol dependence: Likelihood, expression and course. *Drug and Alcohol Dependence,* 112 (1–2): 9–17.

Greenfield, S. F., Brooks, A. J., Gordon, S. M., Green, C. A., Kropp, F., McHugh, R. K., Lincoln, M., Hien, D., Miele, G. M.. (2007) Substance abuse treatment entry, retention, and outcome in women: a review of the literature. *Drug and Alcohol Dependence*, 86:21.

Leonard, K. E. & Eiden, R. D. (2007) Marital and family processes in the context of alcohol use and alcohol disorders. *Annual Review of Clinical Psychology*, 3: 285.

Nolen-Hoeksema, S. (2004) Gender differences in risk factors and consequences for alcohol use and problems. *Clinical Psychology Review*, 24 (8): 981–1010.

West, R. & Hardy, A. (2006) *Theory of addiction*. Oxford: Blackwell.

References

Abbey, A. (2002) Alcohol-related sexual assault: A common problem among college students. *J Stud Alcohol*, Suppl 14:118–128.

Acharyya, S. & Zhang, H. (2003) Assessing sex differences on treatment effectiveness from the drug abuse treatment outcome study (DATOS) *Am J Drug Alcohol Abuse*, 29:415–444. doi: 10.1081/ADA-12002052.

Advisory Council for the Misuse of Drugs (ACMD) (2003). Hidden Harm. Available www.gov.uk/government/uploads/system/uploads/attachment_data/file/120620/hidden-harm-full.pdf.

Agrawal, A., Constantino, A.M., Bucholz, K.K., Glowinski, A., Madden, P.A., Heath, A.C. & Lynskey, M.T. (2013) Characterizing alcohol use disorders and suicidal ideation in young women. *Journal of Studies on Alcohol and Drugs*, 74 (3): 406.

Agrawal, A. & Lynskey, M. T. (2008). Are there genetic influences on addiction: evidence from family, adoption and twin studies. *Addiction*, 103: 1069–1081.

Alcoholics Anonymous (1955). *The big book (second edition.)*. AA World Services.

Alcorn, K. L., O'Donovan, A., Patrick, J., Creedy, D. & Devilly, G. J. (2010) A prospective longitudinal study of the prevalence of post-traumatic stress disorder resulting from childbirth events. *Psychological Medicine*, 40(11): 1849–1859.

Amato, L., Minozzi, S., Vecchi, S., Davoli, M. (2010). Benzodiazepines for alcohol withdrawal. *Cochrane Database Syst Rev*. doi: 10.1002/14651858.CD005063.pub3.

American Psychiatric Association Task Force (1994). *Diagnostic and statistical manual of mental disorders: DSM-IV. 4th Ed.* Washington DC: American Psychiatric Association.

American Psychiatric Association Task Force (2013). *Diagnostic and statistical manual of mental disorders: DSM-5. 5th Ed.* Washington DC: American Psychiatric Association.

Anglin M. D., Hser, Y-I. & McGlothlin, W. H. (1987). Sex differences in addict careers. Becoming addicted. *American Journal of Drug and Alcohol Abuse*, 13(1–2): 59–71. doi: 10.3109/00952998709001500

Back, S. E., Brady, K. T., Jackson, J. L., Salstron. S. & ZinZow, H. (2005) Gender differences in stress reactivity among cocaine-dependent individuals. *Psychopharmacology* 180: 169–176.

Back, S. E., Payne, R. L., Simpson, A. N. & Brady, K. T. (2010) Gender and prescription opioids: Findings from the National Survey on Drug Use and Health. *Addictive Behaviors*, 35(11): 1001–1007.

Baker, A. L., Kavanagh, D. J., Kay-Lambkin, F. J., Hunt, S. A., Lewin, T. J., Carr, V. J. & Connolly, J. (2010) Randomized controlled trial of cognitive–behavioural therapy for coexisting depression and alcohol problems: short-term outcome. *Addiction*, 105(1):87–99. doi: 10.1111/j.1360-0443.2009.02757.x.

Balfour, D.K.J. (2004). The neurobiology of tobacco dependence: a preclinical dependence: a preclinical perspective on the role of the dopamine projections to the nucleus acumbens. *Nicotine Tob Res*, 6(6): 899–912.

Bandura, A. (1971) *Social learning theory*. New York: General Learning Press.

Bandura, A. (1977). Self-efficacy: toward a unifying theory of behavioural change. *Psychological Review*, 84(2):191–215.

Baumeister, R. F., Heatherton, T. F. et al. (1994). *Losing control: How and why people fail at self-regulation*. San Diego: Academic Press.

Bawor, M., Dennis, B. B., Anglin, R., Steiner. M., Thabane, L. & Samaan, Z. (2014). Sex differences in outcomes of methadone maintenance treatment for opioid addiction: a systematic review protocol. *Syst Rev*, 16(3):45. doi: 10.1186/2046-4053-3-45.

Becker, G. S. & Murphy, K. M. (1988). A theory of rational addiction. *Journal of Political Economy*, 96: 675–700.

Becker, J. B. & Hu, M. (2008). Sex differences in drug abuse. *Frontiers in Neuroendocrinology*, 29(1): 36–37.

Becker, J. B., Perry, A. N. & Westenbroek, C. (2012). Sex differences in the neural mechanisms mediating addiction: a new synthesis and hypothesis. *Biology of Sex Differences*, 3: 14.

Benowitz, N. L. (1998) Gender differences in the pharmacology of nicotine addiction. *Addiction Biology*, 3: 383–404.

Bickel, W. K., DEGrandpre, R. J. et al. (1995). The behavioural economics of concurrent drug reinforcers: a review and reanalysis of drug self-administration research. *Psychopharmacology (Berl)*, 118(3): 250–259.

Bobzean. S. A. M., DeNobrega A. K., & Perrotti, L. I. (2014). Sex differences in the neurobiology of drug addiction. *Experimental Neurology*, 259: 64–74.

Boniface, S. & Shelton, N. (2013) How is alcohol consumption affected if we account for under-reporting? A hypothetical scenario. *The European Journal of Public Health* [Online], doi: 10.1093/eurpub/ckt016.

Bradley, K., Boyd-Wickizer, J., Powell, S. & Burman, M. (1998) Alcohol screening questionnaires in women: a critical review. *JAMA: The Journal of the American Medical Association*, 280(2): 166–171.

Brady, K. T., Grice, D. E., Dustan, L., et al. (1993). Gender differences in substance use disorders. *Am J Psychiatry*, 150:1707–1711.

Brady, K. T. & Randall, C. L. (1999). Gender differences in substance use disorders. *Psychiatric Clinics of North America*, 22: 241–252. Available from http://www.ncbi.nlm.nih.gov/pubmed/10385931 [Accessed October 2014].

Breese, G. R., Chu, K., Dayas, C. V., Funk, D., Knapp, D. J., Koob, G. F., Le, D. A., O'Dell. L. E., Overstreet, D. H., Roberts, A. J., Sinha, R., Valdez, G. R., & Weiss, F. (2005). Stress enhancement of craving during sobriety: a risk for relapse. *Alcoholism: Clinical and Experimental Research*, 29:185–195.

Brickman, P., Rabinowitz, V. C., Coates, D., Cohn, E., & Kidder L. (1982). Models of helping and coping. *Am. Psychol*, 37:364–384.

British Crime Survey for England and Wales (2013). Available from www .gov.uk/government/publications/ drug-misuse-findings-from-the- 2012-to-2013-csew/drug-misuse- findings-from-the-2012-to-2013- crime-survey-for-england-and- wales

Brooner, R. K., King, V. L., Kidorf, M., et al. (1997). Psychiatric and substance comorbidity among treatment-seeking opioid abusers. *Arch Gen Psychiatry*, 54:71–80.

Brown, S. A. (2011). Standardized measures for substance use stigma. *Drug and Alcohol Dependence*, 116(1–3):137–141.

Busch, D., McBride, A. B., & Benaventura, L. M. (1986). Chemical dependency in women: the link to OB/GYN problems. *Psychosoc Nurs* 24:2&30.

Carroll, M. E. & Anker, J. J. (2010). Sex differences and ovarian hormones in animal models of drug dependence. *Hormones and Behaviour*, 58:44–56.

Chang, G. (2002). Brief interventions for problem drinking and women. *J Subst Abuse Treat*, 23(1):1–7.

Chatham, L. R., Hiller, M. L., Rowan-Szal, G. A., Joe, G. W. & Simpson, D. D. (1999). Gender differences at admission and follow-up in a sample of methadone maintenance clients. *Subst Use Misuse*, 34:1137–1165. doi: 10.3109/ 10826089909039401

Christiansen, B. A. & Goldman, M. S. (1983). Alcohol-related expectancies versus demographic/background variables in the prediction of adolescent drinking. *J Consult Clin Psychol*, 51(2):249–257.

Cleaver, H., Unell, I. & Aldgate, J. (2011) *Children's needs – parenting capacity – child abuse: Parental mental illness, learning disability, substance misuse, and domestic violence. 2nd edition.* London: The Stationery Office.

Clements, T. M. (1996) Prostitution and the American health care system: Denying access to a group of women in need. *Berkeley Women's Law Journal*, 11:50–98.

Cloninger, C. R. (1987). A systematic method for clinical description and classification of personality variants. A proposal. *Arch Gen Psychiatry*, 44(6):573–588.

Copeland, J., & Hall, W. (1992). A comparison of women seeking drug and alcohol treatment in a specialist women's and two traditional mixed-sex treatment services. *British Journal of Addiction*, 87:1293–1302.

Copeland, J., Hall, W., Didcott, P., et al. (1993). A comparison of a specialist women's alcohol and other drug treatment service with two traditional mixed-sex services: Client characteristics and treatment outcome. *Drug and Alcohol Dependence*, 32:81–92.

Culberson, J. M. & Ziska, M. (2008). Prescription drug misuse/abuse in the elderly. *Geriatrics* 63(9):22–31.

Davies, J. B. (1992). *The myth of addiction: An application of the Psychological Theory of Attribution to illicit drug use.* Chur, Switzerland: Philadelphia, Harvard Academic Publishers.

Dawson, D. A., Goldstein, R. B., Moss, H. B., Li, T. K. & Grant, B. F. (2010) Gender differences in the relationship of internalizing and externalizing psychopathology to alcohol dependence: Likelihood, expression and course. *Drug and Alcohol Dependence*, 112(1–2):9–17.

Degenhardt, L., Ferrari, A. J., Calabria, B., Hall, W. D., Norman, R. E., McGrath, J., Flaxman, A. D., Engell, R. E., Freedman, G. D., Whiteford, H. A. & Vos, T. (2013). The global epidemiology and contribution of cannabis use and dependence to the global burden of disease: Results from the GBD 2010 study. *PLoS One*, doi: 10.1371/journal. pone.0076635.

Dempsey, D., Jacob, P. III & Benowitz, N. L. (2002). Accelerated metabolism in nicotine and contine in women smokers. *Pharmacology and Experimental Therapeutics*, 301: 594–598.

de Visser, R., Smith, J., Abraham, C. & Wheeler, Z. (2012). Gender, alcohol, and interventions. Available from: http://alcoholresearchuk.org/ downloads/finalReports/ FinalReport_0092.pdf [Accessed July 2011].

Diehl, A., Croissant, B., Batra, A., Mundle, G., Nakovics, H. & Mann, K. (2007). Alcoholism in women: is it different in onset and outcome compared to men? *European Archives of Psychiatry and Clinical Neuroscience*, 257(6): 344–351.

Drummond, D. C., Cooper, T. et al. (1990). Conditioned learning in alcohol dependence: implications for cue exposure treatment. *Br J Addict* 85(6):725–743.

Eagon, P. K. (2010). Alcoholic liver injury: Influence of gender and hormones. *World Journal of Gastroenterology*, 16(11):1377–1384.

Edwards, G. & Gross, M.M. (1976). Alcohol dependence: provisional description of a clinical syndrome. *British Medical Journal*, 1 (6017):1058–1061.

European Monitoring Centre for Drugs and Drug Addiction (EMCDDA) (2014). European Drug Report. Trends and Developments. Available from www.emcdda .europa.eu/publications/edr/trends- developments/2014.

Fattore, L. & Fratta, W. (2010). How important are sex differences in cannabinoid action? *British Journal of Pharmacology*, 160: 544–548.

Field, M., Mogg, K. et al. (2004). Cognitive bias and drug craving in recreational cannabis users. *Drug and Alcohol Dependence*, 74(1):105–111.

Fillmore, K. M., Golding, J. M., Leino, E. V., Motoyoshi, M., Shoemaker, C., Terry, H., Ager, C. R. & Ferrer, H. P. (1997). Patterns and trends in women's and men's drinking. In *Gender and alcohol*. Wilsnack, R. W., & Wilsnack, S. (eds). Piscataway, NJ: Rutgers Center of Alcohol Studies.

Franken, I. H., Stam. C. J. et al. (2003). Neurophysiological evidence for abnormal cognitive processing of drug cues in heroin dependence. *Psyhopharmacology (Berl)*, 170(2):205–212.

Frezza, M., di Padova, C. & Pozzato, G. (1990). High blood alcohol levels in women: the Role of Decreased Gastric Alcohol Dehydrogenase Activity and First Pass Metabolism. *New England Journal of Medicine*, 322 (2):95–99.

Gibbon, M., Spitzer, R. L. & First, M. B. (1997). *User's guide for the structured clinical interview for DSM-IV axis II personality disorders: SCID-II*. Washington: American Psychiatric Press Inc.

Gilchrist, G., Moskalewicz, J., Slezakova, S., Okruhlica, L., Torrens, M., Vajd, R. & Baldacchino, A. (2011). Staff regard towards working with substance users: a European multi-centre study. *Addiction*, 106 (2011):1114–1125.

Goldstein, P. J., Bellucci, P. A., Spunt, B. J. & Miller T. (1991). Volume of cocaine use and violence: A comparison between men and women. *Journal of Drug Issues*, 21(2): 345–367.

Golka, K. & Wiese, A. (2004). Carbohydrate-deficient transferrin (CDT)–a biomarker for long-term alcohol consumption. *J Toxicol Environ Health B Crit Rev*, 7(4):319–337.

Gossop, M., Powis, B., Griffiths, P., & Strang, J. (1994). Sexual behaviour and its relationship to drug-taking among prostitutes in south London. *Addiction*, 89(8): 961–970.

Gowing, L. R., Farrell, M., Bornemann, R., Sullivan, L. E. & Ali, R. L. (2006). Brief report: Methadone treatment of injecting opioid users for prevention of HIV infection. *J Gen Intern Med*, 21(2):193–195. Epub Dec 7, 2005.

Grana, R., Benowitz, N. & Glantz, S. A. (2013). *Background paper on e-cigarettes (Electronic Nicotine Delivery Systems). WHO report*. Geneva: World Health Organization. Available from http://escholarship.org/uc/item/13p2b72n and http://www.arizonansconcernedaboutsmoking.com/201312e-cig_report.pdf

Grant, B. F., Stinson, F. S., Dawson, D. A., Chou, S. P., Dufour, M. C., Compton, W., Pickering, R. P. & Kaplan, K. (2004). Prevalence and co-occurrence of substance use disorders and independent mood and anxiety disorders: results from the National Epidemiologic Survey on Alcohol and Related Conditions. *Archives of General Psychiatry*, 61(8):807.

Greenfield, S. F., Back, S. E., Lawson, K. & Brady, K. T. (2010). Substance abuse in women. *Psychiatr Clin North Am*, 33(2):339–355.

Greenfield, S. F., Brooks, A. J., Gordon, S. M., et al. (2007). Substance abuse treatment entry, retention, and outcome in women: a review of the literature. *Drug and Alcohol Dependence*, 86:1–21.

Greenfield, S. F. & Grella, C. E. (2009). Alcohol & drug abuse: what is "women-focused" treatment for substance use disorders? *Psychiatr Serv*, 60:880–882.

Griffin, M. L., Weiss, R. D., Mirin, S. M., et al. (1989). A comparison of male and female cocaine abusers [see comments]. *Arch Gen Psychiatry*, 46:122–126.

Hamdani, N., Ades, J. et al. (2006). Heritability and candidate genes in tobacco use. *Encephale*, 32(6 Pt1):966–975.

Hammen, C. (2007). *Depression (2nd Edition) (Clinical Psychology: A Popular Course)*. Psychology Press.

Hammond, S. K. (2009). Global patterns of nicotine and tobacco consumption. *Handb Exp Pharmacol*, 192:3–28. doi: 10.1007/978-3-540-69248-5_1.

Harris, R. E., Zang, E. A., Anderson, J. I. & Wynder, E. L. (1993). Race and sex difference in lung cancer risk associated with cigarette smoking. *International Journal of Epidemiology*, 22(4):592–599.

Harwin. J., Alrouh. B., Ryan, M. & Tunnard, J. (2014). Family Drug and Alcohol Court (FDAC) – Evaluation Research Study. Available from www.brunel.ac.uk/__data/assets/pdf_file/0007/366370/FDAC_May2014_FinalReport_V2.pdf

Hay, G., Gannon, M., Casey, J. & Millar, T. (2010). Estimates of the Prevalence of Opiate Use and/or Crack Cocaine Use, 2009/10: Sweep 6 report. The Centre for Drug Misuse Research, University of Glasgow. Available from www.nta.nhs.uk/uploads/prevalencestats2009-10fullreport.pdf

Hebebrand, J., Albayrak, O., Adan, R., Antel, J., Dieguez, C., de Jong, J., Leng, G., Menzies, J., Mercer, J. G., Murphy, M., van der Plasse, G. & Dickson, S. L. (2014). "Eating addiction", rather than "food addiction", better captures addictive-like eating behavior. *Neurosci Biobehav Rev*, pii: S0149-7634(14)00214-0.

Heise, L. L. (2011). What Works to Prevent Partner Violence An Evidence Overview. London School of Hygiene and Tropical Medicine. STRIVE research [Online], Available from http://r4d.dfid.gov.uk/Output/189039/Default.aspx [Accessed May 2013].

Hernandez-Avila, C. A., Rounsaville, B. J. & Kranzler, H. R. (2004). Opioid, cannabis and alcohol dependent women show more rapid progression to substance abuse treatment. *Drug and Alcohol Dependence*, 74:265–272.

Howell, H. B., Brawman-Mintzer, O., Monnier, J. & Yonkers, K. A. (2001). Generalized anxiety disorder in women. *Psychiatr Clin North Am*, 24(1):165–178.

Howell, K. K., Lynch, M. E., Platzman, K. A., Smith, G. H. & Coles, C. D. (2006). Prenatal alcohol exposure and ability, academic achievement, and school functioning in adolescence: A longitudinal follow-up. *Journal of Pediatric Psychology*, 31(1): 116–126.

HSCIC (Health and Social Care Information Centre) (2014). Statistics on Alcohol England 2014. Available from www.hscic.gov.uk/catalogue/PUB14184/alc-eng-2014-rep.pdf

HSCIC (Health and Social Care Information Centre) (2010). Infant Feeding Survey. Available from www.hscic.gov.ukpubs/infantfeeding10final.

Hser, Y. I., Anglin, M. D. & McGlothlin, W. (1987). Sex differences in addict careers. 1. Initiation of use. *The American Journal of Drug and Alcohol Abuse*, 13(1–2):33–57.

Innamorati, M., Lester, D., Amore, M., Girardi, P., Tatarelli, R. & Pompili, M. (2010). Alcohol consumption predicts the EU suicide rates in young women aged 15–29 years but not in men: analysis of trends and differences among early and new EU countries since 2004. *Alcohol*, 44(5):463–469.

Jellinek, E. M (1960). *The disease concept of alcoholism*. New Haven: Hillhouse.

Jones, L., Bates, G., Bellis, M., Beynon, C., Duffy, P., Evans-Brown, M., Mackridge, A., McCoya, E., Sunall, H. & McVeigh, J. (2011). A summary of the health harms of drugs. Available from www.gov.uk/government/uploads/system/uploads/attachment_data/file/215470/dh_129674.pdf.

Jones, L., Bellis, M. A., Dedman, D., Sumnall, H. & Tocque, K. (2008). Alcohol-attributable fractions for England: alcohol-attributable mortality and hospital admissions. Available from www.nwph.net/nwpho/publications/alcoholattributablefractions.pdf.

Kachadourian, L. K., Pilver, C. E. & Potenza, M. N. (2014). Trauma, PTSD, and binge and hazardous drinking among women and men: findings from a national study. *J Psychiatr Res*, 55:35–43. doi: 10.1016/j.jpsychires.2014.04.018.

Kandel, D. B., Yamaguchi, K. et al. (1992). Stages of progression in drug involvement from adolescence to adulthood: further evidence for the gateway theory. *J Stud Alcohol*, 53(5):447–457.

Kaner, E., Heather, N., Brodie, J., Lock, C. A. & Mcavoy, B. R. (2001). Patient and practitioner characteristics predict brief alcohol intervention in primary care. *The British Journal of General Practice*, 51(471):822.

Kaplan, M. S., Mcfarland, B. H., Huguet, N., Conner, K., Caetano, R., Giesbrecht, N. & Nolte, K. B. (2013). Acute alcohol intoxication and suicide: a gender-stratified analysis of the National Violent Death Reporting System. *Injury Prevention*, 19:38–43.

Kearney, M. H. & O'Sullivan, J. (2003). Identity shifts as turning points in health behaviour change. *West J Nurs Res*, 25:134–152.

Kerr-Corrêa, F., Igami, T. Z., Hiroce, V. & Tucci, A. M. (2007). Patterns of alcohol use between genders: a cross-cultural evaluation. *Journal of Affective Disorders*, 102(1):265–275.

Khantzian, E. J. (1997). The self-medication hypothesis of substance use disorders: a reconsideration and recent applications. *Harvard Review of Psychiatry*, 4(5): 231–244.

Knibbe, R. A., Derickx, M., Kuntsche, S., Grittner, U. & Bloomfield, K. (2006) A comparison of the Alcohol Use Disorder Identification Test (AUDIT) in general population surveys in nine European countries. *Alcohol and Alcoholism*, 41(suppl 1):19–25.

Leonard, K. E. & Eiden, R. D. (2007). Marital and family processes in the context of alcohol use and alcohol disorders. *Annual Review of Clinical Psychology*, 3:285.

Lex, B. W., Goldberg, M. E., Mendelsen, J. H. et al. (1994). Components of anti-social personality disorder amongst women convicted for drunk driving. *Annals of the New York Academy of Sciences*, 708:49–55.

Lubman, D. I., Yucel, M. et al. (2004). Addiction, a condition of compulsive behaviour? Neuroimaging and neuropsychological evidence of inhibitory dysregulation. *Addiction*, 99(12):1491–1502.

Mackay, J. & Amos, A. (2003). Women and tobacco. *Respirology*, 8:123–130.

Marlett, G. A. (1979). A cognitive-behavioural model of the relapse process. *NIDA Res Monogr*, 25:191–200.

Marsden, J., Farrell, M., Bradbury, C., Dale-Perrera, A., Eastwood, B., Roxburgh, M. & Taylor, S. (2008). Development of the treatment outcomes profile. *Addiction*, 103(9):1450–1460. doi: 10.1111/j.1360-0443.2008.02284.x

Marsh, J. C., D'Aunno. T. A. & Smith. B. D. (2000). Increasing access and providing social services to improve drug abuse treatment for women with children. *Addiction*, 95(8):1237–1247.

Matta, S. G. et al. (2007). Guidelines on nicotine dose selection for in vivo research. *Psychopharmacology*, 190:269–319.

Mattson, S. N., Crocker. N. & Nguyen, T. T. (2011). Fetal alcohol spectrum disorders: neuropsychological and behavioural features. *Neuropsychol Rev*, 21(2):81–101.

May, P. A., Gossage, J. P., Kalberg, W. O., Robinson, L. K., Buckley, D., Manning, M. & Hoyme, H. E. (2009). Prevalence and epidemiologic characteristics of FASD from various research methods with an emphasis on recent in-school studies. *Developmental Disabilities Research Reviews*, 15(3):176–192.

McCarthy M. (2013). Opioid overdose deaths rose fivefold among US women in 10 years. *BMJ*, 347:f4415. doi: 10.1136/bmj.f4415.

Mckeganey, N., Neal, J. & Robertson, M. (2005). Physical and sexual abuse among drug users contacting drug treatment services in Scotland. *Drugs: Education, Prevention and Policy*, 12(3):223–232.

McManus, S. M., H. Brugha, T. Bebbington, P. & Jenkins, R. (2009). Adult psychiatric morbidity in England, 2007: Results of a household survey, Appendices and glossary The Health and Social Care Information Centre. Available from www.hscic.gov.uk/pubs/psychiatricmorbidity07 [Accessed November 2010].

McNeill, A., Etter, J-F., Farsalinos, K., Hajek, P., le Houezec, J. & McRobbie, H. (2014). A critique of a WHO-commissioned report and associated article on electronic cigarettes. *Addiction*, 109(12):2128–2134. doi: 10.1111/add.12730

Mohler-Kuo, M., Dowdall, G. W., Koss, M. & Wechsler, H. (2004). Correlates of rape while intoxicated in a national sample of college women. *Journal of Studies on Alcohol*, 65(1):37–45.

Mueller, S. E., Degen, B., Petitjean, S., Wiesbeck, G. A. & Walter, M. (2009). Gender differences in interpersonal problems of alcohol-dependent patients and healthy controls. *Int J Environ Res Public Health*, 6(12):3010–3022.

Mund, M., Louwen, F., Klingelhoefer, D. & Gerber, A. (2013). Smoking and pregnancy–a review on the first major environmental risk factor of the unborn. *Int J Environ Res Public Health*, 10(12):6485–6499. doi: 10.3390/ijerph10126485.

Naimi, T. S., Lipscomb, L. E., Brewer, R. D. & Gilbert, B. C. (2003). Binge drinking in the preconception period and the risk of unintended pregnancy: Implications for women and their children. *Pediatrics*, 111(5):1136–1141.

National Center on Addiction & Substance Abuse at Columbia University (2003). *Food for thought: Substance abuse and eating disorders*. New York: CASA.

NIAAA NIH (National Institute on Alcohol Abuse and Alcoholism) (1998). Alcohol and Aging. Alcohol Alert 40 available from http://pubs.niaaa.nih.gov/publications/aa40.htm

NIAAA (National Institute on Alcohol Abuse and Alcoholism) (2015). Drinking and your pregnancy. Available from http://pubs.niaaa.nih.gov/publications/DrinkingPregnancy_HTML/pregnancy.htm

National Institute on Drug Abuse (1998). NIDA NOTES: Child Abuse and Drug Abuse Volume 13.

National Treatment Agency (2010). Women in Drug Treatment: What the latest figures reveal. Available from www.nta.nhs.uk/uploads/ntawomenintreatment22march2010.pdf [Accessed October 2014].

Neale, J. (2004). Measuring the health of Scottish drug users. *Health and Social Care in the Community*, 12(3):202–211.

Neale, J., Nettleton, S. & Pickering. L. (2013). Gender sameness and difference in recovery from heroin dependence: a qualitative exploration. *International Journal of Drug Policy*, 25:3–12.

Nolen-Hoeksema, S. (2004). Gender differences in risk factors and consequences for alcohol use and problems. *Clinical Psychology Review*, 24(8):981–1010.

O'Brien, C. P. & Childress, A. R. (1992). A learning model of addiction. *Res Publ Assoc Res Nerv Ment Dis*, 70:157–77.

Orford, J. (2001). Addiction as excessive appetite. *Addiction*, 96 (1):15–31.

Paulozzi, L. J. (2012). Prescription drug overdoses: a review. *J Safety Res*, 43 (4):283–289. doi: 10.1016/j.jsr.2012.08.009.

Perkins, K. A. (1996). Sex differences in nicotine vs non-nicotine reinforcement as determinants of tobacco smoking. *Exp Clin Psychopharmalcol*, 11: 199–212.

Perkins, K. A. (2001). Smoking cessation in women: special considerations. *CNS Drugs*. 15:391–411.

Perkins, K. A. & Scott, J. (2008). Sex differences in long-term smoking cessation rates due to nicotine patch. *Nicotine Top Res*, 10(7):1245–1250.

Perkins, K. A., Donny, E. & Caggiula, A. R.(1999). Sex differences in nicotine effects and self-administration: review of human and animal evidence. *Nicotine and Tobacco Research*, 1(301): 315.

Plant, M. L. (1985). Fetal alcohol syndrome: an overview. *Midwifery*, 1 (4): 225–231.

Plant, M. L. & Plant, M. A. (1988). Maternal use of alcohol and other drugs during pregnancy and birth abnormalities: further results from a prospective study. *Alcohol and Alcoholism*, 23(3):229–233.

Plomin, R., DeFries, J.C., Mc Clearn, G.E. & McGuffin, P. (2008). *Behavioral genetics*. Macmillan.

Prochaska, J. O. & DiClemente, C. C. et al. (1985). Predicting change in smoking status for self-changers. *Addict Behav*, 10(4):395–406.

Robinson, T. E. & Berridge, K. C. (1993). The neural basis of drug craving: an incentive-sensitization theory of addiction. *Brain Res Brain Rev*, 18(3):247–291.

Roth, M. E., Cosgrove, K. P. & Carroll, M. E. (2004). Sex differences in the vulnerability to drug abuse: a review of clinical studies. *Neuroscience and Behavioural Reviews*, 28:533–546.

Rounsaville, B. J., Anton, S. F., Carroll, K., et al. (1991). Psychiatric diagnoses of treatment-seeking cocaine abusers. *Arch Gen Psychiatry*, 48:43–51.

Russell, M., Czarnecki, D. M., Cowan, R., Mcpherson, E. & Mudar, P. J. (1991). Measures of maternal alcohol use as predictors of development in early childhood. *Alcoholism: Clinical and Experimental Research*, 15(6):991–1000.

SAMSHA (Substance Abuse and Mental Health Services Administration) (2001). A Provider's Introduction to Substance Abuse Treatment for Lesbian, Gay, Bisexual, and Transgender Individuals. Available from http://store.samhsa.gov/shin/content//SMA12-4104/SMA12-4104.pdf

SAMSHA (Substance Abuse and Mental Health Services Administration) (2013). The TEDS Report: Trends in Substances of Abuse Among Pregnant Women of Childbearing Age in Treatment. Available from www.samhsa.gov/data/sites/default/files/spot110-trends-pregnant-women-2013.pdf

SAMSHA (Substance Abuse and Mental Health Services Administration) (2013). Results from the 2012 National Survey of Drug Use and Health. Summary of national findings. Available from www.samsha.gov/data/NSDUH/2012SummNatFindDetTables/index.aspx?from=carousel&position=1&date=09052013

Saunders, J. B., Aasland, O. G., Babor, T. F. & Grant, M. (1993). Development of the alcohol use disorders identification test (AUDIT): WHO collaborative project on early detection of persons with harmful alcohol consumption-II. *Addiction*, 88(6): 791–804.

Shand, F. L., Gates, J., Fawcett, J. & Mattick, R. P. (2003). *The treatment of alcohol problems: A review of the evidence*. Australia: Department of Health and Ageing.

Shand, F. L., Stafford, J. A., Fawcett, J., Mattick, R. P. (2003). *Guidelines for the treatment of alcohol problems*. Canberra, Australia: Publication Production Unit, ACT.

Shiffman, S., Pillitteri, J. L., Burton, S. L., Rohay, J. M. & Gitchell, J. G. (2001). Smokers' beliefs about "Light" and "Ultra Light" cigarettes. *Tobacco Control*, 10(suppl 1): i17–i23.

Sinha, R. & Rounsaville, B. J. (2002). Sex differences in depressed substance abusers. *The Journal of Clinical Psychiatry*, 63(7):616–627.

Skog. O. J. (2000). Addicts' choice. *Addiction*, 95(9):1309–1314.

Slovic, P., Finucane, M. et al. (2002). The affect heuristic. In *Intuitive judgement: Heuristics and biases*. T. Gilovich, D. Griffin and D. Kahneman (eds.). New York: Cambridge University Press.

Slutske, W. S., Piasecki, T. M., Deutsch, A. R., Statham. D. J. & Martin, N. G. (2014). Telescoping and gender differences in the time course of disordered gambling: evidence from a general population sample. *Addiction*. doi: 10.1111/add.12717 [Epub ahead of print].

Smith. J. P. & Randall. C. L. (2012). Anxiety and alcohol use disorders: Comorbidity and treatment considerations. *Alcohol Research: Current Reviews*, 34(4). Available from http://pubs.niaaa.nih.gov/publications/arcr344/414-431.htm

Sofuoglu, M., Dudish-Poulsen, S., Nelson, D., et al. (1999). Sex and menstrual cycle differences in the subjective effects from smoked cocaine in humans. *Exp Clin Psychopharmacol*, 7(3):274–283.

Solomon, R. L. (1980). The Opponent-Process Theory of Acquired Motivation: The costs of pleasure and the benefits of pain. *American Psychologist*, 35(8):691–712.

Stockwell, T., Murphy, D. & Hodgson, R. (1983). The severity of alcohol dependence questionnaire: its use, reliability and validity. *British Journal of Addiction*, 78(2): 145–155.

Stratton, K., Howe, C. & Battaglia, F. (1996). *Fetal alcohol syndrome: Diagnosis epidemiology prevention and treatment*. Washington, DC: Institute of Medicine, National Academy.

Thomas. A. G., Brodine, S. K., Shaffer, R., Shafer, M. A., Boyer, C. B., Putnam, S., et al. (2001). Chlamydial infection and unplanned pregnancy in women with ready access to health care. *Obstet Gynecol*, 98(6):1117–1123.

Tiffany, S. T. & Conklin, C. A. (2000). A cognitive processing model of alcohol craving and compulsive alcohol use. *Addiction*, 95(Supp 2): s145–s153.

UNODC (United Nations Office of Drugs and Crime) (2014). World Drug Report. Available from www.unodc.org/documents/wdr2014/World_Drug_Report_2014_web.pdf

US Department of Health and Human Services (2001). *Women and smoking: a report of the Surgeon General*. Rockville, MD. Available from www.cdc.gov/tobacco/data_statistics/sgr/2001/index.htm [Accessed Oct 2014]

Vuong, C., Van Uum, S. H., O'Dell, L. E., Lutfy, K. & Friedman, T. C. (2010). The effects of opioids and opioid analogs on animal and human endocrine systems. *Endocr Rev*, 31(1):98–132. doi: 10.1210/er.2009-0009.

Waldrop, A. E., Back, S. E., Verduin, M. L. & Brady, K. T. (2007). Triggers for cocaine and alcohol use in the presence and absence of posttraumatic stress disorder. *Addictive Behaviours*, 32(3):634–663.

Wanigaratne, S. (2006). Psychology of addiction. *Psychiatry* 5(12):455–460.

Weiss, F. & Koob, G. F. (2001). Drug addiction: functional neurotoxicity of the brain reward systems. *Neurotox Res*, 3(1):145–156.

West, R. & Hardy, A. (2006). *Theory of addiction*. Oxford: Blackwell.

White, N. M. (1996). Addictive drugs as reinforcers: multiple partial actions on memory systems. *Addiction*, 91(7):921–949.

White, A. M., Jamieson-Drake, D. W. & Swartzwelder, H. S. (2002). Prevalence and correlates of alcohol-induced blackouts among college students: Results of an e-mail survey. *Journal of American College Health*, 51(3):117–131.

Wilsnack, S. C. & Wilsnack, R. W. (2002). International gender and alcohol research: Recent findings and future directions. *Alcohol Research and Health*, 26(4):245–250.

World Health Organization (1993). *The ICD-10 classification of mental and behavioural disorders: diagnostic criteria for research*. Geneva: World Health Organization.

World Health Organisation (2010). Gender, women and the tobacco epidemic. Available from www.who.int/tobacco/publications/gender/women_tob_epidemic/en/ [Accessed Oct 2014].

World Health Organisation (2014). Global status report on alcohol and health. Available from www.who.int/substance_abuse/publications/global_alcohol_report/en/

World Health Organisation (2011). WHO report on global tobacco epidemic. Available from www.who.int/tobacco/global_report/2011/en/

Zakhari, S. (2006). Overview: how is alcohol metabolized by the body? *Alcohol Research & Health: The Journal of the National Institute on Alcohol Abuse and Alcoholism*, 29(4): 245–255.

Zilberman, M. L., Tavares, H., Blume, S. B. & El-Guebaly, N. (2003). Substance use disorders: sex differences and psychiatric comorbidities. *Canadian Journal of Psychiatry*, 48(1):5–13.

Zilberman, M., Tavares, H. et al. (2003). Gender similarities and differences in the prevalence and course of alcohol- and other substance-related disorders. *J Addict Dis*, 22(4):61–74.

Chapter

16

Body image disorders in women

Serafino G. Mancuso, Andrea Phillipou, Susan L. Rossell and David J. Castle

Within contemporary Western cultures, women are subject to ubiquitous sociocultural factors that are thought to play a central role in the development of body image and eating disorders. These sociocultural pressures comprise the thin body ideal promoted for women, the emphasis of appearance in the female gender-role and the importance of appearance for the societal success of women (Thompson et al., 1999). Not surprisingly, then, there are high rates of body dissatisfaction amongst women, particularly young women, so much so that weight has been described as a "normative discontent" for women (Rodin et al., 1985, p. 267). This chapter sets out to introduce the sociocultural perspective on body image and body image disturbance, and presents body dysmorphic disorder (BDD) and the eating disorders anorexia nervosa (AN), bulimia nervosa (BN) and binge eating disorder (BED) as exemplars of body image disorders in women.

Body image

Body image is a multidimensional construct that represents how an individual thinks, feels and behaves in relation to their physical appearance (Cash, 2002). The body image construct can be further divided into two core facets comprising evaluation and investment. Body image *evaluation* refers to the evaluative thoughts and beliefs a person may have about appearance, such as the degree of satisfaction or dissatisfaction with their body. In contrast, body image *investment* refers to the cognitive and behavioral importance that a person assigns to their physical appearance (Cash et al., 2004), including the extent to which they focus on their physical appearance and engage in behaviors associated with management or enhancement of their appearance, including dieting and exercise. When an individual maintains

disturbances in the cognitive, behavioral and emotional aspects of their body image, however, this may lead to the development and subsequent maintenance of disorders such as BDD, AN, and BN (Hrabosky et al., 2009). The manner in which body image disturbances may arise will be examined within the context of the sociocultural model.

Sociocultural model

The sociocultural model posits that, within a particular culture, there exist societal ideals of beauty that are transmitted via a variety of sociocultural channels, most notably mass media, family and peers (Thompson et al., 1999). These ideals are internalized by individuals such that dissatisfaction with appearance becomes a function of the extent to which individuals do not meet the body image ideal.

Over the last several decades, the weight of idealized women in the Western media has decreased (e.g., Sypeck et al., 2004). In the 1950s, the ideal body for Western women was full-figured with fat on her hips and a waist that was in proportion to large breasts; whereas the contemporary ideal woman is expected to have large breasts despite her slim waist and hips (Murnen, 2011). This Western thin ideal is very difficult for most women to attain without engaging in extreme weight loss efforts (Brownell, 1992) or cosmetic procedures such as breast enhancement.

Unfortunately, the ultra-slim female Western ideal is pervasively portrayed in the media, which then is adopted and internalized by many girls and women (Polivy & Herman, 2002). This then serves as the reference point against which they judge themselves. Females perceiving a discrepancy between their appearance and this thin body ideal may experience body dissatisfaction. In turn, this may lead to dieting and other unhealthy strategies to pursue thinness, potentially resulting in body image or eating disorders (Thompson et al., 1999) as presented in the next section.

Body dysmorphic disorder

According to the *Diagnostic and Statistical Manual of Mental Disorders, 5th edition* (DSM-5; American Psychiatric Association, 2013), BDD is characterized by four criteria. First, the individual is preoccupied with one or more perceived defects in physical appearance that are not observable or appear slight to others. Second, the individual has performed repetitive behaviors or mental acts in response to the concerns about appearance at some point during the course of the disorder. Third, the preoccupation causes clinically significant distress or functional impairment. Fourth, the appearance preoccupation is not better explained by concerns with body fat or weight in an individual whose symptoms meet diagnostic criteria for an eating disorder. The DSM-5 contains a specifier for muscle dysmorphia, which is used when the individual is predominantly preoccupied with the idea that their body build is too small or insufficiently muscular. There is also a specifier to indicate the degree of insight about the BDD beliefs, including those with good or fair insight, those with poor insight, or those with absent insight/delusional beliefs.

Clinical features

Individuals with BDD are preoccupied with a perceived or minor defect in one or more aspects of their appearance. The most common preoccupations concern the hair, nose and skin (e.g., balding, misshapen nose, acne, or skin tone), but any body part can be the focus of concern. Whilst BDD appears to affect women and men roughly equally, women with the condition are particularly likely to be concerned about weight, hips, breasts and excessive body hair (Phillips, Menard, et al., 2006). Some concerns are specific, while others are vague or amount to no more than a general perception of ugliness. The mean number of reported appearance concerns can range from five to seven (Phillips, Menard, et al., 2005). However, this average may be an underestimate, as most patients are too embarrassed or reluctant to disclose specific appearance concerns. The nature of preoccupations can fluctuate over time, either with the addition of defects or substitution of

defects (Fontenelle et al., 2006). The preoccupations are typically difficult to resist or control and, on average, consume 3 to 8 hours daily.

Almost all people with BDD perform compulsive behaviors that serve to examine, improve or hide their perceived defect. Checking the defect in mirrors and other reflective surfaces occurs in almost all patients with BDD, while the remainder will periodically avoid mirrors to try to prevent the distress of seeing their own reflection and the time consumed when using them (Veale & Riley, 2001). Other common behaviors are comparing one's appearance with that of others, touching the body area of concern, excessive grooming, seeking reassurance about the perceived flaw or trying to convince others of its unattractiveness and camouflaging the perceived defect with makeup or clothing (Grant et al., 2006). These behaviors typically occur for several hours a day and are difficult to resist or control. Skin picking can also occur in BDD, notably in women, and usually with a desire to achieve "perfect flat skin." However, these behaviors can lead to skin lesions and infections that are truly unsightly (Castle et al., 2004; Phillips, 2004).

Epidemiology

Because of the lack of large-scale epidemiological studies, exact prevalence rates for BDD remain unclear. Rief and colleagues (2006) administered a self-report diagnostic measure to a large, representative sample of the German population ($N = 2,552$) and reported a prevalence rate of 1.7%. In a large United States (US) nationwide prevalence study ($N = 2,513$), Koran et al. (2008) reported a BDD prevalence rate of 2.4%. In other large community samples, reported rates of BDD were 0.7% (Italy; Faravelli et al., 1997), 1.1% (US; Bienvenu et al., 2000), 0.7% in women aged 36 to 44 (US; Otto et al., 2001) and 2.3% in adolescents (US; Mayville et al., 1999).

In psychiatric settings, reported rates of BDD range from 3.2% to 16.0% (Conroy et al., 2008; Grant et al., 2001; Zimmerman & Mattia, 1998). In these settings, however, BDD is often underdiagnosed or underrepresented because individuals are secretive about their symptoms because of embarrassment or shame (Phillips, 1998). Zimmerman and Mattia (1998), for example, noted that clinicians failed to recognize the 16 (3.2%) of 500 consecutive psychiatric outpatients who fulfilled diagnostic criteria for BDD, despite 11 of them indicating that their BDD symptoms were one of the reasons they were seeking treatment. Comparable results were reported by Grant et al. (2001), who found that although 13.1% of one sample of psychiatric inpatients ($N = 122$) fulfilled criteria for BDD, these patients reportedly did not disclose their BDD symptoms to the clinician unless specifically asked.

Another factor contributing to underdiagnosis of the disorder is that individuals with BDD tend to consult dermatologists, cosmetic surgeons or dentists, rather than seeking psychiatric assistance (Crerand et al., 2006; Sarwer et al., 1998). This trend is highlighted in reported prevalence rates of BDD ranging from 3.2% to 16.6% in cosmetic surgery settings (Altamura et al., 2001; Aouizerate et al., 2003; Bellino et al., 2006; Crerand et al., 2004; Sarwer et al., 1998; Vulink et al., 2006) and from 8.5% to 15% in dermatologic settings (Bowe et al., 2007; Dufresne et al., 2001; Phillips et al., 2000; Uzun et al., 2003; Vulink et al., 2006).

Dermatological, cosmetic and other nonpsychiatric procedures, however, do not appear to improve BDD symptoms. Crerand et al. (2005) found that non-psychiatric treatment was sought by 71% and received by 64% of 200 patients with BDD. However, 91% of individuals receiving such treatments did not experience any improvement in their overall symptoms of BDD. Phillips et al. (2001) similarly reported that although non-psychiatric treatment was sought by 76.4% and received by 66.0% of 289 patients with BDD, these treatments rarely improved BDD symptoms. Indeed, most patients with BDD who do undergo cosmetic procedures are unhappy with the outcome, often returning for repeat procedures and/or suing, threatening or even murdering the cosmetic surgeon (Sarwer & Crerand, 2008)!

Course of the illness

For both women and men, the age of onset of BDD is typically late adolescence at 16 to 18 years of age (Phillips, Grant, et al., 2005), but subclinical BDD (i.e., dislike of one's appearance) can begin at 12 to 14 years of age (Phillips, Menard, et al., 2005) or even earlier. BDD tends to follow a chronic and deteriorating course. Phillips and Diaz (1997), for example, asked 188 patients with BDD to describe retrospectively the course of their BDD symptoms. The mean duration of BDD was 15.7 years ($SD = 11.9$). In most patients (82%), BDD was found to have a chronic course, with less than 1 month of remission since the onset of the disorder, and almost

half of all patients experiencing a deteriorating course of the disorder (49.5%).

In another retrospective study, Phillips et al. (2005) assessed the status of 95 outpatients with BDD by chart review at 6-month intervals over 4 years. At the 6-month and/or 12-month assessments, 24.7% of patients had achieved full remission and 57.8% attained partial of full remission. Over the full 4 years, 58.2% of patients reported full remission and 83.8% had experienced partial or full remission at one or more 6-month assessment points. However, 28.6% of those patients who attained partial or full remission at one or more assessment points had relapsed. At the conclusion of the study, 16.7% of patients were in full remission, 37.8% were in partial remission and 45.6% still met full criteria for BDD. However, the limitations of this study are that retrospective chart review methods were used and that patients received treatment in a BDD specialty program, potentially limiting the ability to generalize these findings to other treatment settings.

Recognizing this limitation, Phillips et al. (2006) prospectively investigated the course of symptoms for 183 patients with BDD over 12 months. Over two-thirds of the sample were women. Over this timeframe, 9% of patients experienced full remission (i.e., minimal or no BDD symptoms) and 21% experienced partial remission (i.e., meeting less than full diagnostic criteria for at least 8 consecutive weeks). The mean proportion of time that the patients met full BDD criteria during the 12-month period was 80%, despite most patients receiving mental health treatment during the follow-up period.

Comparable results were reported by Phillips et al. (2005) in their prospective study of the course of symptoms for 161 patients with BDD over 12 months. Patients with BDD who received psychiatric treatment did not have a greater likelihood of remitting from BDD than those who did not. However, greater BDD severity at intake, longer BDD duration and the presence of a comorbid personality disorder predicted a lower likelihood of remission.

In sum, BDD tends to onset in childhood or adolescence, has a mean duration of about 16 years and remission rates of the disorder are low. The remission rates may not differ between those patients receiving psychiatric treatment for their BDD symptoms and those who are not. However, these rates may be influenced by the severity of and duration of BDD symptoms, and comorbidity with a personality disorder.

BDD in women

Although there are similar BDD prevalence rates for women and men in adult clinical samples, several gender differences in BDD phenomenology have been reported. Phillips and Diaz (1997) examined gender differences in 93 female and 95 male patients with BDD. Men were more likely than women to be concerned with thinning or balding, their genitals and their body build (e.g., muscularity), while women were more likely to be preoccupied with their weight, hips and excessive body hair. Women are also more likely to pick their skin and use cosmetics on their hands for camouflage, whereas men were more likely to use a hat for camouflaging their hair concerns.

Comparable results were reported by Phillips et al. (2006) in their investigation of gender differences in 137 female and 63 male patients with BDD. Women were more likely to have a younger age of subclinical BDD onset than men. Males were more likely to be concerned with their genitals, body build and thinning or balding hair. Females were more likely to be preoccupied with their skin, stomach, weight, breasts, buttocks, thighs, legs, hips, toes and excessive body hair. Women were also more likely to check mirrors excessively, change their clothes often and pick their skin, whereas men were more likely to lift weights excessively.

In sum, women with BDD tend to have an earlier age of subclinical BDD onset and to be preoccupied with their skin, stomach, weight, breasts, buttocks, thighs, legs, hips, toes and excessive body hair. They are also likely to engage in mirror checking, clothes changing and skin picking; and to use cosmetics to camouflage their perceived appearance flaws.

Eating disorders

Although eating disorders and body image concerns are often regarded as a recent phenomenon, their existence has been documented throughout history (Brumberg, 2000). The eating disorders include three relatively distinct illnesses: anorexia nervosa (AN), bulimia nervosa (BN) and binge eating disorder (BED). The first description of AN was provided by Gull in 1868 at the annual meeting of the British Medical Association in Oxford, whereas BN was first described in 1979 by Russell as an "ominous variant of AN." BED has long been recognized by clinicians, but entered the DSM as a distinct entry only in its fifth revision (DSM-5; American Psychiatric Association, 2013).

Anorexia nervosa
Clinical features

According to DSM-5, AN is characterized by three criteria: restriction of energy intake relative to requirements, leading to significantly low body weight; the experience of intense fear of weight gain or persistent behavior that interferes with weight gain; and a disturbance in the experience of one's body weight or shape, or a persistent lack of recognition of the seriousness of the current low weight (American Psychiatric Association, 2013). Two subtypes of AN are delineated, namely a restricting type (AN-R) and a binge-eating purging (AN-BP) type (American Psychiatric Association, 2013). AN-R is distinguished by weight loss accomplished through dieting, fasting and/or excessive exercise, and not through regular engagement in purging (American Psychiatric Association, 2013). In contrast, AN-BP is characterized by regular binging and/or purging aiming to achieve and retain low body weight. The method of purging can take the form of self-induced vomiting, or the misuse of laxatives, diuretics or enemas (American Psychiatric Association, 2013). Though AN can be categorized into these two subtypes, the distinction is not always clear and individuals with AN often alternate between the two over the course of the illness (Eddy et al., 2008a). Individuals with AN are also likely to transition to or from BN, usually within the first 5 years of the illness (Tozzi et al., 2005).

Epidemiology

In 2011, an annual survey carried out by Mission Australia (2011), the National Survey of Young Australians, collected information from close to 46,000 young people aged 11–24 years. The results from the survey indicated that body image concerns were one of the top three issues of personal concern for young people, with 33.1% of respondents expressing the concern, an increase of 7.6% over the previous 3 years. Though body image concerns appear to be on the increase, the incidence of AN does not appear necessarily to be following this trend (Fombonne, 1995; Pawluck & Gorey, 1998). Various studies have reported an increase in the incidence of AN in recent times (Eagles et al., 1995; Hoek, 2006; Hoek & Van Hoeken, 2003; Lucas et al., 1991), particularly for those aged in their 20s and 30s (Pawluck & Gorey, 1998), though the authors do not discount other plausible explanations such as increasing awareness of the condition and improved case detection. However, a comprehensive review of the literature conducted by Hoek & Van Hoeken (2003) reported the incidence of AN increased over the past century until the 1970s, but has since remained relatively stable. Incidence and prevalence rates can also be difficult to estimate due to the nature of the condition as AN is often associated with a high level of denial about the illness and individuals with the condition often do not seek medical attention independently (Strober, 2004; Vandereycken, 2006). Furthermore, incidence rates based on admissions into mental health care or general hospitals may not truly reflect the incidence of AN in the community (Hoek & Van Hoeken, 2003).

The 12-month prevalence of AN is 0.4% among females and approximately one-tenth of that among males (American Psychiatric Association, 2013). The crude mortality rate of individuals admitted into university hospitals with AN is around 5% per decade and is most commonly due to medical complications associated with the physical consequences of the condition or from suicide (American Psychiatric Association, 2013). This is among the highest mortality rate of any psychiatric disorder (Harris & Barraclough, 1998; Sullivan, 1995). The prevalence of AN appears to be much greater in individuals with an upper or upper-middle social status (Crisp et al., 1976; McClelland & Crisp, 2001), and in industrialized societies where there is an abundance of food and where a slim physique is promoted as an attractive physical trait (Keel & Klump, 2003; Miller & Pumariega, 2001). Although AN may be more prevalent in Western cultures, the condition is not only seen in societies promoting a thin ideal, having been described in countries such as Kenya and Iran (Buhrich, 1981; Lee, 1991; Njenga & Kangethe, 2004; Nobakht & Dezhkam, 2000).

Course of the illness

Though the onset of the AN can occur at any age, the typical age of onset is in mid to late adolescence, and rarely occurs in individuals over 40 years (American Psychiatric Association, 2013; Lucas et al., 1991). Within the first few years of onset, many individuals alternate between the AN-R and AN-BP subtypes, with many shifting to the diagnosis of BN (Eddy et al., 2008a; Eddy et al., 2002; Tozzi et al., 2005). There is great variability in the course and outcome of

AN, with some individuals making a full recovery after a single episode, others fluctuating between weight gain and relapse, others who experience the illness chronically over many years, yet others who die from the physical consequences of the illness or suicide (Norring & Sohlberg, 1993; Steinhausen, 2002; Strober et al., 1997). Additionally, AN is associated with exceptionally high relapse rates (Eckert et al., 1995; Löwe et al., 2001; Norring & Sohlberg, 1993; Strober et al., 1997; Zipfel et al., 2000). A major contributing factor for the high rates of morbidity and mortality experienced by individuals with this condition is that the cause or causes of the illness are not clear, and although treatment modalities such as cognitive behavior therapy and family therapy have emerging evidence for efficacy, many patients remain under- or unresponsive.

Bulimia nervosa
Clinical features

BN is characterized by the experience of recurrent episodes of binge eating and recurrent inappropriate compensatory behavior to prevent weight gain, both of which occur on average at least once a week for 3 months; self-evaluation influenced unduly by body shape and weight; and the disturbance does not occur during an episode of AN (American Psychiatric Association, 2013). Unlike AN, individuals with BN are not typically underweight and usually fall within the normal weight or overweight body ranges (American Psychiatric Association, 2013).

Epidemiology

Like AN, the incidence and prevalence of BN can be difficult to estimate because of the concealing nature of the condition and their avoidance in seeking treatment. Whether rates of BN have been on the rise in the last several years is also difficult to establish, in part as a result of its late inclusion as a diagnostic category in 1980. However, the incidence of BN had been found to be decreasing between 1980s and 1990s to approximately 6.6 per 100,000 from incidence rates as high as 13.5 per 100,000 (Currin et al., 2005; Hoek et al., 1995; Soundy et al., 1995). Yet, the incidence of BN may actually be higher than reported in epidemiological studies as a large majority of individuals with the condition may never seek treatment (Hudson et al., 2007).

The 12-month prevalence of BN is 1–1.5% among young women, and like AN, the prevalence among men is approximately one-tenth of that among women (American Psychiatric Association, 2013). The crude mortality rate of BN is somewhat lower than in AN at approximately 2% per decade (American Psychiatric Association, 2013). The incidence of BN is higher in industrialized areas (Hoek et al., 1995), typically affecting more individuals from Western cultures (Makino et al., 2004), particularly Caucasian people (Striegel-Moore et al., 2003).

Course of the illness

BN is similar to AN with the onset typically during adolescence or young adulthood and rarely before puberty. Increasingly, women are presenting in later adulthood after the age of 40 (American Psychiatric Association, 2013). The binge-eating behaviors often begin during or following an episode of dieting (American Psychiatric Association, 2013). The course of the illness may be chronic or intermittent with many patients alternating between remission and recurrences of illness symptoms. Relapse rates as high as 43% have been reported and rates as high as 67% have been reported for individuals who continue to meet diagnostic criteria for BN at long-term follow-up (Keel & Mitchell, 1997). Furthermore, a small percentage will transition into AN, though this crossover occurs much less frequently than the transition from AN to BN (Eddy et al., 2008b; Tozzi et al., 2005).

Binge eating disorder
Clinical features

BED is characterised by recurrent episodes of binge eating, where an "episode" is described as eating an amount of food within a discrete period of time (usually less than 2 hours) that would be considered considerably larger than what most people would eat in a similar period of time and in similar circumstances; importantly, this behavior is associated with a sense of lack of control over eating during the episode. Episodes are also associated with three or more of the following features: eating much more rapidly than normal; eating until feeling uncomfortably full; eating large amounts of food when not feeling hungry; eating alone because of embarrassment about how much one is eating; feeling depressed and very guilty or disgusted with oneself following the binge.

The individual experiences marked distress from the binge eating and the binge eating occurs at least once a week for 3 months. The binge eating is also not associated with inappropriate compensatory behavior as in BN, and does not exclusively occur during a course of BN or AN (American Psychiatric Association, 2013). BED typically occurs in healthy-weight, overweight and obese individuals, but is distinct from obesity *per se* as most obese individuals do not partake in recurrent episodes of binge eating (American Psychiatric Association, 2013).

Epidemiology

The 12-month prevalence of BED among US adults is 0.8% among men, half the rate of that among women at 1.6% (American Psychiatric Association, 2013). Unlike AN and BN, BED does not appear to have a higher prevalence among Caucasian women from Western cultures, but may occur equally among diverse racial and ethnic groups (Striegel-Moore & Franko, 2003; Grucza et al., 2007).

Course of the illness

As BED has only recently received official recognition in the DSM-5, it is the most understudied of the eating disorders and relatively little is known about the course of the illness. However, like the other eating disorders, BED typically begins in adolescence or young adulthood (Mitchell & Mussell, 1995; Spurrell et al., 1997). It is a relatively persistent condition, with an illness course, severity and duration similar to that of BN, though remission rates are considerably higher than BN or AN, with a greater tendency to be episodic in nature (Fairburn et al., 2000). Unlike the crossover often reported between AN and BN, the crossover from BED to the other eating disorders in uncommon (American Psychiatric Association, 2013).

Comorbid BDD and eating disorders

Although DSM-5 criteria suggest that the presence of an eating disorder precludes a diagnosis of BDD (American Psychiatric Association, 2013), an individual can have a comorbid eating disorder with BDD. In fact, many eating disorder patients are preoccupied with nonweight-related physical attributes such as the skin, hair, teeth, jaw, nose, ears and height (Gupta & Gupta, 2001; Gupta & Johnson, 2000; Kollei et al.,

2013), while some patients with BDD are preoccupied with body weight and body shape (Kittler et al., 2007).

Traditionally, there has been far greater public awareness and media attention for both anorexia and bulimia nervosa. The severity of disability and poor life outcomes associated with BDD is increasingly recognized by the clinical and research communities. Comorbid BDD is highlighted by lifetime prevalence rates of AN or BN amongst patients with BDD, which range from 10% to 19% (Gunstad & Phillips, 2003; Ruffolo et al., 2006; Zimmerman & Mattia, 1998). The clinical correlates of eating disorder comorbidity in a BDD patient sample was investigated by Ruffolo et al. (2006), who compared 65 patients with BDD with a comorbid eating disorder to 135 patients with BDD without a comorbid eating disorder. Amongst the comorbid group, 63.1% developed BDD before the onset of their eating disorder, while only 20% developed BDD after the onset of an eating disorder. Although the comorbid group reported greater dissatisfaction with general appearance, both groups most frequently endorsed the skin as their most disliked body area. Relative to patients without a comorbid eating disorder, those with a comorbid eating disorder were more likely to be women, have greater body image disturbance, suffer from a higher number of other comorbid disorders and have received more psychiatric treatment.

Conversely, the prevalence and clinical correlates of BDD comorbidity amongst 41 female AN inpatients was examined by Grant et al. (2002). The lifetime prevalence rate of comorbid BDD was found to be 39%. The 16 patients with comorbid BDD were then compared to the 25 without comorbid BDD. In almost all of patients with comorbid BDD, the onset of BDD preceded anorexia nervosa symptoms and BDD was considered their "biggest" or "major" problem. Relative to the patients without comorbid BDD, the comorbid patients with BDD were more severely ill, with poorer psychosocial functioning, greater appearance preoccupation and likelihood of experiencing delusional ideation, twice the number of psychiatric hospitalizations and up to three times the number of suicide attempts.

Problems of chronicity and BDD comorbidity are now well-described. Dingemans et al. (2012) examined the prevalence of BDD in 154 female and 4 male patients with an eating disorder and found an overall 45% prevalence rate of BDD, including 46% for AN

patients, 54% for BN patients and 38% for patients with an eating disorder not otherwise specified (EDNOS). Compared to the 87 patients with an eating disorder only, the 71 patients with both BDD and an eating disorder had significantly higher dysmorphic appearance concerns, more psychopathology and were dissatisfied with a larger number of body parts even after controlling for severity of eating disorder psychopathology.

Research by Rabe-Jablonska and Sobow (2000) provides additional support for the observation that BDD may precede the onset of an eating disorder (Grant et al., 2002). In a sample of 36 female patients with anorexia nervosa, a BDD prevalence rate of 25% was reported. Those patients with comorbid anorexia nervosa and BDD had BDD symptoms for an average of 14 months prior to the onset of their eating disorder.

In sum, BDD is a distinct comorbid disorder in up to half of patients with an eating disorder. The literature suggests that BDD symptoms usually precede the onset of an eating disorder by over 12 months. Eating disorder patients with comorbid BDD tend to have more severe psychopathology and poorer psychosocial functioning. Therefore, it is important to recognize and treat BDD in patients with an eating disorder.

Summary

Body image dissatisfaction is commonly experienced by women and girls, in part related to evolutionary pressures, in part sociocultural factors, and fuelled by the proliferation of the thin body ideal by the mass media especially in Western cultures. Women who idealize this archetype and then perceive a discrepancy between it and their actual appearance may diet and perform other dysfunctional behaviors to pursue this ideal. Some women may then develop an eating disorder such as AN, BN or BED. Others develop broader body image concerns and might manifest BDD. While it is not uncommon for BDD symptoms to manifest before the onset of a full-threshold eating disorder, up to half of individuals with an eating disorder will have comorbid BDD. Because these individuals will likely have more severe psychiatric symptoms and functional impairment, it is important to recognize and treat BDD in eating disorder settings.

References

Altamura, C., Paluello, M. M., Mundo, E., Medda, S., & Mannu, P. (2001). Clinical and subclinical body dysmorphic disorder. *European Archives of Psychiatry and Clinical Neuroscience*, 251(3), 105–108.

American Psychiatric Association. (2013). *Diagnostic and statistical manual of mental disorders, 5th edition*. Washington, DC: American Psychiatric Association.

Aouizerate, B., Pujol, H., Grabot, D., Faytout, M., Suire, K., Braud, C., ... Tignol, J. (2003). Body dysmorphic disorder in a sample of cosmetic surgery applicants. *European Psychiatry*, 18(7), 365–368.

Bellino, S., Zizza, M., Paradiso, E., Rivarossa, A., Fulcheri, M., & Bogetto, F. (2006). Dysmorphic concern symptoms and personality disorders: A clinical investigation in patients seeking cosmetic surgery. *Psychiatry Research*, 144(1), 73–78.

Bienvenu, O. J., Samuels, J. F., Riddle, M. A., Hoehn-Saric, R., Liang, K. Y., Cullen, B.A.M., ... Nestadt, G. (2000). The relationship of obsessive–compulsive disorder to possible spectrum disorders: Results from a family study. *Biological Psychiatry*, 48(4), 287–293.

Bowe, W. P., Leyden, J. J., Crerand, C. E., Sarwer, D. B., & Margolis, D. J. (2007). Body dysmorphic disorder symptoms among patients with acne vulgaris. *Journal of the American Academy of Dermatology*, 57(2), 222–230.

Brownell, K. D. (1992). Dieting and the search for the perfect body: Where physiology and culture collide. *Behavior Therapy*, 22(1), 1–12.

Brumberg, J. (2000). *Fasting girls: The history of anorexia nervosa*. New York: Vintage.

Buhrich, N. (1981). Frequency of presentation of anorexia nervosa in Malaysia. *Australasian Psychiatry*, 15(2), 153–155.

Cash, T. F. (2002). Cognitive-behavioral perspectives on body image. In T. F. Cash & T. Pruzinsky (Eds.), *Body image: A handbook of theory, research, and clinical practice* (pp. 38–46). New York: The Guilford Press.

Cash, T. F., Melnyk, S. E., & Hrabosky, J. I. (2004). The assessment of body image investment: An extensive revision of the appearance schemas inventory. *International Journal of Eating Disorders*, 35(3), 305–316. doi: 10.1002/eat.10264

Castle, D. J., Phillips, K. A., & Dufresne, R. G. (2004). Body dysmorphic disorder and cosmetic dermatology: More than skin deep. *Journal of Cosmetic Dermatology*, 3(2), 99–103.

Conroy, M., Menard, W., Fleming-Ives, K., Modha, P., Cerullo, H., & Phillips, K.A. (2008). Prevalence and clinical characteristics of body dysmorphic disorder in an adult inpatient setting. *General Hospital Psychiatry*, 30(1), 67–72.

Crerand, C. E., Franklin, M. E., & Sarwer, D. B. (2006). Body dysmorphic disorder and cosmetic surgery. *Plastic and Reconstructive Surgery*, 118(7).

Crerand, C. E., Phillips, K. A., Menard, W., & Fay, C. (2005). Nonpsychiatric medical treatment of body dysmorphic disorder. *Psychosomatics*, 46(6), 549–555. doi: 10.1176/appi.psy.46.6.549

Crerand, C. E., Sarwer, D. B., Magee, L., Gibbons, L. M., Lowe, M. R., Bartlett, S. P., ... Whitaker, L. A. (2004). Rate of body dysmorphic disorder among patients seeking facial plastic surgery. *Psychiatric Annals*, 34(12), 958–965.

Crisp, A. H., Palmer, R. L., & Kalucy, R. S. (1976). How common is anorexia nervosa? A prevalence study. *British Journal of Psychiatry*, 128(6), 549–554.

Currin, L., Schmidt, U., Treasure, J., & Jick, H. (2005). Time trends in eating disorder incidence. *British Journal of Psychiatry*, 186(2), 132–135.

Dingemans, A. E., van Rood, Y. R., de Groot, I., & van Furth, E. F. (2012).

Body dysmorphic disorder in patients with an eating disorder: Prevalence and characteristics. *International Journal of Eating Disorders*, 45(4), 562–569.

Dufresne, R. G., Phillips, K. A., Vittorio, C. C., & Wilkel, C. S. (2001). A screening questionnaire for body dysmorphic disorder in a cosmetic dermatologic surgery practice. *Dermatologic Surgery*, 27(5), 457–462.

Eagles, J. M., Johnston, M. I., Hunter, D., & Lobban, M. (1995). Increasing incidence of anorexia nervosa in the female population of northeast Scotland. *American Journal of Psychiatry*, 152(9), 1266–1271.

Eckert, E. D., Halmi, K. A., Marchi, P., Grove, W., & Crosby, R. (1995). Ten-year follow-up of anorexia nervosa: Clinical course and outcome. *Psychological Medicine*, 25(1), 143–156.

Eddy, K. T., Keel, P. K., Dorer, D. J., Delinsky, S. S., Franko, D. L., & Herzog, D. B. (2002). Longitudinal comparison of anorexia nervosa subtypes. *International Journal of Eating Disorders*, 31(2), 191–201.

Eddy, K. T., Dorer, D. J., Franko, D. L., Tahilani, K., Thompson-Brenner, H., & Herzog, D. B. (2008). Diagnostic crossover in anorexia nervosa and bulimia nervosa: Implications for DSM-V. *American Journal of Psychiatry*, 165(2), 245.

Fairburn, C. G., Cooper, Z., Doll, H. A., Norman, P., & O'Connor, M. (2000). The natural course of bulimia nervosa and binge eating disorder in young women. *Archives of General Psychiatry*, 57(7), 659–665.

Faravelli, C., Salvatori, S., Galassi, F., Aiazzi, L., Drei, C., & Cabras, P. (1997). Epidemiology of somatoform disorders: A community survey in Florence. *Social Psychiatry and Psychiatric Epidemiology*, 32(1), 24–29.

Fombonne, E. (1995). Anorexia nervosa. No evidence of an increase. *British Journal of Psychiatry*, 166(4), 462–471.

Fontenelle, L. F., Telles, L. L., Nazar, B. P., Menezes, G., Nascimento, A., Mendlowicz, M. V., & Versiani, M. (2006). A sociodemographic, phenomenological, and long-term follow-up study of patients with body dysmorphic disorder in brazil. *The International Journal of Psychiatry in Medicine*, 36(2), 243–259.

Grant, J. E., Kim, S., & Crow, S. J. (2001). Prevalence and clinical features of body dysmorphic disorder in adolescent and adult psychiatric inpatients. *The Journal of Clinical Psychiatry*, 62(7), 517–522.

Grant, J. E., Kim, S. W., & Eckert, E. D. (2002). Body dysmorphic disorder in patients with anorexia nervosa: Prevalence, clinical features and delusionality of body image. *International Journal of Eating Disorders*, 32(3), 291–300.

Grant, J. E., Menard, W., & Phillips, K. A. (2006). Pathological skin picking in individuals with body dysmorphic disorder. *General Hospital Psychiatry*, 28(6), 487–493.

Grucza, R. A., Przybeck, T. R., & Cloninger, C. R. (2007). Prevalence and correlates of binge eating disorder in a community sample. *Comprehensive Psychiatry*, 48(2), 124–131.

Gull, W. W. (1868). The address in medicine delivered before the annual meeting of the british medical association at oxford. *The Lancet*, 92(2345), 171–176. doi: 10.1016/s0140-6736(01)13059-x

Gunstad, J., & Phillips, K. A. (2003). Axis i comorbidity in body dysmorphic disorder. *Comprehensive Psychiatry*, 44(4), 270–276.

Gupta, M. A., & Gupta, A. K. (2001). Dissatisfaction with skin appearance among patients with eating disorders and non-clinical controls. *British Journal of Dermatology*, 145(1), 110–113.

Gupta, M. A., & Johnson, A. M. (2000). Nonweight-related body image concerns among female eating-disordered patients and nonclinical controls: Some preliminary observations. *International Journal of Eating Disorders*, 27(3), 304–309.

Harris, E. C., & Barraclough, B. (1998). Excess mortality of mental disorder. *British Journal of Psychiatry*, 173(1), 11–53.

Hoek, H. W. (2006). Incidence, prevalence and mortality of anorexia nervosa and other eating disorders. *Current Opinion in Psychiatry*, 19(4), 389.

Hoek, H. W., Bartelds, A.I.M., Bosveld, J.J.F., & van der Graaf, Y. (1995). Impact of urbanization on detection rates of eating disorders. *American Journal of Psychiatry*. 152: 1272–1278.

Hoek, H. W., & Van Hoeken, D. (2003). Review of the prevalence and incidence of eating disorders. *International Journal of Eating Disorders*, 34(4), 383–396.

Hrabosky, J. I., Cash, T. F., Veale, D., Neziroglu, F., Soll, E. A., Garner, D. M., . . . Phillips, K. A. (2009). Multidimensional body image comparisons among patients with eating disorders, body dysmorphic disorder, and clinical controls: A multisite study. *Body Image*, 6(3), 155–163.

Hudson, J. I., Hiripi, E., Pope Jr., H. G., & Kessler, R. C. (2007). The prevalence and correlates of eating disorders in the national comorbidity survey replication. *Biological Psychiatry*, 61(3), 348–358.

Keel, P. K., & Klump, K. L. (2003). Are eating disorders culture-bound syndromes? Implications for conceptualizing their etiology. *Psychological Bulletin*, 129(5), 747.

Keel, P. K., & Mitchell, J. E. (1997). Outcome in bulimia nervosa. *American Journal of Psychiatry*.

Kittler, J. E., Menard, W., & Phillips, K. A. (2007). Weight concerns in individuals with body dysmorphic disorder. *Eating Behaviors*, 8(1), 115–120.

Kollei, I., Schieber, K., de Zwaan, M., Svitak, M., & Martin, A. (2013). Body dysmorphic disorder and nonweight-related body image concerns in individuals with eating disorders. *International Journal of Eating Disorders*, 46(1), 52–59.

Koran, L. M., Abujaoude, E., Large, M. D., & Serpe, R. T. (2008). The prevalence of body dysmorphic disorder in the United States adult population. *CNS Spectrums*, 13(4), 312–322.

Lee, S. (1991). Anorexia nervosa in Hong Kong: A Chinese perspective. *Psychological Medicine*, 21(3), 703–711.

Löwe, B., Zipfel, S., Buchholz, C., Dupont, Y., Reas, D. L., & Herzog, W. (2001). Long-term outcome of anorexia nervosa in a prospective 21-year follow-up study. *Psychological Medicine*, 31(05), 881–890.

Lucas, A. R., Beard, C. M., O'Fallon, W. M., & Kurland, L. T. (1991). 50-year trends in the incidence of anorexia nervosa in Rochester, Minn.: A population-based study. *The American Journal of Psychiatry*, 148(7), 917–922.

Makino, M., Tsuboi, K., & Dennerstein, L. (2004). Prevalence of eating disorders: A comparison of western and non-western countries. *Medscape General Medicine*, 6(3), 49.

Mayville, S., Katz, R. C., Gipson, M. T., & Cabral, K. (1999). Assessing the prevalence of body dysmorphic disorder in an ethnically diverse group of adolescents. *Journal of Child and Family Studies*, 8(3), 357–362.

McClelland, L., & Crisp, A. (2001). Anorexia nervosa and social class. *International Journal of Eating Disorders*, 29(2), 150–156.

Miller, M. N., & Pumariega, A. J. (2001). Culture and eating disorders: A historical and cross-cultural review. *Psychiatry: Interpersonal and Biological Processes*, 64(2), 93–110.

205

Mission Australia. (2011). *National survey of young Australians*. Sydney, New South Wales: Mission Australia.

Mitchell, J. E., & Mussell, M. P. (1995). Comorbidity and binge eating disorder. *Addictive Behaviors*, 20(6), 725–732.

Murnen, S. K. (2011). Gender and body image. In T. F. Cash & L. Smolak (Eds.), *Body image* (2nd ed., pp. 173–179). New York, NY: The Guilford Press.

Njenga, F. G., & Kangethe, R. N. (2004). Anorexia nervosa in Kenya. *East African Medical Journal*, 81(4), 188–193.

Nobakht, M., & Dezhkam, M. (2000). An epidemiological study of eating disorders in iran. *International Journal of Eating Disorders*, 28(3), 265–271.

Norring, C.E.A., & Sohlberg, S.S. (1993). Outcome, recovery, relapse and mortality across six years in patients with clinical eating disorders. *Acta Psychiatrica Scandinavica*, 87(6), 437–444.

Otto, M. W., Wilhelm, S., Cohen, L. S., & Harlow, B. L. (2001). Prevalence of body dysmorphic disorder in a community sample of women. *American Journal of Psychiatry*, 158(12), 2061–2063. doi: 10.1176/appi.ajp.158.12.2061

Pawluck, D. E., & Gorey, K. M. (1998). Secular trends in the incidence of anorexia nervosa: Integrative review of population-based studies. *International Journal of Eating Disorders*, 23(4), 347–352.

Phillips, K. A. (1998). Body dysmorphic disorder: Clinical aspects and treatment strategies. *Bulletin of the Menninger Clinic*, 62(4), 33–48.

Phillips, K. A. (2004). Treating body dysmorphic disorder using medication. *Psychiatric Annals*, 34(12), 945–953.

Phillips, K. A., & Diaz, S. (1997). Gender differences in body dysmorphic disorder. *Journal of Nervous and Mental Disease*, 185(9), 570–577.

Phillips, K. A., Dufresne, R. G., Wilkel, C. S., & Vittorio, C. C. (2000). Rate of body dysmorphic disorder in dermatology patients. *Journal of the American Academy of Dermatology*, 42(3), 436–441.

Phillips, K. A., Grant, J., Siniscalchi, J., & Albertini, R. S. (2001). Surgical and nonpsychiatric medical treatment of patients with body dysmorphic disorder. *Psychosomatics*, 42(6), 504–510. doi: 10.1176/appi.psy.42.6.504

Phillips, K. A., Grant, J. E., Siniscalchi, J. M., Stout, R., & Price, L. H. (2005). A retrospective follow-up study of body dysmorphic disorder. *Comprehensive Psychiatry*, 46(5), 315–321.

Phillips, K. A., Menard, W., & Fay, C. (2006). Gender similarities and differences in 200 individuals with body dysmorphic disorder. *Comprehensive Psychiatry*, 47(2), 77–87.

Phillips, K. A., Menard, W., Fay, C., & Weisberg, R. (2005). Demographic characteristics, phenomenology, comorbidity, and family history in 200 individuals with body dysmorphic disorder. *Psychosomatics: Journal of Consultation Liaison Psychiatry*, 46(4), 317–325.

Phillips, K. A., Pagano, M. E., Menard, W., Fay, C., & Stout, R. L. (2005). Predictors of remission from body dysmorphic disorder: A prospective study. *Journal of Nervous and Mental Disease*, 193(8), 564–567.

Phillips, K. A., Pagano, M. E., Menard, W., & Stout, R. L. (2006). A 12-month follow-up study of the course of body dysmorphic disorder. *American Journal of Psychiatry*, 163(5), 907–912. doi: 10.1176/appi.ajp.163.5.907

Polivy, J., & Herman, C. P. (2002). Causes of eating disorders. *Annual Review of Psychology*, 53(1), 187–213.

Rabe-Jablonska, J., & Sobow, T. M. (2000). The links between body dysmorphic disorder and eating disorders. *European Psychiatry*, 15(5), 302–305.

Rief, W., Buhlmann, U., Wilhelm, S., Borkenhagen, A.D.A., & Brähler, E. (2006). The prevalence of body dysmorphic disorder: A population-based survey. *Psychological Medicine*, 36(06), 877–885.

Rodin, J., Silberstein, L., Striegel-Moore, R., Sonderegger, T. B., & Anastasi, A. (1985). Psychology and gender: Nebraska symposium on motivation, 1984. In T. Sonderegger (Ed.), *Psychology and gender* (pp. 267–307). Lincoln: University of Nebraska Press.

Ruffolo, J. S., Phillips, K. A., Menard, W., Fay, C., & Weisberg, R. B. (2006). Comorbidity of body dysmorphic disorder and eating disorders: Severity of psychopathology and body image disturbance. *International Journal of Eating Disorders*, 39(1), 11–19.

Russell, G. (1979). Bulimia nervosa: An ominous variant of anorexia nervosa. *Psychological Medicine*, 9(3), 429–448.

Sarwer, D. B., & Crerand, C. E. (2008). Body dysmorphic disorder and appearance enhancing medical treatments. *Body Image*, 5(1), 50–58.

Sarwer, D. B., Wadden, T. A., Pertschuk, M. J., & Whitaker, L. A. (1998). Body image dissatisfaction and body dysmorphic disorder in 100 cosmetic surgery patients. *Plastic and Reconstructive Surgery*, 101(6), 1644–1649.

Soundy, T. J., Lucas, A. R., Suman, V. J., & Melton, L. J. (1995). Bulimia nervosa in Rochester, Minnesota from 1980 to 1990. *Psychological Medicine*, 25(5), 1065–1072.

Spurrell, E. B., Wilfley, D. E., Tanofsky, M. B., & Brownell, K. D. (1997). Age of onset for binge eating: Are there different pathways to binge eating?. *International Journal of Eating Disorders*, 21(1), 55–65.

Steinhausen, H. C. (2002). The outcome of anorexia nervosa in the

20th century. *American Journal of Psychiatry*, 159(8), 1284–1293.

Striegel-Moore, R. H., Dohm, F. A., Kraemer, H. C., Taylor, C. B., Daniels, S., Crawford, P. B., & Schreiber, G. B. (2003). Eating disorders in white and black women. *American Journal of Psychiatry*, 160(7), 1326–1331.

Strober, M. (2004). Managing the chronic, treatment-resistant patient with anorexia nervosa. *International Journal of Eating Disorders*, 36(3), 245–255.

Strober, M., Freeman, R., & Morrell, W. (1997). The long-term course of severe anorexia nervosa in adolescents: Survival analysis of recovery, relapse, and outcome predictors over 10–15 years in a prospective study. *International Journal of Eating Disorders*, 22(4), 339–360.

Sullivan, P. F. (1995). Mortality in anorexia nervosa. *American Journal of Psychiatry*, 152(7), 1073–1074.

Sypeck, M. F., Gray, J. J., & Ahrens, A. H. (2004). No longer just a pretty face: Fashion magazines' depictions of ideal female beauty from 1959 to 1999. *International Journal of Eating Disorders*, 36(3), 342–347.

Thompson, J. K., Heinberg, L. J., Altabe, L., & Tantleff-Dunn, S. (1999). *Exacting beauty.* Washington, DC: American Psychological Association.

Tozzi, F., Thornton, L. M., Klump, K. L., Fichter, M. M., Halmi, K. A., Kaplan, A. S., . . . Mitchell, J. (2005). Symptom fluctuation in eating disorders: Correlates of diagnostic crossover. *American Journal of Psychiatry*, 162(4), 732–740.

Uzun, Ö., Başoğlu, C., Akar, A., Cansever, A., Özşahin, A., Çetin, M., & Ebrinç, S. (2003). Body dysmorphic disorder in patients with acne. *Comprehensive Psychiatry*, 44(5), 415–419.

Vandereycken, W. (2006). Denial of illness in anorexia nervosa – a conceptual review: Part 1 diagnostic significance and assessment. *European eating disorders review*, 14(5), 341–351.

Veale, D., & Riley, S. (2001). Mirror, mirror on the wall, who is the ugliest of them all? The psychopathology of mirror gazing in body dysmorphic disorder. *Behaviour Research and Therapy*, 39(12), 1381–1393.

Vulink, N.C.C., Sigurdsson, V., Kon, M., Bruijnzeel-Koomen, C.A.F.M., Westenberg, H.G.M., & Denys, D. (2006). Body dysmorphic disorder in 3-8% of patients in outpatient dermatology and plastic surgery clinics. *Ned Tijdschr Geneeskd*, 150(2), 97–100.

Zimmerman, M., & Mattia, J. I. (1998). Body dysmorphic disorder in psychiatric outpatients: Recognition, prevalence, comorbidity, demographic, and clinical correlates. *Comprehensive Psychiatry*, 39(5), 265–270.

Zipfel, S., Löwe, B., Reas, D. L., Deter, H. C., & Herzog, W. (2000). Long-term prognosis in anorexia nervosa: Lessons from a 21-year follow-up study. *The Lancet*, 355(9205), 721–722.

17

Post-traumatic stress disorder in women

Darryl Wade, Susan Fletcher, Jessica Carty and Mark Creamer

The diagnosis of post-traumatic stress disorder (PTSD) has been the focus of considerable attention since it first appeared in the diagnostic nomenclature in 1980. Since that time, the diagnostic criteria have been refined, with both DSM-5 (American Psychiatric Association, 2013) and ICD-10 (World Health Organization, 1993) recognizing the condition. In recent years, a major focus of research and debate has been the impact of gender on the risk of developing PTSD and related conditions following traumatic exposure. In general, the available evidence suggests that there is a two-fold risk of PTSD among women compared with men (Tolin & Foa, 2006); there has been considerable interest in developing theories and models to explain this gender difference (Christiansen & Elklit, 2013; Olff, Langeland, Draijer, & Gersons, 2007). The purpose of this chapter is to provide an overview of key issues regarding PTSD in women.

The nature of PTSD

According to DSM-5 (American Psychiatric Association, 2013), the first criterion to be met for a diagnosis of PTSD is the experience of a traumatic event (criterion A), defined as involving actual or threatened physical threat to the self or others. Four broad clusters of symptoms characterize the disorder and are required in some form for a diagnosis. First, evidence of reexperiencing the trauma is required (known as the B criteria). This is likely to take the form of intrusive memories, images or perceptions that invade consciousness; dreams; flashbacks; and emotional distress or physical reactions on reminders of the traumatic event. These symptoms are very distressing and the next symptom group (C criteria) is often conceptualized as a way of trying to prevent their return. The

C criteria include evidence of active avoidance, often with a phobic quality (such as attempts to avoid people, places, situations, thoughts, feelings and conversations associated with the trauma). The D criteria include alterations in mood or cognitions, sometimes thought of as "passive avoidance," with characteristic symptoms of social withdrawal; loss of interest; persistent negative emotions or inability to experience positive emotions; distorted beliefs about the cause or consequences of the event; exaggerated negative beliefs about oneself or the world; and psychogenic amnesia. The E criteria are those of persistent hyperarousal, characterized by sleep disturbance; anger and irritability; poor concentration; hypervigilance; exaggerated startle response; and reckless or self-destructive behavior. The symptoms must have been present for at least 1 month before a diagnosis of PTSD can be made, and must be associated with significant distress and/or impairment of social or occupational functioning.

Many symptoms of PTSD overlap with those of other diagnoses. There is also ample evidence that PTSD is often comorbid with a range of other Axis I and Axis II (personality) disorders (Chapman et al., 2012; Kessler et al., 1995; Pietrzak et al., 2011). Thus, the clinical presentation in both women and men is often quite complex. In more chronic cases, the disorder is associated with progressively deteriorating social and occupational functioning, often confronting the clinician with a myriad of psychosocial problems in addition to the primary symptom set.

Prevalence of PTSD

Epidemiological studies from several countries have indicated that, while women are less likely than men to be exposed to traumatic events, the prevalence of

Comprehensive Women's Mental Health, ed. David J. Castle and Kathryn M. Abel. Published by Cambridge University Press.
© Cambridge University Press 2016.

PTSD within the community is significantly higher among women (Breslau et al., 1998; Chapman et al., 2012; de Vries & Olff, 2009; Kessler et al., 1995; Norris et al., 2003; Pietrzak et al., 2011; Stein et al., 1997). One of the most influential of those studies, the National Comorbidity Study (NCS), estimated that the lifetime prevalence of trauma exposure was 51% for women and 61% for men; however, lifetime rates of PTSD were estimated at 10% for women and 5% for men (Kessler et al., 1995).

In Norway, Amstadter and colleagues (2013) found that the lifetime rate of trauma exposure was 23% for women and 32% for men, whilst the rate of lifetime PTSD was roughly 4 times higher among women compared with men (15% versus 4%). Similarly, a national survey of Australian adults found that although an equal proportion of women and men reported trauma exposure (76% and 74% respectively) (Mills et al., 2011), the 12-month prevalence of PTSD was significantly greater in women than men (9.7% versus 4.7%) (Chapman et al., 2012).

Environmental and cultural factors

It is worth noting that the prevalence of PTSD generally, as well as the differential rates of PTSD in women and men, may vary according to environmental and cultural factors. In a comparative study across four post-conflict, low-income countries, de Jong and colleagues found equal rates of PTSD in women and men in Ethiopia, higher rates among women in Algeria and Cambodia, and higher rates among men in Gaza (de Jong et al., 2001). In some settings, it is possible that gender differences may be obscured by the disproportionately high rates of post-traumatic symptomatology that characterize populations exposed to extreme prolonged trauma (Atwoli et al., 2013; Norris et al., 2002). For example, elevated rates of PTSD, depression and anxiety were reported for Armenian communities exposed to either extreme earthquake trauma or severe political violence 4 years later, regardless of gender or trauma type (Goenjian et al., 2000).

There is some evidence that the gender difference in the prevalence of PTSD may be particularly evident in cultural groups that emphasize traditional gender roles. Norris and colleagues (2001) compared gender differences in the rate of PTSD in Mexican, African-American and Anglo-American samples following hurricanes in Mexico and the United States

and found that the gender difference was greatest in the Mexican sample and least in the African-American sample, with the Anglo-American sample falling in between. The authors suggested that these rates may reflect differences in gender roles in Mexico and the United States; the discouragement of emotional expression in Mexican men may exacerbate gender differences in the diagnosis of PTSD and related disorders, whilst these differences may be reduced in African-American communities, which are considered to have a more egalitarian approach to gender role expectations.

In a similar vein, the process of socialization in different cultures may produce gender differences in coping style, which may mediate response to stressful life events. Gavranidou and colleagues (2003) have suggested that, as a result of cultural expectations, women are more likely to practice emotion-focused coping whereas men are more likely to use problem-focused coping, with the latter often associated with better outcome. Similarly, Foster and colleagues (2004) suggested that gender differences in PTSD may reflect socialization processes, whereby women are taught to internalize and men to externalize negative emotions in accordance with accepted feminine and masculine roles (see also Chapter 1). Thus, women and men may respond differently to trauma, with women more likely to internalize emotions in the form of anxiety and depression, and men more likely to externalize in the form of aggression and substance use. If this is the case, then a tendency to internalize may result in higher rates of PTSD diagnoses in women.

Developmental context

While relatively few epidemiological studies have considered trauma exposure and response across the life span, preliminary evidence suggests that gender differences may manifest from a relatively early age. Similar to adult studies, a number of epidemiological studies of adolescents have found an elevated risk for PTSD among females compared with males (Giaconia et al., 1995; Landolt et al., 2013; McLaughlin et al., 2013). Landolt and colleagues (2013) did not find gender differences in rates of exposure to any traumatic event among Swiss adolescents, but did find that female gender, not living with both biological parents, lower parental education and exposure to multiple traumatic events were significant risk factors for PTSD. In the United States, McLaughlin and colleagues (2013) found that adolescent females were more likely to develop PTSD than males, even after controlling for type of trauma exposure. In addition, and consistent with the extant literature (Brewin et al., 2000; Ozer et al., 2003), the results indicated that prior trauma exposure was associated with increased vulnerability to PTSD among adolescents regardless of gender.

Exposure to traumatizing events at an early developmental stage potentially has serious implications for the way in which individuals deal with stress and trauma in later life, and this may be particularly true for females. Breslau and colleagues (1997) found some evidence of differential traumatic stress reactions among women and men depending on the timing of the trauma, with gender differences in the rate of PTSD more marked if first exposure to trauma occurred at or before age 15. While women remained at higher risk following first exposure that occurred later, the gender difference was less pronounced, suggesting that women's greater vulnerability to PTSD may be greater if exposure occurs during childhood.

Although beyond the scope of this chapter, it is important to note that the long-term effects of prolonged exposure to childhood trauma may not be best conceptualized as PTSD. The contribution of prolonged and severe developmental trauma to the development of Axis II personality disorders, especially the B cluster such as borderline and antisocial personality disorder, has been the subject of considerable debate in the literature (e.g., McLean & Gallop, 2003; Yen et al., 2002). In an attempt to develop a more etiologically useful clinical description of these effects, several authors have proposed the existence of a new diagnostic category variously known as complex PTSD or DESNOS – disorders of extreme stress not otherwise specified – characterized by disturbances in affective, self, and interpersonal capacities (Herman, 1992; Zlotnick et al., 1996). Although not formally accepted in DSM as a diagnostic category, emerging evidence supports the proposed inclusion of complex PTSD in ICD-11 as a "sibling" disorder to PTSD (Cloitre et al., 2013; Maercker et al., 2013).

There is somewhat less research to inform our understanding of gender and traumatic stress at the other end of the life span. In a reanalysis of one of the few studies to include individuals over the age of 55, Norris and colleagues (2002) found that age interacted with gender to predict current PTSD. Although higher prevalence rates of PTSD were apparent for

women aged 18–55 compared to men in that age range, rates did not differ by gender for those over 55. Interestingly, and perhaps not surprisingly, the higher levels of trauma exposure routinely reported for males only applied to the population under 30 years of age. From approximately 30 onwards, rates of trauma exposure did not differ between women and men. In a comparison of older and younger women, Acierno et al. (2002) found that women over the age of 55 reported fewer physical and sexual assaults, as well as a reduced risk of trauma-related morbidity following interpersonal violence, than women aged 18–34. Finally, Creamer and Parslow (2008) found a clear trend of reduced prevalence of current PTSD over the life span in both women and men, with the highest rates in young adults and negligible rates in those over the age of 65. Indeed, those rates were so low that meaningful gender comparisons were not possible.

In summary, it appears that women are more vulnerable to developing PTSD from a relatively young age, with this gender difference persisting through middle adulthood but being less apparent in the older adulthood period during which there is a reduced rate of PTSD for both genders.

Possible explanations for gender differences in PTSD

A review of epidemiological research thus indicates that women are more vulnerable to the development of PTSD than males. While this might to some extent be influenced by environmental and cultural factors and early childhood experiences, these factors cannot fully account for the differential rates. This section describes a number of other factors that may interact to mediate the relationship between gender, trauma exposure and PTSD vulnerability.

Assessment and phenomenology

It is conceivable that gender differences in the prevalence of PTSD may, in part, be simply an artifact of the diagnostic criteria and assessment procedures. Several studies have reported gender-related differences in patterns of PTSD symptomatology that may increase the likelihood that women will meet criteria for PTSD. More women, for example, have been found to endorse avoidance symptoms in both DSM- (Breslau et al., 1999; Fullerton et al., 2001) and ICD-defined PTSD (Peters et al., 2006). Avoidance and numbing symptoms are relatively infrequently endorsed (e.g., Foa et al., 1995; North et al., 1999); hence, the presence of this symptom criterion substantially increases the likelihood of a PTSD diagnosis. Of note, a latent class analysis conducted on data collected from individuals with PTSD found no evidence of gender-related differential symptom reporting in each of three classes of PTSD-related disturbance: no, intermediate and pervasive disturbance (Chung & Breslau, 2008). The finding that proportionally more women than men experienced pervasive disturbance led the authors to conclude that this is likely to reflect a substantive difference between women and men in their vulnerability to develop PTSD rather than a gender-related reporting bias.

Peritraumatic dissociation, including time distortion, reduced awareness, emotional numbing, amnesia and derealization experienced at the time or soon after the trauma, has been found to be an important risk factor for PTSD (Ozer et al., 2003). There is some evidence that the presence of peritraumatic dissociation predicts PTSD more accurately in women than in men (e.g., Bryant & Harvey, 2003; Fullerton et al., 2001; Irish et al., 2011). For example, Irish and colleagues (2011) found that peritraumatic dissociation contributed to gender differences in PTSD symptoms among MVA victims at 6 months. The mechanisms underlying this relationship require further investigation, although a range of pre- and post-trauma factors are likely to be involved. However, it is difficult to disentangle this finding from the role of prior trauma; adverse early childhood experiences may promote the use of dissociation as a coping strategy in response to stress and trauma, thereby increasing vulnerability to subsequent PTSD.

Importantly, gender differences are not limited to the prevalence of PTSD: women are also more likely than men to be diagnosed with other anxiety and depressive disorders (Kessler et al., 2005; Kessler et al., 1994; Korten & Henderson, 2000; Oakley Browne et al., 2006; Slade et al., 2009). Estimates of PTSD prevalence may be complicated by the substantial overlap of symptoms between PTSD and other anxiety and depressive disorders. Thus, increased rates of PTSD in women may reflect a broader vulnerability to negative affect or at least a willingness to acknowledge and report emotional distress. While elevated rates of PTSD, as well as anxiety and depression in women may reflect a heightened vulnerability to emotional disorders, they may also reflect biases in the diagnostic criteria and assessment processes (see for example Martin et al., 2013 for a discussion of the influence of diagnostic criteria on the

prevalence of depression in women and men. Also see Chapters 8, 19, and 20).

Trauma type

A second, and highly plausible, explanation for the higher PTSD prevalence among women is that women and men are prone to experience different types of trauma. Epidemiological studies and systematic reviews have consistently found that girls and women are more likely to report sexual assault, rape and childhood sexual abuse; whereas boys and men are more likely to experience nonsexual physical assault, combat, accidental injury and witnessing someone being badly injured or killed (Amstadter et al., 2013; Breslau et al., 1999; Breslau et al., 1997; Creamer, et al, 2001; Kessler et al., 1995; McLaughlin et al., 2013; Tolin & Foa, 2006). There is a large body of evidence indicating that exposure to traumas involving interpersonal violence carries a high risk of subsequent psychological adjustment problems (e.g., Creamer et al., 2001; Kessler et al., 1995). It is also reasonable to assume that some types of interpersonal violence (and even some types of sexual assault) are especially "psychopathogenic" and more likely to result in poorer psychological adjustment when, for example, the attacker is known to, and previously trusted by, the victim and/or when the level of perceived threat is very high. As a result, it is conceivable that a higher rate of these types of trauma among women might contribute to gender differences in the prevalence of PTSD.

One way to test this hypothesis is to examine whether there are gender differences in the prevalence of PTSD among both women and men who have experienced the same type of event (i.e., control for the type of trauma). If similar rates of PTSD are found for both genders, then this finding would indicate that it is the differences in the types of trauma that men and women report being exposed to that represents the main contributor to PTSD risk. However, if gender differences are evident, then alternative explanations for the higher rates of PTSD in women compared to men are required.

To this end, Tolin and Foa (2006) undertook a meta-analysis of gender differences in trauma and PTSD and found that overall women were more likely to meet criteria for PTSD and reported greater severity of PTSD symptoms compared to men for all types of trauma. Of note, the few available studies that investigated adult sexual assault or child sexual assault did not find gender differences in rates of PTSD, although for child sexual assault significant differences did emerge under certain methodological conditions (e.g., assessment of lifetime versus current PTSD; use of diagnostic interviews versus self-report questionnaires). However, for traumas experienced more frequently by men – such as nonsexual assault, combat, accidental injury and witnessing someone being badly injured or killed – women were more likely to meet criteria for PTSD and reported greater severity of PTSD than men. Taken together, these findings indicate that the higher prevalence of PTSD in women is not simply the result of increased exposure to certain types of trauma. Interestingly, the results of the meta-analysis showed that the greatest gender difference in conditional risk for PTSD was for nonsexual physical assault. Betts and colleagues (2013) also found that women were at a much greater risk of partial and full PTSD after experiencing physical assault, but did not find any gender-related difference in risk of PTSD resulting from other types of traumas. It may be speculated that these findings can at least in part be explained by the type of assaultive violence women experience; that is, women are more likely to be assaulted by someone they know (and, perhaps, trust), while men are more likely to be assaulted by a stranger (for example, in a bar room brawl). Clearly, the former event type is more likely to shatter fundamental assumptions about the self and the world, particularly those relating to trust and safety, creating greater challenges for subsequent adjustment.

Social and material support

It has been suggested that loss of resources in the aftermath of trauma, including both social and material support, may help to explain the development of PTSD and, further, that women are more vulnerable to such resource loss than men (Hobfoll, Johnson, Ennis, & Jackson, 2003). In a sample of 714 inner city women, Hobfoll and colleagues (2003) found that resource loss and worsening economic circumstances had a greater negative impact than resource gain and improving economic circumstances had a positive impact, suggesting the greater saliency of loss than gain. Perhaps the most important "resource" following trauma is that of social support, with lack of social support a powerful predictor of PTSD (Brewin et al., 2000; Ozer et al., 2003). Although measurement of social support is notoriously difficult, it usually

encompasses several aspects such as availability, use and perceived benefits of both practical and emotional support. However, an important distinction has been drawn between positive and negative social support. In a sample of crime victims, Andrews and her colleagues (2003) found that perceived positive social support had a protective effect, while perceived negative response from friends and family had a detrimental effect on self-reported PTSD symptoms at 6 months. While women and men reported comparable levels of positive support and support satisfaction, women reported higher levels of negative support (even after controlling for trauma type). Furthermore, the benefits of support satisfaction and the adverse effects of negative support were far more influential on 6-month PTSD symptoms for women than men. This factor contributed substantially to the explanation of gender differences in symptom severity, and is clearly an important direction for future research. Another issue that requires further study is potential gender differences in the source and context of social support that facilitates recovery. For example, research conducted with military personnel found that for men, social support from within the military was associated with lower levels of post-traumatic stress, while support from outside the military (i.e., from family and friends) had no effect. For female personnel, the reverse was true (Smith et al., 2013). In summary, the available evidence suggests that social support, and particularly negative social support, is likely to interact with acute symptom severity to influence the course of recovery following trauma.

Cognitive factors

Epidemiological studies, such as those described earlier, often focus on objective trauma type and severity. It is widely recognized, however, that the individual's perception or appraisal of threat level is a powerful predictor of subsequent adjustment (Ehlers & Clark, 2000). There is some evidence to suggest that women may perceive traumatic events as more aversive than men who experience the same event. Norris and colleagues (2002) noted that comparable proportions of women and men meet the DSM-IV Criterion A2 (powerful emotional reactions to trauma), despite the fact that men report a higher prevalence of objective trauma exposure. Goenjian and colleagues (2001) found that Nicaraguan adolescent girls reported significantly higher subject-ive levels of exposure than adolescent boys, despite no difference in their objective experience of Hurricane Mitch. Thus, girls and women may tend subjectively to experience traumatic events as more aversive, with these negative appraisals increasing vulnerability to PTSD. In some circumstances, it is understandable that women may feel more threatened by a traumatic event, particularly if the experience involves inten-tional harm. For example, it is plausible that a woman who is a victim of nonsexual assault by a male perpet-rator may also fear that the perpetrator will rape her. Thus, an assault of the same objective severity may at times be considerably more frightening for a woman than for a man. Another cognitive factor that may contribute to the development of PTSD is negative appraisal of acute symptoms following trauma, including beliefs that the symptoms signify personal weakness or impending madness (McNally, 2003). At present, however, there is a lack of empirical data on gender differences in how women and men interpret acute trauma symptoms.

The important role of cognitive factors in the development of PTSD has strong theoretical support, as discussed by Tolin and Foa (2002). These authors build on the emotional processing theory described by Foa and her colleagues (e.g., Foa & Rothbaum, 1998) to explore differential patterns of cognitive processing between women and men that may serve to increase PTSD vulnerability. Emotional processing theory proposes that the development of traumatic stress symptoms is dependent upon an individual's prior perception of the self and the world, as well as the degree to which these views change as a conse-quence of trauma. Tolin and Foa (2002) reviewed the literature and found preliminary evidence to support the proposition of gender differences in patterns of cognitive processing, memory of the event, and the effect of trauma on cognitive schemas. Self-blame was more prevalent in women than men following trauma, as were negative self-beliefs and perceptions of the world as a dangerous place. It is, of course, difficult to separate the influence of trauma type from cognitive appraisals; traumas that are objectively more severe are also likely to be appraised more negatively. It was noted earlier, however, that trauma type accounted for only a limited amount of the variance in post-traumatic stress levels, suggesting that cognitive processing patterns may mediate vulnerability to PTSD. Again, the underlying

mechanisms that explain these gender differences in processing of information associated with the trauma remain a matter for speculation (Olff et al., 2007). Presumably, the difference is accounted for by a com-plex interaction between a range of influences.

Biological factors

Few studies have investigated psychophysiological dif-ferences between men and women in acute reactions to threat that may serve as potential mediators for PTSD vulnerability. A review of the empirical data by Pierce and colleagues (2002) suggested that there was little evidence for gender-specific differences in physio-logical responses (such as cardiovascular and skin con-ductance reactivity) to threat-related stimuli. They acknowledged, however, that studies are lacking and that those that exist have methodological limitations. A more recent review reported that any evidence for gender differences in physiological reactivity seemed to depend on how it was operationalized in particular studies (McLean & Anderson, 2009).

Greater support has been found for the impact of hormone fluctuations across the life span in medi-ating response to stress cues and vulnerability to anxiety disorders. Piggott (1999) reported that estro-gen and progesterone have been associated with the regulation of neurotransmitters that mediate the anxiety response. These include the locus coeruleus-noradrenaline and serotonergic systems, as well as the y-aminobutyric acid (GABA) benzodiazepine receptor complex. Higher levels of estrogen are pro-posed to be stress-protective while progesterone may have the reverse effect. Fluctuations in these hor-mones during a woman's menstrual and reproductive cycle may influence the degree of reactivity to stress cues and the course of symptomatology. A review by Kajantie and Phillips (2006) concluded that adult women between puberty and menopause tend to be less physiologically reactive to stress than men, are more reactive during the luteal phase of the menstrual cycle, and less reactive during pregnancy and after menopause. Consistent with this summary, more recent research suggests that the luteal phase and the associated increase in progesterone is predictive of enhanced recall of negative events (Felmingham et al., 2012), and increased risk of flashbacks (Bryant et al., 2011). Thus, it would seem that gender differ-ences in physiological reactivity are influenced by women's hormonal status (see Chapter 8).

In summary, it is likely that several factors interact to explain the higher rates of PTSD among women. These include cultural and societal pressures and expectations (see Chapter 1), the types of trauma to which women are more likely to be exposed, the reaction of loved ones and associates to their experience, and hormonal levels. It is likely that these factors combine to influence cognitive processing and appraisals of the trauma, which, in turn, affect the course of recovery. While it is possible that the diagnostic criteria and common assessment strategies serve to inflate artificially the reported prevalence of PTSD, this seems an unlikely and unhelpful explanation. Rather than denying the existence of these elevated rates, a more productive approach is to focus upon what can be done to address the causes of this differential vulnerability and how best to treat those affected.

Treatment

While few studies have specifically investigated gender differences in PTSD treatment outcomes, the literature suggests that women may have a slightly better response rate when compared to men (Foa et al., 2000). Gender-based comparisons are problematic, however, since many treatment studies comprise either female sexual assault victims or male combat veterans. Thus, gender differences in treatment efficacy may be obscured by several confounding variables, including trauma type.

Psychological interventions

The majority of studies investigating the efficacy of psychotherapy in the treatment of PTSD have fallen under the broad rubric of cognitive behavior therapy (CBT). A descriptive review by Blain and colleagues (2010) concluded that the available research shows support for equivalent outcomes on primary PTSD symptoms for women and men, although the authors acknowledged significant limitations of their review including its descriptive and qualitative nature and that it was limited to studies reporting the effects of gender. A review by Cason and colleagues (2002) examined effect sizes of psychological interventions for PTSD from mixed-gender, female-only and male-only controlled studies and concluded that women fared as well if not better than men in reduction of PTSD symptoms. Interestingly, a recent study by Felmingham and Bryant (2012) found no differences between women and men with PTSD at post-treatment following exposure therapy, but men showed reduced maintenance of treatment gains at follow-up. They had lower rates of relapse, however, if exposure therapy was combined with cognitive therapy. Galovski and colleagues (2013) evaluated the response to CBT for PTSD following interpersonal assault, and found that women and men demonstrated similar improvement in symptoms during treatment and at follow-up, although there were nonsignificant differences favoring women.

Pharmacotherapy

A mounting body of empirical research has supported the efficacy of certain types of psychotropic medication in the treatment of PTSD. Specifically, there is a relatively large body of evidence supporting the use of selective serotonin reuptake inhibitors (SSRIs), with some promising findings for serotonin noradrenaline reuptake inhibitors (SNRIs) and atypical antipsychotics (Ipser & Stein, 2012). The pharmacotherapy of choice in PTSD, however, remains the SSRIs due to their relatively low side-effect burden and good tolerability (Australian Centre for Posttraumatic Mental Health, 2013). Large-scale randomized controlled trials have indicated that both sertraline and paroxetine significantly improve all three PTSD symptom clusters, as well as ameliorating comorbid symptoms (e.g., Brady et al., 2000; Davidson et al., 2001; Tucker et al., 2001).

Some evidence suggests that women have a somewhat greater response than men to SSRIs and SNRIs, which raises the possibility that antidepressants may work somewhat differently in women and men (Khan et al., 2005). However, recent evidence on pharmacotherapy for PTSD from multiple trials suggests that gender is unlikely to be a significant determinant of treatment outcome (Ipser & Stein, 2012; Rothbaum et al., 2008). Consideration should be given to reproductive status and whether or not women are planning to become pregnant when considering SSRI use (see Chapter 9).

In summary, although the data are not strong, it does appear that women may be somewhat more responsive than men to psychological, and possibly pharmacological, treatments for PTSD. This is despite their greater vulnerability for developing the disorder. Indeed, it may be that at least some of those factors that increase vulnerability (for example, greater emotional expression) may be positive characteristics when it comes to psychological treatment. Along the same lines, the type of comorbid disorders occurring with chronic PTSD may differ between women and men. For example, it can be speculated that substance use disorders, more common in men (Creamer et al., 2001; Kessler et al., 1995), are more disruptive to therapeutic efficacy. There is also evidence that women are more likely to seek treatment following traumatic exposure (Livanou et al., 2002). This may, of course, simply be a function of the higher prevalence of PTSD and related reactions in females. It may also, however, be a function of social and cultural influences that support emotional expression and accept vulnerability in women but not men.

Summary

The evidence reviewed in this chapter strongly suggests that women are at greater risk than men for the development of PTSD following exposure to a traumatic experience. Most community-based epidemiological studies attest to this increased risk, suggesting that women are roughly twice as likely to be diagnosed with PTSD.

The mechanisms underlying this apparently increased vulnerability remain largely a matter of speculation. Sociocultural factors appear to be of significance, particularly in regard to gender role socialization. These social processes may affect willingness to acknowledge distress, as well as the pattern of symptomatology expressed by men and women. They may also influence access to, and the impact of, trauma on, social and material support. The nature and severity of post-traumatic morbidity is strongly influenced by the type of traumatic event. Women are more likely than men to experience interpersonal

trauma, such as sexual assault, which is associated with high rates of PTSD, although the higher prevalence of PTSD in women is not likely to be due simply to increased exposure to certain types of trauma. Cognitive appraisals are a crucial mediating factor between exposure and psychological adjustment, with research suggesting a tendency for women to experience the same trauma as more aversive than men. While strong evidence is lacking at this stage, gender-specific biological mechanisms, such as hormonal fluctuations across a woman's menstrual and life cycle, may also be mediating factors. Finally, while women may be at greater risk for the development of psychiatric sequelae following trauma, preliminary findings from treatment outcome studies indicate that they may benefit from PTSD interventions to a greater extent than men. While further research is required, it may be speculated that many of the same gender-specific mechanisms that increase women's vulnerability to PTSD may also facilitate treatment response.

While this review has discussed a range of issues regarding the relationship between gender and PTSD, no single factor provides a sufficient explanation as to why women are more likely to be diagnosed with the disorder. Psychological adjustment following trauma is determined by a complex interaction of many factors. It is likely that these mechanisms affect both men and women, but may have differential influence on adjustment according to gender. Future theoretical and empirical elaboration of these issues will contribute not only to our understanding of the relationship between gender and PTSD, but also to the identification of those at risk following trauma. In the long run, the goal will be to enhance early identification and intervention practices in order to reduce the debilitating effects of PTSD and related mental health sequelae of trauma.

References

Acierno, R., Brady, K., Gray, M., Kilpatrick, D. G., Resnick, H., & Best, C. L. (2002). Psychopathology following interpersonal violence: A comparison of risk factors in older and younger adults. *Journal of Clinical Geropsychology*, 8(1), 13–23.

American Psychiatric Association. (2013). *Diagnostic and Statistical Manual of Mental Disorders*

(5th ed.). Washington DC: American Psychiatric Association.

Amstadter, A. B., Aggen, S. H., Knudsen, G. P., Reichborn-Kjennerud, T., & Kendler, K. S. (2013). Potentially traumatic event exposure, posttraumatic stress disorder, and Axis I and II comorbidity in a population-based study of Norwegian young adults. *Social Psychiatry and Psychiatric*

Epidemiology, 48(2), 215–223. doi: 10.1007/s00127-012-0537-2.

Andrews, B., Brewin, C. R., & Rose, S. (2003). Gender, social support, and PTSD in victims of violent crime. *Journal of Traumatic Stress*, 16(4), 421–427.

Atwoli, L., Stein, D. J., Williams, D. R., Mclaughlin, K. A., Petukhova, M., Kessler, R. C., & Koenen, K. C. (2013). Trauma and posttraumatic stress disorder in South Africa:

Analysis from the South African Stress and Health Study. *BMC Psychiatry*, 13. doi: 10.1186/1471-244x-13-182.

Australian Centre for Posttraumatic Mental Health. (2013). *Australian Guidelines for the Treatment of Acute Stress Disorder and Posttraumatic Stress Disorder.* Melbourne, Victoria: ACPMH.

Betts, K. S., Williams, G. M., Najman, J. M., & Alati, R. (2013). Exploring the female specific risk to partial and full PTSD following physical assault. *Journal of Traumatic Stress*, 26(1), 86–93. doi: 10.1002/Jts.21776.

Blain, L. M., Galovski, T. E., & Robinson, T. (2010). Gender differences in recovery from posttraumatic stress disorder: A critical review. *Aggression and Violent Behavior*, 15(6), 463–474. doi: 10.1016/j.avb.2010.09.001.

Brady, K. T., Pearlstein, T., Asnis, G. M., Baker, D. G., Rothbaum, B., Sikes, C. R., & Farfel, G. M. (2000). Efficacy and safety of sertraline treatment of posttraumatic stress disorder: A randomized controlled trial. *Journal of the American Medical Association*, 283(14), 1837–1844.

Breslau, N., Chilcoat, H. D., Kessler, R. C., Peterson, E. L., & Lucia, V. C. (1999). Vulnerability to assaultive violence: Further specification of the sex difference in post-traumatic stress disorder. *Psychological Medicine*, 29, 813–821.

Breslau, N., Davis, G. C., Andreski, P., Peterson, E. L., & Schultz, L. R. (1997). Sex differences in posttraumatic stress disorder. *Archives of General Psychiatry*, 54(11), 1044–1048.

Breslau, N., Kessler, R. C., Chilcoat, H. D., Schultz, L. R., Davis, G. C., & Andreski, P. (1998). Trauma and posttraumatic stress disorder in the community. *Archives of General Psychiatry*, 55(7), 626–632.

Brewin, C. R., Andrews, B., & Valentine, J. D. (2000). Meta-analysis of risk factors for posttraumatic stress disorder in trauma-exposed adults. *Journal of Consulting and Clinical Psychology*, 68(5), 748–766. doi: 10.1037/0022-006X.68.5.748.

Bryant, R. A., Felmingham, K. L., Silove, D., Creamer, M., O'Donnell, M., & McFarlane, A. C. (2011). The association between menstrual cycle and traumatic memories. *Journal of Affective Disorders*, 131(1–3), 398–401. doi: 10.1016/j.jad.2010.10.049.

Bryant, R. A., & Harvey, A. G. (2003). Gender differences in the relationship between acute stress disorder and posttraumatic stress disorder following motor vehicle accidents. *Australian and New Zealand Journal of Psychiatry*, 37(2), 226–229.

Cason, D., Grubaugh, A., & Resick, P. (2002). Gender and PTSD treatment: Efficacy and effectiveness. In R. Kimerling, P. Ouimette, & J. Wolfe (Eds.), *Gender and PTSD* (pp. 305–334). New York: Guilford Press.

Chapman, C., Mills, K., Slade, T., McFarlane, A. C., Bryant, R. A., Creamer, M., . . . Teesson, M. (2012). Remission from post-traumatic stress disorder in the general population. *Psychological Medicine*, 42(8), 1695–1703. doi: 10.1017/S0033291711002856.

Christiansen, D., & Elklit, A. (2013). Sex differences in PTSD. In E. Ovuga (Ed.), *Posttraumatic stress disorders in a global context* (pp. 113–142). InTech.

Chung, H., & Breslau, N. (2008). The latent structure of post-traumatic stress disorder: Tests of invariance by gender and trauma type. *Psychological Medicine*, 38(4), 563–573.

Cloitre, M., Garvert, D. W., Brewin, C. R., Bryant, R. A., & Maercker, A. (2013). Evidence for proposed ICD-II PTSD and complex PTSD: A latent profile analysis. *European Jouranl of Psychotraumatology*, 4(20706). doi: 10.3402/ejpt.v4i0.20706.

Creamer, M., Burgess, P., & McFarlane, A. C. (2001). Post-traumatic stress disorder: Findings from the Australian National Survey of Mental Health and Well-being. *Psychological Medicine*, 31(7), 1237–1247.

Creamer, M., & Parslow, R. (2008). Trauma exposure and posttraumatic stress disorder in the elderly: A community prevalence study. *American Journal of Geriatric Psychiatry*, 16(10), 853–856.

Davidson, J., Rothbaum, B. O., van der Kolk, B. A., Sikes, C. R., & Farfel, G. M. (2001). Multicenter, double-blind comparison of sertraline and placebo in the treatment of posttraumatic stress disorder. *Archives of General Psychiatry*, 58(5), 485–492.

de Jong, J., Komproe, I. H., Van Ommeren, M., El Masri, M., Araya, M., Khaled, N., . . . Somasundaram, D. (2001). Lifetime events and posttraumatic stress disorder in 4 postconflict settings. *Journal of the American Medical Association*, 286(5), 555–562.

de Vries, G. J., & Olff, M. (2009). The lifetime prevalence of traumatic events and posttraumatic stress disorder in the Netherlands. *Journal of Traumatic Stress*, 22(4), 259–267.

Ehlers, A., & Clark, D. M. (2000). A cognitive model of posttraumatic stress disorder. *Behaviour Research and Therapy*, 38(4), 319–345.

Felmingham, K. L., & Bryant, R. A. (2012). Gender differences in the maintenance of response to cognitive behavior therapy for posttraumatic stress disorder. *Journal of Consulting and Clinical Psychology*, 80(2), 196–200. doi: 10.1037/a0027156.

Felmingham, K. L., Fong, W. C., & Bryant, R. A. (2012). The impact of progesterone on memory consolidation of threatening images in women. *Psychoneuroendocrinology*, 37(11),

1896–1900. doi: 10.1016/j.psyneuen.2012.03.026.

Foa, E. B., Keane, T. M., & Friedman, M. J. (2000). *Effective treatments for PTSD: Practice guidelines from the International Society for Traumatic Stress Studies.* New York: Guilford Press.

Foa, E. B., Riggs, D. S., & Gershuny, B. S. (1995). Arousal, numbing, and intrusion: Symptom structure of PTSD following assault. *American Journal of Psychiatry,* 152(1), 116–120.

Foa, E. B., & Rothbaum, B. O. (1998). *Treating the trauma of rape: Cognitive-behavioral therapy for PTSD.* New York: Guilford Press.

Foster, J. D., Kuperminc, G. P., & Price, A. W. (2004). Gender differences in posttraumatic stress and related symptoms among inner-city minority youth exposed to community violence. *Journal of Youth and Adolescence,* 33(1), 59–69.

Fullerton, C. S., Ursano, R. J., Epstein, R. S., Crowley, B., Vance, K., Kao, T. C., . . . Baum, A. (2001). Gender differences in posttraumatic stress disorder after motor vehicle accidents. *American Journal of Psychiatry,* 158(9), 1486–1491.

Galovski, T., Blain, L., Chappuis, C., & Fletcher, T. (2013). Sex differences in recovery from PTSD in male and female interpersonal assault survivors. *Behaviour Research and Therapy,* 51(6), 247–255.

Gavranidou, M., & Rosner, R. (2003). The weaker sex? Gender and post-traumatic stress disorder. *Depression and Anxiety,* 17(3), 130–139.

Giaconia, R. M., Reinherz, H. Z., Silverman, A. B., Pakiz, B., Frost, A. K. & Cohen, E. (1995). Traumas and posttraumatic stress disorder in a community population of older adolescents. *Journal of the American Academy of Child and Adolescent Psychiatry,* 34(10), 1369–1380.

Goenjian, A. K., Molina, L., Steinberg, A. M., Fairbanks, L. A., Alvarez, M. L., Goenjian, H. A., & Pynoos, R. S. (2001). Posttraumatic stress and depressive reactions among Nicaraguan adolescents after hurricane mitch. *American Journal of Psychiatry,* 158(5), 788–794.

Goenjian, A. K., Steinberg, A. M., Najarian, L. M., Fairbanks, L. A., Tashjian, M., & Pynoos, R. S. (2000). Prospective study of posttraumatic stress, anxiety, and depressive reactions after earthquake and political violence. *American Journal of Psychiatry,* 157(6), 911–916.

Herman, J. L. (1992). *Trauma and recovery: The aftermath of violence from domestic abuse to political terror.* New York: Basic Books.

Hobfoll, S. E., Johnson, R. J., Ennis, N., & Jackson, A. P. (2003). Resource loss, resource gain, and emotional outcomes among inner city women. *Journal of Personality and Social Psychology,* 84(3), 632–643.

Ipser, J. C., & Stein, D. J. (2012). Evidence-based pharmacotherapy of post-traumatic stress disorder (PTSD). *International Journal of Neuropsychopharmacology,* 15(6), 825–840. doi: 10.1017/S1461145711001209.

Irish, L. A., Fischer, B., Fallon, W., Spoonster, E., Sledjeski, E. M., & Delahanty, D. L. (2011). Gender differences in PTSD symptoms: An exploration of peritraumatic mechanisms. *Journal of Anxiety Disorders,* 25(2), 209–216. doi: 10.1016/j.janxdis.2010.09.004

Kajantie, E., & Phillips, D. I. W. (2006). The effects of sex and hormonal status on the physiological response to acute psychosocial stress. *Psychoneuroendocrinology,* 31(2), 151–178. doi: 10.1016/j.psyneuen.2005.07.002

Kessler, R. C., Berglund, P., Demler, O., Jin, R., & Walters, E. E. (2005). Lifetime prevalence and age-of-onset distributions of DSM-IV disorders in the National Comorbidity Survey Replication. *Archives of General Psychiatry,* 62(6), 593–602.

Kessler, R. C., McGonagle, K. A., Zhao, S., Nelson, C. B., Hughes, M., Eshleman, S., . . . Kendler, K. S. (1994). Lifetime and 12-month prevalence of DSM-III-R psychiatric disorders in the United States. *Archives of General Psychiatry,* 51, 8–19.

Kessler, R. C., Sonnega, A., Hughes, M., & Nelson, C. B. (1995). Posttraumatic stress disorder in the National Comorbidity Survey. *Archives of General Psychiatry,* 52(12), 1048–1060.

Khan, A., Broadhead, A., Schwartz, K. A., Kolts, R. L., & Brown, W. A. (2005). Sex differences in antidepressant response in recent antidepressant clinical trials. *Journal of Clinical Psychopharmacology,* 25(4), 318–324.

Korten, A., & Henderson, S. (2000). The Australian National Survey of Mental Health and Well-Being. *British Journal of Psychiatry,* 177, 325–330.

Landolt, M. A., Schnyder, U., Maier, T., Schoenbucher, V., & Mohler-Kuo, M. (2013). Trauma exposure and posttraumatic stress disorder in adolescents: A national survey in Switzerland. *Journal of Traumatic Stress,* 26(2), 209–216. doi: 10.1002/jts.21794

Livanou, M., Basoglu, M., Salcioglu, E., & Kalender, D. (2002). Traumatic stress responses in treatment-seeking earthquake survivors in Turkey. *Journal of Nervous & Mental Disease,* 190(12), 816–823.

Maercker, A., Brewin, C. R., Bryant, R. A., Cloitre, M., Reed, G. M., van Ommeren, M., . . . Saxena, S. (2013). Proposals for mental disorders specifically associated with stress in the International Classification of Diseases-11. *Lancet,* 381(9878), 1683–1685. doi: 10.1016/s0140-6736(12)62191-6

Martin, L. A., Neighbors, H. W., & Griffith, D. M. (2013). The experience of symptoms of depression in men vs women: Analysis of the National Comorbidity Survey Replication. *JAMA Psychiatry*, Early online publication. doi: 10.1001/jamapsychiatry.2013.1985

McLaughlin, K. A., Koenen, K. C., Hill, E. D., Petukhova, M., Sampson, N. A., Zaslavsky, A. M., & Kessler, R. C. (2013). Trauma exposure and posttraumatic stress disorder in a national sample of adolescents. *Journal of the American Academy of Child & Adolescent Psychiatry*, 52(8), 815–830. doi: 10.1016/j.jaac.2013.05.011

McLean, C. P., & Anderson, E. R. (2009). Brave men and timid women? A review of the gender differences in fear and anxiety. *Clinical Psychology Review*, 29(6), 496–505. doi: 10.1016/j.cpr.2009.05.003

McLean, L. M., & Gallop, R. (2003). Implications of childhood sexual abuse for adult borderline personality disorder and complex posttraumatic stress disorder. *American Journal of Psychiatry*, 160(2), 369–371.

McNally, R. J. (2003). Psychological mechanisms in acute response to trauma. *Biological Psychiatry*, 53(9), 779–788.

Mills, K. L., McFarlane, A. C., Slade, T., Creamer, M., Silove, D., Teesson, M., & Bryant, R. (2011). Assessing the prevalence of trauma exposure in epidemiological surveys. *Australian and New Zealand Journal of Psychiatry*, 45(5), 407–415. doi: 10.3109/00048674.2010.543654

Norris, F. H. (1992). Epidemiology of trauma: Frequency and impact of different potentially traumatic events on different demographic groups. *Journal of Consulting and Clinical Psychology*, 60(3), 409–418.

Norris, F. H., Foster, J. D., & Weisshaar, D. L. (2002). The epidemiology of gender differences in PTSD across developmental,

societal, and research contexts. In R. Kimerling, P. Ouimette & J. Wolfe (Eds.), *Gender and PTSD* (pp. 3–42). New York: Guilford Press.

Norris, F. H., Murphy, A. D., Baker, C. K., Perilla, J. L., Rodriguez, F. G., & Rodriguez, J. D. (2003). Epidemiology of trauma and posttraumatic stress disorder in Mexico. *Journal of Abnormal Psychology*, 112(4), 646–656.

Norris, F. H., Perilla, J. L., & Murphy, A. D. (2001). Postdisaster stress in the United States and Mexico: A cross-cultural test of the multicriterion conceptual model of posttraumatic stress disorder. *Journal of Abnormal Psychology*, 110(4), 553–563.

North, C. S., Nixon, S. J., Shariat, S., Mallonee, S., McMillen, J. C., Spitznagel, E. L., & Smith, E. M. (1999). Psychiatric disorders among survivors of the Oklahoma City bombing. *Journal of the American Medical Association*, 282(8), 755–762.

Oakley Browne, M. A., Wells, J. E., Scott, K. M., McGee, M. A., & New Zealand Mental Health Survey Research Team. (2006). Lifetime prevalence and projected lifetime risk of DSM-IV disorders in Te Rau Hinengaro: The New Zealand Mental Health Survey. *Australian and New Zealand Journal of Psychiatry*, 40(10), 865–874. doi: 10.1111/j.1440-1614.2006.01905.x

Olff, M., Langeland, W., Draijer, N., & Gersons, B.P.R. (2007). Gender differences in posttraumatic stress disorder. *Psychological Bulletin*, 133(2), 183–204.

Ozer, E. J., Best, S. R., Lipsey, T. L., & Weiss, D. S. (2003). Predictors of posttraumatic stress disorder and symptoms in adults: A meta-analysis. *Psychological Bulletin*, 129(1), 52–73. doi: 10.1037/0033-2909.129.1.52

Peters, L., Issakidis, C., Slade, T., & Andrews, G. (2006). Gender differences in the prevalence of DSM-IV and ICD-10 PTSD.

Psychological Medicine, 36(1), 81–89.

Pierce, J. M., Newton, T. L., Buckley, T. C., & Keane, T. M. (2002). Gender and psychophysiology of PTSD. In R. Kimerling, P. Ouimette & J. Wolfe (Eds.), *Gender and PTSD* (pp. 177–204). New York: Guilford Press.

Pietrzak, R. H., Goldstein, R. B., Southwick, S. M., & Grant, B. F. (2011). Prevalence and Axis I comorbidity of full and partial posttraumatic stress disorder in the United States: Results from Wave 2 of the National Epidemiologic Survey on Alcohol and Related Conditions. *Journal of Anxiety Disorders*, 25(3), 456–465. doi: 10.1016/j.janxdis.2010.11.010.

Pigott, T. A. (1999). Gender differences in the epidemiology and treatment of anxiety disorders. *Journal of Clinical Psychiatry*, 60(Suppl 18), 4–15.

Rothbaum, B. O., Davidson, J. R. T., Stein, D. J., Pedersen, R., Musgnung, J., Tian, X. W., ... Baldwin, D. S. (2008). A pooled analysis of gender and trauma-type effects on responsiveness to treatment of PTSD with venlafaxine extended release or placebo. *Journal of Clinical Psychiatry*, 69(10), 1529–1539.

Slade, T., Johnston, A., Oakley-Browne, M. A., Andrews, G., & Whiteford, H. (2009). 2007 National Survey of Mental Health and Wellbeing: Methods and key findings. *Australian and New Zealand Journal of Psychiatry*, 43(7), 594–605. doi: 10.1080/00048670902970882

Smith, B. N., Vaughn, R. A., Vogt, D., King, D. W., King, L. A., & Shipherd, J. C. (2013). Main and interactive effects of social support in predicting mental health symptoms in men and women following military stressor exposure. *Anxiety, Stress, and Coping*, 26(1), 52–69. doi: 10.1080/10615806.2011.634001

Stein, M. B., Walker, J. R., Hazen, A. L., & Forde, D. R. (1997). Full and partial posttraumatic stress disorder: Findings from a community survey. *American Journal of Psychiatry*, 154, 1114–1119.

Tolin, D. F., & Foa, E. B. (2002). Gender and PTSD: A cognitive model. In R. Kimerling, P. Ouimette, & J. Wolfe (Eds.), *Gender and PTSD* (pp. 76–97). New York: Guilford Press.

Tolin, D. F., & Foa, E. B. (2006). Sex differences in trauma and posttraumatic stress disorder: A quantitative review of 25 years of research. *Psychological Bulletin*, 132(6), 959–992.

Tucker, P., Zaninelli, R., Yehuda, R., Ruggiero, L., Dillingham, K., & Pitts, C. D. (2001). Paroxetine in the treatment of chronic posttraumatic stress disorder: Results of a placebo-controlled, flexible-dosage trial. *Journal of Clinical Psychiatry*, 62(11), 860–868.

World Health Organization. (1993). *The ICD-10 Classification of Mental and Behavioural Disorders: Diagnostic criteria for research.* Geneva: World Health Organization.

Yen, S., Shea, M. T., Battle, C. L., Johnson, D. M., Zlotnick, C., Dolan-Sewell, R., ... McGlashan, T. H. (2002). Traumatic exposure and posttraumatic stress disorder in borderline, schizotypal, avoidant, and obsessive-compulsive personality disorders: Findings from the collaborative longitudinal personality disorders study. *Journal of Nervous & Mental Disease*, 190(8), 510–518.

Zlotnick, C., Zakriski, A. L., Shea, M. T., & Costello, E. (1996). The long-term sequelae of sexual abuse: Support for a complex posttraumatic stress disorder. *Journal of Traumatic Stress*, 9(2), 195–205.

Chapter

18

Anxiety disorders in women

Kimberly A. Yonkers, Heather Howell, Katherine Sevar and David J. Castle

Anxiety is a common human experience, and varies in depth and intensity. The experience most typically occurs in response to life stressors and may be temporary. However, many people experience anxiety symptoms that comprise a diagnosable mental illness. Individuals with an anxiety disorder are functionally impaired by the condition that is beyond a reasonable temporary response to trauma, stress or danger.

Anxiety disorders are highly prevalent and persist, frequently with periods of remission and relapse across the life-course (Yonkers, 2003). They are universally reported to be more common in women than men. For example, Australian data from the Australian Survey of Mental Health and Wellbeing, conducted in 2007, estimated the weighted 12-month prevalence of any anxiety disorder, diagnosable using DSM-IV criteria, as 14.6% for women and 8.9% for men (McEvoy et al., 2011).

The US National Comorbidity Survey (NCS), a community prevalence study, found the following risk factors to be associated with a lifetime anxiety disorder: lower income, less education, living in the northeast and female sex. The likelihood of developing an anxiety disorder was 85% higher in women than men. In a prospective, longitudinal, population-based study of 643 women, psychosocial variables were examined to evaluate whether it was possible to predict the onset of a new anxiety disorder or the recurrence of an existing disorder. The presence of anxiety disorders was assessed every 6 months over a 3-year period, using the Structured Clinical Interview for the Diagnostic Statistical Manual for Mental Disorders (SCID) and significant predictors of anxiety were found to include a history of anxiety, increased anxiety sensitivity (meaning the fear of anxiety-related sensations) and increased neuroticism (Calkins et al., 2009). The

prevalence over 12 months of specific types of anxiety disorders in women (Kessler et al., 2012) were recorded as follows: specific phobia 12.1%, social phobia 7.4%, post-traumatic stress disorder 3.7%, generalized anxiety disorder 2.0%, separation anxiety disorder 1.2%, panic disorder 2.4%, agoraphobia 1.7%, and obsessive-compulsive disorder 1.2%.

Anxiety disorders often exist comorbidly with major depressive disorder and the lifetime prevalence in a sample of (n=1970) Chinese patients surveyed to assess the association between major depressive disorder and comorbid anxiety disorders found the lifetime prevalence rate for any type of comorbid anxiety disorder was 60%, which is consistent with findings from European and American studies (Li et al., 2012).

The degree of disability women experience as a result of anxiety disorders was explored by McLean and colleagues (2011) in a pooled data set of 20,000 adults from the Collaborative Psychiatric Epidemiology Studies (CPES). Women had higher rates of a lifetime diagnosis for each of the anxiety disorders (aside from social anxiety disorder) and were more likely to be diagnosed with more than one anxiety disorder. Anxiety disorders were associated with a greater illness burden in women than men.

The gender difference in the prevalence of anxiety symptoms is evident even during childhood (Hayward et al., 2000; Lewinsohn et al., 1998; Wittchen et al., 1998). Boys and girls begin to experience the onset of pathological anxiety at about the same age (Lewinsohn et al., 1998; Wittchen et al., 1998) but girls are more vulnerable.

In this chapter, we review sex differences in the epidemiology, clinical characteristics and illness course for the anxiety disorders, excluding post-traumatic stress disorder (this is the focus of Chapter 17 in this

Comprehensive Women's Mental Health, ed. David J. Castle and Kathryn M. Abel. Published by Cambridge University Press.
© Cambridge University Press 2016.

book). Additionally, we discuss the influence of the premenstruum as well as gestation and delivery on the expression of anxiety disorders, but treatment of anxiety disorders is not addressed in this chapter.

Generalized anxiety disorder

Generalized anxiety disorder (GAD) is defined as excessive worry about a number of events or issues that is difficult to control. Worry is experienced for at least 6 months and may be accompanied by restlessness, fatigue, difficulty concentrating, irritability, muscle tension and sleep disturbance. The worry cannot be limited to a core feature of another syndrome, for example, worry about having a panic attack or gaining weight because in that case, it would be supportive of the other condition and not GAD.

In the Epidemiological Catchment Area Study (ECA), the prevalence of GAD was determined using DSM-III criteria, which stipulates only 1, rather than 6 months of illness (DSM-III-R and DSM-IV) (Blazer et al., 1991). The 12-month prevalence rate in women was about twice as high as it was for men (2.4% in men and 5.0% in women). Those at greatest risk were African-American women under 30 and Hispanic women aged 45–64; the rates in both of these groups was greater than the rate in Caucasian women (Blazer et al., 1991).

According to the NCS, 3.6% (se=0.5) of men and 6.6% (se=0.5) of women will meet criteria for DSM-III R GAD at some point in their lives (Wittchen et al., 1994). In that dataset, women were 63% more likely to develop GAD than were men (Wittchen et al., 1994).

Women with generalized anxiety disorder report intrusive, pervasive worries that affect their function and quality of life across many domains (Grant et al., 2005). The majority of people with generalized anxiety disorder are diagnosed and managed within primary care, with many people initially presenting with physical symptoms, rather than the psychological symptoms. Physical symptoms can include fatigue, muscle tension, palpitations, and a sensation of constricted breathing or be associated with a tremor or sleep disturbance. These physical symptoms can cause significant distress and functional impairment.

Generalized anxiety disorder usually has an onset prior to 25 years of age and most often has a chronic course (Stein et al., 2005). In a US study, generalized anxiety disorder was second only to substance abuse in terms of population prevalence (Fricchione et al.,

2004). Individuals with generalized anxiety disorder have a significantly increased risk of developing subsequent depression (Hettema et al., 2006) with up to 75% of sufferers developing a major depressive episode in their lifetime. Individuals with comorbid generalized anxiety disorder and depression are more disabled than those with either disorder alone (Grant et al., 2005).

Risk factors for the development of generalized anxiety disorder include a family history of generalized anxiety disorder, as well as stress and trauma. A neurobiological model of generalized anxiety disorder suggests that the early life experience of elevations of adrenaline and cortisol, as a result of exposure to stressful situations, may upregulate and hypersensitize the HPA axis in adulthood (see also Chapter 17). The possible transgenerational transmission of generalized anxiety disorder is worth considering in this context given that the infants of women with anxiety disorders in pregnancy are more likely to be exposed to greater circulating levels of adrenaline in-utero, meaning that they are more vulnerable to developing anxiety disorders in childhood if exposed to early life trauma. Social stressors may have a divergent impact on the risk of depression and anxiety in men and women (Cameron & Hill, 1989). In a 3-year longitudinal study of English women, danger predicted later anxiety, while loss predicted depression (Brown et al., 1996); a combination of loss and danger led to comorbid anxiety and depression. External support did not modify the effect of these events.

Clinical course

Generalized anxiety disorder has a generally chronic course throughout the lifetime for both women and men (Pigott, 1999) although comorbidity decreases the chance of recovery particularly if there are comorbid personality disorders from either cluster B or cluster C (Yonkers et al., 2000). The majority of adults with GAD experience the illness for over 5 years (Blazer et al., 1991), and women and men have approximately the same likelihood of experiencing a remission (probability 0.46 in women and 0.56 in men; Log rank χ^2 = 1.39 (df=1); p=0.24) (Yonkers et al., 2003).

Comorbidity

GAD is most often comorbid with other conditions, with the US National Comorbidity Survey discovering that over 90% of people diagnosed with GAD had a comorbid diagnosis, including dysthymia, depression, somatization, other anxiety disorders, bipolar disorder or substance abuse. In their longitudinal study, Yonkers et al. (1996) found that 23% of GAD subjects had two, and 16% had three or more other anxiety disorders active at initial assessment. GAD can also occur comorbidly with eating disorders; a systematic review, considering two observational studies ($n=55$), found a lifetime prevalence of GAD among people with anorexia nervosa of between 24% and 31% (Dyck et al., 2001).

Comorbidity of depression and GAD is particularly common (Angst & Vollrath, 1991). Some research suggests shared inheritance of these disorders (Kendler et al., 1992). Both women and men who have anxiety coupled with depression have a poorer outcome (Angst & Vollrath, 1991; Durham et al., 1997). There is also evidence that a history of GAD predisposes individuals to develop major depression (Parker et al., 1997), although this effect may not be limited to GAD amongst the anxiety disorders (Breslau et al., 1995). Another possibility is that an anxiety disorder increases the risk for a mood disorder and vice-versa (Hayward et al., 2000; Kessler et al., 2003).

Comorbidity between anxiety disorders and alcohol abuse and dependence disorders is also very common (Massion et al., 1993; Yonkers et al., 1996). Anxious symptoms may increase the susceptibility to alcohol consumption (Fischer & JW, 1998). Men are overall more likely to abuse drugs and alcohol, but moderate anxiety in depressed women seems to increase their risk for alcohol abuse (Fischer & JW, 1998). Other work has found an association between alcoholism and anxiety disorders that is greater for phobias than for panic or generalized anxiety (Merikangas et al., 1998).

Some authors propose that the expression of anxiety in depressed women may differ from anxiety in depressed men (Katz et al., 1993; Parker et al., 1997). For example, highly anxious depressed women may express their anxious-depressive symptoms through motor retardation and vagueness, with less evident body movement, while men may show hostility and increased visible body agitation (Katz et al., 1993).

Panic disorder

Panic disorder is a pattern of brief but intense, recurrent and usually unanticipated episodes of fear or discomfort that occur without a notable precipitant. In DSM-5, panic disorder remains classified as an anxiety disorder and the diagnostic criteria specify that episodes of panic must be present for over 1 month and that an individual must experience a continual fear of having future attacks and display avoidance of certain situations in an attempt to prevent further attacks.

A change in DSM-5, in comparison to DSM-IV, is that panic disorder was previously classified as occurring with, or without, agoraphobia, while in DSM-5, agoraphobia is listed as a separate condition. In practice though, co-occurring panic disorder and agoraphobia will remain prevalent given that panic disorder leads to functional impairment in patients predominantly through the limitations on their lifestyle engendered by fear of future panic attacks.

The physical symptoms associated with panic attacks are driven by overactivation of the sympathetic nervous system and include palpitations, sweating, feeling short of breath or a choking sensation, nausea or abdominal discomfort, feeling dizzy, having a sense of unreality, numbness or tingling, chills or hot flushes, and a fear of dying or losing control (APA, 1994). The cognitive features may include acute fear of dying, losing control, going mad and a need to escape from the current situation, and there can also be a feeling of depersonalisation or derealization.

Estimates suggest 1–2% of the adult population suffer panic disorder (Yates, 2009). Common risk factors for the development of panic disorder include female gender, low socioeconomic status and anxious childhood temperament. Panic disorder is associated with an elevated risk of suicide as well as all-cause mortality and cardiovascular disease. It ranks highest among the anxiety disorders in terms of disease burden.

Women and men with panic disorder tend to experience their symptoms somewhat differently. Data from the NCS show that, compared to men, women were more likely to endorse shortness of breath, nausea and a perception of being smothered; men were more likely to identify difficulties with sweating and stomach pain (Sheikh et al., 2002). The greater proclivity for women to develop respiratory symptoms is interesting in light of results from provocation studies. Women with panic may have greater sensitivity to panic-inducing respiratory challenge than their male counterparts (Papp et al., 1997; Papp & Gorman, 1988; Sheikh et al., 2002). Work by one group found that women have a higher resting breathing rate and lower end-tidal CO_2 that may increase anxiety sensitivity (Papp et al., 1997; Papp & Gorman, 1988).

There has been interest in the conceptualization of anxiety disorders as resulting from psychopathology during childhood, in particular in relation to the presence of separation anxiety disorder in childhood. A meta-analysis of 20 studies indicated that children with separation anxiety disorder were more likely to develop panic disorder in adulthood (odds ratio=3.45; 95% CI=2.37–5.03). Additionally, there were five studies which suggested that a childhood diagnosis of separation anxiety disorder increased the overall risk of the development of future anxiety disorders in adulthood (odds ratio=2.19; 95% CI=1.40–3.42) (Kossowsky et al., 2013).

There has been particular interest in the effectiveness of MAO inhibitors in the treatment of panic disorder given previous studies of MAO inhibitors in animal models of panic disorder (Reif et al., 2012). Recent research focused on the gene encoding monoamine oxidase A (MAOA) in women. A meta-analysis of four studies with a pooled sample size of (n=1,115 patients and n=1,260 controls) reported a significant female-specific association when calculating an allelic model in panic disorder, leading the authors to suggest that "this sex-specific effect might be explained by a gene-dose effect causing higher MAOA expression in females." Furthermore, they hypothesize that high-expression MAOA-uVNTR alleles significantly increase the risk of women developing panic disorder. This finding will require further replication in larger samples, but may be a lead in the appreciation of female vulnerability to the development of panic disorder (Reif et al., 2012).

In a prospective study 2,325 female twins were examined using structural modelling to determine how genes, childhood, past-year environmental stressors, personality and episodes of major depression and generalized anxiety disorder influence an etiological model for symptoms of anxiety and depression (Kendler et al., 2010). The model that fit the data best revealed two etiological pathways. The first, a "trait-like" pathway reflects personality vulnerabilities that were mediated by genetic and early environmental risk factors. The second was mediated through episodes of major depression, or generalized anxiety disorder, recent environmental adversities and "trait-like" factors that influence exposure to stressful events and increase the probability of the onset of a depressive or anxiety disorder. Chen et al. (2010) found that women with panic disorder who experienced panic attacks during pregnancy carry an increased risk of having small-for-gestational-age infants, and the adjusted odds ratio for having a preterm delivery was 2.54 (95% CI=1.09–5.93). It appeared from this study though that it was only if the symptoms were experienced during the pregnancy, and for those women with a historical diagnosis of panic disorder there were no adverse outcomes noted (Chen, Lin, & Lee, 2010).

Clinical course

In panic disorder, women and men have approximately equal rates of remission but women have a much greater likelihood of relapse of their condition. In a study evaluating the course of panic disorder, the relapse rate over 8 years of follow up was 3-fold higher in women compared to men (Yonkers et al., 2003). This relapsing course of illness in women may be caused by higher anxiety sensitivity, even after treatment is instituted and remission is attained. In some instances, this vulnerability may be mediated by biological differences in respiratory mechanics between men and women (Sheikh et al., 2002) or by the increased prevalence of comorbid psychiatric illness, such as depression, in women (Hayward et al., 2000).

Agoraphobia

Agoraphobia is the fear of being in a closed space or an area from which escape may be difficult. This typically leads to a modification of behavior in an attempt to avoid panic attacks. Bekker (1996) offers a thorough review of gender and agoraphobia, finding the illness more prevalent in women than in men, across both clinical and community samples. Specifically, data from the NCS found that when panic disorder is accompanied by agoraphobia, the 1-month prevalence rate for men is 0.4% (sd=0.2) while 1.0% (sd=0.3) of women meet criteria (Eaton et al., 1994). Agoraphobia without panic is somewhat more common and the lifetime prevalence rate in men is 3.5% (se=0.4) and in women is 7% (se=0.6) (Eaton et al., 1994).

In DSM-5, agoraphobia is now listed as a separate condition, a change from DSM-IV where it was listed as accompanying panic disorder in some individuals. The new diagnostic criteria for agoraphobia include the experience of intense fear or anxiety in at least two agoraphobic situations, for example, using public transport, being outside the home alone, being in open spaces, being in public places (e.g., shopping centers), being in crowds or standing in a line with other people, or a combination of two or more of these scenarios. An essential part of the diagnosis of agoraphobia is that the individual also has to exhibit avoidance behavior that occurs due to the fear of experiencing a panic attack or anxiety-related symptoms in a situation where it would be difficult to escape or seek help. Overall, it is the avoidance behavior itself that most seriously affects the quality of life and functioning of people with agoraphobia as their world gradually reduces until, at its most severe, they are unable to leave the home.

Women tend to adapt to their agoraphobia by limiting excursions outside of the home, especially without a companion, significantly more than men (Bourdon et al., 1988; Starcevic et al., 1998). It is notable that this is often more culturally acceptable, in that women can work inside the home while men tend to work outside the home and thus are less likely to function adequately if they are homebound. There is also evidence to suggest women report a significantly greater reduction in quality of life as a result of their agoraphobia in comparison to men (Starcevic et al., 1998). This is consistent with other data showing that panic disorder with agoraphobia is a more severe condition in women than in men (Turgeon et al., 1998). Women expressed greater avoidance severity, more catastrophic fears and more frequent comorbidity of another anxiety disorder, most notably social phobia or post-traumatic stress disorder.

Comorbidity

Among a group of anxiety-disordered individuals presenting in a clinical setting, 72% of whom were female, there were no significant sex differences in psychiatric comorbidity (Apfeldorf et al., 2000). Other work has found that women are more likely than males to have a co-occurring anxiety disorder, namely social phobia or post-traumatic stress disorder (PTSD) (Turgeon et al., 1998). PTSD comorbidity did not predict higher agoraphobic avoidance.

Alcohol dependence is a significant comorbidity in agoraphobia and men with agoraphobia are more likely than their female counterparts to suffer from alcoholism (Bibb & Chambless, 1986; Starcevic et al.,

1998; Yonkers et al., 1998). Although this may reflect the overall higher rate of hazardous alcohol use in men compared to women (Kessler et al. 1994) some work finds a higher rate of alcohol abuse in male agoraphobics compared to male non-agoraphobics (Bibb & Chambless, 1986). In evaluating these sex differences, it is also important to consider the gender-specific social implications of agoraphobic self-disclosure. Men may be less inclined to acknowledge agoraphobic tendencies than women because it discredits male strength and bravery (Barlow, 1988). This is believed by some to contribute to the disparate rates of agoraphobia diagnoses in men and women, and it is presumed that there is a group of "hidden male agoraphobics" who tend to present with alcoholism. There is some empirical support for this. In a study of gender-specific alcohol use in agoraphobic individuals, there were significant sex differences in the ways in which each gender described the experience of the anxiety disorder (Cox et al., 1993): males consumed significantly more alcohol than females and they described their drinking as a specific coping strategy for the anxiety. Turgeon and colleagues (1998) did not confirm this quantitative difference and found comparable alcohol consumption in male and female samples. However, in both studies, males and not females directly reported drinking as a way to decrease agoraphobic inhibition (Cox et al., 1993; Turgeon et al., 1998).

Social phobia

Social anxiety disorder (SAD) affects the sexes almost equally with approximately 15% of women and 11% of men affected across the life-course. (Kessler et al., 2005). SAD usually begins in childhood or early adolescence and maintains a chronic course throughout adulthood. The clinical features include experiencing extreme anxiety in social scenarios due to a fear of embarrassment. The feared situation is either endured with difficulty or avoided altogether, and the fear and avoidance behavior leads to disability in functioning. Sufferers often manifest physical signs such as blushing and stuttering if asked to speak in public. They may become avoidant of social situations and there is some difference between with sexes with women stating that they have more distress when speaking in public or meeting strangers (Turk et al. 1998).

In the NCS, the 1-year prevalence of social phobia was 6.6% (se=0.4) in men and 9.1% (se=0.7) in women

(Kessler et al., 1994). The lifetime risk for males was 11.1% (se=0.8) while for females it was 15.5% (se=1.0). Slightly lower lifetime rates (13.7%) were found in an epidemiological study from Ontario, Canada, but a 2:1 ratio for females compared to males was noted (DeWit, 1999). A community study in Australia found that women were only slightly more likely than men to develop the illness (Lampe et al., 2003).

Possible sex differences in the expression of social phobia have been investigated in clinical cohorts. Male (*n*=108) and female (*n*=104) subjects with social phobia differed somewhat in the fearful situations they endorsed (Turk et al., 1998). Severity was significantly greater for women compared to men for the following tasks: talking to an authority, acting or speaking in front of an audience, being observed at work, entering into a room while others were seated, being the center of attention, expressing disagreement and giving a party (Turk et al., 1998). Men had significantly more difficulty with urinating in public and returning goods to a store. An independent study also found that socially phobic women had more difficulty than men with speaking in public (Pollard & Henderson, 1988).

One small study suggests sex differences in the psychophysiological response to stress among people with social phobia (Grossman et al., 2001). Women with social phobia were more likely than men with the disorder to show an increase in heart rate and both diastolic and systolic blood pressure in response to speech stress.

Comorbidity

Social phobia is commonly comorbid with other conditions, particularly panic disorder, generalized anxiety disorder, major depressive disorder, obsessive-compulsive disorder and agoraphobia (Yonkers, 2001). In most instances, social phobia is temporally primary (Yonkers et al., 2001).

Clinical course

Social phobia typically begins during adolescence (~age 16) with a predominance of girls over boys (Compton et al., 2000). Several studies document the chronicity associated with the condition (DeWit et al., 1999; Yonkers et al., 2001). The clinical course appears to be similar in men and women (Yonkers et al., 2001); however, those individuals with an early age of onset are less likely to recover than those with a later onset.

Obsessive-compulsive disorder

Obsessive-compulsive disorder (OCD) is characterized by intrusive thoughts (obsessions) and compulsive activities that attenuate (at least in the short term) the level of anxiety associated with the obsession. The condition is associated with considerable distress and impairment of daily activities, with (by definition) at least 1 hour per day being expended on rituals.

Increasingly, OCD is recognized as a fairly common and disabling condition, estimated to have been the fifth leading cause of disability for women aged 15–44 years, in developed countries in 1990 (Murray & Lopez, 1996). Most epidemiological surveys suggest that the condition afflicts women at a somewhat higher rate than men. Bebbington (1990) reviewed population-based studies of OCD, and found a female:male ratio varying from 0.9:1 (Puerto Rico) to 3.4:1 (Christchurch, New Zealand). He concluded that overall females appear somewhat more prone to the condition, with an overall relative risk of 1.5, compared to men. Clinical samples tend to show a somewhat less marked female excess, perhaps a reflection of the rather more severe illness course in men or differences in help-seeking behavior (Castle et al., 1995; Lensi et al., 1996; Noshirvani et al., 1991).

What certainly seems consistent in the literature is that males tend to have an earlier onset of OCD than their female counterparts. For example, in a clinical series of 307 OCD patients (55% female), onset of illness for males was 21 while it was 24 years for females (p<0.01) (Noshirvani et al., 1991). Similar discrepancies in onset have been reported by other researchers (Castle et al., 1995; Lensi et al., 1996; Lochner et al., 2004). What is also consistent is that early-onset samples of OCD show a preponderance of males. In a review of eight studies of child- and adolescent-onset OCD, there was a total of 174 boys and 70 girls, yielding a gender ratio of 5:2 (Noshirvani et al., 1991).

This is also reflected in case series across all ages of onset; for example, Castle et al. (1995) found males were overrepresented amongst patients with an onset of illness before 16 years (26% vs. 12% of females; p=0.01).

In terms of symptom profile, women with OCD are generally more likely that men to manifest contamination fears and cleaning rituals, while males are more prone to aggressive and sexual obsessions, and symmetry concerns (Lensi et al., 1996; Bogetto et al., 1999).

Women with OCD often report that symptoms first appear or exacerbate during reproductive cycle events and recent research has demonstrated the relationship between OCD and the reproductive cycle in women. A meta-analysis (Russell et al., 2013) found that the prevalence of OCD increased during pregnancy (mean = 2.07%) and even more so in the postpartum period (mean = 2.43%) compared with the general population (mean = 1.08%). Additionally, both pregnant (mean = 1.45) and postpartum (mean = 2.38) women were at greater risk of experiencing OCD compared to the general female population, with an aggregate risk ratio of 1.79 (Russell et al., 2013).

Further research has focused on OCD across the reproductive cycle including at menarche, premenstruum, pregnancy, postpartum and at menopause (Gulielmi et al., 2014). In a survey of 542 women (United States, $n=352$; Netherlands, $n=190$) using a self-report questionnaire of symptoms across time, a significant relationship between exacerbations of OCD and various phases of the reproductive cycle was found. OCD onset occurred within 12 months of menarche in 13.0% of participants, during pregnancy in 5.1%, postpartum in 4.7% and at menopause in 3.7%. It was evident that worsening of preexisting OCD occurred at reproductive cycle stages with 37.6% of women reporting worsening of symptoms at premenstruum, 33.0% during pregnancy, 46.6% in postpartum period, and 32.7% at menopause. Furthermore, OCD during a first pregnancy was significantly associated with exacerbation in a second pregnancy (OR = 10.82, 95% CI 4.48–26.16); similarly, postpartum exacerbation in a first pregnancy was associated with an elevated risk in ensuing pregnancies (OR = 6.86, 95% CI 3.27–14.36). These findings reinforce the importance of clinical vigilance during these phases of the reproductive cycle (Guglielmi et al., 2014).

Comorbidity

Females with OCD are more likely than their male counterparts to suffer from depression or eating disorders, but males appear more vulnerable to later hypomania (Lensi et al., 1996; Bogetto et al., 1999). Furthermore, males with OCD, and particularly those with an early onset illness, are more likely to exhibit motor tics and neurological "soft signs" (see Blanes & McGuire, 1997).

Clinical course

Most (though not all; Lensi et al., 1996) case series suggest a more benign longitudinal course for OCD amongst women, with a more abrupt onset and more episodic course (Bogetto et al., 1999). Women with OCD are also more likely to be married and to have less impairment of psychosocial functioning.

Whether the relatively more benign course of illness in women is due to the late mean age at onset, or is a reflection of a male vulnerability to a particularly pernicious subtype of the illness, is not clear. One hypothesis is there is a male-predominant "neurodevelopmental" subtype of OCD, characterized by an early onset of illness, neurological soft signs, motor tics and a poor treatment response to serotonergic antidepressants (see Blanes & McGuire, 1997)

Another interesting line of enquiry has been into the possibility that genetic factors might play a differential role between the sexes, in terms of OCD. For example, Enoch et al. (2001) reported the frequency of 5-HT2A promoter polymorphism 1438G>A to be higher among OCD women but not men, versus a comparison group. Of interest is that this polymorphism had been found previously to be associated with anorexia nervosa, believed by some researchers to be part of an OCD spectrum of disorders. Lochner et al. (2004) found that Caucasian females (but not males) with OCD were more likely than those in a comparison group to have the high activity T allele of the EcoRV variant of the monoamine oxidase A gene. These lines of genetic enquiry need to be pursued further and to be intergrated into broader explanatory models of gender differences in OCD.

Influences of the menstrual cycle on anxiety symptoms

Several researchers note high rates of anxiety disorders in their patients with Premenstrual Dysphoric Disorder (PMDD) (Facchinetti et al., 1992; Fava et al., 1992) with the most common diagnosis being panic disorder. Sexual trauma history seems prevalent in PMDD patients. In one study of 42 women (Golding et al., 2000), 95% had experienced sexual trauma at least once; upon further assessment, 65% were diagnosed with PTSD.

Worsening of panic during the premenstrual week is endorsed by many women with panic disorder. However, research has failed to confirm worsening panic when daily calendars are used to evaluate menstrual cycle symptoms prospectively (Cameron et al., 1988; Cook et al., 1990; Stein et al., 1989). However, some studies have identified anxiety as a key problematic symptom prior to the onset of menses (Stein et al., 1989). PMDD is clinically categorized as a depressive mood disorder, but further evaluation is required to understand the anxious quality of the disorder better (see also Chapter 10).

There is additional information suggesting a link between premenstrual conditions and anxiety disorders. In a study of women seeking treatment for premenstrual dysphoria (n=206), they prospectively rated their daily symptoms (Bailey and Cohen, 1999). According to the Structured Clinical Interview for DSM (SCID), 7.3% (n=15) were diagnosed with solely an anxiety disorder. A further 8.2% (n=17) had both an anxiety and a mood disorder; by far the most common diagnosis was panic disorder (n=18). Furthermore, 20 undiagnosed women were already receiving treatment for a mood or anxiety disorder, possibly minimizing identification of current illness. In a clinical sample of female patients presenting for treatment for PMDD, approximately 20% had a co-occurring Axis I anxiety disorder (Yonkers, unpublished data, 2004).

Perinatal anxiety disorders

Early studies of pregnant patients with a history of panic disorder observed an overall improvement in the illness during pregnancy (Levine et al., 2003). Studies are limited and subsequent studies have mixed findings. Retrospective studies find that the course of illness had an equal likelihood of improving, worsening or remaining unchanged during the course of pregnancy (Cohen et al., 1994, 1996; and see Chapter 10); the postpartum period offers no greater certainty of symptom abatement, and in fact is a time when some women experience the first manifestation of panic disorder. Indeed, new onset of postpartum panic disorder seems to afflict between 11 and 33% of pregnant women (Levine et al., 2003). On the other hand, recent retrospective work suggests improvement in panic over the course of pregnancy (Yonkers, unpublished data, 2014). A review found that postpartum improvement in panic episodes was most notably due to medication treatment (Levine et al., 2003). In one cohort of patients with panic disorder, 90% were symptomatic in the immediate postpartum

period (Cohen et al., 1996); the asymptomatic 10% of patients were all taking medication to treat their panic disorder.

Research that assessed rates of panic disorder and PTSD in a prenatal sample (n=387) in primary care found a rate of panic disorder during pregnancy was 2%, and the rate of PTSD, 3% (Smith et al., 2004). Rates of detection by these women's obstetricians were low, although rates of treatment were high, such that at the time of the study's contact with the anxious patients, all of the women with panic disorder (n=9) were currently or had previously been engaged in treatment, while 50% of the women with PTSD (n=5) were currently or had previously been treated. While these sample sizes are small, the rates of participation in treatment are encouraging.

As noted earlier, pregnancy and the postpartum period can be times of worsening or onset of OCD (Brandes et al., 2004; Levine, et al., 2003). Current data suggest that an OCD patient has little hope for symptomatic reprieve during pregnancy or postpartum (Altshuler et al., 1998; Levine et al., 2003). Of particular concern in the postpartum population are intrusive and unwanted thoughts, impulses and images of harming the infant. These thoughts could occur as symptoms of OCD and/or as indicators of postpartum depression, raising particular challenges for clinicians (see Chapter 10).

Pregnancy is protective against the continuous expression of symptoms of GAD (Buist et al, 2011). Nearly one-half of women with GAD in the 6 months prior to pregnancy experienced a remission in pregnancy (Buist et al 2011). Women were less likely to remit if they were older than age 35 as compared to 25–34, had a college education as compared to high school degree, experienced multiple prior episodes of GAD, had low social support and a history of child abuse.

A study of self-reported anxiousness during the postpartum period (not diagnosable anxiety disorder per se) suggested a common occurrence of comorbid anxiety and depression in the postpartum period (Stuart et al., 1998). The sample consisted of 107 community volunteers, primarily Caucasian, married and employed. Self-reported anxiety increased over time in this sample, reaching 8.7% at 14 weeks postpartum and increasing to 16.8% at 30 weeks. One could loosely parallel this to generalized anxiety, although no formal axis I diagnoses were made. It is unknown for this sample whether their anxiety was being treated, and/or whether they had a history of anxiety or depressive disorder during pregnancy or perhaps even prior to gestation. The findings do suggest, however, a high index of suspicion amongst clinicians working with postpartum women, such that anxiety symptoms are recognized and appropriately dealt with. For a more detailed discussion, the reader is referred to Chapter 10.

Anxiety disorders in older women

Anxiety disorders tend to show a reduction in prevalence as people age, but rates remain higher in women than in men (Byers et al., 2010). For women in midlife, a history of anxiety is a most significant predictor of reduced quality of life, an effect that is not explained by the sleep disturbance associated with these disorders (Joffe et al., 2012).

In a recent systematic review, examining 19 studies conducted between 1960 and 2011, Bryant et al. (2012) evaluated the prevalence of anxiety disorders during the menopausal transition to ascertain whether there was any utility in the diagnosis of "menopausal anxiety" as a discrete category. The review examined the relationship between the vasomotor symptoms of menopause, for example "hot flushes," and anxiety states and they suggested that

in studying these symptoms it is essential that physiological and psychological symptoms are not confounded through the use of inappropriate outcome measures. The authors determined that there is no current evidence to suggest that there is an increased prevalence of anxiety disorders during menopause, nor the emergence of an anxiety disorder specifically determined by menopause.

For a discussion about anxiety disorders in postmenopausal women, the reader is referred to Chapter 20 of this book.

Conclusions

Women are disproportionally afflicted by all the anxiety disorders and as yet there are few firm findings as to why women remain more susceptible than men. Research concentrating on the relationship between early life traumatic events, heritable genetic predisposition to anxiety disorders and the influence of the menstrual cycle on anxiety disorders are all areas that require further elaboration. Given the early onset of anxiety disorder, studies evaluating gender and risk will need to include investigations in children and adolescents. Further work is also required into gender-informed treatments across the life-course.

References

Altshuler, L., Hendrick, V. & Cohen, L. (1998) Course of mood and anxiety disorders during pregnancy and the postpartum period. *Journal of Clinical Psychiatry*, 59(Suppl 2), 29–33.

American Psychiatric Association (APA). (1994) *Diagnostic and Statistical Manual of Mental Disorders-DSM-IV* (Fourth edn). Washington, DC: American Psychiatric Association.

Andrews, B., Brewin, C. & Rose, S. (2003) Gender, Social Support, and PTSD in victims of violent crime. *Journal of Traumatic Stress*, 16(4), 421–427.

Angst, J. & Vollrath, M. (1991) The natural history of anxiety disorders. *Acta Psychiatrica Scandinavica (Copenhagen)*, 84, 446–452.

Apfeldorf, W., Spielman, L., Cloitre, M., et al. (2000) Morbidity of comorbid psychiatric diagnoses in the clinical presentation of panic disorder. *Depression and Anxiety*, 12, 78–84.

Bailey, J. & Cohen, L. (1999) Prevalence of mood and anxiety disorders in women who seek treatment for premenstrual syndrome. *Journal of Women's Health & Gender-Based Medicine*, 8(9), 1181–1184.

Barlow, D. H. (1988) *Anxiety and its disorders: The nature and treatment of anxiety and panic*. New York: Guilford Press.

Bebbington P. E. (1990) Population surveys of psychiatric disorder and the need for treatment. *Social Psychiatry and Psychiatric Epidemiology*, 25(1), 33–40.

Bekker, M. H. J. (1996) Agoraphobia and gender: A review. *Clinical Psychology Review*, 16(2), 129–146.

Blanes, T. & McGuire, P. (1997). Heterogeneity within obsessive-compulsive disorder: evidence for primary and neurodevelopmental subtypes. *Neurodevelopmental Models of Psychopathology*, 206–213.

Bibb, J. L. & Chambless, D. L. (1986) Alcohol use and abuse among diagnosed agoraphobics. *Behaviour Research and Therapy*, 24(1), 49–58.

Blazer, D. G., Hughes, D., George, L. K., et al. (1991) Generalized anxiety disorder. In *Psychiatric Disorders in America* (eds. L. N. Robins & D. A. Regier), 1st edn, pp. 181–203. New York, New York: Free Press.

Bogetto, F., Venturello, S., Albert, U. et al. (1999) Gender-related clinical differences in obsessive-compulsive disorder. *European Psychiatry*, 14(8), 434–441.

Bourdon, K. H., Boyd, J. H., Rae, D. S., et al. (1988) Gender differences in phobias: Results of the ECA community survey. *Journal of Anxiety Disorders*, 2, 227–241.

Brandes, M., Soares, C. & Cohen, L. (2004) Postpartum onset obsessive-compulsive disorder: Diagnosis and management. *Archives of Women's Mental Health*, 7, 99–110.

Breslau, N. & Davis, G. (1992) Posttraumatic stress disorder in an urban population of young adults: Risk factors for chronicity. *American Journal of Psychiatry*, 149, 671–675.

Breslau, N., Davis, G. C., Andreski, P., et al. (1997) Sex differences in posttraumatic stress disorder. *Archives of General Psychiatry*, 54, 1044–1048.

Breslau, N., Schultz, L. & Peterson, E. (1995) Sex differences in depression: A role for preexisting anxiety. *Psychiatry Research*, 58, 1–12.

Bromet, E., Sonnega, A. & Kessler, R. C. (1998) Risk factors for DSM-III-R Posttraumatic Stress Disorder: Findings from the National Comorbidity Survey. *American Journal of Epidemiology*, 147, 353–361.

Brown, G., Harris, T. & Eales, M. (1996) Social factors and comorbidity of depressive and anxiety disorders. *British Journal of Psychiatry*, 168(suppl. 30), 50–57.

Bryant, C., Judd, F. K., & Hickey, M. (2012). Anxiety during the menopausal transition: A systematic review. *Journal of Affective Disorders*, 139(2), 141–148.

Buist, A., Gotman, N., & Yonkers, K. A. (2011) Generalized anxiety disorder: Course and risk factors in pregnancy. *Journal of Affective Disorders*, 131(1), 277–283.

Byers, A. L., Yaffe, K., Covinsky, K. E. et al. (2010) High occurrence of mood and anxiety disorders among older adults: The National Comorbidity Survey Replication. *Archives of General Psychiatry*, 67(5), 489–496.

Calkins, A. W., Otto, M. W., Cohen, L. S. et al. (2009) Psychosocial predictors of the onset of anxiety disorders in women: Results from a prospective 3-year longitudinal study. *Journal of Anxiety Disorders*, 23(8), 1165–1169. doi: 10.1016/j.janxdis.2009.07.022.

Cameron, O. G. & Hill, E. M. (1989) Women and anxiety. *Psychiatric Clinics of North America*, 12, 175–186.

Cameron, O. G., Kuttesch, D., McPhee, K., et al. (1988) Menstrual fluctuation in the symptoms of panic anxiety. *Journal of Affective Disorders*, 15, 169–174.

Castle, D. J., Deale, A. & Marks, I. M. (1995) Gender differences in obsessive compulsive disorder. *Australian and New Zealand Journal of Psychiatry*, 29, 114–117.

Chen, Y. H., Lin, H. C., & Lee, H. C. (2010). Pregnancy outcomes among women with panic disorder – do panic attacks during pregnancy matter? *Journal of Affective Disorders*, 120(1–3), 258–262.

Cohen, L. S., Sichel, D. A., Dimmock, J. A., et al. (1994) Impact of pregnancy on panic disorder: A case series. *Journal of Clinical Psychiatry*, 55, 284–289.

Cohen, L., Sichel, D., Faraone, S., et al. (1996) Course of panic disorder during pregnancy and the puerperium: A preliminary study. *Biological Psychiatry*, 39, 950–954.

Compton, S., Nelson, A. & March, J. (2000) Social phobia and separation anxiety symptoms in community and clinical samples of children and adolescents. *Journal of the American Academy of Child and Adolescent Psychiatry*, 39(8), 1040–1046.

Cook, B. L., Noyes, R., Garvey, M. J., et al. (1990) Anxiety and the menstrual cycle in panic disorder. *Journal of Affective Disorders*, 19, 221–226.

Cox, B. J., Swinson, R. P., Shulman, I. D., et al. (1993) Gender effects and alcohol use in panic disorder with agoraphobia. *Behaviour Research and Therapy*, 31(4), 413–416.

DeWit, D. J., Ogborne, A., Offord, D. R., et al. (1999) Antecedents of the risk of recovery from DSM-III-R social phobia. *Psychological Medicine*, 29(3), 569–582.

Durham, R. C., Allan, T. & Hackett, C. A. (1997) On predicting improvement and relapse in generalized anxiety disorder following psychotherapy. *British Journal of Clinical Psychology*, 36, 101–119.

Dyck, I. R., Phillips, K. A., Warshaw, M. G., et al. (2001). Patterns of personality pathology in patients with generalized anxiety disorder, panic disorder with and without agoraphobia, and social phobia. *Journal of Personality Disorders*, 15(1), 60–71.

Eaton, W. W., Kessler, R. C., Wittchen, H. U., et al. (1994) Panic and panic disorder in the United States. *American Journal of Psychiatry*, 151, 413–420.

Enoch, M. A., Greenberg, B. D., Murphy, D. L., & Goldman, D. (2001). Sexually dimorphic relationship of a 5-HT 2A promoter polymorphism with obsessive-compulsive disorder. *Biological Psychiatry*, 49(4), 385–388.

Facchinetti, F., Romano, G., Fava, M., et al. (1992) Lactate infusion induces panic attacks in patients with premenstrual syndrome. *Psychosomatic Medicine*, 54, 288–296.

Fava, M., Pedrazzi, F., Guaraldi, G. P., et al. (1992) Comorbid anxiety and depression amont patients with late luteal phase dysphoric disorder. *Journal of Anxiety Disorders*, 6, 325–335.

Fischer, E. H. & JW, G. (1998) Anxiety and alcohol abuse in patients in treatment for depression. *American Journal Drug Alcohol Abuse*, 24(3), 453–463.

Freedman, S., Gluck, N., Tuval-Mashiach, R., et al. (2002) Gender differences in responses to traumatic events: A Prospective Study. *Journal of Traumatic Stress*, 15(5), 407–413.

Fricchione, G. (2004). Clinical practice. Generalized anxiety disorder. *New England Journal of Medicine*, 351(7), 675–682. doi: 10.1056/NEJMcp022342.

Fullerton, C. S., Ursano, R. J., Epstein, R. S., et al. (2001) Gender differences in posttraumatic stress disorder after motor vehicle accidents. *American Journal Psychiatry*, 158, 1486–1491.

Golding, J., Taylor, D., Menard, L., et al. (2000) Prevalence of sexual abuse history in a sample of women seeking treatment for premenstrual syndrome. *Journal of Psychsomatic Obstetrics and Gynecology*, 21, 69–80.

Grant, B. F., Hasin, D. S., Stinson, F. S. et al. (2005) Co-occurrence of 12-month mood and anxiety disorders and personality disorders in the US: Results from the national epidemiologic survey on alcohol and related conditions. *Journal of Psychiatric Research*, 39(1), 1–9.

Green, B. (2003) Post-traumatic stress disorder: Symptom profiles in men and women. *Current Medical Research and Opinion*, 19, P1–P5.

Grossman, P., Wilhelm, F., Kawachi, I., et al. (2001) Gender differences in psychophysiological responses to speech stress among older social phobics: Congruence and incongruence between self-evaluative and cardiovascular reactions. *Psychosomatic Medicine*, 63, 765–777.

Guglielmi, V., Vulink, N. C., Denys, D. et al., (2014). Obsessive-compulsive disorder and female reproductive cycle events: Results from the OCD and Reproduction Collaborative Study. *Depression and Anxiety*, 31(12), 979–987.

Hayward, C., Killen, J. D., Kraemer, H. C., et al. (2000) Predictors of panic attacks in adolescents. *Journal of the American Academy of Child and Adolescent Psychiatry*, 39(2), 207–214.

Hettema, J. M., Kuhn, J. W., Prescott, C. A., & Kendler, K. S. (2006) The impact of generalized anxiety disorder and stressful life events on risk for major depressive episodes. *Psychological Medicine*, 36(6), 789–795. doi: 10.1017/S0033291706007367.

Holbrook, T. L., Hoyt, D. B., Stein, M. B., et al. (2002) Gender difference in long-term Posttraumatic Stress Disorder outcomes after major trauma: Women are at higher risk of adverse outcomes than men. *The Journal of Trauma*, 53(5), 882–888.

Joffe, H., Chang, Y., Dhaliwal, S. et al. (2012) Lifetime history of depression and anxiety disorders as a predictor of quality of life in midlife women in the absence of current illness episodes. *Archives of General Psychiatry*, 69(5), 484–492.

Katz, M., Wetzler, S., Cloitre , M., et al. (1993) Expressive characteristics of anxiety in depressed men and women. *Journal of Affective Disorders*, 28, 267–277.

Kendler, K. S., Aggen, S., Knudsen, G. P., et al. (2010) The structure of genetic and environmental risk factors for syndromal and subsyndromal common DSM-IV axis I and all axis II personality disorders. *American Journal of Psychiatry*, 168(1), 29–39.

Kendler, K., Neale, M., Kessler, R., et al. (1992) Major Depression and Generalized Anxiety Disorder: Same genes, (partly) different environments? *Archives of General Psychiatry*, 49, 716–722.

Kessler, R., Berglund, P., Demler, O., et al. (2003) The epidemiology of major depressive disorder. *Journal of the American Medical Association*, 289(23), 3095–3105.

Kessler, R. C., McGonagle, K. A., Nelson, C. B., et al. (1994) Sex and depression in the National Comorbidity Survey. II: Cohort effects. *Journal of Affective Disorders*, 30, 15–26.

Kessler, R., McGonagle, K., Zhao, S., et al. (1994) Lifetime and 12-month prevalence of DSM-III-R psychiatric disorders in the United States. *Results from the National Comorbidity Survey*. *Archives of General Psychiatry*, 51, 8–19.

Kessler, R. C., Petukhova, M., Sampson, N. A., Zaslavsky, A. M., & Wittchen, H. U. (2012) Twelve-month point prevalence and lifetime morbid risk of anxiety and mood disorders in the United States. *International Journal of Methods in Psychiatric Research*, 21(3), 169–184. doi: 10.1002/mpr.1359.

Kessler, R. C., Sonnega, A., Bromet, E., et al. (1995) Posttraumatic stress disorder in the National Comorbidity Survey. *Archives of General Psychiatry*, 52, 1048–1060.

Kossowsky, J., Pfaltz, M. C., Schneider, S., Taeymans, J., Locher, C., & Gaab, J. (2013). The separation anxiety hypothesis of panic disorder revisited: A meta-analysis. *American Journal of Psychiatry*, 170(7), 768–781. doi: 10.1176/appi.ajp.2012.12070893.

Lampe, L., Slade, T., Issakidis, C., et al. (2003) Social phobia in the Australian National Survey of Mental Health and Well-Being (NSMHWB). *Psychological Medicine*, 33, 637–646.

Lensi, P., Cassano, G. B., Correddu, G., et al. (1996) Obsessive-compulsive disorder. Familial-developmental history, symptomatology, comorbidity and course with special reference to gender-related differences. *British Journal of Psychiatry*, 169, 101–107.

Levine, R. E., Oandasan, A. P., Primeau, L. A., et al. (2003) Anxiety disorders during pregnancy and postpartum. *American Journal of Perinatology*, 20(5), 239–248.

Lewinsohn, P., Lewinsohn, M., Gotlib, I., et al. (1998) Gender differences in anxiety disorders and anxiety symptoms in adolescents. *Journal of Abnormal Psychology*, 107(1), 109–117.

Li, Y., Shi, S., Yang, F., et al. (2012) Patterns of co-morbidity with anxiety disorders in Chinese women with recurrent major depression. *Psychological Medicine*, 42(6), 1239–1248. doi: 10.1017/S003329171100273X.

Lochner, C., Hemmings, S., Kinnear, C., et al. (2004) Gender in obsessive-compulsive disorder: Clinican and genetic findings. *Suropean Neuropsychopharmacology*, 14, 105–113.

Massion, A., Warshaw, M. & Keller, M. (1993) Quality of life and psychiatric morbidity in panic disorder versus generalized anxiety disorder. *American Journal of Psychiatry*, 150, 600–607.

McEvoy, P. M., Grove, R., & Slade, T. (2011) Epidemiology of anxiety disorders in the Australian general population: findings of the 2007 Australian National Survey of Mental Health and Wellbeing. *Australian and New Zealand Journal of Psychiatry*, 45(11), 957–967. doi: 10.3109/00048674.2011.624083.

McLean, C. P., Asnaani, A., Litz, B. T., & Hofmann, S. G. (2011) Gender differences in anxiety disorders: Prevalence, course of illness, comorbidity and burden of illness. *Journal of Psychiatric Research*, 45(8), 1027–1035.

Merikangas, K., Stevens, D., Fenton, B., et al. (1998) Co-morbidity and familial aggregation of alcoholism and anxiety disorders. *Psychological Medicine*, 28, 773–788.

Murray, C.J. & Lopez, A. D. (1996) The incremental effect of age-weighting on YLLs, YLDs, and DALYs: A response. *Bulletin of the World Health Organization* , 74(4), 445–446.

North, C. S., Smith, E. M. & Spitznagel, E. L. (1997) One-year follow-up of a mass shooting. *American Journal of Psychiatry*, 154, 1696–1702.

Noshirvani, H. F., Kasvikis, Y., Marks, I. M., et al. (1991) Gender-divergent etiological factors in obsessive-compulsive disorder. *British Journal of Psychiatry*, 158, 260–263.

Papp, L. A. & Gorman, J. M. (1988) Sex differences in panic disorder. *American Journal of Psychiatry*, 145(6), 766.

Papp, L., Martinez, J., Klein, D., et al. (1997) Respiratory psychophysiology of panic disorder: three respiratory challenges in 98 subjects. *American Journal of Psychiatry*, 154, 1557–1565.

Parker, G., Wilhelm, K. & Asghari, A. (1997) Early onset depression: The relevance of anxiety. *Social Psychiatry And Psychiatric Epidemiology*, 32(1), 30–37.

Pigott, T. (1999) Gender differences in epidemiology and treatment of anxiety disorders. *Journal of Clinical Psychiatry*, 60(Suppl 18), 4–15.

Pollard, C. A. & Henderson, J. G. (1988) Four types of social phobia in a community sample. *Journal of Nervous and Mental Disease*, 176, 440–444.

Reif, A., Weber, H., Domschke, K. et al. (2012) Meta-analysis argues for a female-specific role of MAOA-uVNTR in panic disorder in four European populations. *American Journal Of Medical Genetics. Part B, Neuropsychiatric Genetics: The Official Publication Of The International Society Of Psychiatric Genetics*, 159B(7), 786–793.

Russell, E. J., Fawcett, J. M., & Mazmanian, D. (2013) Risk of obsessive-compulsive disorder in pregnant and postpartum women: A meta-analysis. *Journal of Clinical Psychiatry*, 74(4), 377–385.

Sheikh, J., Leskin, G. & Klein, D. (2002) Gender Differences in Panic Disorder: Findings from the National Comorbidity Survey. *American Journal of Psychiatry*, 159, 55–58.

Smith, M. V., Cavaleri, M. A., Howell, H. B., et al. (2004) Screening for and detection of depression, panic disorder, and PTSD in public-sector obstetrical clinics. *Psychiatric Services*, 55(4), 407–414.

Sonne, S., Back, S., Zuniga, C., et al. (2003) Gender differences in individuals with comorbid alcohol dependence and Post-traumatic Stress Disorder. *American Journal on Addiction*, 12, 412–423.

Starcevic, V., Djordjevic, A., Latas, M., et al. (1998) Characteristics of agoraphobia in women and men with panic disorder and agoraphobia. *Depression and Anxiety*, 8, 8–13.

Stein, M. B., Roy-Byrne, P. P., Craske, M. G., et al. (2005) Functional impact and health utility of anxiety disorders in primary care outpatients. *Medical Care*, 43(12), 1164–1170.

Stein, M. B., Schmidt, P. J., Rubinow, D. R., et al. (1989) Panic disorder and the menstrual cycle: Panic disorder patients, healthy control subjects, and patients with premenstrual syndrome. *American Journal of Psychiatry*, 146(10), 1299–1303.

Stuart, S., Couser, G., Schilder, K., et al. (1998) Postpartum anxiety and depression: Onset and comorbidity in a community sample. *Journal Of Nervous And Mental Disease*, 186(7), 420–424.

Turgeon, L., Marchand, A. & Dupuis, G. (1998) Clinical features in panic disorder with agoraphobia: A comparison of men and women. *Journal of Anxiety Disorders*, 12(6), 539–553.

Turk, C., Heimberg, R., Orsillo, S., et al. (1998) An investigation of gender differences in social phobia. *Journal of Anxiety Disorders*, 12, 209–223.

Wittchen, H.-U., Reed, V. & Kessler, R. C. (1998) The relationship of agoraphobia and panic in a community sample of adolescents and young adults. *Archives of General Psychiatry*, 55, 1017–1024.

Wittchen, H.-U., Zhao, S., Kessler, R. C., et al. (1994) DSM-III-R generalized anxiety disorder in the National Comorbidity Survey. *Archives of General Psychiatry*, 51, 355–364.

Yates, W. R. (2009). Phenomenology and epidemiology of panic disorder. *Annuals of Clinical Psychiatry*, 21(2), 95–102.

Yonkers, K. A., Bruce, S., Dyck, I., et al. (2003) Chronicity, relapse and illness – Course of panic disorder, social phobia, and generalized anxiety disorder: Findings in men and women from 8 years

of follow-up. *Depression and Anxiety*, 17, 173–179.

Yonkers, K. A., Dyck, I. R. & Keller, M. B. (2001) An eight year longitudinal comparison of clinical course and characteristics of social phobia among men and women. *Psychiatric Services*, 52(5), 637–643.

Yonkers, K., Dyck, I., Warshaw, M., et al. (2000) Factors predicting the clinical course of generalised anxiety disorders. *British Journal of Psychiatry*, 176, 544–550.

Yonkers, K. A., Warshaw, M. G., Massion, A. O., et al. (1996)

Phenomenology and course of generalised anxiety disorder. *British Journal of Psychiatry*, 168, 308–313.

Yonkers, K. A., Zlotnick, C., Allsworth, J., et al. (1998) Is the course of panic disorder the same in women and men? *American Journal of Psychiatry*, 155, 596–602.

Zlotnick, C., Zimmerman, M., Wolfsdorf, B. A., et al. (2001) Gender differences in patients with posttraumatic stress disorder in a general psychiatric practice. *American Journal of Psychiatry*, 158, 1923–1925.

Chapter

19

Depression
Special issues in women

John Kelly and Timothy G. Dinan

Introduction

By 2020, the World Health Organization (WHO) has predicted that unipolar depression will be second only to cardiovascular disease in the leading causes of total disease burden worldwide. Women have a higher lifetime prevalence of depression in high-, middle- and low-income countries (WHO, 2008), and this higher prevalence is due to high risk of first onset of depression and not to persistence or recurrence (Kessler, 2003). The higher prevalence is not limited to depression, as women have higher rates of other stress-related disorders (Weich et al., 2001). The higher rates of depression and anxiety in women have implications for future generations as maternal depression has negative effects on perinatal outcomes (Grigoriadis et al., 2013).

Stressful life events are strongly associated with depression and the vast majority of first episodes of depression are preceded by such events (Kendler and Gardner, 2010). There is conflicting evidence regarding gender differences in exposure to stressful life events; however, it is clear that women are at an increased risk of experiencing physical and sexual abuse during their lifetime, and may be more likely to become depressed following stressful life events (Maciejewski et al., 2001). The cause for this is multifactorial, but could partially be explained by sex differences in stress responsivity and reactivity of the hypothalamic-pituitary-adrenal axis (HPA) (Kudielka and Kirschbaum, 2005). Sex hormones can modulate the HPA axis, and the evidence that women have twice the rate of depression only after the onset of puberty (Chapter 7) with an equalization after menopause suggests that the female sex hormones contribute to the female preponderance in rates of depression.

The concept of "reproductive depression" has been proposed to account for the association between hormonal changes and mood during the female reproductive cycle. Clinically, reproductive depression is manifested as premenstrual depression, postnatal depression and perimenopausal depression (Studd and Nappi, 2012). Although not a subcategory of depression in current classification systems, a subsection of women may be vulnerable to this type of depression (Craig, 2013). See also Chapters 8, 9, 10.

Clearly the etiology underlying gender differences in depression is complex and not completely understood. Reduction to a single explanatory paradigm would be overly simplistic. Rather, an understanding of the modulating role of the female sex hormones and the interaction between genetic configuration and environmental influences is necessary to advance our understanding of the gender differences in depression.

In this chapter we discuss sex differences in the serotonergic system, the HPA axis, neuroimaging, reproductive depression and finally the medical implications of depression as they relate to women.

Sex differences in serotonergic neurotransmitters

The serotonergic system develops early in the course of embryogenesis and modulates the development of specific brain areas (Kinast et al., 2013). In animal studies it has been shown to be involved in the modulation of anxiety-like behavior, conditioned fear, stress responses and reward-related behaviors (Asan et al., 2013). The serotonergic system projects from the dorsal raphe nuclei in the brainstem to the forebrain. The modulation of the circuit that connects the dorsal

Comprehensive Women's Mental Health, ed. David J. Castle and Kathryn M. Abel. Published by Cambridge University Press.
© Cambridge University Press 2016.

raphe nucleus, the prefrontal cortex and the amygdala is of particular importance in mood disorders.

Serotonin is synthesized from L-tryptophan and the rate limiting step in the pathway is controlled by tryptophan hydroxylase (TPH), which converts tryptophan to 5-hydroxytryptophan. The monoamine oxidases (MAOs) breakdown serotonin into 5-hydroxyindoleacetic acid (5-HIAA), a step that is inhibited by the monoamine oxidase inhibitor (MAOI) class of antidepressants. There are 15 subtypes of serotonin (5-HT) receptors, and in addition to the central nervous system serotonin is produced in the gastrointestinal tract and in platelets. The serotonin transporter (SERT) reuptakes 5-HT from the synaptic cleft into the presynaptic neuron, and selective serotonin reuptake inhibitor (SSRI) antidepressants act by inhibiting the SERT, resulting in an increase in 5-HT in the extracellular space. The presynaptic 5-HT1A autoreceptors detect serotonin in the extracellular space and modulate the activity of the serotonin neuron (Celada et al., 2004).

Under normal physiological conditions, approximately 99% of tryptophan is metabolized to kynurenine in the liver by tryptophan 2,3-dioxygenase (TDO). However, proinflammatory cytokines such as interferon-γ, C-reactive protein, IL-1, IL-6 and TNF-α, can induce the enzyme indoleamine-2,3-dioxygenase (IDO), which is found in macrophages and microglia cells. IDO is the first and rate limiting step in the kynurenine pathway of tryptophan catabolism. Kynurenine is metabolized to hydroxykynurenine (3-HK), 3-hydroxyanthranilic acid (3-HAA) and quinolinic acid (QUIN), which are neurotoxic. Additionally, this process diverts tryptophan from the synthesis of serotonin, and could potentially result in decreased availability of serotonin. In the competing kynurenine pathway, kynurenine is metabolized to kynurenic acid, which blocks the neurotoxic effects of QUIN (Geng and Liu, 2013). The kynurenine pathway has important implications for neuropsychiatric disorders, including depression, as kynurenine can cross the blood brain barrier to increase central levels, and when metabolized could result in neurotoxic metabolites (Myint and Kim, 2013).

There is a polymorphism in the 5-HTT gene promoter region, which has been extensively studied for its links with neuropsychiatric disorders. A recent meta-analysis showed a small but significant association between 5-HTTLPR genotype and HPA-axis reactivity to acute psychosocial stress. The homozygous carriers of the short allele had increased cortisol

reactivity compared to individuals with the s/l and l/l genotype, though there was no association with gender (Miller et al., 2013).

The sex steroids can alter serotonin (5HT) homeostasis (Sanders, 2012) and therefore have important implications for the regulation of mood. The primary female sex hormones (estradiol and progesterone) regulate the serotonergic system and affect serotonin transporter promotion region expression (Michopoulos et al., 2011). Estrogens can increase the expression and activity of tryptophan hydroxylase (TPH) gene expression, thereby increasing 5HT availability (Smith et al., 2004) and can modulate 5HT1A and 5HT2A receptors (Moses-Kolko et al., 2003). Positron emission tomography (PET) studies have shown differences in the binding potential of the 5HT1A receptor in the raphe nuclei in women with premenstrual dysphoric disorder compared to controls (Jovanovic et al., 2006). Ovarian hormones also regulate serotonin reuptake transporter gene (SERT) protein expression (Lu et al., 2003) and modulate gene expression of adhesion molecules in serotonin neurons that are important for synapse assembly (Bethea and Reddy, 2012).

Estrogen can decrease MAO A gene expression, which is the primary enzyme involved in serotonin breakdown (Gundlah et al., 2002). A PET study (N=15) investigated the link between reduced levels of estrogen in the postpartum period and monoamine oxidase A levels in the prefrontal cortex, anterior cingulate cortex, anterior temporal cortex, thalamus, dorsal putamen, hippocampus and midbrain. MAO A levels were significantly elevated, which indicated a monoamine lowering effect was occurring postpartum (Sacher et al., 2010).

Sex differences in neuroendocrine system

Stress can be physical or psychological and has been defined as a state where homeostasis is threatened or perceived to be threatened (Bradley and Dinan, 2010). The hypothalamic pituitary adrenal axis (HPA) is the core endocrine stress system, and when the brain perceives a threat, the HPA in conjunction with the sympathetic adrenal medullary (SAM) axis is activated. The paraventricular nucleus (PVN) in the hypothalamus regulates the neuroendocrine response whereas the amygdala regulates the majority of the autonomic and behavioral stress reactions in the brain (Kovacs, 2013). At the molecular level corticotropin releasing hormone (CRH) and arginine vasopressin (AVP) regulate HPA activity, both of which are synthesized in the PVN. These hormones act on the anterior pituitary gland and cause the release of adrenocorticotropic hormone (ACTH). ACTH stimulates the release of glucocorticoids (cortisol) from the adrenal cortex, which bind with specific intracellular receptors called the mineralocorticoid and glucocorticoid receptors, which are located in multiple tissues in the body. This system works as a negative feedback loop, whereby glucocorticoids modulate their own secretion by acting at various levels of the HPA axis, such as the hypothalamus and pituitary.

The HPA axis has been extensively studied and there is robust evidence that dysfunction of the HPA axis is associated with stress-related disorders including depression (Stetler and Miller, 2011). Indeed, this HPA axis dysfunction may extend beyond the mood disorders into psychotic disorders, and a recent finding from the North American longitudinal study (N=256) showed higher cortisol levels in subjects who meet clinical high risk (CHR) criteria for psychosis (Walker et al., 2013).

Animal studies have shown that females have higher glucocorticoid levels after HPA axis stimulation (Yoshimura et al., 2003), but in humans the effect is inconsistent. Overall the evidence suggests that there are higher cortisol responses in young men than in young women after exposure to acute real-life psychological stress whereas females tend to display an enhanced stress response to pharmacological challenge tests (Kudielka and Kirschbaum, 2005). This appears contradictory given the higher rates of stress-related disorders in women, but there are several hypothetical reasons for the differences.

The discordance may be attributable to the different pathways that lead to the activation of the paraventricular nucleus (PVN) in the hypothalamus. Psychological stress activates the PVN via the prefrontal cortex, hippocampus and amygdala (limbic circuit), whereas physiological and pharmacological stress may bypass the limbic circuit to activate the PVN directly (Herman and Cullinan, 1997). Interestingly the sex differences in the HPA axis reactivity persist even under induced hypogonadal conditions (Roca et al., 2005).

It is postulated that different types of psychological stress affect women and men differently. It has been shown that women have a greater cortisol response to rejection stress (Stroud et al., 2002), whereas men react more to achievement challenges. The Trier Social Stress Test (TSST) is a 15-minute psychosocial stress protocol involving 5 minutes of anticipatory stress, 5 minutes of public speaking and 5 minutes of mental arithmetic performed in front of a panel of evaluators. It therefore contains elements of uncontrollability and social evaluative threat and it elicits a greater ACTH and free cortisol response in men compared to women (Allen et al., 2013). Marin et al. (2012) randomly assigned 30 women and 30 men to either real neutral news or real negative news excerpts for 10 minutes. Then all subjects were exposed to the TSST. Only in women did the reading of negative news result in a significant increase in salivary cortisol levels in the TSST. One day later a free recall of the news was performed and women were better able to remember the negative news excerpts compared to men (Marin et al., 2012).

Early traumatic events, such as sexual or physical abuse increase the risk of psychiatric disorders in later life (Dube et al., 2001, Banyard et al., 2001, Faravelli et al., 2012). Childhood sexual abuse is more common in girls (Stoltenborgh et al., 2011). These traumatic early life events can adversely affect the development of the brain and HPA axis. Although not the only factor involved, dysregulation of the HPA axis associated with childhood trauma is an important mechanism underlying the increased rate of depression experienced by women who have been abused during childhood (Weiss et al., 1999). Women who experience childhood abuse may be more susceptible to alterations in HPA axis reactivity, and this may have implications for the increased vulnerability to depression in later life (DeSantis et al., 2011, Heim et al., 2000, Bremner et al., 2003). Traumatic events in adulthood do not have the same impact on the HPA axis, indicating that traumatic events during the period of brain development may result in persistent changes in the reactivity of the HPA axis (Klaassens, 2010, Klaassens et al., 2009). Furthermore, the persistent alteration in the HPA axis reactivity of women with a history of childhood sexual abuse can have implications for their offspring. Infants born to mothers with a history of childhood abuse have altered HPA reactivity in the postpartum period (Brand et al., 2010). Early life trauma can therefore be transferred to the next generation via HPA axis reactivity and thus highlights the profound negative effect of childhood trauma on the future development of stress-related disorders.

In addition to HPA axis dysregulation, studies show brain changes in women with a history of childhood abuse. The most consistent finding in this group of women is of smaller hippocampal volumes

(Stein et al., 1997, Vythilingam et al., 2002, Rao et al., 2010), although other brain changes have also been demonstrated. A recent study found decreased gray matter volumes in the right middle cingulate gyrus in healthy young adults with a history of childhood trauma, and this was associated with increased levels of awakening cortisol (Lu et al., 2013).

HPA axis dysfunction has been linked to other stress-related disorders. The functional somatic disorders (FSDs), which compromise chronic fatigue syndrome, fibromyalgia and irritable bowel syndrome (IBS), are more common in women (Lovell and Ford, 2012). IBS is characterized by an overactivity of the HPA axis and an increase in proinflammatory cytokines (Dinan et al., 2006) and it is well established that these disorders are associated with higher rates of depression and anxiety (Henningsen et al., 2003). Recent evidence suggests that cognitive performance is also affected in IBS patients (Kennedy et al., 2013). However, a recent meta-analysis of 85 studies investigating HPA axis activity and functional somatic disorders reported that there was insufficient evidence to suggest that IBS was a hypocortisolemic disorder, but did find a significant reduction in basal cortisol in females with fibromyalgia (Tak et al., 2011).

Sex differences in neuroimaging

The Human Connectome Project (HCP) is a major project that aims to construct a map of the complete structural and functional neural connections *in vivo* within and across individuals (Van Essen and Ugurbil, 2012). This will certainly add to the evidence that there are significant differences in the structure and functioning of female and male brains and more specifically in those brain regions that control emotion.

Sex differences in functional magnetic resonance imaging (fMRI), diffusion tensor imaging (DTI) and positron emission tomography (PET) studies have recently been reviewed (Sacher et al., 2013). In structural MRI studies, women have smaller total brain volumes (Cosgrove et al., 2007), a higher ratio of grey to white matter thickness (Luders et al., 2005) and increased cortical depth (Im et al., 2006). They have increased grey matter volume in dorsal anterior, posterior and ventral cingulated cortices and in the right inferior parietal lobe (Chen et al., 2007) with greater regional density and volume in dorsal and ventral stream regions (Keller and Menon, 2009).

It is hypothesized that sex steroids may account for the sex differences in grey matter volumes (Witte et al., 2010). In addition to chromosomal makeup, sex steroids are involved in sex differentiation in early development (Tokarz et al., 2013) and have an organizational role in the structure and function of the developing human brain (Peper et al., 2009).

Diffusion tensor imaging has shown gender differences in white matter connectivity between many brain regions, including the thalamus, cingulum, corpus callosum (Menzler et al., 2011), frontooccipital fasciculus, parahippocampal gyrus, bilateral internal capsule, medial frontal gyrus, hippocampus, insula, post central gyrus, frontal and temporal lobes (Sacher et al., 2013). A diffusion tensor imaging study of 8–22-year-old males and females (N=949) demonstrated sex specific differences in connectivity during the course of development. Male brains are structured to facilitate connectivity between perception and coordinated action, and female brains are structured to facilitate communication between analytical and intuitive processing (Ingalhalikar et al., 2013).

In MRI resting state functional studies there are hemisphere-related differences (Tian et al., 2011) and differences within the dorsolateral prefrontal cortex, the amygdala (Zuo et al., 2010) and periaqueductal grey (Kong et al., 2010) areas, which are involved in mood and emotion regulation.

Most PET studies show a higher rate of global glucose utilization in females, particularly in the orbital-frontal area (Andreason et al., 1994). This can change with different phases of the menstrual cycle (Reiman et al., 1996). PET studies investigating gender differences in the serotonergic and dopaminergic systems are inconsistent (Sacher et al., 2013) so it is difficult to draw firm conclusions.

A meta-analysis demonstrated that women have greater activation than men in the left amygdala, left thalamus, hypothalamus, mammillary bodies, left caudate and medial prefrontal cortex in response to negative emotions. This valence specificity was most marked for the amygdala (Stevens and Hamann, 2012). This is in keeping with earlier studies showing that women experience the remembering of emotional events in more detail and with greater intensity than men (Seidlitz and Diener, 1998). Yuan et al. (2009) compared event-related potentials in men and women in response to images of different emotional valence (rated high negative, moderately negative or neutral) and found that females are more susceptible to negative stimuli of lesser salience and this susceptibility was not seen for positive stimuli.

In an fMRI study using a working memory task and an emotional distraction, women had increased sensitivity to emotional distraction in brain areas associated with "hot" emotional processing, whereas men showed increased sensitivity in areas associated with "cold" executive processing. There was a sex-related dorsal-ventral hemispheric dissociation in the lateral prefrontal cortex (PFC) related to coping with emotional distraction, with women showing a positive correlation with working memory performance in the left ventral PFC and men showing similar effects in the right dorsal PFC (Iordan et al., 2013).

In a recent study by Holsen et al. (2013), 15 women with recurrent major depressive disorder (rMDD) and 15 healthy controls were MRI scanned during neutral and negative stimuli. Women with rMDD demonstrated higher anxiety ratings, increased cortisol levels and hyperactivation in the amygdala and hippocampus. Amygdala activation was negatively related to cortisol changes and positively associated with the duration of remission.

Reproductive depression

Prepubescent boys have slightly higher rates of depression than prepubescent girls (Twenge and Nolen-Hoeksema, 2002). This pattern reverses during mid-puberty and rates of depression remain higher in women until after menopause (Cyranowski et al., 2000). Pubertal changes in sex hormones contribute to this divergence in mid-puberty, as they modulate the HPA and may sensitize girls to stressful life events and therefore potentially result in higher rates of depression during this period (Young and Altemus, 2004). That stress responses are influenced by female sex steroids is now beyond doubt.

A recent study using the Avon Longitudinal study of parents and children cohort in the United Kingdom demonstrated that early menarche is associated with an increase in depressive symptoms in early to mid-adolescence (Joinson et al., 2013). Indeed the menstrual cycle continues to be problematic for a subsection of women who experience premenstrual syndrome (PMS). This includes a wide variety of physical, psychological and cognitive symptoms that occur recurrently and cyclically during the luteal phase of the menstrual cycle and disappear soon after the onset of menstruation (Allais et al., 2012). Up to

20% of women with premenstrual symptoms are severe enough to require treatment (Halbreich, 2004).

At the cognitive level there are changes in the integration of emotional and cognitive processing in women with PMS. A recent pilot study demonstrated an increase in the mean reaction time for resolving emotional conflict from the follicular to the luteal cycle phase in all women, but only women with PMS showed an increase in physiological (salivary cortisol) and subjective stress measures during the luteal phase (Hoyer et al., 2013). Salivary cortisol is an easily accessible and reliable measure of HPA activity.

Five percent of women of reproductive age will experience a severe form of PMS called premenstrual dysphoric disorder (PMDD) (Brown et al., 2009), which has a heritability of approximately 50% (Kendler et al., 1998). Although symptoms are not associated with defined concentrations of any specific sex or nonsex hormone (Rapkin and Akopians, 2012), hormonal changes during the late luteal phase of the menstrual cycle are thought to contribute to this disorder. Interestingly these symptoms are effectively eliminated by ovarectomy or by treatment with a gonadotropin releasing hormone antagonist (Eriksson et al., 2012) – again supporting a link between female sex steroids and depression.

The underlying pathophysiology of PMS, although not fully clear, is thought to be linked to the interaction between the sex hormones and the GABAergic and serotonergic systems with involvement of the HPA. Progesterone is produced in the ovaries in the corpus luteum and its metabolites 3α,5α-tetrahydrodeoxycorticosterone (THDOC) and 3α-hydroxy-5α-pregnane-20-one (allopregnanolone) are neuroactive steroids and modulators of GABA-A receptors (Zorumski and Mennerick, 2013). Allopregnanolone can augment the function of GABA-A and has similar effects to benzodiazepines, barbiturates and alcohol (Akk et al., 2007, Paul and Purdy, 1992), substances known to induce mood effects at low dosages in humans and animals. In addition to GABAergic modulation, certain neurosteroids modulate glutamate receptors particularly N-methyl-D-aspartate receptors (Zorumski et al., 2013). Although meta-analysis has shown that progesterone is not an effective treatment for PMS (Ford et al., 2012), its derivatives acting as GABAergic and glutamatergic modulators may have potential as future treatments in certain subtypes of mood disorders.

In addition to modulating GABA and glutamate NMDA receptors, sex hormones interact with the serotonergic system and may contribute to altering mood during the menstrual cycle. Indeed the lowering of serotonin can give rise to PMS-like symptoms (Rapkin and Akopians, 2012) and meta-analysis has demonstrated that SSRIs are effective in the treatment of PMS if taken only in the luteal phase or continuously throughout the cycle (Marjoribanks et al., 2013).

The menstrual cycle is associated with inflammatory changes (Berbic and Fraser, 2013). Innate immune inflammatory responses are associated with depression, with most consistent findings for elevations in the cytokines interleukin-6 (IL-6), tumor necrosis factor-a (TNF-a), and C-reactive protein in those diagnosed with depression (Dowlati et al., 2010). Cytokines can activate HPA and induce the production of CRH, ACTH and cortisol (Pariante and Miller, 2001). Increased levels of cytokines in the periphery can affect the brain, via permeable or leaky blood brain barrier, activation of vagal fibers or active transport by cytokine specific transporters (Miller et al., 2009). One part of the innate immune system is comprised of pattern recognition receptors (PRR), a subtype of which are the Toll like receptors (TLRs) (McCusker and Kelley, 2013). Activation of the TLRs can result in the production and release of cytokines. A study investigating the TLRs during the menstrual cycle demonstrated that the responsivity of these receptors change during the course of the menstrual cycle (Dennison et al., 2012). Although increased levels of cytokines are found in certain subgroups of depressed patients, the implications of inflammatory changes during the menstrual cycle for mood are not fully elucidated.

The next stage in the female reproductive cycle is the perinatal period (see also Chapter 10). Mild depressive symptoms are common in the postpartum period, with up to 50–80% of women experiencing such symptoms in the early postpartum period (Workman et al., 2012). There is an increased risk of depression and psychiatric admission during the postpartum period (Munk-Olsen et al., 2006) with up to 20% of women meeting the criteria for a depressive episode in the first postpartum year (Wisner et al., 2013) with most of the episodes occurring in the first 3 months postpartum (Gavin et al., 2005).

For those women with a history of mood disorders, the perinatal period is a time of significant relapse risk. The risk of having a major affective episode if there is a history of recurrent major depression is approximately 40% and in those women with a history of bipolar disorder it is 50% (Di Florio et al., 2013).

There are considerable changes in biological parameters during the postpartum period, particularly in the neuroendocrine system. During delivery estriol, progesterone and CRH levels decrease rapidly, with modest decreases in cortisol. It has been shown that depressive symptom scores positively correlate with ACTH and negatively correlate with estriol and CRH levels (O'Keane et al., 2011). Although depressive symptoms may be associated with neuroendocrine changes, estrogen replacement alone is not effective in the treatment of postpartum depression (Craig, 2013) highlighting the multifactorial nature of this condition.

Due to the high risk of affective disorders during the perinatal period, thorough screening of women with a particular emphasis on monitoring those women with a history of mood disorders is necessary. The optimal management of mood disorders during pregnancy and the postpartum period has even greater consequence, as it may affect mother-child bonding with resultant negative effects on brain development in the offspring (Chapter 11). Preclinical studies highlight the detrimental impact of these early events and explore potential mechanisms. Mice subjected to chronic and unpredictable maternal separation in the postpartum period show depressive-like behaviors as adults. Epigenetic alterations in separated mice affect the germline, which has implications for the transgenerational transfer of stress-related disorders (Franklin et al., 2010). Furthermore, recent evidence shows that maternal care can result in alterations in the epigenetic regulation of hormone receptor levels (Pena et al., 2013). Preclinical and clinical studies indicate that the provision of adequate maternal care during the critical postpartum period is necessary for the normal development of brain circuits involved in emotion regulation.

The perimenopausal period is marked by a decline in ovarian function with associated fluctuations in estrogen levels (Wharton et al., 2012) and changes in the estrogen–androgen balance (McConnell et al., 2012). Clinically this stage consists of psychological, psychosomatic, sexual and vasomotor symptoms, and it is well established that perimenopausal women are at an increased risk of developing a depressive disorder and are more vulnerable to cognitive decline compared to premenopausal women (Weber et al., 2013). Interestingly, in addition to the SSRI's effectiveness in treating perimenopausal depression, a recent meta-analysis of 11 randomized controlled trials showed that SSRIs also result in a modest improvement in vasomotor symptoms (Shams et al., 2013), which can affect up to 39% of perimenopausal women (Grigoriou et al., 2013).

The sex differences in depression equalize in the elderly population (Chapter 20). However, there may be higher rates of anxiety in elderly females (Vadla et al., 2013). In a recent cross-sectional analysis of survivors in the population-based Faenza study that included 359 subjects aged 74 years or older, an overall prevalence of depression of 25.1% was found with no evidence of gender differences (Forlani et al., 2013). Like postpartum depression, studies have shown estradiol to be ineffective in the treatment of depression in the postmenopausal stage (Morrison et al., 2004). Although hormone replacement is not an effective therapeutic agent in the treatment of depression, it is clear that female sex hormones play an important role in mood regulation. They accomplish this by modulating the HPA and the neurotransmitter systems involved in mood.

Interestingly, in contrast to the biological theories for the epidemiological sex differences in rates of depression, it has been hypothesized that women and men experience depression differently (Addis, 2008). Men are more likely to react with anger or self-destructive behavior, and engage in substance abuse with lower levels of impulse control compared to women (Winkler et al., 2005). In a recently published secondary analysis of the National Comorbidity Survey Replication, men reported higher rates of anger, aggression, substance use and risk taking compared to women, and when this is taken into account men and women met criteria for depression in equal proportions: 30.6% of men and 33.3% of women (Martin et al., 2013). Although an interesting prospect, further research would be required to validate these findings.

Implications of depression in women

Depression has a detrimental impact on quality of life and ability to function, but is also associated with a number of medical comorbidities. Cardiovascular disease (CVD) is the leading cause of mortality in women, and although rates of CVD have decreased in men in recent decades, similar reductions in women have not occurred. Men develop heart disease earlier than women, though the rates in women exceed those in men by the mid-40s (Go et al., 2013). Although the cardiac risk factors for men and women are the same, sex hormone changes during menopause and their impact on hypertension, lipid concentrations and central adiposity may contribute to the increased risk of cardiovascular disease in women during this period (Banos et al., 2011).

Depression is an independent risk factor for cardiac morbidity and mortality (Versteeg et al., 2013, Larsen et al., 2013), and the prevalence of depression in cardiac disease is 15–20% (Celano and Huffman, 2011). The relationship between cardiac disease and depression is bidirectional, as depression can increase the risk of cardiovascular disease and cardiovascular disease can increase the risk of depression (Plante, 2005). The etiology is multifactorial and involves the interaction of the autonomic nervous system, the neuroimmune, the neuroendocrine and the vascular systems. Depression is associated with overactivity of the HPA and SAM axes, both of which can result in vascular endothelial cell damage (Joynt et al., 2003). Inflammation is the principal pathophysiological process that occurs in cardiovascular disease, and oxidative stress and neuroinflammation have been linked to neurovascular dysfunction in depression (Najjar et al., 2013). Chronic stress can result in a proinflammatory state, and the increase of proinflammatory cytokines can result in platelet aggregation and contribute to atherosclerosis (Elsenberg et al., 2013). As mentioned earlier, cytokines can decrease the availability of serotonin postsynaptically, and enhance IDO activity resulting in decreased levels of tryptophan and potentially lead to serotonin deficiency (Halaris, 2013).

Several large trials have investigated the role of SSRIs in the treatment of depression in cardiovascular disease. The Sertraline treatment of major depression in patients with acute myocardial infarction or unstable angina (SADHART) demonstrated that sertraline was a safe and effective in the treatment of depression in CVD (Glassman et al., 2002, Glassman et al., 2009). The Enhancing Recovery in Coronary Heart Disease (ENRICHD) trial showed that there was an association with a lower risk of cardiac morbidity and mortality in the subgroup of patients taking SSRI antidepressants, though the effect was found in men only (Taylor et al., 2005, Jaffe et al., 2006). The Canadian Cardiac Randomized Evaluation of Antidepressant Psychotherapy Efficacy (CREATE) trial showed that citalopram was effective in the treatment of depression in CVD, and found that the addition of interpersonal therapy did not improve outcomes further (Lesperance et al., 2007). The Women's Ischemia Syndrome Evaluation (WISE) study investigated subcategories of depressive symptoms in women with suspected myocardial ischemia as predictors of adverse cardiac outcomes, and found that somatic symptoms but not cognitive or affective symptoms predicted worse outcomes (Linke et al., 2009).

Although a direct causal link between depression and CVD has not been established, screening for depression in women with CVD is important, as depression should be viewed as an additional modifiable risk factor for the prevention of adverse cardiac events in women of all ages, but particularly in the perimenopausal stage.

An additional medical comorbidity associated with depression of particular importance in women is osteoporosis. Female gender, advancing age, estrogen and calcium deficiencies, limited physical activity, glucocorticoid treatment and smoking are established risk factors for this disorder. An estimated 22 million women in Europe have osteoporosis, which is 3 times higher than the rate in men, and is a major risk for fractures (Svedbom et al., 2013). A meta-analysis of 23 studies involving 2,327 depressed patients and 21,141 nondepressed subjects, showed that women that were diagnosed as depressed by a psychiatrist using DSM criteria had significantly lower bone mineral densities (BMD) (Yirmiya and Bab, 2009).

Recent evidence has raised concerns regarding antidepressant use and associated bone loss and fractures (Rizzoli et al., 2012). A meta-analysis of 12 observational studies showed a higher risk of fractures in those using SSRI medication (Eom et al., 2012), and another study showed an increase in fractures in elderly women using SSRIs (Diem et al., 2011). A recent study investigating a 12-week course of the serotonin and noradrenaline reuptake inhibitor venlafaxine in an elderly group of depressed patients found an increase in serum C-terminal cross linking telopeptide of type I collagen (ß-CTX), (used as a marker of bone resorption) in the venlafaxine group. However, the increase in ß-CTX was only significant in patients whose depression did not remit, suggesting attribution to venlafaxine is overly simplistic (Shea et al., 2013). Indeed, in a multicenter prospective cohort trial involving 1,972 middle-age women, antidepressants were not associated with an increased rate of bone loss, suggesting the risk is age dependent (Diem et al., 2013).

The interaction between depression, serotonin and bone metabolism is complex. Depression can result in lower bone mineral densities and fractures, and SSRIs can result in similar effects, particularly in elderly women. High-risk groups may require BMD screening and appropriate treatment to reduce the risk of fractures. Treating psychiatrists should take these factors into account when managing depression in this subgroup of women.

Conclusion

It is established that women experience more depression than men. However, the precise reasons for this are not fully understood. The interaction between genes and the environment is further influenced by the female sex hormones, which impact on the development of the brain and result in structural and functional brain differences as demonstrated by neuroimaging. The sex hormones modulate neurotransmitters and the HPA axis, which play important roles in emotional regulation. Fluctuations in the sex hormones during the female reproductive cycle and the related mood and cognitive changes can result in reproductive depression in a certain subgroup of women. Depression has medical implications for women as it is associated with an increased risk of comorbidities such as cardiovascular disease and osteoporosis. Indeed, the detrimental effects of depression in women are not limited to the individual as maternal depression in the perinatal period has important implications for the development of stress-related disorders in the next generation. Clinicians should take these important factors into account when managing depression in women.

References

ADDIS 2008. Gender and depression in men. *Clin Psychol Sci Prac*, 153–168.

Akk, G., Covey, D. F., Evers, A. S., Steinbach, J. H., Zorumski, C. F. & Mennerick, S. 2007. Mechanisms of neurosteroid interactions with GABA(A) receptors. *Pharmacol Ther*, 116, 35–57.

Allais, G., Castagnoli Gabellari, I., Burzio, C., Rolando, S., de Lorenzo, C., Mana, O. & Benedetto, C. 2012. Premenstrual syndrome and migraine. *Neurol Sci*, 33 Suppl 1, S111–S115.

Allen, A. P., Kennedy, P. J., Cryan, J. F., Dinan, T. G. & Clarke, G. 2013. Biological and psychological markers of stress in humans: focus on the Trier Social Stress Test. *Neurosci Biobehav Rev.*, 38, 94–124.

Andreason, P. J., Zametkin, A. J., Guo, A. C., Baldwin, P. & Cohen, R. M. 1994. Gender-related differences in regional cerebral glucose metabolism in normal volunteers. *Psychiatry Res*, 51, 175–183.

Asan, E., Steinke, M. & Lesch, K. P. 2013. Serotonergic innervation of the amygdala: targets, receptors, and implications for stress and anxiety. *Histochem Cell Biol*, 139, 785–813.

Banos, G., Guarner, V. & Perez-Torres, I. 2011. Sex steroid hormones, cardiovascular diseases and the metabolic syndrome. *Cardiovasc Hematol Agents Med Chem*, 9, 137–146.

Banyard, V. L., Williams, L. M. & Siegel, J. A. 2001. The long-term mental health consequences of child sexual abuse: an exploratory study of the impact of multiple traumas in a sample of women. *J Trauma Stress*, 14, 697–715.

Berbic, M. & Fraser, I. S. 2013. Immunology of normal and abnormal menstruation. *Womens Health (Lond Engl)*, 9, 387–395.

Bethea, C. L. & Reddy, A. P. 2012. Effect of ovarian steroids on gene expression related to synapse assembly in serotonin neurons of macaques. *J Neurosci Res*, 90, 1324–1334.

Bradley, A. J. & Dinan, T. G. 2010. A systematic review of hypothalamic-pituitary-adrenal axis function in schizophrenia: implications for mortality. *J Psychopharmacol*, 24, 91–118.

Brand, S. R., Brennan, P. A., Newport, D. J., Smith, A. K., Weiss, T. &

Stowe, Z. N. 2010. The impact of maternal childhood abuse on maternal and infant HPA axis function in the postpartum period. *Psychoneuroendocrinology*, 35, 686–693.

Bremner, J. D., Vythilingam, M., Anderson, G., Vermetten, E., Mcglashan, T., Heninger, G., Rasmusson, A., Southwick, S. M. & Charney, D. S. 2003. Assessment of the hypothalamic-pituitary-adrenal axis over a 24-hour diurnal period and in response to neuroendocrine challenges in women with and without childhood sexual abuse and posttraumatic stress disorder. *Biol Psychiatry*, 54, 710–718.

Brown, J., O'Brien, P. M., Marjoribanks, J. & Wyatt, K. 2009. Selective serotonin reuptake inhibitors for premenstrual syndrome. *Cochrane Database Syst Rev*, CD001396.

Celada, P., Puig, M., Amargos-Bosch, M., Adell, A. & Artigas, F. 2004. The therapeutic role of 5-HT1A and 5-HT2A receptors in depression. *J Psychiatry Neurosci*, 29, 252–265.

Celano, C. M. & Huffman, J. C. 2011. Depression and cardiac disease: a review. *Cardiol Rev*, 19, 130–142.

Chen, X., Sachdev, P. S., Wen, W. & Anstey, K. J. 2007. Sex differences in regional gray matter in healthy individuals aged 44-48 years: a voxel-based morphometric study. *NeuroImage*, 36, 691–699.

Cosgrove, K. P., Mazure, C. M. & Staley, J. K. 2007. Evolving knowledge of sex differences in brain structure, function, and chemistry. *Biol Psychiatry*, 62, 847–855.

Craig, M. C. 2013. Should psychiatrists be prescribing oestrogen therapy to their female patients? *Br J Psychiatry*, 202, 9–13.

Cyranowski, J. M., Frank, E., Young, E. & Shear, M. K. 2000. Adolescent onset of the gender difference in lifetime rates of major depression: a theoretical model. *Arch Gen Psychiatry*, 57, 21–27.

Dennison, U., Mckernan, D. P., Scully, P., Clarke, G., Cryan, J. & Dinan, T. 2012. Menstrual cycle influences Toll-like receptor responses. *Neuroimmunomodulation*, 19, 171–179.

Desantis, S. M., Baker, N. L., Back, S. E., Spratt, E., Ciolino, J. D., Moran-Santa Maria, M., Dipankar, B. & Brady, K. T. 2011. Gender differences in the effect of early life trauma on hypothalamic-pituitary-adrenal axis functioning. *Depress Anxiety*, 28, 383–392.

di Florio, A., Forty, L., Gordon-Smith, K., Heron, J., Jones, L., Craddock, N. & Jones, I. 2013. Perinatal episodes across the mood disorder spectrum. *JAMA Psychiatry*, 70, 168–175.

Diem, S. J., Blackwell, T. L., Stone, K. L., Cauley, J. A., Hillier, T. A., Haney, E. M. & Ensrud, K. E. 2011. Use of antidepressant medications and risk of fracture in older women. *Calcif Tissue Int*, 88, 476–484.

Diem, S. J., Ruppert, K., Cauley, J. A., Lian, Y., Bromberger, J. T., Finkelstein, J. S., Greendale, G. A. & Solomon, D. H. 2013. Rates of bone loss among women initiating antidepressant medication use in midlife. *J Clin Endocrinol Metab*, 98, 4355–4363.

Dinan, T. G., Quigley, E. M., Ahmed, S. M., Scully, P., O'Brien, S., O'Mahony, L., O'Mahony, S., Shanahan, F. & Keeling, P. W. 2006. Hypothalamic-pituitary-gut axis dysregulation in irritable bowel syndrome: plasma cytokines as a potential biomarker? *Gastroenterology*, 130, 304–311.

Dowlati, Y., Herrmann, N., Swardfager, W., Liu, H., Sham, L., Reim, E. K. & Lanctot, K. L. 2010. A meta-analysis of cytokines in major depression. *Biol Psychiatry*, 67, 446–457.

Dube, S. R., Anda, R. F., Felitti, V. J., Chapman, D. P., Williamson, D. F. & Giles, W. H. 2001. Childhood abuse, household dysfunction, and the risk of attempted suicide throughout the life span: findings from the Adverse Childhood Experiences Study. *JAMA*, 286, 3089–3096.

Elsenberg, E. H., Sels, J. E., Hillaert, M. A., Schoneveld, A. H., van den Dungen, N. A., van Holten, T. C., Roest, M., Jukema, J. W., van Zonneveld, A. J., de Groot, P. G., Pijls, N., Pasterkamp, G. & Hoefer, I. E. 2013. Increased cytokine response after toll-like receptor stimulation in patients with stable coronary artery disease. *Atherosclerosis*, 231, 346–351.

Eom, C. S., Lee, H. K., Ye, S., Park, S. M. & Cho, K. H. 2012. Use of selective serotonin reuptake inhibitors and risk of fracture: a systematic review and meta-analysis. *J Bone Miner Res*, 27, 1186–1195.

Eriksson, O., Landen, M., Sundblad, C., Holte, J., Eriksson, E. & Naessen, T. 2012. Ovarian morphology in premenstrual dysphoria. *Psychoneuroendocrinology*, 37, 742–751.

Faravelli, C., Lo Sauro, C., Godini, L., Lelli, L., Benni, L., Pietrini, F., Lazzeretti, L., Talamba, G. A., Fioravanti, G. & Ricca, V. 2012. Childhood stressful events, HPA axis and anxiety disorders. *World J Psychiatry*, 2, 13–25.

Ford, O., Lethaby, A., Roberts, H. & Mol, B. W. 2012. Progesterone for premenstrual syndrome. *Cochrane Database Syst Rev*, 3, CD003415.

Forlani, C., Morri, M., Ferrari, B., Dalmonte, E., Menchetti, M., de Ronchi, D. & Atti, A. R. 2013. Prevalence and gender differences in late-life depression: a population-based study. *Am J Geriatr Psychiatry*. doi: 10.1016/j.jagp.2012.08.015.

Franklin, T. B., Russig, H., Weiss, I. C., Graff, J., Linder, N., Michalon, A., Vizi, S. & Mansuy, I. M. 2010. Epigenetic transmission of the impact of early stress across generations. *Biol Psychiatry*, 68, 408–415.

Gavin, N. I., Gaynes, B. N., Lohr, K. N., Meltzer-Brody, S., Gartlehner, G. &

Swinson, T. 2005. Perinatal depression: a systematic review of prevalence and incidence. *Obstet Gynecol*, 106, 1071–1083.

Geng, J. & Liu, A. 2013. Heme-Dependent Dioxygenases in Tryptophan Oxidation. *Arch Biochem Biophys*. doi: 10.1016/j. abb.2013.11.009.

Glassman, A. H., Bigger, J. T., JR. & Gaffney, M. 2009. Psychiatric characteristics associated with long-term mortality among 361 patients having an acute coronary syndrome and major depression: seven-year follow-up of SADHART participants. *Arch Gen Psychiatry*, 66, 1022–1029.

Glassman, A. H., O'Connor, C. M., Califf, R. M., Swedberg, K., Schwartz, P., Bigger, J. T., JR., Krishnan, K. R., van Zyl, L. T., Swenson, J. R., Finkel, M. S., Landau, C., Shapiro, P. A., Pepine, C. J., Mardekian, J., Harrison, W. M., Barton, D. & Mclvor, M. 2002. Sertraline treatment of major depression in patients with acute MI or unstable angina. *JAMA*, 288, 701–709.

Go, A. S., Mozaffarian, D., Roger, V. L., Benjamin, E. J., Berry, J. D., Borden, W. B., Bravata, D. M., Dai, S., Ford, E. S., Fox, C. S., Franco, S., Fullerton, H. J., Gillespie, C., Hailpern, S. M., Heit, J. A., Howard, V. J., Huffman, M. D., Kissela, B. M., Kittner, S. J., Lackland, D. T., Lichtman, J. H., Lisabeth, L. D., Magid, D., Marcus, G. M., Marelli, A., Matchar, D. B., Mcguire, D. K., Mohler, E. R., Moy, C. S., Mussolino, M. E., Nichol, G., Paynter, N. P., Schreiner, P. J., Sorlie, P. D., Stein, J., Turan, T. N., Virani, S. S., Wong, N. D., Woo, D. & Turner, M. B. 2013. Executive summary: heart disease and stroke statistics–2013 update: a report from the American Heart Association. *Circulation*, 127, 143–152.

Grigoriadis, S., Vonderporten, E. H., Mamisashvili, L., Tomlinson, G., Dennis, C. L., Koren, G., Steiner,

M., Mousmanis, P., Cheung, A., Radford, K., Martinovic, J. & Ross, L. E. 2013. The impact of maternal depression during pregnancy on perinatal outcomes: a systematic review and meta-analysis. *J Clin Psychiatry*, 74, e321–41.

Grigoriou, V., Augoulea, A., Armeni, E., Rizos, D., Alexandrou, A., Dendrinos, S., Panoulis, K. & Lambrinoudaki, I. 2013. Prevalence of vasomotor, psychological, psychosomatic and sexual symptoms in perimenopausal and recently postmenopausal Greek women: association with demographic, life-style and hormonal factors. *Gynecol Endocrinol*, 29, 125–128.

Gundlah, C., Lu, N. Z. & Bethea, C. L. 2002. Ovarian steroid regulation of monoamine oxidase-A and-B mRNAs in the macaque dorsal raphe and hypothalamic nuclei. *Psychopharmacology (Berl)*, 160, 271–282.

Halaris, A. 2013. Inflammation, heart disease, and depression. *Curr Psychiatry Rep*, 15, 400.

Halbreich, U. 2004. The diagnosis of premenstrual syndromes and premenstrual dysphoric disorder–clinical procedures and research perspectives. *Gynecol Endocrinol*, 19, 320–334.

Heim, C., Newport, D. J., Heit, S., Graham, Y. P., Wilcox, M., Bonsall, R., Miller, A. H. & Nemeroff, C. B. 2000. Pituitary-adrenal and autonomic responses to stress in women after sexual and physical abuse in childhood. *JAMA*, 284, 592–597.

Henningsen, P., Zimmermann, T. & Sattel, H. 2003. Medically unexplained physical symptoms, anxiety, and depression: a meta-analytic review. *Psychosom Med*, 65, 528–533.

Herman, J. P. & Cullinan, W. E. 1997. Neurocircuitry of stress: central control of the hypothalamo-pituitary-adrenocortical axis. *Trends Neurosci*, 20, 78–84.

Holsen, L. M., Lancaster, K., Klibanski, A., Whitfield-Gabrieli, S., Cherkerzian, S., Buka, S. & Goldstein, J. M. 2013. HPA-axis hormone modulation of stress response circuitry activity in women with remitted major depression. *Neuroscience*, 250, 733–742.

Hoyer, J., Burmann, I., Kieseler, M. L., Vollrath, F., Hellrung, L., Arelin, K., Roggenhofer, E., Villringer, A. & Sacher, J. 2013. Menstrual cycle phase modulates emotional conflict processing in women with and without premenstrual syndrome (PMS)–a pilot study. *PLoS One*, 8, e59780.

Im, K., Lee, J. M., Lee, J., Shin, Y. W., Kim, I. Y., Kwon, J. S. & Kim, S. I. 2006. Gender difference analysis of cortical thickness in healthy young adults with surface-based methods. *NeuroImage*, 31, 31–38.

Ingalhalikar, M., Smith, A., Parker, D., Satterthwaite, T. D., Elliott, M. A., Ruparel, K., Hakonarson, H., Gur, R. E., Gur, R. C. & Verma, R. 2013. Sex differences in the structural connectome of the human brain. *Proc Natl Acad Sci USA*. doi: 10.1073/pnas.1316909110.

Jaffe, A. S., Krumholz, H. M., Catellier, D. J., Freedland, K. E., Bittner, V., Blumenthal, J. A., Calvin, J. E., Norman, J., Sequeira, R., O'Connor, C., Rich, M. W., Sheps, D. & Wu, C. 2006. Prediction of medical morbidity and mortality after acute myocardial infarction in patients at increased psychosocial risk in the Enhancing Recovery in Coronary Heart Disease Patients (ENRICHD) study. *Am Heart J*, 152, 126–135.

Joinson, C., Heron, J., Araya, R. & Lewis, G. 2013. Early menarche and depressive symptoms from adolescence to young adulthood in a UK cohort. *J Am Acad Child Adolesc Psychiatry*, 52, 591–598 e2.

Iordan, A. D., Dolcos, S., Denkova, E. & Dolcos, F. 2013. Sex differences in the response to emotional distraction: an event-related fMRI investigation. *Cogn Affect Behav Neurosci*, 13, 116–134.

Jovanovic, H., Cerin, Å., Karlsson, P., Lundberg, J., Halldin, C. & NordstrÖM, A.-L. 2006. A PET study of 5-HT1A receptors at different phases of the menstrual cycle in women with premenstrual dysphoria. *Psychiatry Research: Neuroimaging*, 148, 185–193.

Joynt, K. E., Whellan, D. J. & O'Connor, C. M. 2003. Depression and cardiovascular disease: mechanisms of interaction. *Biol Psychiatry*, 54, 248–61.

Keller, K. & Menon, V. 2009. Gender differences in the functional and structural neuroanatomy of mathematical cognition. *NeuroImage*, 47, 342–352.

Kendler, K. S. & Gardner, C. O. 2010. Dependent stressful life events and prior depressive episodes in the prediction of major depression: the problem of causal inference in psychiatric epidemiology. *Arch Gen Psychiatry*, 67, 1120–1127.

Kendler, K. S., Karkowski, L. M., Corey, L. A. & Neale, M. C. 1998. Longitudinal population-based twin study of retrospectively reported premenstrual symptoms and lifetime major depression. *Am J Psychiatry*, 155, 1234–1240.

Kennedy, P. J., Clarke, G., O'Neill, A., Groeger, J. A., Quigley, E. M., Shanahan, F., Cryan, J. F. & Dinan, T. G. 2013. Cognitive performance in irritable bowel syndrome: evidence of a stress-related impairment in visuospatial memory. *Psychol Med*. doi: 10.1017/S0033291713002171.

Kessler, R. C. 2003. Epidemiology of women and depression. *J Affect Disord*, 74, 5–13.

Kinast, K., Peeters, D., Kolk, S. M., Schubert, D. & Homberg, J. R. 2013. Genetic and pharmacological manipulations of the serotonergic system in early life: Neurodevelopmental underpinnings of autism-related behaviour. *Frontiers in Cellular Neuroscience*, 7, 72.

Klaassens, E. R. 2010. Bouncing back-trauma and the HPA-axis in healthy adults. *Eur J Psychotraumatol*, 1. doi: 10.3402/ejpt.v1i0.5844.

Klaassens, E. R., van Noorden, M. S., Giltay, E. J., van Pelt, J., van Veen, T. & Zitman, F. G. 2009. Effects of childhood trauma on HPA-axis reactivity in women free of lifetime psychopathology. *Prog Neuropsychopharmacol Biol Psychiatry*, 33, 889–894.

Kong, J., Tu, P.-C., Zyloney, C. & Su, T.-P. 2010. Intrinsic functional connectivity of the periaqueductal gray, a resting fMRI study. *Behavioural Brain Research*, 211, 215–219.

Kovacs, K. J. 2013. CRH: The link between hormonal-, metabolic- and behavioral responses to stress. *J Chem Neuroanat.*, 54, 25–33.

Kudielka, B. M. & Kirschbaum, C. 2005. Sex differences in HPA axis responses to stress: a review. *Biol Psychol*, 69, 113–132.

Larsen, K. K., Christensen, B., Sondergaard, J. & Vestergaard, M. 2013. Depressive symptoms and risk of new cardiovascular events or death in patients with myocardial infarction: a population-based longitudinal study examining health behaviors and health care interventions. *PLoS One*, 8, e74393.

Lesperance, F., Frasure-Smith, N., Koszycki, D., Laliberte, M. A., van Zyl, L. T., Baker, B., Swenson, J. R., Ghatavi, K., Abramson, B. L., Dorian, P. & Guertin, M. C. 2007. Effects of citalopram and interpersonal psychotherapy on depression in patients with coronary artery disease: the Canadian Cardiac Randomized Evaluation of Antidepressant and Psychotherapy Efficacy (CREATE) trial. *JAMA*, 297, 367–379.

Linke, S. E., Rutledge, T., Johnson, B. D., Vaccarino, V., Bittner, V., Cornell, C. E., Eteiba, W., Sheps, D. S., Krantz, D. S., Parashar, S. &

Bairey Merz, C. N. 2009. Depressive symptom dimensions and cardiovascular prognosis among women with suspected myocardial ischemia: a report from the National Heart, Lung, and Blood Institute-sponsored Women's Ischemia Syndrome Evaluation. *Arch Gen Psychiatry*, 66, 499–507.

Lovell, R. M. & Ford, A. C. 2012. Effect of gender on prevalence of irritable bowel syndrome in the community: systematic review and meta-analysis. *Am J Gastroenterol*, 107, 991–1000.

Lu, N. Z., Eshleman, A. J., Janowsky, A. & Bethea, C. L. 2003. Ovarian steroid regulation of serotonin reuptake transporter (SERT) binding, distribution, and function in female macaques. *Mol Psychiatry*, 8, 353–360.

Lu, S., Gao, W., Wei, Z., Wu, W., Liao, M., Ding, Y., Zhang, Z. & Li, L. 2013. Reduced cingulate gyrus volume associated with enhanced cortisol awakening response in young healthy adults reporting childhood trauma. *PLoS One*, 8, e69350.

Luders, E., Narr, K. L., Thompson, P. M., Woods, R. P., Rex, D. E., Jancke, L., Steinmetz, H. & Toga, A. W. 2005. Mapping cortical gray matter in the young adult brain: effects of gender. *NeuroImage*, 26, 493–501.

Maciejewski, P. K., Prigerson, H. G. & Mazure, C. M. 2001. Sex differences in event-related risk for major depression. *Psychol Med*, 31, 593–604.

Marin, M. F., Morin-Major, J. K., Schramek, T. E., Beaupre, A., Perna, A., Juster, R. P. & Lupien, S. J. 2012. There is no news like bad news: women are more remembering and stress reactive after reading real negative news than men. *PLoS One*, 7, e47189.

Marjoribanks, J., Brown, J., O'Brien, P. M. & Wyatt, K. 2013. Selective serotonin reuptake inhibitors for premenstrual syndrome. *Cochrane Database Syst Rev*, 6, CD001396.

Martin, L. A., Neighbors, H. W. & Griffith, D. M. 2013. The experience of symptoms of depression in men vs women: analysis of the National Comorbidity Survey Replication. *JAMA Psychiatry*, 70, 1100–1106.

Mcconnell, D. S., Stanczyk, F. Z., Sowers, M. R., Randolph, J. F., JR. & Lasley, B. L. 2012. Menopausal transition stage-specific changes in circulating adrenal androgens. *Menopause*, 19, 658–663.

Mccusker, R. H. & Kelley, K. W. 2013. Immune-neural connections: how the immune system's response to infectious agents influences behavior. *J Exp Biol*, 216, 84–98.

Menzler, K., Belke, M., Wehrmann, E., Krakow, K., Lengler, U., Jansen, A., Hamer, H. M., Oertel, W. H., Rosenow, F. & Knake, S. 2011. Men and women are different: diffusion tensor imaging reveals sexual dimorphism in the microstructure of the thalamus, corpus callosum and cingulum. *NeuroImage*, 54, 2557–2562.

Michopoulos, V., Berga, S. L. & Wilson, M. E. 2011. Estradiol and progesterone modify the effects of the serotonin reuptake transporter polymorphism on serotonergic responsivity to citalopram. *Exp Clin Psychopharmacol*, 19, 401–408.

Miller, A. H., Maletic, V. & Raison, C. L. 2009. Inflammation and its discontents: the role of cytokines in the pathophysiology of major depression. *Biol Psychiatry*, 65, 732–741.

Miller, R., Wankerl, M., Stalder, T., Kirschbaum, C. & Alexander, N. 2013. The serotonin transporter gene-linked polymorphic region (5-HTTLPR) and cortisol stress reactivity: a meta-analysis. *Mol Psychiatry*, 18, 1018–1024.

Morrison, M. F., Kallan, M. J., Ten Have, T., Katz, I., Tweedy, K. & Battistini, M. 2004. Lack of efficacy of estradiol for depression in postmenopausal women: a randomized, controlled trial. *Biol Psychiatry*, 55, 406–412.

Moses-Kolko, E. L., Berga, S. L., Greer, P. J., Smith, G., Cidis Meltzer, C. & Drevets, W. C. 2003. Widespread increases of cortical serotonin type 2A receptor availability after hormone therapy in euthymic postmenopausal women. *Fertil Steril*, 80, 554–559.

Munk-Olsen, T., Laursen, T. M., Pedersen, C. B., Mors, O. & Mortensen, P. B. 2006. New parents and mental disorders: a population-based register study. *JAMA*, 296, 2582–2589.

Myint, A. M. & Kim, Y. K. 2013. Network beyond IDO in psychiatric disorders: revisiting neurodegeneration hypothesis. *Prog Neuropsychopharmacol Biol Psychiatry*. doi: 10.1016/j.pnpbp.2013.08.008.

Najjar, S., Pearlman, D. M., Devinsky, O., Najjar, A. & Zagzag, D. 2013. Neurovascular unit dysfunction with blood–brain barrier hyperpermeability contributes to major depressive disorder: a review of clinical and experimental evidence. *J Neuroinflammation*, 10, 142.

O'Keane, V., Lightman, S., Patrick, K., Marsh, M., Papadopoulos, A. S., Pawlby, S., Seneviratne, G., Taylor, A. & Moore, R. 2011. Changes in the maternal hypothalamic-pituitary-adrenal axis during the early puerperium may be related to the postpartum 'blues'. *J Neuroendocrinol*, 23, 1149–1155.

Pariante, C. M. & Miller, A. H. 2001. Glucocorticoid receptors in major depression: relevance to pathophysiology and treatment. *Biol Psychiatry*, 49, 391–404.

Paul, S. M. & Purdy, R. H. 1992. Neuroactive steroids. *FASEB J*, 6, 2311–2322.

Pena, C. J., Neugut, Y. D. & Champagne, F. A. 2013. Developmental timing of the effects of maternal care on gene expression and epigenetic regulation of hormone receptor levels in female rats. *Endocrinology*, 154, 4340–4351.

Peper, J. S., Brouwer, R. M., Schnack, H. G., van Baal, G. C., van Leeuwen, M., van den Berg, S. M., Delemarre-Van DE WAAL, H. A., Boomsma, D. I., Kahn, R. S. & Hulshoff Pol, H. E. 2009. Sex steroids and brain structure in pubertal boys and girls. *Psychoneuroendocrinology*, 34, 332–342.

Plante, G. E. 2005. Depression and cardiovascular disease: a reciprocal relationship. *Metabolism*, 54, 45–48.

Rao, U., Chen, L. A., Bidesi, A. S., Shad, M. U., Thomas, M. A. & Hammen, C. L. 2010. Hippocampal changes associated with early-life adversity and vulnerability to depression. *Biol Psychiatry*, 67, 357–364.

Rapkin, A. J. & Akopians, A. L. 2012. Pathophysiology of premenstrual syndrome and premenstrual dysphoric disorder. *Menopause Int*, 18, 52–59.

Reiman, E. M., Armstrong, S. M., Matt, K. S. & Mattox, J. H. 1996. The application of positron emission tomography to the study of the normal menstrual cycle. *Hum Reprod*, 11, 2799–2805.

Rizzoli, R., Cooper, C., Reginster, J. Y., Abrahamsen, B., Adachi, J. D., Brandi, M. L., Bruyere, O., Compston, J., Ducy, P., Ferrari, S., Harvey, N. C., Kanis, J. A., Karsenty, G., Laslop, A., Rabenda, V. & Vestergaard, P. 2012. Antidepressant medications and osteoporosis. *Bone*, 51, 606–613.

Roca, C. A., Schmidt, P. J., Deuster, P. A., Danaceau, M. A., Altemus, M., Putnam, K., Chrousos, G. P., Nieman, L. K. & Rubinow, D. R. 2005. Sex-related differences in stimulated hypothalamic-pituitary-adrenal axis during induced gonadal suppression. *J Clin Endocrinol Metab*, 90, 4224–4231.

Sacher, J., Neumann, J., Okon-Singer, H., Gotowiec, S. & Villringer, A. 2013. Sexual dimorphism in the human brain: evidence from neuroimaging. *Magn Reson Imaging*, 31, 366–375.

Sacher, J., Wilson, A. A., Houle, S., Rusjan, P., Hassan, S., Bloomfield, P. M., Stewart, D. E. & Meyer, J. H. 2010. Elevated brain monoamine oxidase A binding in the early postpartum period. *Arch Gen Psychiatry*, 67, 468–474.

Sanders, B. K. 2012. Flowers for Algernon: steroid dysgenesis, epigenetics and brain disorders. *Pharmacol Rep*, 64, 1285–1290.

Seidlitz, L. & Diener, E. 1998. Sex differences in the recall of affective experiences. *J Pers Soc Psychol*, 74, 262–271.

Shams, T., Firwana, B., Habib, F., Alshahrani, A., Alnouh, B., Murad, M. H. & Ferwana, M. 2013. SSRIs for hot flashes: a systematic review and meta-Analysis of randomized trials. *J Gen Intern Med*. doi: 10.1007/s11606-013-2535-9.

Shea, M. L., Garfield, L. D., Teitelbaum, S., Civitelli, R., Mulsant, B. H., Reynolds, C. F., 3RD, Dixon, D., Dore, P. & Lenze, E. J. 2013. Serotonin-norepinephrine reuptake inhibitor therapy in late-life depression is associated with increased marker of bone resorption. *Osteoporos Int*, 24, 1741–1749.

Smith, L. J., Henderson, J. A., Abell, C. W. & Bethea, C. L. 2004. Effects of ovarian steroids and raloxifene on proteins that synthesize, transport, and degrade serotonin in the raphe region of macaques. *Neuropsychopharmacology*, 29, 2035–2045.

Stein, M. B., Koverola, C., Hanna, C., Torchia, M. G. & Mcclarty, B. 1997. Hippocampal volume in women victimized by childhood sexual abuse. *Psychol Med*, 27, 951–959.

Stetler, C. & Miller, G. E. 2011. Depression and hypothalamic-pituitary-adrenal activation: a quantitative summary of four decades of research. *Psychosom Med*, 73, 114–126.

Stevens, J. S. & Hamann, S. 2012. Sex differences in brain activation to emotional stimuli: a meta-analysis of neuroimaging studies. *Neuropsychologia*, 50, 1578–1593.

Stoltenborgh, M., van Ijzendoorn, M. H., Euser, E. M. & Bakermans-Kranenburg, M. J. 2011. A global perspective on child sexual abuse: meta-analysis of prevalence around the world. *Child Maltreat*, 16, 79–101.

Stroud, L. R., Salovey, P. & Epel, E. S. 2002. Sex differences in stress responses: social rejection versus achievement stress. *Biol Psychiatry*, 52, 318–327.

Studd, J. & Nappi, R. E. 2012. Reproductive depression. *Gynecol Endocrinol*, 28 Suppl 1, 42–45.

Svedbom, A., Hernlund, E., Ivergard, M., Compston, J., Cooper, C., Stenmark, J., Mccloskey, E. V., Jonsson, B. & Kanis, J. A. 2013. Osteoporosis in the European Union: a compendium of country-specific reports. *Arch Osteoporos*, 8, 137.

Tak, L. M., Cleare, A. J., Ormel, J., Manoharan, A., Kok, I. C., Wessely, S. & Rosmalen, J. G. 2011. Meta-analysis and meta-regression of hypothalamic-pituitary-adrenal axis activity in functional somatic disorders. *Biol Psychol*, 87, 183–194.

Taylor, C. B., Youngblood, M. E., Catellier, D., Veith, R. C., Carney, R. M., Burg, M. M., Kaufmann, P. G., Shuster, J., Mellman, T., Blumenthal, J. A., Krishnan, R. & Jaffe, A. S. 2005. Effects of antidepressant medication on morbidity and mortality in depressed patients after myocardial infarction. *Arch Gen Psychiatry*, 62, 792–798.

Tian, L., Wang, J., Yan, C. & He, Y. 2011. Hemisphere- and gender-related differences in small-world brain networks: a resting-state functional MRI study. *NeuroImage*, 54, 191–202.

Tokarz, J., Moller, G., Hrabe de Angelis, M. & Adamski, J. 2013. Zebrafish and steroids: what do we know and what do we need to know? *J Steroid Biochem Mol Biol*, 137, 165–173.

Twenge, J. M. & Nolen-Hoeksema, S. 2002. Age, gender, race, socioeconomic status, and birth cohort differences on the children's depression inventory: a meta-analysis. *J Abnorm Psychol*, 111, 578–588.

Vadla, D., Bozikov, J., Blazekovic-Milakovic, S. & Kovacic, L. 2013. Anxiety and depression in elderly-prevalence and association with health care. *Lijec Vjesn*, 135, 134–138.

van Essen, D. C. & Ugurbil, K. 2012. The future of the human connectome. *NeuroImage*, 62, 1299–1310.

Versteeg, H., Hoogwegt, M. T., Hansen, T. B., Pedersen, S. S., Zwisler, A. D. & Thygesen, L. C. 2013. Depression, not anxiety, is independently associated with 5-year hospitalizations and mortality in patients with ischemic heart disease. *J Psychosom Res*, 75, 518–525.

Vythilingam, M., Heim, C., Newport, J., Miller, A. H., Anderson, E., Bronen, R., Brummer, M., Staib, L., Vermetten, E., Charney, D. S., Nemeroff, C. B. & Bremner, J. D. 2002. Childhood trauma associated with smaller hippocampal volume in women with major depression. *Am J Psychiatry*, 159, 2072–2080.

Walker, E. F., Trotman, H. D., Pearce, B. D., Addington, J., Cadenhead, K. S., Cornblatt, B. A., Heinssen, R., Mathalon, D. H., Perkins, D. O., Seidman, L. J., Tsuang, M. T., Cannon, T. D., Mcglashan, T. H. & Woods, S. W. 2013. Cortisol levels and risk for psychosis: initial findings from the north american prodrome longitudinal study. *Biol Psychiatry*, 74, 410–417.

Weber, M. T., Maki, P. M. & Mcdermott, M. P. 2013. Cognition and mood in perimenopause: a systematic review and meta-analysis. *J Steroid Biochem Mol Biol*.

Weich, S., Sloggett, A. & Lewis, G. 2001. Social roles and the gender difference in rates of the common mental disorders in Britain: a 7-year, population-based cohort study. *Psychol Med*, 31, 1055-64. doi: 10.1016/j.jsbmb.2013.06.001.

Weiss, E. L., Longhurst, J. G. & Mazure, C. M. 1999. Childhood sexual abuse as a risk factor for depression in women: psychosocial and neurobiological correlates. *Am J Psychiatry*, 156, 816–828.

Wharton, W., Gleason, C. E., Olson, S. R., Carlsson, C. M. & Asthana, S. 2012. Neurobiological Underpinnings of the Estrogen-Mood Relationship. *Curr Psychiatry Rev*, 8, 247–256.

WHO 2008. The Global Burden of Disease 2004 update.

Winkler, D., Pjrek, E. & Kasper, S. 2005. Anger attacks in depression-evidence for a male depressive syndrome. *Psychother Psychosom*, 74, 303–307.

Wisner, K. L., Sit, D. K., Mcshea, M. C., Rizzo, D. M., Zoretich, R. A., Hughes, C. L., Eng, H. F., Luther, J. F., Wisniewski, S. R., Costantino, M. L., Confer, A. L., Moses-Kolko, E. L., Famy, C. S. & Hanusa, B. H. 2013. Onset timing, thoughts of self-harm, and diagnoses in postpartum women with screen-positive depression findings. *JAMA Psychiatry*, 70, 490–498.

Witte, A. V., Savli, M., Holik, A., Kasper, S. & Lanzenberger, R. 2010. Regional sex differences in grey matter volume are associated with sex hormones in the young adult human brain. *NeuroImage*, 49, 1205–1212.

Workman, J. L., Barha, C. K. & Galea, L. A. 2012. Endocrine substrates of cognitive and affective changes during pregnancy and postpartum. *Behav Neurosci*, 126, 54–72.

Yirmiya, R. & Bab, I. 2009. Major depression is a risk factor for low bone mineral density: a meta-analysis. *Biol Psychiatry*, 66, 423–432.

Yoshimura, S., Sakamoto, S., Kudo, H., Sassa, S., Kumai, A. & Okamoto, R. 2003. Sex-differences in adrenocortical responsiveness during development in rats. *Steroids*, 68, 439–445.

Young, E. A. & Altemus, M. 2004. Puberty, ovarian steroids, and stress. *Ann N Y Acad Sci*, 1021, 124–133.

Yuan, J., Luo, Y., Yan, J. H., Meng, X., Yu, F. & Li, H. 2009. Neural correlates of the females' susceptibility to negative emotions: an insight into gender-related prevalence of affective disturbances. *Hum Brain Mapp*, 30, 3676–3686.

Zorumski, C. F. & Mennerick, S. 2013. Neurosteroids as therapeutic leads in psychiatry. *JAMA Psychiatry*, 70, 659–660.

Zorumski, C. F., Paul, S. M., Izumi, Y., Covey, D. F. & Mennerick, S. 2013. Neurosteroids, stress and depression: potential therapeutic opportunities. *Neurosci Biobehav Rev*, 37, 109–122.

Zuo, X. N., Kelly, C., di Martino, A., Mennes, M., Margulies, D. S., Bangaru, S., Grzadzinski, R., Evans, A. C., Zang, Y. F., Castellanos, F. X. & Milham, M. P. 2010. Growing together and growing apart: regional and sex differences in the lifespan developmental trajectories of functional homotopy. *J Neurosci*, 30, 15034–15043.

Chapter

20

Anxiety and depression in women in old age

Robert C. Baldwin and Jane Garner

One is not born a woman: one becomes one.
Simone de Beauvoir, Le Deuxieme Sexe (1949)

Introduction

Gender, age, ethnicity and class are major dimensions of social inequality in human societies (see Chapter 1). Mental illness adds to this inequality and to stigmatization. Gender and age, although with roots in biology, are both understood within a social context. Women in later life may be seen as comprising the negative myths that surround both the feminine and old age.

In classical mythology, the three Fates were conceived of as old women at a spinning wheel determining men's life spans and destinies. Clotho draws out the thread of life; Lachesis measures it out; Atropos cuts it off. This duality of women, the weaker sex, but with a dark and powerful side, is evident in religions, pseudoscience, art and literature. Old age similarly attracts fables that emerge from and influence deeply ingrained fears and attitudes. Old age rarely attracts positive epithets, usually they are denigratory or patronizing – grumpy old, boring old, sweet old ... We praise old people not for aging well but for seeming younger than their years.

This negative perception is reflected in the way older people view themselves. Aging is a wound to one's narcissism and self-esteem. To counteract it, it is possible to enumerate many who have overcome the barriers and handicaps of age, but an idealization of a few biographies (Garner & Ardern 1998) does not adequately redress the balance in a culture where most would fail by comparison with the youth-centered norm. Elders are defined as a "minority" group, except of course numerically where the expectation is that

services will be overwhelmed and the (younger) taxpayer will be burdened by this tide of need and dependence. Stereotypes of masculinity and femininity change with advancing years. The loss of "men are strong and women are beautiful" simplicities may be felt as a personal blow to the older person who struggles to seem younger. The inequalities between the genders may seem more unfair to older women. The Jungian Archetype "senex" (Hubback, 1996) seems very male. Old women do not command the adjective "wise." The mature man will be seen as having character lines, the old woman wrinkles. The lusty old man with an eye for the ladies is admired for his energy and continued libido, the elderly woman with sexual interests is seen perjoratively. The dominant cultural storyline is of asexual older women (Jones, 2002).

Old people, being part of society, have incorporated these concepts into their own view of themselves. Few clinicians have questioned the prevailing myths about women, old age and even psychological disorders. Freud regarded the feminine as a lack of a penis and old age as the castration of youth: old women associated with images of absence.

Psychiatrists have not been immune from myths and misconceptions regarding clinical disorders in old age. It is thought that depression in later life is symptomatically different, more common, more chronic, more difficult to treat and more often caused by psychological factors. The evidence does not bear this out. Levels of depression in later life are typically lower than for adults in middle age and younger adulthood (Blazer, 2010). However, these ideas, untruths, among lay and professional people continue to generate a pessimism that does a disservice to older people suffering from depression. The majority of women in late life are not depressed

Comprehensive Women's Mental Health, ed. David J. Castle and Kathryn M. Abel. Published by Cambridge University Press.
© Cambridge University Press 2016.

but still the doctor may say or think "you are old, widowed, arthritic, living on only a pension – what do you expect?" As for any "minority" group it is easy to categorize them together with general descriptions, to stereotype older women rather than look at the unique individual personal history and experience each brings to their current situation. Old women are more than their age and their gender.

Old-age psychiatrists see people born over four decades with inevitably different experiences and cohort effects. External socioeconomic factors leave their psychological mark in the internal world. Contemporary postmodern western society with its self-absorbed emphasis on youth, beauty, fashion, lifestyle and individuality is a difficult place to be old, particularly old and ill (Garner, 2004). The increased sexualization of society does no favors to older women, who are supposed to be asexual, but nevertheless may be struggling with unmet needs (Garner & Bacelle 2004). In younger life when thinking about old age, there will have been anticipated roles and activities. However, rapid societal changes, social mobility for family members, marital problems in retirement, becoming a carer, widowhood or financial problems may change and upset plans. The prospect of some freedom in later life will also be blighted if the woman herself becomes ill. Chronic and multiple handicaps may accumulate, either increasing isolation or forcing a change of accommodation.

When does old age begin? The popular saying is that a man is as old as he feels, a woman as old as she looks. Junkers (2006) observes that the period when people are called old has been extended by more than 20 years since the early twentieth century. Women are consistently viewed as aging more rapidly and sooner than men (Covey, 1992). Psychiatry services for older people tend to be organized around the age of 65 and above.

Psychological development and old age

Psychological development poses a number of challenges and opportunities that can trigger depression or mitigate it. This section considers this in the context of old age.

For Freud development was a childhood task only. Jung (1931) spoke of the "morning" of life being different from the "afternoon" of life, which was governed by distinct principles, a focus on culture and spirituality and the necessity of giving serious attention to the self to achieve individuation. Erikson (1959) also saw development continuing beyond early

libidinal stages throughout the life cycle with specific tasks to be negotiated in each of the eight phases he described. His framework was the person's attitude to and interaction with the world emphasizing cultural as well as intrapsychic factors; the life cycle is charted through social science and psychoanalysis. The final developmental stage is of "ego-integrity versus despair and disgust." The person with integrity sees his or her personal life and history to be as it had to be: his or her route through life was the only possible one for him or her. The one without emotional integration is despairing that there is no more time to try out different paths now death is near; the fear is of "not being" rather than valuing the experiences one has had. In addition to this task, the mark left by the previous seven stages may be stimulated by the exigencies of old age.

The challenges of later life for women particularly involve accepting bodily changes with equanimity; reconsidering the marital relationship in retirement, the children having left; perhaps feeling one has failed as a mother, paradoxically worse for those who are childless; coming to terms with increasing dependency, perhaps also forced dependency in residential or nursing home care; retirement, which may or may not live up to expectations; widowhood; financially straitened circumstances, particularly if she had been dependent on her husband to make pension contributions on her behalf; the cultural expectation of an asexual old age; and the sexism and agism that is a part of sociocultural existence.

The assumption that older women do not have libido is just that. Of a surveyed group of reasonably healthy women, ranging in age from 80 to 102, 70% still fantasized about intimacy with men, 64% engaged in touching and caressing men, 40% masturbated and 25% had a regular sexual partner (Bretschneider & McCoy, 1989). If women do experience a decline in libido this tends to start at or around menopause rather than late in life. Subsequent to this, sexual interest is influenced less by age than health, medication and availability of a partner (Bretschneider & McCoy, 1989). Sexual needs across the lifespan may not differ dramatically, although older women voice more concerns about their partner's sexual difficulties (Nusbaum et al., 2004). Even these contemporary findings date quickly in societies where attitudes to same-sex relationships are undergoing rapid change, a subject hardly touched when considering later-life partnerships. Many older women would welcome the opportunity to discuss sexual concerns at consultation but few physicians seem willing to initiate this (Nusbaum et al., 2004). Perhaps things are changing for the better. In a Swedish study (Beckman et al., 2008) the quantity and quality of sexual experiences of 70-year-olds had improved over a 30-year period. There is no reason why sexuality should not continue to develop in old age and for wider society to accept and encourage this aspect of a healthy old age.

Positive factors in old age are predominantly the adaptive personality traits, strengths and coping strategies one brings into the senium; for those with sufficient internal resources, aging itself may be a creative process in developmental adaptation (Garner, 2004). Other positive factors include an increased diversity, greater individuality, a capacity for delayed gratification and being a resource for others (Garner, 2009). Coming to terms with one's own inevitable death is a task for middle age (Knight, 1986), which, if successfully accomplished, eases later years. The capacity to make mutual and sharing relationships with family, but particularly with friends, will help women deal with this time of their life. Fooken (1994) suggests that sexuality promotes health in later life. For those whose pension is sufficient, the removal of the pressure for paid employment may be helpful but only if sufficient activity of some sort fills the available time; exercising body and mind extends the span of healthy life.

Epidemiology

Depression

Nearly twice as many women as men suffer from major depressive disorder. This difference continues into extreme old age but the differential decreases (see Chapter 7). The higher prevalence of depression among women is due to a higher risk of first onset rather than differential persistence/chronicity or recurrence (Kessler, 2003). The cause of the gender difference in rates is not known but speculation covers cognitive styles, psychosocial and economic stress, an increased rate of abuse in childhood and in the work place, an increase in the incidence of hypothyroidism, and other biological factors related to the effects of endogenous and exogenous gonadal steroids (there is no sex difference in incidence before adolescence). For a fuller exposition of these factors, the reader is referred to Chapters 1, 7, and 19 of this book. However, these differences only pertain to unipolar depression. For bipolar disorder, the male/

female ratio is equal (Blehar et al. 1998) although women tend to have more depressive and fewer manic episodes (see also Chapter 21).

The rate of depressive disorder in residential and nursing homes where the population is predominantly female is 2 to 3 times higher than in community surveys. There may be a number of reasons why this is so. Inevitably, this population will have many with physical illness and handicaps; there may also be comorbidity with dementia.

Anxiety

There are difficulties in arriving at estimates of prevalence for anxiety disorders in later life. First, the most widely used classificatory systems for psychiatric disorder are hierarchical and tend to subsume symptoms of anxiety under depressive disorder. Second, judging whether symptoms of anxiety are "understandable" is not easy. What may start as an appropriately cautious response to threat, for example, fear of falling or fear of crime, can spiral into disabling fear and phobic avoidance. Fear of falling has even been proposed as a form of agoraphobia in the elderly (Kay, 1988).

Lindesay et al. (1989), in a community survey of elderly individuals in the UK, found that the prevalence of generalized anxiety disorder was 3.7% and of phobias 10%. Among the latter, specific phobias were often longstanding and agoraphobia associated with physical disability. Save for specific phobias, which were equally distributed between the sexes, the rates for women were 2 to 3 times those of men. Using a symptom check-list, a more recent study found that 15% of older people were anxious, rising to 43% in those who were concurrently depressed (Mehta et al., 2003). Again women predominated.

Classification and diagnosis

With the exception of increased hypochondriasis and a greater preoccupation with poor memory, the symptoms of major depression do not alter dramatically over the adult life span (Baldwin, 2008). An unanswered question, though, is whether the term major depression adequately encompasses all clinically relevant forms of mood disorder in later life. A clue comes from epidemiological studies, which show that for every older woman with major depression between two to four more have "subthreshold" symptoms (Beekman et al., 1999). There is no perfect way to classify these syndromes but terms such as "minor" depression and "subsyndromal" depression are used. "Minor" depression is not trivial depression; it is associated with considerable morbidity (Katon et al., 2003).

A factor analysis using a depression rating scale in 14 European countries identified two that represented the main classes seen in older people. One was called "affective suffering," characterized by depression, tearfulness and a wish to die; this was associated with the female gender. The second was a "motivation" factor, comprising loss of interest, poor concentration and anhedonia; this showed a positive correlation with age but not gender. Speculatively, this may be linked to the emerging concept of vascular depression, a form of late-onset depression associated with vascular disease and more "deficit" depressive symptoms such as poor motivation (Alexopoulos et al., 1997).

These modest, age-related differences in symptoms are outweighed by more general factors, which may mask the presentation or detection of late-life depression. These include poor health, alcohol misuse, medication effects and comorbid psychiatric disorder, notably dementia (Baldwin, 2008).

Detection can be difficult. Medical comorbidity may obscure interpretation of physical depressive symptoms such as appetite change or reduced energy. It is unusual for a neurosis to present *de novo* in later life. Where marked symptoms of anxiety, obsessive-compulsive symptoms or phobia newly present, the underlying cause is usually depressive disorder. Hysteria, the latter-day classical condition of women, is rare in old age. Most "hysterical" symptoms in later life arise from organic disorders or depression.

Burden of depression

Depression is predicted to be the second leading illness associated with negative impact and disease burden by 2020 (Lopez & Murray, 1998). As a cause of morbidity, depression ranks alongside most major disabling medical conditions (Wells et al., 1989). It is now recognized that "subthreshold" depression constitutes an important public health problem as its prevalence is high and it is associated with almost as much impairment of quality of life and function as major depression (Blazer, 2003). It is also a risk factor for major depression.

After a decline lasting several decades, the suicide rate for people aged 65 years and over rose 9% between 1980 and 1992 (CDC, 1996). The increase was most dramatic for women and men aged 80–84 years, the fastest growing segment of the population, for whom the rate rose over 35% during this 12-year period. Among young adults, those who commit suicide have a heterogeneous mixture of psychotic, mood and substance use disorders. In middle age, affective and addictive disorders predominate. Older people who kill themselves constitute a more homogeneous population in which nonaffective psychoses are rare, addictive disorders are less common and late-onset major depression is the rule (Conwell et al., 1996). Substance misuse, whilst less common than among younger adults who kill themselves, is not rare. In the survey of Conwell et al. (1996) of older adults, almost half of those who killed themselves had both depressive disorder and substance (mainly alcohol) misuse. Chui et al. (2010) note that all the major mental disorders of late life increase the risk of completed suicide.

Depressive disorder adds to disability from physical disorder when present and is associated with greater physical decline (Penninx et al., 2000). There is a strong relationship between mental health and physical health. This influence works in both directions with inextricable linkage (Royal College of Psychiatrists, 2013). Depressed older women are at increased risk of hip fracture (Whooley et al., 1999). They are less likely to adhere to medical treatments (Dimatteo et al., 2000). Conversely, poorer health is associated with a worse prognosis for depression (Lyness et al., 1999), again emphasizing the two-way nature of the interaction. This is a complex subject, involving putative mechanisms such as immune function, hypothalamic hormones, turnover of substances such as homocysteine, cytokines and vascular processes, and is beyond the scope of this chapter. To give a flavor, though, a group of older adults (mean age 71 years) were rated for depressive symptoms before being given an influenza vaccination and afterwards. Those with even a modest number of depressive symptoms had a significantly greater and longer inflammatory response (assessed by interleukin 6 levels) compared to those who were not depressed (Glaser et al., 2003).

Depressive symptoms in older women are associated with both poorer cognitive function and subsequent cognitive decline (Yaffe et al., 1999); and female gender is a risk factor for both depression and Alzheimer's disease. In a study of 2000 patients with Alzheimer's disease (the MIRAGE study; Green et al., 2003), depression contributed significantly to the risk for up to 25 years, even after controlling for other factors.

Mortality is increased in older patients with depressive disorder (Murphy et al., 1988). Although much of this is due to comorbid physical disorder, depression is an independent risk factor (Blazer, 2003). However, in one study women with subthreshold depression, as opposed to depressive disorder or no depression, had significantly reduced mortality (Hybels et al., 2002). This counterintuitive finding may accord with suggestions that some forms of depression may be adaptive (Nesse, 2000). Speculatively, in women, this may reflect in women a biological drive to retreat from external threats in order to focus on more immediate protective functions (Hybels et al., 2002).

The economic health burden of depression in late life is high. In a large study of older people living at home, the total outpatient costs were 43% to 52% higher and combined inpatient and outpatient costs 47% to 51% higher in depressed compared with nondepressed elderly patients after adjustment for chronic medical illness. This increase was seen in every component of health care costs, with only a small percentage due to mental health treatment. No differences in costs were seen between those with subthreshold depressive syndromes compared to those with major depression (Katon et al., 2003).

Risk and protective factors

Predisposing factors

Age alone is not a risk factor for women in the development of depression or anxiety, nor is family history (Baldwin, 2008). A history of depression, suicide attempts or other psychiatric disorders increases the likelihood of a further depressive episode. Comorbid medical illness is a major risk factor in late onset depression. Up to 50% of general hospital patients may also be depressed, and there is an association with a variety of systemic medical and neurological disorders as well as medication (Szewczyk & Chennault 1997) (Table 20.1). Depression may mimic dementia, herald it or increase the risk of developing it (Barnes et al., 2012; Green et al., 2003).

In refining the impact of physical illness as a risk factor for depression, Prince et al. (1998) identified handicap, the social disadvantage that accompanies disability, as an important determinant. Two older women may share a similar degree of disability from arthritis. If one has inadequate local transport then she is the more handicapped. The concept of handicap lends itself to practical remedies.

Table 20.1 Medical conditions and central-acting drugs that may cause organic depression

MEDICAL CONDITIONS	CENTRAL-ACTING DRUGS
Endocrine / metabolic	**Anti-hypertensive drugs**
Hypo / hyperthyroidism	Beta-blockers
Cushing's disease	Methyldopa
Hypercalcemia	Reserpine (rarely used)
Pernicious anemia	Clonidine
Organic brain disease	Nifedipine
Stroke	Digoxin
CNS tumors	**Steroids / analgesic drugs**
Parkinson's disease	Opioids
Alzheimer's disease and	Indomethacin
vascular dementia	**Anti-Parkinson's**
Multiple sclerosis	L-dopa preparations
Systemic lupus	Amantadine
erythematosus (SLE)	Tetrabenazine
Occult carcinoma	**Psychiatric drugs**
Pancreas	Neuroleptics
Lung	Benzodiazepines
Chronic infections	**Miscellaneous**
Neurosyphilis	Sulphonamides
Brucellosis	
AIDS	

Widowhood, divorce, stressful life events and poor social support are also risk factors (Lepine & Bouchez 1998; Kivela et al., 1998b). Social isolation and a lack of a close confiding relationship predispose to late-life depression. The latter appears to reflect personality traits rather than simply a lack of opportunity (Murphy, 1982). Early loss, maternal loss among men and an early loss of the father among women are risk factors for depression (Kivela et al., 1998a). Poverty and lower social class are linked to depression but probably via poorer health, itself a major risk factor (Murphy, 1982).

Whether age-related brain changes increase the susceptibility to depression in later life is of great interest. Some, but by no means all, brain biochemical changes associated with aging are similar to those seen in depression. For example, both are associated with decreased brain concentrations of serotonin, dopamine, noradrenaline and their metabolites, and increased MAO-B activity (Veith & Raskind, 1988). A variety of neuroendocrine changes are associated with aging (Veith & Raskind, 1988). Aging is associated with increasing cortisol levels and cortisol non-suppression (Alexopoulos, et al., 1984). It seems likely that normal aging is associated with enhanced limbic-HPA axis activity, perhaps related to neuronal degeneration in the hippocampus; this may be exacerbated by raised glucocorticoid secretion, caused either by depression or repeated stressful life events or both (the "feed-forward cascade"; Sapolsky et al., 1986).

However, the much-touted term "age-related" is probably inaccurate. Many, perhaps most, geriatric syndromes are due to pathology rather than age. Research into the relationship between late-onset depression and vascular pathology supports this (Baldwin & O'Brien, 2002).

Changes in estrogen levels are associated with depression. Although the perimenopausal period is associated with an increase in depressive symptoms there is no definite evidence of a rise in depressive disorder (Cutter et al., 2003).

Risk factors for suicide in later life include depression, chronic illness, social isolation and alcohol misuse. Older women with depression and longstanding anxiety may also be at increased risk (Waern et al., 2002).

Personality and coping styles are important. As already mentioned, many older women begin to acknowledge their own mortality in mid-life, so for them negotiating death may be a less difficult task in later years. For others, death is a persecutory or depressive anxiety (Carvalho, 2008). If this anxiety is great enough life may be over before death (Quinodoz, 2010). Turner (1992) sees death as a longitudinal issue: if one fears death when young, one also fears it when old. As old age is not an event but a process, it will depend on the whole of a preceding life and how individuality and particularity have been molded. The most vulnerable older adults are those who have to date focused on a single sphere of activity: work-centered men and child-centered women in role-divided marriages; these marriages tend, also, to be less intimate and sexually unfulfilled (Thompson, 1993).

Precipitating factors

Loss life events often precipitate depression in susceptible individuals. In later life, especially for women, the major example is the loss of a life partner. However, other painful losses include health deterioration, loss of function, death of a pet, role changes at retirement, children or friends moving away and the loss of one's home. Some losses may reawaken earlier grief.

Among the long-term widowed, rates of depression decline, suggesting that a majority of elderly widows do eventually adjust. However, this may take a number of years (Turvey et al., 1999).

Going into a residential or nursing home may seem to others the right and logical decision but to the older person it often signifies a loss of independence, choice, privacy and the familiarities of one's own home, street and neighborhood. Moving homes is immensely stressful (Holmes & Rahe, 1967) and particularly if it is seen as the last move one will make or if becoming more physically dependent reawakens childhood failures or leads to overidentification with the frailties of one's own parents (Martindale, 2007). If clinical assessments prior to the move are not comprehensive, failure to function at home may not be recognized as depression. Achterberg et al. (2003) found that low social engagement was very common in newly admitted nursing home residents in the Netherlands and that depression was an important independent risk factor.

The role of less obviously catastrophic life events ("daily hassles") are greater than is generally realized, especially if occurring close to other significant losses (Murdock et al., 1998).

As both a risk factor and a precipitant, caregiving deserves a special mention. By virtue of traditional roles and because of their longevity, women are often the main caregivers. A high proportion of those caring for someone with dementia will become depressed and the majority are women (Ballard et al., 1996). Female carers attract less formal and informal support than male ones. Women as Carers are considered fully in Chapter 3 of this book.

Protective factors

True to the stereotype of old age as uniformly bleak, little has been written about factors that are likely to be protective against depression such as the arrival of grandchildren, improved financial security or "fresh start" experiences including new friendships and relationships. Although retirement is usually greeted with mixed feelings (Kelly & Barratt, 2007; Boyd-Carpenter, 2010), for those who do not see work as the whole of life, the increased time and rekindled energy can be used to increase existing skills or acquire new ones.

Whether or not a woman's marital state is a risk or protective factor is a matter of much debate.

It would seem that marital dissatisfaction is uniquely related to major depression and post-traumatic stress disorder for women (Whisman, 1999). Protective factors include the ability to make confiding relationships and friendships and being able to maintain them over time. This includes having the ability to accept appropriate help when increasing difficulties occur, as well as to make relationships with formal and informal carers. Having a religious conviction has been shown to be protective from depression in later life (Blazer, 2003). Older women may take on particular roles in different religions. The ability to maintain a meaningful life focus may be crucial (Thompson, 1993).

The higher rate of depression in older women than men is found across cultures. The prevalence of depression in African American and Hispanic women is twice that in men. Major depression seems to be diagnosed less frequently in African American women and more frequently in Hispanic than in Caucasian women. Different groups may express depression and anxiety in different ways. Harralson et al. (2002) explored similarities and differences in depression among black and white nursing home residents in Philadelphia, Pennsylvania, United States. White residents were more likely to report psychological symptoms and blacks to report somatic symptoms. Functional disability was an important predictor of depression in both groups.

Ego integrity (Erikson, 1959), with the internal knowledge that it implies, will facilitate resilience in later life, perhaps having had containing and dependable early care opening the possibility of accepting dependency in later life with some equanimity (Garner, 2013).

Compared to depression, less is known about risk factors for anxiety disorders in later life, but women are more at risk than men (Kay, 1988). As with depression, white race is associated with greater risk than black (Mehta et al, 2003). Several physical disorders may cause anxiety. The more common include thyroid disorder, chronic obstructive pulmonary disease, pulmonary embolism, Meniere's disease, hypoglycaemia and paroxysmal tachyarrhythmias (Kay, 1988). In women urinary incontinence is a neglected cause (Mehta et al., 2003). Hypochondriasis is closely linked to depression but in Europe is also classified separately as one of the somatoform disorders. In psychotic depression hypochondriacal delusions are common (Baldwin, 2008). Interestingly, in older women hypochondriasis does not correlate with the degree of physical illness present (Kramer-Ginsberg et al, 1989).

Management
Depression
Assessment

Until recently, rating scales to measure depression were not ideally suited to older adults. Perhaps the most widely used, the Hamilton Rating Scale for Depression (Hamilton, 1960), contains a number of somatic symptoms that may be hard to interpret in the older adult. The Montgomery Asberg Depression Rating Scale is perhaps more appropriate (Mottram et al., 2000). The Geriatric Depression Scale (GDS) is specifically designed for older people (Yesavage et al., 1983). This self- or assisted-rated tool is available in versions from 4 to 30 items and has been translated into a number of languages, most of which can be found on a free website (http://stanford.edu/~yesavage/GDS.html). The GDS works reasonably well in cases of mild to moderate dementia but loses sensitivity in patients with severe dementia (Baldwin, 2008). The GDS is reproduced in Table 20.2. It can be completed online. The Cornell Depression Rating Scale (Alexopoulos et al., 1988) has been developed to detect depression in those with dementia. It utilizes information from a caregiver as well as the patient.

Bearing in mind the earlier discussion about sexuality in later life, of the three scales mentioned, only the Hamilton rates libido and under the unsatisfactory item "genital symptoms," which includes "menstrual disturbance."

Screening for depression using rating scales is useful but is not a substitute for clinical skills. The history should include medical illness, medication (including over-the-counter drugs such as analgesics), alcohol intake and information about recent life events. Modifications to the clinical interview (shorter sessions, slower pace) may be required if there is sensory impairment, poor health or pain. A cognitive assessment should be included. This can be undertaken by using the Montreal Cognitive Assessment (MoCA; Nasredinne et al., 2005) or the briefer 6-item Orientation-Memory-Concentration (OMC; Brooke & Bullock, 1999). The MoCa can be downloaded from: www.mocatest.org/default.asp along with scoring instructions. Provided it is used for clinical purposes, copyright permission is not required.

Table 20.2 Geriatric Depression Scale

Instructions: Choose the best answer for how you have felt over the past week.

*1. Are you basically satisfied with your life? No

*2. Have you dropped many of your activities and interests? Yes

3. Do you feel your life is empty? Yes

4. Do you often get bored? Yes

5. Are you hopeful about the future? No

6. Are you bothered by thoughts you can't get out of your head? Yes

7. Are you in good spirits most of the time? No

*8. Are you afraid something bad is going to happen to you? Yes

*9. Do you feel happy most of the time? No

10. Do you often feel helpless? Yes

11. Do you often get restless and fidgety? Yes

12. Do you prefer to stay at home, rather than going out and doing new things? Yes

13. Do you frequently worry about the future? Yes

14. Do you feel you have more problems with your memory than most? Yes

15. Do you think it is wonderful to be alive now? No

16. Do you often feel down-hearted and blue (sad)? Yes

17. Do you feel pretty worthless the way you are? Yes

18. Do you worry a lot about the past? Yes

19. Do you find life very exciting? No

20. Is it hard for you to start on new projects (plans)? Yes

21. Do you feel full of energy? No

22. Do you feel that your situation is hopeless? Yes

23. Do you think most people are better off (in their lives) than you are? Yes

24. Do you frequently get upset over little things? Yes

25. Do you frequently feel like crying? Yes

26. Do you have trouble concentrating? Yes

27. Do you enjoy getting up in the morning? No

28. Do you prefer to avoid social gatherings (get-togethers)? Yes

29. Is it easy for you to make decisions? No

30. Is your mind as clear as it used to be? No

Notes (1) Answers refer to responses which score '1'; (2) bracketed phrases refer to alternative ways of expressing the questions; (3) questions in bold comprise the 15-item version. Cut-off scores for *possible* depression: 10/11 (GDS30); 5/6 (GDS15); 1/2 (GDS4). *= 4-item GDS questions

At the time of writing, the Mini-Mental State Examination (Folstein et al., 1975) is subject to copyright and therefore payment.

A physical examination should be conducted. As mentioned, ill-health is often the trigger for severe depression (Table 20.1) and so is linked closely to prognosis. Laboratory investigation should include hemoglobin, full blood count, biochemical profile, B_{12} and folate levels. Severe depression can rapidly lead to undernutrition. Elderly people have less physiological reserve than younger adults. In a frail 80-year-old woman it may lead to serious metabolic derangement in a short time.

Specialist referral should be considered for patients where dementia is suspected; when depression is severe, as evidenced by psychotic depression or suicidality; where risk is present through failure to eat or drink; or when patients have not responded to first-line treatment.

Treatment principles

The treatment of late-life depression should be multimodal and multidisciplinary. General principles are outlined in Table 20.3. Full remission (no symptoms) rather than improvement is the goal. There is evidence of efficacy for antidepressants (compared to placebo) (Nelson et al., 2008); psychological treatments, notably Cognitive Behavior Therapy (CBT; Laidlaw, 2010) and Inter-Personal Therapy (van Shaik et al., 2008); and psychosocial interventions.

Shedler (2010) compared effect sizes for different types of therapy and antidepressant medication from meta-analyses of recent outcome studies. Effect sizes for dynamic psychotherapy were as large as those reported for other treatments. Further, there is good evidence that older people have outcomes from different kinds of psychotherapy at least equal to those for younger patients (Woods & Roth, 1996).

Antidepressants

There is no difference between women and men in terms of antidepressant response (Quitkin et al.,

Table 20.3 Management goals

Goal	Ways to achieve
Risk reduction – of suicide or harm from self-neglect	• A risk assessment and monitoring of risk • Prompt referral of urgent cases to a specialist
Remission of all depressive symptoms	• Providing appropriate treatment (usually an antidepressant and/or a psychological treatment) • Giving the patient and his/her supporters timely education about depression and its treatment
To help the patient achieve optimal function	• Enable practical support • Ensure access to appropriate agencies that can help
To treat the whole person, including somatic problems	• Treat co-existing physical health problems • Reduce wherever possible the effects of handicap caused by factors such as chronic disease, sensory impairment and poor mobility • Review medication and withdraw unnecessary ones
To prevent relapse and recurrence	• Educate the patient about staying on medication once recovered • Continuation of treatment (12 months after recovery, see text) • Maintenance treatment (preventive treatment, see text)

2002); nor is it true that older patients respond less well to antidepressants although attaining remission may be harder (Kok et al., 2012) and it may take 2 to 4 weeks longer to recover (Nelson et al., 2008). Selective Serotonin Reuptake Inhibitors (SSRIs) are nowadays usually the first-line choice. They are as effective as tricylics antidepressants and somewhat better tolerated. However, there has been some concern about an increased risk of upper gastrointestinal bleeding in older patients prescribed SSRIs who are taking aspirin or non-steroidal anti-inflammatory drugs (de Abajo et al., 1999). There is a greater likelihood of the Syndrome of Inappropriate Anti-Diuretic Hormone (SIADH) with SSRIs than other antidepressants.

Altered pharmacodyamics and kinetics coupled with frailty mean that initial antidepressant dosages may be half those recommended for younger adults. The adage "start low, go slow" is appropriate. A recent warning of effects on prolonging the ECG QT interval, with an increased risk of arrhythmia, with citalopram and escitalopram has led to revisions of the upper dose recommendations, to 20 mg and 10 mg respectively. The use of these drugs with antipsychotic drugs (as in psychotic depression or augmentation treatment) is not recommended, as antipsychotics are themselves pro-arrhythmic.

Antidepressants are effective in patients with comorbidity such as stroke, heart disease and chronic obstructive pulmonary disease (COPD) and are tolerated satisfactorily by patients in nursing homes, although no adequate trials of efficacy have been conducted. Unfortunately evidence shows that they are often ineffective in treating depression complicating Alzheimer's disease (Banerjee et al., 2011).

Average starting and therapeutic dosages for elderly patients, along with side effect profiles, are shown in Table 20.4.

Psychological and psychotherapeutic interventions

Psychological treatments are as effective as antidepressants for mild and moderate depressive disorder (Baldwin et al., 2003) and may be preferred by older patients over medication (Unűtzer et al., 2002). However, they are seldom readily available and a belief that medicine alone will eradicate depression may increase feelings of helplessness and dependence with poor long-term effects (Heifner, 1996). In fact there is increasing evidence that psychotherapy may produce neurobiological change in the patient (Shore, 1997). For example, there is a significant effect on serotonin metabolism (Viinamaki et al., 1998) and serotonin receptors (Karlsson, 2011). There is also evidence that attachment styles have physical and neural effects (Ciechanowski et al., 2001; Buchheim et al., 2011). In this sense, Freud the neurologist was correct in anticipating reconciliation between neurology and psychology.

Table 20.4

Drug	Main mode of action	Main side effects	Starting dosage (mg)	Average daily dose (mg)
Amitriptyline	NA++ 5HT+	Sedation Anticholinergic, postural hypotension, tachycardia / arrhythmia	25–50	75–100(*)
Imipramine	NA++ 5HT+	As for amitriptyline but less sedation	25	75–100(*)
Nortripyline	NA++ 5HT+	As for amitriptyline but less sedation, anticholinergic effects and hypotension	10 tds	75–100(*)
Dothiepin	NA++ 5HT+	As for amitripyline	50–75	75–150(*)
Lofepramine	NA++ 5HT+	As for amitriptyline but less sedation, anticholinergic effects, hypotension and cardiac problems	70–140	70–210
Trazodone	$5HT_2$	Sedation, dizziness, headache	100	300–400
Citalopram	5HT	Nausea, vomiting, dyspepsia, abdominal pain, diarrhea, headache, sexual dysfunction; risk of gastric bleeding; inappropriate ADH secretion	20	20
Sertraline	5HT	As for citalopram	50	100–200
Fluoxetine	5HT	As for citalopram but insomnia and agitation more common	20	20*
Paroxetine	5HT	As for citalopram but sedation and anticholinergic effects may occur	20	20
Fluvoxamine	5HT	As for citalopram but nausea more common	50–100	100–200
Escitalopram	5HT	As for citalopram	5	10
Moclobemide	MAO	Sleep disturbance, nausea, agitation	300	300–400
Venlafaxine	NA 5HT	Nausea, insomnia, dizziness, dry mouth, somnolence, hyper- and hypotension	75	150(**)
Duloxetine	NA 5HT	Nausea, insomnia, dizziness	30	60–90
Mirtazapine	α_2 blocking selective antagonist of $5HT_2$ and $5HT_3$ receptors	Increased appetite, weight gain, somnolence, headache	15	30–45
Bupropion	Noradrenaline / dopamine re-uptake inhibition	Seizures, hypertension; not sedative and less likely to cause weight gain or sexual side effects	150 bd (as extended release)	300 mg
Agomelatine	Melatonergic agonist (MT 1& 2 receptors); $5HT_{2c}$ antogonist	Dizziness, sickness, somnolence	25	25–50

* These are average doses. Some patients will require higher dosages depending on response and tolerability
** Titration up to higher dosages is common in specialist care
NA=noradrenaline; 5HT=serotonin; MAO=monoamine oxidase inhibitor
'+' indicates relative strength of monoamine effect

There are few studies examining the psychotherapies with older people and the results are rarely distinguished by gender. The most common theme is loss. Losses accumulate with age although each one is particular and specific (Knight & Satre, 1999). Pollack (1982) writes of the psychodynamic work in mourning leading to liberation and the possibilities of future freedoms. However, it may be impossible to recover from some losses, for example the loss of a child.

Other analysts too have eschewed Freud's (1905) dictum that people over 50 are no longer educable and have drawn on the work of Erikson (1959) and King (1974, 1980). In the UK, Hildebrand (1982) pioneered workshops aimed at helping younger therapists see patients who were struggling with the developmental tasks and difficulties of later life. Good supervision helps the therapist deal with powerful countertransferential feelings evoked by working with older, possibly disabled patients (Garner, 2004). The biological and social realities of the patients' lives need to be acknowledged. Physical pain and disability will not be alleviated by psychotherapy but the effects on the patient's life and relationships may be understood and changed. There are a number of accounts of group psychotherapy with older patients (Evans, 2004). This modality can diminish a sense of isolation, failure and shame (Garland, 2007). In a group, denial of age becomes less possible, helping patients to accept approaching death and the process of dying (Canete et al., 2000; Evans, 2004).

The lack of social interaction in nursing and residential homes is a potential focus for psychosocial interventions. Although the task may feel overwhelming, something can be done about the level of social engagement. Jones (2003) writes of the success of a nurse-led group, using a modified reminiscence technique, on the level of depression in elderly women in long-term care. Reminiscence therapy, as well as being a treatment in its own right, also increases the engagement and contact between staff and residents. Perhaps more attention needs to be given to admitting friends together (Dayson et al., 1998), as well as to increase the emotional engagement and understanding of the staff (Garner, 1998).

In a large-scale meta-analysis of psychosocial and psychotherapeutic interventions with older adults, Pinquart and Sorensen (2001) found CBT improved depression and subjective well-being, an effect that was greater if the therapist had had specialized training in work with older adults. CBT is now a mainstream treatment for depression and anxiety in later life (Laidlaw, 2008; Wilson et al., 2008), with evidence for its efficacy in primary care (Serfaty et al., 2009) and among the oldest old (Gallagher-Thompson & Thompson, 2010). Patients often attribute to aging – to being old – the signs and symptoms of depression. The attitude to aging needs to be a focus in all types of psychological treatments with older women (Laidlaw, 2010; Garner & Evans, 2010).

Life review is involved in many psychotherapeutic models and particularly in modifications that may be made for older adults. Creatively reminiscing, the patient may constructively reevaluate failures, achievements and relationships. Reminiscence can of itself be adaptive, helping to maintain a sense of permanence and continuity of the self. In a comparison of a life-review group and a cognitive therapy group, both treatments were equally effective, as measured by the Beck Depression Inventory and Life Satisfaction in the Elderly Scale; this also held true for the old-old group (Weiss, 1994).

Miller et al. (1994) used Interpersonal Psychotherapy (IPT) to spousal bereavement-related-depression in late life with some success, and IPT may hold promise in the treatment of dysthymia.

Resistant depression

Resistant depression should be approached in the same way as for younger patients (see Chapter 19), although in older adults white matter disease of the brain may be an additional factor in poor treatment response (Baldwin & O'Brien, 2002). The steps to consider are: optimize the dose; switch to an antidepressant from another class; combine two antidepressants from different classes; augment with a non-antidepressant. Lithium augmentation has a reasonable (albeit incomplete) evidence base (Baldwin, 2003), but is often not well tolerated by older people. Combining an antidepressant with an atypical antipsychotic drug is increasingly popular and has an evidence base (Nelson et al., 2009), but there is a real risk of precipitating the metabolic syndrome over time. For that reason, unless the combination is specifically to treat psychotic depression, the atypical agent should be reviewed at 4–6 months with a view to gradual discontinuation. Lipids, glucose, weight and waist circumference should be monitored. Age should not be a barrier to Electroconvulsive Therapy (ECT) in the right cases (generally to save life or prevent serious deterioration). It is generally well tolerated (Tew et al., 1999) but relapse rates are high. Combining medication with a psychological intervention gives the best results (Reynolds et al., 1999).

As yet, there is no definitive evidence that Hormone Replacement Therapy either protects against depression in older women or can be successfully used to treat it (Whooley et al., 2000; Cutter et al., 2003). Looking to the future, novel agents such as ketamine can induce short-term remission in resistant depression and is attracting research interest (see Chapter 19).

As with all clinical work, using psychological mindedness in interactions will be to the benefit of older patients with chronic resistant low mood and to their caregivers and staff endeavoring to look after them (Garner, 2008). Negative reactions among staff and caregivers toward patients with resistant symptoms are common and difficult to discuss but need to be addressed.

Anxiety

As at other ages, for panic disorder, generalized anxiety disorder, obsessive compulsive disorder (rare *de novo* in older people) and agoraphobia, first-line treatment is CBT with SSRIs the second-line choice. For more details the reader is referred to Chapter 18 of this book.

The anxieties of old age are not so different from universal anxieties such as loss, abandonment and loss of autonomy but the realities of later life may enhance a person's fear. Likewise, those with compensated disorders of personality, such as narcissism and dependency, can lapse into marked anxiety when facing such critical issues.

The Geriatric Anxiety Inventory (Pachana et al., 2007) was specifically developed for use with older people, and differentiates between anxiety and depression and anxiety related to physical symptoms of medical comorbidities.

Anxiolytic drugs

Used in the lowest possible dose for the shortest period of time benzodiazepines are highly effective in the short-term treatment of moderate-to-severe symptoms of anxiety. Treatment beyond 2 to 4 weeks risks dependency. As with antidepressants, starting dosages and therapeutic dosages are roughly half that of the younger adult (Table 20.5). Falls, sedation and

ataxia may occur in older adults and some may even develop a reversible dementia. Benzodiazepines are contraindicated in patients with respiratory depression, sleep apnea and severe hepatic impairment.

Buspirone is thought to act on $5HT_{1A}$ receptors and has a low risk of dependence but may take a number of days before it is effective. It does not counteract benzodiazepine withdrawal. Beta-blockers reduce somatic symptoms of anxiety but can be problematic in older patients because there is a risk of aggravating underlying physical problems such as bronchospasm, hypotension, heart failure and diabetes. Water-soluble beta-blockers such as atenolol are less likely to cross the blood-brain barrier and may be associated with fewer central nervous system side effects such as sleep disturbance and nightmares. Atenolol is also more cardioselective. The use of low-dose phenothiazines in the treatment of anxiety in older women is not recommended because of the risk of tardive dyskinesia. Pregabalin, an antiepileptic drug, is licensed for the treatment of anxiety and has an evidence base for later life (Montgomery et al., 2008).

Nonpharmacological interventions

In a large US survey of prescriptions, 7.5% of older people were prescribed anxiolytic drugs (Aparasu et al., 2003) while in Europe 15% were taking benzodiazepines even though they had no diagnosed mental disorder (Kirby et al., 1999). Higher prescription rates have been reported among widows and those who are socially isolated (Hartikainen et al., 2003) and older women are significantly more likely to be prescribed antianxiety drugs than are men (Aparasu et al., 2003). Older women taking such medication are 1.5 times more likely to have falls than nonusers, with no evidence that shorter-acting anxiolytics are safer in this regard (Ensrud et al., 2002).

There is, therefore, growing interest in nonpharmacological approaches to the treatment of anxiety disorders in older women. Evidence is best for CBT, which is skills-enhancing and problem-focused for patients fearful of being overwhelmed by fearful thoughts. Barrowclough et al. (2001) demonstrated sustained benefit for CBT over counseling for anxiety in older adults living at home. Single-session CBT was effective in reducing symptoms of anxiety and depression in older patients with chronic obstructive pulmonary disease (Kunik et al., 2001). Using CBT, patients with panic disorder achieve a decrease in

Table 20.5 Drugs used in anxiety

Drug	Mode of action or class	Important interactions or precautions	Starting dosage (mg)	Average therapeutic dosage (mg)
Diazepam	Long-acting benzodiazepine	- Sedation (enhanced with antidepressants and antipsychotics) - Ulcer healing drugs (may inhibit benzodiazepines) - May impair epilepsy control	2 bd	6–15
Alprazolam	Medium half life benzodiazepine	Ditto	0.25 bd	0.25 bd or tds
Oxazepam	Short-acting benzodiazepine	Ditto plus greater risk of withdrawal	10	20
Lorazepam	Short-acting benzodiazepine	Ditto plus greater risk of withdrawal	0.5 bd	1–2
Buspirone	Specific $5HT_{1A}$ agonist	- Diltiazem, verapamil (may enhance effect of buspirone) - Does not prevent benzodiazepine withdrawal	5 bd	15–30
Propranolol	Non-selective beta-blocker	- Co-prescription with chlorpromazine enhances concentration of both drugs - Hypotension with tricyclics and some antipsychotics	40	80–120
Atenolol	Water-soluble beta-blocker	Generally fewer central nervous system side effects	25–50	50–100
Pregabalin	Anti-epileptic	Dizziness, drowsiness	75 mg	150–600 mg (dependent on renal function – check Glomerular Filtration Rate [GFR])

symptoms and in physiological arousal (Swales et al., 1996). A randomized controlled trial (Stanley et al., 2009) showed good outcomes with CBT for late-life anxiety in primary care. Last, a psychoeducational program was effective in reducing both anxiety and depressive symptoms in older women (Schimmel-Spreeuw et al., 2000). The course included relaxation training.

Prognosis

In specialist mental health services about 60% of older women with major depression recover completely or recover but have further treatable relapses. The remainder either stay unwell or recover only partially. Ill-health is a major adverse predictor (Cole & Bellavance, 1997). The prognosis in community settings and in medical wards is poorer than this (Cole & Bellavance, 1997), with low rates of treatment an important factor.

Barriers to care

Depression and anxiety are undertreated in old age to the extent that it presents a serious public health problem but depressed or anxious older women are unlikely to create a political or public relations furor about it. The undertreatment occurs for a number of reasons. Depression impairs the ability to seek help by inducing a lack of energy and motivation and feelings of worthlessness. Old people are less likely to report feelings of worthlessness and dysphoria or attribute them to the aging process – as do the doctors. Evans (1998) writes of elderly patients mirroring others' attitude to them – they are quite aware of society's prejudice and stereotyping, which they share and project onto other older people.

The rapid throughput in primary care may mitigate against a thorough assessment; those who are old and those who are depressed need time to express themselves. Clinicians may regard the signs and symptoms of depression as "normal aging" or attribute them to the "inevitable decline of dementia" or they may have the diagnosis veiled by the psychosocial situation, multiple losses, deteriorating physical health or sensory impairment. Depression may amplify physical symptoms and so increase attention given to them at the expense of detecting underlying depressive disorder. The clinician may correctly diagnose depression in an elderly woman but is prevented from doing anything about it either by ignorance or attitude.

Knight (2010), in writing of clinical supervision, mentions barriers needing attention in psychotherapeutic work. There is a need for cohort competency, for cultural competency and the ability to be able to handle questions about the clinician's age, which is likely to be less than that of the patient. All working in this field are aware of the need to confront sensitively the older patient who is avoiding particular topics. Both patient and clinician may have anxiety about the end of therapy, linking discharge with death. Practical problems of lack-of-transport flexibility for attendance and family interference are further potential barriers.

As well as societal stereotypes of aging there are also societal values. Children would always command sympathetic and active care and treatment whereas the old woman "has had her innings." The Age Concern (2007) Inquiry in the UK into mental health and well-being in later life notes age discrimination as a fundamental problem, a view endorsed by older people themselves. Some political groups claim that discrimination is greatest for older women. The report names it as a barrier to much-needed improvements in the funding, planning and provision of services and support for older people with mental ill-health. Improving Access to Psychological Therapies (IAPT, 2008) is an initiative from the Department of Health for England and Wales, and is to be warmly welcomed but so far a small minority of patients referred are over aged 65. So far IAPT has not delivered in respect to older people.

Dartington (2010) writes movingly about the dynamics of care, exploring the lack of compassion, the splitting between health and social care, which seems to be the societal response to vulnerability and long-term dependence.

Organizational and financial barriers are erected to continuing care in a society where independence is prized and dependence treated with contempt (Bell, 1996). Policy makers are undoubtedly influenced by personal and societal attitudes and no doubt the wish for a quiet life. Depressed old women are likely to create less bother than young men with forensic problems. It is up to clinicians to endeavor to redress the balance.

Prevention: primary and secondary

Until relatively recently the prevention of depression amounted merely to advice about "healthy living." Epidemiology shows that both selective primary prevention (targeting individuals at risk of but not expressing depression) and indicated prevention (those identified with subthreshold depression) are effective ways to prevent a significant proportion of later-life depressive disorders. Thus far, there is evidence that some depressions in the setting of disorders such as stroke and macular degeneration can be prevented either with antidepressant medication or a psychological intervention such as Problem-solving Treatment. Unfortunately, despite some well-designed studies, depression associated with hip fracture has not proved preventable in this way (summarized by Baldwin, 2010). Although the prevention and treatment of depression associated with dementia has not borne fruit, prevention of depression among caregivers does have evidence, using psychological approaches centered on family interventions (Baldwin, 2010). Likewise, if individuals with mild symptoms of depression are identified – often by applying a screening questionnaire to those at risk, such as older women with functional impairment of whatever cause – then again a proportion of cases can be prevented from becoming full-blown depressive disorders (Baldwin, 2010).

Mental attitude is also important. Those who see growing older as positive may be less likely to succumb to the exigencies of aging. It is easy to adopt a loss-deficit approach to old age; a different, more positive view is the maturity model (Patrick, 2006), which may account for levels of depression being lower in old age. Quinodoz (2010) makes the point that it is possible to "lose everything without losing oneself" and that growing old can be an enriching experience borne out of our own internal life history. This echoes some of the thinking of Erikson (1959) and of Limentani (1995). Perhaps we end as the fruit of our own creation. We can look at our life as a coherence or as a series of events without links and internal meaning.

Continuation therapy after major depression should be for a minimum of 12 months in older patients. Both tricyclics and SSRIs have been proven effective in the prevention of relapse and recurrence (Baldwin et al., 2008). Longer-term treatment should be considered, after discussion with the patient, for those experiencing their third or more recurrence (Baldwin et al., 2003). Importantly, of older people who kill themselves, a majority will have consulted their primary care physician recent to the act (Harwood et al., 2001). The correct identification of depression in primary care therefore offers a prospect of influencing suicide rates among older people.

Cuijpers and van Lammeren (2001) studied secondary prevention of depressive symptoms in elderly residents of residential homes. Staff were trained in detecting depression and in supporting depressed residents. Information was given to residents and their relatives and group interventions offered. Their results suggest that general approaches within a residential home are capable of influencing depressive symptoms in the residents. Early intervention seems to be successful and avoids the need for more extensive treatment.

Looking to the future and to unanswered questions

Societies need to consider how to react positively to major demographic change and to be more accepting and embracing of diversity that increases with age. From the point of view of research, there is a need to consider why so little is known about anxiety in old age. Charting physiological changes in emotion in aging may illuminate mood disorders and anxiety in older people. Prevention research is needed throughout the life cycle. Gender differences in depression in late life are poorly understood. Something may be learned from the biological, psychological and social situation of women in considering the higher suicide rate in men and the greater incidence of vascular depression in older males. The narrowing of the gender gap in the incidence of depression in old age needs to be understood as well as the intriguing suggestion (Hybels et al., 2002) that older women with subthreshold depression are more likely to live longer than those who are not depressed.

One would be hard-pressed to produce evidence that the new antidepressants developed over the past 20 years have led to any improvement in the outcome of depression in older women. Rather, attention is turning to new ways of delivering existing treatments, as well as to improve their uptake. Combining treatments offers considerable advantages over single modalites. In primary care, collaborative management offers significant advantages for outcome over usual care. The key components are a care manager based in primary care and timely access to specialist advice. The data are encouraging (Unützer et al, 2002).

Consideration is needed as to why despite professionals' avowed adherence to evidence-based medicine myths about old age, women and mental disorders persist. An attitude needs to be promoted that makes the world and its health and social services a reasonable place for today's young women to grow old.

References

de Abajo, F. J., Garcia Rodríguez, L. A., & Montero, D. (1999) Association between selective serotonin reuptake inhibitors and upper gastrointestinal bleeding: population based case-control study. *BMJ* 319: 1106–1109.

Achterberg, W., Pot, A. M., Kerkstra. A., Ooms, M., Muller, M., & Ribbe, M. (2003) The effects of depression on social engagement in newly admitted Dutch nursing home residents. *Gerontologist* 43: 213–218.

Age Concern (2007) *Improving services and support for older people with mental health problems. Second report from the UK Inquiry into mental health and well-being in later life.* London: Age Concern.

Alexopoulos, G. S., Abrams, R. C., Young, R. C. (1988) Cornell Scale for Depression in Dementia. *Biological Psychiatry* 23:271–284.

Alexopoulos, G. S., Meyers, B. S., Young, R. C., Campbell, S., Silbersweig, D., & Charlson, M. (1997) 'Vascular depression' hypothesis. *Archives of General Psychiatry* 54:915–922.

Aparasu, R. R., Mort, J. R., & Brandt, H. (2003) Psychotropic prescription use by community-dwelling elderly in the United States. *Journal of the American Geriatrics Society* 51: 671–677.

Alexopoulos, G. S., Young, R. C., Kocsis, J. H.. (1984) Dexamethasone suppression test in geriatric depression. *Biological Psychiatry* 19:1567–1571.

Baldwin, R. C. (2008) Depressive Illness. In R. Jacoby, C. Oppenheimer, T, Dening, A, Thomas (Eds.), *Oxford Textbook of Old Age Psychiatry*, 4th edition. Oxford, England: Oxford University Press.

Baldwin, R. C. (2010) Preventing late-life depression: a clinical update. *International Psychogeriatrics* 22:1216–1224. doi:10.1017/S1041610210000864.

Baldwin, R., Anderson, D., Black, S., Evans, S., Jones, S., Wilson, K., & Iliffe, S. (2003) Guideline for the management of late-life depression in primary care. *International Journal of Geriatric Psychiatry* 18:829–838.

Baldwin, R. C., & O'Brien, J. (2002) Vascular basis of late-onset depressive disorder. *British Journal of Psychiatry* 180:157–160.

Ballard, C. G., Eastwood, C., & Gahir, M. (1996) A follow-up study of depression in carers of dementia sufferers. *BMJ* 312:947.

Banerjee, S., Hellier, J., Dewey, M., Romeo, R., Ballard, C., Baldwin, R., Bentham, P., Fox, C., Holmes, C., Katona, C., Knapp, M., Lawton, C., Lindesay, J., Livingston, G., McCrae, N., Moniz-Cook, E., Murray, J., Nurock, S., Orrell, M., O'Brien, J., Poppe, M., Thomas, A., Walwyn, R., Wilson. K., Burns, A. et al. (2011) Sertraline or mirtazapine for depression in dementia (HTA-SADD): a randomised, multicentre, double-blind, placebo-controlled trial. *Lancet* 378: 403–411.

Barnes, D. E., Yaffe, K., Byers, A. L., McCormick, M., Schaefer, C., & Whitmer, R. A. (2012) Midlife vs late-life depressive symptoms and risk of dementia differential effects for Alzheimer Disease and Vascular Dementia. *Archives of General Psychiatry* 69(5):493–498.

Barrowclough. C., King, P., Colville, J., Russell, E., Burns, A., & Tarrier. N. (2001) A randomized trial of the effectiveness of cognitive-behavioral therapy and supportive counseling for anxiety symptoms in older adults. *Journal of Consulting & Clinical Psychology.* 69:756–762.

Beckman, N., Waern, M., Gustafson, D., & Skoog, I. (2008) Secular trends in self reported sexual activity and satisfaction in Swedish 70 year olds: cross sectional survey of four populations, 1971-2001. *BMJ* 337(7662):151–154.

Beekman, A. T., Copeland, J. R., & Prince, M. J. (1999) Review of community prevalence of depression in later life. *British Journal of Psychiatry* 174:307–311.

Bell. D. (1996). Primitive mind of state. *Psychoanalytic Psychotherapy* 10:45–57.

Blazer, D. G. (2003) Depression in late life: review and commentary. *Journal of Gerontology: Medical Sciences* 58A:249-265.

Blazer, D. (2010) Protection from depression. *International Psychogeriatrics* 22:171–173.

Blehar. M., De Paulo, R., Gershon, E., Reich, T., Simpson, S., & Nurnberger, J. (1998) Women with bipolar disorder: findings from the NIMH genetics initiative sample. *Psychopharmacology Bulletin*, 34(3):239–243.

Boyd-Carpenter, M. (2010) Reflections on retirement. *Psychodynamic Practice* 16(1):89–94.

Bretschneider, J., & McCoy, N. (1989) Sexual interest and behavior in healthy 80- to 102-year-olds. *Our Sexuality Update.* Benjamin/Cummings Publishing, pp. 5–6.

Brooke, P., & Bullock, R. (1999) Validation of the 6 Item Cognitive Impairment Test. *International Journal of Geriatric Psychiatry* 14:936–940.

Buchheim, A., Viviani, R., Geage, C., Kächele, H., & Walters, H. (2011) Neural correlates of emotion,

cognition and attachment in borderline personality disorder In R. A. Levy, J. S. Ablon & H. Kächele (Eds.), *Psychodynamic psychotherapy research: Practice-based evidence and evidence-based practice* (pp. 239–256). New York: Humana Press.

Canete, M., Stormont, F., & Ezquero, A. (2000) Group analytic psychotherapy with the elderly. *British Journal of Psychotherapy* 17:94–105.

Carvalho, R. (2008) The final challenge: ageing, dying, individuation. *Journal of Psychoanalytic Psychology* 53:1–18.

CDC (1996) Suicide among older persons-United States, 1980–1992. *Morbidity and Mortality Weekly Report* 45:3–6.

Chui, H., Chan, S., & Tsoh, J. (2010) Suicide in later life. In N. Pachana, K. Laidlaw, & B. Knight (Eds.), *Casebook of clinical geropsychology: International Perspectives on Practice.* Oxford, England: Oxford University Press.

Ciechanowski, P. S., Katon, W. J., Russo, J. E., & Walker, E. A. (2001) The patient provider relationship: attachment theory and adherence to treatment in diabetes. *American Journal of Psychiatry* 158:29–35.

Cole, M. G., & Bellavance, F. (1997) The prognosis of depression in old age. *American Journal of Geriatric Psychiatry* 5:4–14.

Conwell, Y., Duberstein. P. R., Cox, C., Herrmann, J. H., Forbes, N. T., & Caine, E. D. (1996) Relationships of age and Axis I diagnoses in victims of completed suicide: a psychological autopsy study. *American Journal of Psychiatry* 153:1001–1008.

Covey H.S. (1992) The definitions of the beginnings of old age in history. *International Journal of Aging and Human Development* 34(4):325–337.

Cuijpers P, van Lammeren, P. (2001) Secondary prevention of depressive symptoms in elderly inhabitants of residential homes. *International Journal of Geriatric Psychiatry* 16:702–708.

Cutter, W. J., Norbury, R,, & Murphy, D.G.M. (2003) Oestrogen, brain function, and neuropsychiatric disorders *Journal of Neurology, Neurosurgery & Psychiatry* 74:837–840.

Dartington, T. (2010) *Managing vulnerability: the underlying dynamics of systems of care.* The Tavistock Clinic series. London: Karnac Books.

Dayson, D., Lee-Jones, R., Chahal, K. K. & Leff, J. (1998) The TAPS project 32: social networks of two group homes . . . 5 years on. *Social Psychiatry and Psychiatric Epidemiology* 33:438–444.

Dimatteo, M. R., Lepper, H. S., & Croghan, T. W. (2000) Depression is a risk factor for noncompliance with medical treatment: meta-analysis of the effects of anxiety and depression on patient adherence. *Archives of Internal Medicine* 160:2101–2107.

Ensrud, K. E., Blacwell, T. E., Mangione, C. M., Bowman, P. J., Whooley, M. A., & Bauer, D. C. (2002) Central nervous system-active medications and risk of falls in older women. *Journal of the American Geriatrics Society* 50:1629–1637.

Erikson, E. H. (1959) *Identity and the life cycle.* Psychological Issues Monograph No. 1. New York: International Universities Press.

Evans. S. (1998) Beyond the mirror: a group analytic exploration of late life and depression. *Ageing and Mental Health* 2, 94–99.

Evans, S. (2004) Group psychotherapy: Foulkes, Yalom, Bion and others. Chapter 7 in S. Evans & J. Garner (Eds.), *Talking over the years: a handbook of psychodynamic psychotherapy with older adults.* London: Brunner-Routledge.

Folstein, M. F., Folstein, S. E., & McHugh, P. R. (1975) 'Mini-Mental State': a practical method for grading the cognitive state of patients for the clinician. *Journal of Psychiatric Research* 12:189–198.

Fooken, I. (1994) Sexuality in the later years – the impact of health and body image in a sample of older women. *Patient Education and Counselling* 23: 227–233.

Freud S. (1905) *On psychotherapy.* Standard Edition 7.

Gallagher-Thompson, D. & Thompson, L. (2010) Effectively using cognitive behavioural therapy with the oldest-old: case examples and issues for consideration. In N. A. Pachana, K. Laidlaw & B. G. Knight (Eds.), *Casebook of clinical geropsychology* (pp. 227–241). Oxford, England: Oxford University Press.

Garland, C. (2007) "Tragical-comical-historical-pastoral": groups and group psychotherapy in the third age. In R. Davenhill (Ed.), *Looking into Later Life: a psychoanalytic approach to depression and dementia in old age.* The Tavistock Clinic series. London: Karnac.

Garner, J. (1998) Open letter to Director General of Fair Trading. APP Newsletter. *Psychoanalytic Psychotherapy,* 22:4–5.

Garner, J. (2008) Wot! No psychotherapist. *APP Newsletter, special older adults edition* 40:7–8.

Garner, J. (2009) Considerably better than the alternative: positive aspects of getting older. *Quality in Ageing and Older Adults* 10(1):5–8.

Garner, J. (2013) Psychodynamic therapy. In T. Dening and A. Thomas (Eds.), *Oxford Textbook of Old Age Psychiatry, 2nd Edition.* Oxford: Oxford University Press.

Garner, J., & Ardern, M. (1998) Reflections on old age. *Aging and Mental Health* 2: 92–93.

Garner, J., & Bacelle, L. (2004) Sexuality. Chapter 17 in S. Evans and J. Garner (Eds.), *Talking over*

the years: a handbook of psychodynamic psychotherapy with older adults.* London: Brunner-Routledge.

Garner, J. & Evans, S. (2010) Psychodynamic approaches to the challenges of ageing. In N. A. Pachana, K. Laidlaw & B. G. Knight, (Eds.), *Casebook of clinical geropsychology* (pp. 55–72). Oxford, England: Oxford University Press.

Glaser, R., Robles, T. F., Sheridan, J., Malarkey, W. B., & Kiecolt-Glaser, J. K. (2003) Mild depressive symptoms are associated with amplified and prolonged inflammatory responses after influenza virus vaccination in older adults. *Archives of General Psychiatry* 60:1009–1014.

Green, R. C., Cupples, A., Kurz, A., Auerbach, S., Go, R., Sadovnick, D., Duara, R., Kukull, W. A., Chui, H., Edeki, T., Griffith, P. A., Friedland, R. P., Bachman, D., & Farrer, L. (2003) Depression as a risk factor for Alzheimer Disease: The MIRAGE Study. *Archives of Neurology* 60:753–759.

Hamilton, M. (1960) A rating scale for depression. *Journal of Neurology, Neurosurgery and Psychiatry* 23:56–62.

Harralson. T., White, T., Regenberg, A., Kallan, M., Have, T. T., Parmelee, P., & Johnson, J. (2002) Similarities and differences in depression among black and white nursing home residents. *American Journal of Geriatric Psychiatry* 10:175–184.

Hartikainen, S., Rahkonen, T., Kautiainen, H., Sulkava, R. (2003) Kuopio 75+ study: does advanced age predict more common use of psychotropics among the elderly? *International Clinical Psychopharmacology* 18(3):163–167.

Harwood, D., Hawton, K., Hope, T., & Jacoby, R. (2001) Psychiatric disorder and personality factors associated with suicide in older people: a descriptive and case-control study. *International*

Journal of Geriatric Psychiatry 16: 155–165.

Heifner, C. A. (1996) Women, depression and biological psychiatry: implications for psychiatric nursing. *Perspectives in Psychiatric Care* 32:4–9.

Hildebrand, H. P. (1982) Psychotherapy with older patients. *British Journal of Medical Psychology* 55, 19–28.

Holmes, T. H. & Rahe, R. H. (1967) The social readjustment rating scale. *Journal of Psychosomatic Research* 11:213–218.

Hubback, J. (1996) The archetypal senex: an explanation of old age. *Journal of Analytic Psychology* 41(1): 3–18.

Hybels, C. F., Pieper, C. F. & Blazer, D. G. (2002) Sex differences in the relationship between subthreshold depression and mortality in a community sample of older adults. *American Journal of Geriatric Psychiatry* 10:283–291.

Improving Access to Psychological Therapies (2008) *The IAPT Pathfinders: achievements and challenges*. London, England: Department of Health.

Jones, E. D. (2003) Reminiscence therapy for older women with depression. Effects of nursing intervention classification in assisted-living long term care. *Journal of Gerontological Nursing* 29:26–33.

Jones, R. (2002) That's very rude, I shouldn't be telling you that: older women talking about sex. *Narrative Inquiry* 12: 121–142.

Jung, C. G. (1931) The stages of life. *Collected works*, vol. 8, 387–403.

Junkers, G. (2006) *Is it too late? Key papers on psychoanalysis and ageing*. London: Karnac.

Karlsson, H. (2011) Psychotherapy increases the amount of serotonin receptors in the brains of patients with major depressive disorder. In R. A. Levy, J. S. Ablon & H. Kächele (Eds.), *Psychodynamic*

psychotherapy research: Practice-based evidence and evidence-based practice (pp. 233–238). New York: Humana Press.

Katon, W. J., Lin, E., Russo, J. & Unützer, J. (2003) Increased medical costs of a population-based sample of depressed elderly patients. *Archives of General Psychiatry* 60:897–903.

Kay, D.W.K. (1988) Anxiety in the elderly. In R. Noyes, M. Roth, G. D. Burrows (Eds.), *Handbook of Anxiety vol. 2: Classification, etiological factors and associated disturbances*. Elsevier Science Publications BV.

Kelly, M. & Barratt, G. (2007) Retirement: phantasy and reality – dying in the saddle or facing up to it? Psychodynamic practice: individuals. *Groups and Organisations* 13(2):197–202.

Kessler, R. C. (2003) Epidemiology of women and depression. *Journal of Affective Disorders* 74:5–13.

King. P.H.M. (1974) Notes on the psychoanalysis of older patients. *Journal of Analytical Psychology* 19, 22–37.

King P.H.M. (1980) The life-cycle as indicated by the transference in the psychoanalysis of the middle aged and elderly. *International Journal of Psychoanalysis* 61:153–160.

Kirby. M., Denihan, A., Bruce, I., Radic, A., Coakley, D. & Lawlor, B. A. (1999) Benzodiazepine use among the elderly in the community. *Int J Geriat Psychiatry* 14:280–284.

Kivela, S. L., Luukinen, H., Koski, K., Viramo, P. & Pahkala, K. (1998a) Early loss of mother or father predicts depression in old age. *International Journal of Geriatric Psychiatry* 13(8):527–530.

Kivela, S-L, Pahkala, K, Laippala. P. (1988b) Prevalence of depression in an elderly Finnish population. *Acta Psychiatrica Scandinavica* 78:401–13.

Knight B. G. (1986) *Psychotherapy with Older Adults*. London: Sage.

Knight, B. G. (2010) Clinical supervision for psychotherapy with older adults. In N. A. Pachana, K. Laidlaw & B. G. Knight (Eds.), *Casebook of clinical geropsychology* (pp. 107–116). Oxford, England: Oxford University Press.

Knight B. G. & Satre D. D. (1999). Cognitive behavioural psychotherapy with older adults. *Clinical Psychology: Science and Practice* 6:188–203.

Kok, R. M., Nolen, W. A., & Heeren, T. J. (2012) Efficacy of treatment in older depressed patients: a systematic review and meta-analysis of double-blind randomized controlled trials with antidepressants. *Journal of Affective Disorders* 141:103–115.

Kramer-Ginsberg, E., Greenwald, B. S., Aisen, P. S., Brod-Miller, C. (1989) Hypochondriasis in the elderly depressed. *Journal of the American Geriatrics Society* 37:507–510.

Kunik, M. E., Braun, U., Stanley, M. A. Wristers, K., Molinari, V., Stoebner, D. & Orengo, C. A. (2001) One session cognitive behavioural therapy for elderly patients with chronic obstructive pulmonary disease. *Psychological Medicine* 31:717–723.

Laidlaw, K. (2008) Cognitive behaviour therapy. In R. T. Woods & L. Clare (Eds.), *Handbook of the clinical psychology of ageing*, 2nd Edition. Chichester, West Sussex, UK: John Wiley & Sons.

Laidlaw, K. (2010) Enhancing CBT with older people using gerontological theories as vehicles for change. In N. A. Pachana, K. Laidlaw & B. G. Knight (Eds.), *Casebook of clinical geropsychology* (pp. 17–31). Oxford, England: Oxford University Press.

Lepine, J. P. & Bonchez, S. (1998) Epidemiology of depression in the elderly. *International Clinical Psychopharmacology* 13(suppl 5): S7–S12.

Limentani, A. (1995) Creativity and the Third Age. *International Journal of Psychoanalysis* 76:825–833.

Lindesay, J., Briggs, K., & Murphy, E. (1989) The Guy's/Age Concern survey. Prevalence rates of cognitive impairment, depression and anxiety in an urban elderly community. *British Journal of Psychiatry* 155:317–329.

Lopez, A. D. & Murray, C. C. (1998) The global burden of disease, 1990–2020. *Nature Medicine* 4:1241–1243.

Lyness, J. M., King, D. A., Cox, C., Yoediono, Z. & Caine, E. D. (1999) The importance of subsyndromal depression in older primary care patients: prevalence and associated functional disability. *Journal of the American Geriatrics Society* 47:647–652.

Martindale, B. (2007) Resilience and vulnerability in later life. *British Journal of Psychotherapy* 23(2):205–216.

Medicines and Healthcare products Regulatory Agency (MHRA) (2011) *Citalopram and escitalopram: QT interval prolongation—new maximum daily dose restrictions (including in elderly patients), contraindications, and warnings.* Volume 5, Issue 5, www.mhra.gov.uk/Safetyinformation/DrugSafetyUpdate/CON137769

Mehta, K. M., Simonssick, E. M., Penninx, B.W.J.H., Schultz, S., Rubin, S. M., Satterfield, S. & Yaffe, K. (2003) Prevalance and correlates of anxiety symptoms in well-functioning older adults: findings from the Health Aging and Body Composition study. *Journal of the American Geriatrics Society* 51:499–504.

Miller, M., Frank, E. & Cornes, C. (1994) Applying interpersonal psychotherapy to bereavement – related depression following loss of a spouse in late life. *Journal of Psychotherapeutic Practise Research* 3:149–162.

Montgomery, S., Chatamra, K., Pauer, L., Whalen, E., & Baldinetti, F.

(2008) Efficacy and safety of pregabalin in elderly people with generalised anxiety disorder. *British Journal of Psychiatry* 193(5):389–394.

Mottram, P., Wilson, K., & Copeland, J. (2000) Validation of the Hamilton Depression Scale and Montgomery and Asberg rating scales in terms of AGECAT depression cases. *International Journal of Geriatric Psychiatry* 15:1113–1119.

Murdock, M. E., Guarnaccia, C. A., Hayslip, B. Jr. & McKibbin, C. L. (1998) The contribution of small life events to the psychological distress of married and widowed older women. *Journal of Women & Aging* 10:3–22.

Murphy, E. (1982) Social origins of depression in old age. *British Journal of Psychiatry* 141:135–142.

Murphy, E., Smith, R., Lindesay, J. & Slattery, J. (1988) Increased mortality rates in late-life depression. *British Journal of Psychiatry* 152:347–353.

Nasreddine, Z. S., Phillips, N. A., Bédirian, V., Charbonneau, S., Whitehead, V., Collin, I., Cummings, J. L. & Chertkow, H. (2005) The Montreal Cognitive Assessment (MoCA): a brief screening tool for mild cognitive impairment. *Journal of the American Geriatrics Society* 53:695–699.

Nelson, J .C., Delucchi, K. L. & Schneider, L. S. (2008) Efficacy of second generation antidepressants in late-life depression: a meta-analysis of the evidence. *American Journal of Geriatric Psychiatry* 16(7):558–567.

Nelson, J. C. & Papakostas, G. I. (2009) Atypical antipsychotic augmentation in major depressive disorder: a meta-analysis of placebo-controlled randomized trials. *American Journal of Psychiatry* 166:980–991.

Nesse, R. M. (2000) Is depression an adaptation? *Archives of General Psychiatry* 57:14–20.

Nusbaum, M.R.H., Singh, A.R. & Pyles, A. A. (2004) Sexual healthcare needs of women aged 65 and older. *Journal of the American Geriatrics Society* 52:117–122.

Pachana, N., Byrne, G., Siddle, H., Koloski, N., Harley, E. & Arnold, E. (2007) Development and validation of the Geriatric Anxiety Inventory. *International Psychogeriatrics* 19:103–114.

Patrick, E. (2006) Older, wise and unlikely to present. *Therapy Today* 17(3)4–8.

Penninx, B. W., Deeg, D. J., van Eijk, J.t., Beekman, A. T. & Gurainik, J. M. (2000) Changes in depression and physical decline in older adults: a longitudinal perspective *Journal of Affective Disorders* 61:1–12.

Pinquart, M. & Sorensen, S. (2001). How effective are psychotherapeutic and other psychosocial interventions with older adults? *A Meta-analysis Journal of Mental Health and Aging* 7: 207–243.

Pollack, G. (1982). On ageing and psychoanalysis. *International Journal of Psychoanalysis* 63: 275–281.

Prince, M. J., Harwood, R. H., Thomas, A. & Mann, A. H. (1998) A prospective population-based cohort study of the effects of disablement and social milieu on the onset and maintenance of late-life depression. *The Gospel Oak Project VII Psychological Medicine* 28:337–350.

Quinodoz, D. (2010) *Growing old: a journey of self discovery.* Translated D. Alcorn. Hove: Routledge.

Quitkin, F. M., Stewart, J. W., McGrath, P. J., Taylor, B. P., Tisminetzky, M. S., Petkova, E., Chen, Y., Ma, G. & Klein, D. F. (2002) Are there differences between women's and men's antidepressant responses? *American Journal of Psychiatry* 159:1848–1854.

Reynolds, III, C. F., Frank, E., Perel, J. M., Imber, S. D., Cornes, C.,

Miller, M. D., Mazumdar, S., Houck, P. R., Dew, M. A., Stack, J. A., Pollock, B. G., & Kupfer, D. J. (1999) Nortriptyline and interpersonal psychotherapy as maintenance therapies for recurrent major depression: a randomized controlled trial in patients older then 59 years. *Journal of the American Medical Association* 281:39–45.

Royal College of Psychiatrists (2013) *OP88. Whole-person Care: from rhetoric to reality (Achieving parity between mental and physical health).* London: Royal College of Psychiatrists.

Sapolsky, R., Krey, L., McEwen, B. (1986) The neuroendocrinology of stress and aging: the glucocorticoid cascade hypothesis. *Endocrine Rev* 7:284–301.

Schimmel-Spreeuw, A., Linssen, A. C., Heeren, T. J. (2000) Coping with depression and anxiety: preliminary results of a standardized course for elderly depressed women. *International Psychogeriatrics,* 12:77–86.

Serfaty, M., Howarth, D., Blanchard, M., Buszewicz, M., Murad, S., & King, M. (2009) Clinical effectiveness of individual cognitive behavioural therapy for depressed older people in primary care: a randomized controlled trial. *Archives of General Psychiatry* 66:1332–1340.

Shedler, J. (2010) The efficacy of psychodynamic psychotherapy. *American Journal of Psychiatry* 65:98–109.

Shore, A. N. (1997) A century after Freud's project: is a rapprochement between psychoanalysis and neurobiology at hand? *Journal of the American Psychoanalytic Association* 45:807–840.

Stanley, M. A., Wilson, N. L. & Novy, D. M. (2009) Cognitive Behaviour Therapy for generalized anxiety disorder among older adults in primary care: a randomized controlled trial. *Journal of the*

American Medical Association 301:1460–1467.

Swales, P., Solfvin, J. & Sheikh, J. (1996) Cognitive-behavioural therapy in older panic disorder patients. *American Journal of Geriatric Psychiatry,* 4: 46–60.

Szewczyk, M. & Chennault, S. (1997) Depression and related disorders. *Primary Care (Women's Health)* 24: 83–101.

Terry, P. (1997). *Counselling the elderly and their carers.* London: Macmillan Press.

Tew, J. D., Mulsant, B. H., Haskett, R. F., Prudic, J., Thase, M. E., Crowe, R. R., Dolata, D., Begley, A. E., Reynolds III, C. F., & Sackeim, H. A. (1999) Acute efficacy of ECT in the treatment of major depression in the Old-Old. *American Journal of Psychiatry* 156:1865–1870.

Thompson, P. (1993) 'I don't feel old': the significance of the search for meaning in later life. *International Journal of Geriatric Psychiatry* 8:685–692.

Turner, M. S. (1992) Individual psychodynamic psychotherapy with older adults: perspective from a nurse psychotherapist. *Archives of Psychiatric Nursing,* 6:266–274.

Turvey, C. L., Carney, C., Arndt, S., Wallace, R. B. & Herzog, R. (1999) Conjugal loss and syndromal depression in a sample of elders aged 70 years or older. *American Journal of Psychiatry,* 156:1596–1601.

Unützer, J., Katon, W., Callahan, C., Williams, J. W., Hunkeler, E., Harpole, L., Hoffing, M., Della Penna, R. D., Noel, P. H., Lin, E.H.B., Arean, P., Hegel, M., Tang, L., Belin, T. R., Oishi, S., & Langston, C. (2002) Collaborative care management of late-life depression in the primary care setting. *Journal of the American Medical Association* 288:2836–2845.

Van Scaik, A., van Marwijk, H., Ader, H., van Dyck, R., de Haan, M., & Penninx, B. (2008) Inter-personal

psychotherapy for elderly patients in primary care. *American Journal of Geriatric Psychiatry* 14:777–786.

Veith, R. C., Raskind, M. A. (1988) The neurobiology of aging: does it predispose to depression? *Neurobiology of Aging* 9:101–117.

Viinamaki, H., Kuikka, J., Tilhonen, J. & Lehtonen, J. (1998) Change in monoamine transporter density in related to clinical recovery: a case control study. *Nordic Journal of Psychiatry* 52:39–44.

Waern, M., Runeson, B. S., Allebeck, P., Beskow, J., Rubenowitz, E., Skoog, I. & Wilhelmsson, K. (2002) Mental disorder in elderly suicides: a case-control study. *American Journal of Psychiatry* 159:450–455.

Weiss J. C. (1994) Group therapy for older adults in long term care settings, research and clinical cautions and recommendations. *Journal for Specialists in Group Work,* 19:22–29.

Wells, K. B., Stewart, A. & Hays, R. D. (1989) The functioning and well being of depressed patients: results from the Medical Outcomes Study. *Journal of the American Medical Association,* 262:914–919.

Whisman, M. A. (1999) Marital dissatisfaction and psychiatric disorders: results from the National Comorbidity Survey. *Journal of Abnormal Psychology* 108:701–706.

Whooley, M. A., Grady, D. & Cauley, J. A. (2000) Postmenopausal estrogen therapy an depressive symptoms in older women. *Journal of General Internal Medicine* 15:535–541.

Whooley, M. A., Kip, K. E., Cauley, J. A., Ensrud, K. E., Nevitt, M. C. & Browner, W. S. (1999) Depression, falls and risk of hip fracture in older women. *Archives of Internal Medicine* 159:484–490.

Wilson, K.C.M., Mottram, P.G. & Vassilas, C. A. (2008) Psychotherapeutic treatments for older depressed people. *Cochrane*

Database of Systematic Reviews, Issue 1. Art. No.: CD004853. doi: 10.1002/14651858.CD004853.pub2.

Woods, R. T. & Roth, A. (1996) Effectiveness of psychological interventions with older people. In A. D. Roth & P. Fonagy (Eds.), *What works for whom? A critical*

Review of Psychotherapy Research, 2nd Edition (pp. 425–446). New York: Guilford.

Yaffe, K., Blackwell, T., Gore, R., Sands, L., Reus, V. & Browner, W. S. (1999) Depressive symptoms and cognitive decline in nondemented elderly women: a prospective study.

Archives of General Psychiatry 56:425–430.

Yesavage, J. A., Brink, T. L., Rose, T. L. & Lum, O. (1983) Development and validation of a geriatric depression screening scale: a preliminary report *Journal of Psychiatric Research* 17:37–49.

Bipolar disorders
Special issues for women

Shaila Misri, Jasmin Abizadeh and Arjun Nanda

The stigma, struggle and suffering associated with bipolar illness in a childbearing woman has been known to clinicians for centuries. It is only in the last two or three decades that recognition of the illness with its attendant impairment has led to scientific research and management. As yet, a totally safe mode of treating acutely ill bipolar mothers has proved to be challenging. With increasing knowledge, the bipolar-related disorders (BD) are in a constant state of evolution. During pregnancy, childbirth and breastfeeding the clinician is faced with the unique challenge of treating not only the mother, but also the developing baby. Irrespective of whether this illness begins in pregnancy or after childbirth, management of the disease in the context of maternal fetal wellness should be the central goal for every treating clinician.

This chapter includes prevalence rates, gender differences, screening, symptom profile, comorbidity and risk factors. We provide a discussion regarding the contribution of paternal mood to the course of the illness in the mother. Management is then discussed.

Gender differences in bipolar disorder

The combined lifetime prevalence of BD in the United States has been reported to be as high as 1.8% (American Psychiatric Association, 2013). Others have reported individual prevalence rates, with Bipolar I Disorder (BD I) accounting for 1.0%, Bipolar II Disorder (BD II) for 1.1% and subthreshold BD for 2.4% (Merikangas et al., 2011). The 12-month prevalence in the United States is estimated to be 0.6% for BD I and 0.8% for BD II (American Psychiatric Association, 2013; Merikangas et al., 2007). Whilst women and men are equally affected by BD, the expression of this condition and course of illness differs between the sexes (Arnold, 2003; DiFlorio & Jones, 2010; Yang et al., 2013).

The mean age of onset of BD has been reported to be later in women than in men (Hendrick et al., 2000; Baldessarini et al., 2010) with one study showing that the onset of BD was a mean 3.2 years later in women than in men (Viguera et al., 2001).

The relationship between rapid cycling and gender is well established. The *Diagnostic and Statistical Manual of Mental Disorders, Fifth Edition* (DSM-5) reports that rapid cycling – along with mixed states and depressive episodes – is more likely to occur in females (American Psychiatric Association, 2013). Rapid cycling is also more common in patients with BD II (Baek et al., 2011), which women are 1.6 times more likely to develop (Viguera et al., 2001; Baldessarini et al., 2010). Rapid cycling is a marker of severity and poor treatment response (Anderson et al., 2012). In addition, women with BD appear to have frequent episodes and possibly mixed mania (Kupka et al., 2005; Nivoli et al., 2011; Vieta & Moralla, 2010).

Viguera et al., (2001) found that the period between the onset of BD and starting treatment was 24.4 months longer for females, likely due to initial misdiagnosis of unipolar depression (Viguera et al., 2001), especially those with BD II diagnosis (Suominen et al., 2009). The impact of delayed or misdiagnosis may lead to untimely or inappropriate treatment, for example, prescribing an antidepressant – which then induces a switching phenomenon (Ghaemi et al., 2005; Sharma, 2009). A higher risk of hospitalization, psychosocial impairment, suicide attempts and an increase in mixed and rapid states have also been associated with misdiagnosis (Goldberg & Ernst, 2002; Sharma, 2009).

Comprehensive Women's Mental Health, ed. David J. Castle and Kathryn M. Abel. Published by Cambridge University Press.
© Cambridge University Press 2016.

Symptoms of peripartum bipolar disorders I and II

The postpartum period is a time of increased risk for the onset and exacerbation of BD I and BD II (see Chapter 8). If the onset of mania, hypomania or major depression occurs in pregnancy and in the four weeks following delivery, these mood episodes are described as having peripartum onset (American Psychiatric Association, 2013).

Bipolar disorder I

BD I is characterized by the occurrence of a manic episode, which may be preceded or followed by major depressive episodes (American Psychiatric Association, 2013). A manic episode is identifiable by feelings of euphoria, "excessively cheerful, high, or feeling on top of the world"; individuals may shift between periods of euphoria, dysphoria and irritability, leading to marked impairment in social and occupational functioning (American Psychiatric Association, 2013). These shifts in mood may occur on a rapid basis and over a brief period of time. During a manic episode, a person with BD may experience inflated self-esteem, a decreased need for sleep, rapid speech, racing thoughts, increased sociability and excessive engagement in plans and activities. Poor insight often accompanies acute mania (Anderson et al., 2012). The depressive episodes are characterized by low mood, sadness, lack of energy, sleep and appetite change, with negative ruminating thoughts.

DSM-5 does not use the term "postpartum psychosis," but rather makes reference to mood episodes presenting either with or without psychotic features (American Psychiatric Association, 2013). This definition fits most closely with the definition proposed by Kendell and colleagues (1987). Irrespective of the diagnostic status, symptoms of postpartum psychosis closely resemble that of BD in the postpartum period.

There has been significant debate about whether postpartum psychosis is a distinct psychiatric condition or a time- and situation-specific expression of BD, for which the trigger is childbirth. In a review of the relationship between BD and postpartum psychosis, Chaudron and Pies (2003, p. 1286) commented that "postpartum psychosis is not a discrete nosologic entity, but a postpartum presentation of an underlying mood disorder. In many, if not most cases, this underlying disorder appears to be in the bipolar spectrum." Another study by Munk-Olsen et al. (2012) suggested

that "an early postpartum onset of illness has prognostic implications and raises the chance of subsequent conversion to a diagnosis of bipolar disorder."

The incidence of postpartum psychosis ranges between 1 in 500 to 1 in 1000 and may be more common in primiparous women (American Psychiatric Association, 2013). It is treated as a psychiatric emergency because of its associated high risk of suicide and infanticide. Women with a history of BD have an increased risk for recurrence of psychosis in subsequent pregnancies (25–50% versus 0.1–0.25% in the general population) (Jones & Craddock, 2001). DSM-5 has specified the risk of recurrence with each subsequent delivery as even higher (30–50%) for women with a previous postpartum episode with psychotic features (American Psychiatric Association, 2013). The risk of postpartum episodes with psychotic features is particularly elevated for women with prior postpartum mood episodes, those with a history of depressive or bipolar disorder (especially BD I) and for those with a family history of bipolar disorders (American Psychiatric Association, 2013). Jones and Craddock (2001) reported that 74% of women with puerperal psychosis had a history of postpartum psychosis in first-degree relatives. It is unclear whether the development and/or recurrence of postpartum psychosis is due to biological stressors of genetic predisposition, primiparity, pregnancy/delivery complications, previous episodes (Valdimarsdóttir et al., 2009; Pfuhlmann et al., 2002; Sharma et al., 2004) or psychological stressors associated with the early postpartum period (Pfuhlmann et al., 2002).

The risk of bipolar relapse is highest in the immediate postpartum period, with the onset most often occurring within 72 hours (Sit et al., 2006). Patients can manifest symptoms of a manic, depressed or mixed state (Porter & Gavin, 2010). Risk continues to be elevated for years thereafter. Kendell et al. (1987) reported the relative risk of psychiatric admission 30 days from birth to be 6.0, while for primiparae the risk was 10.9.

Sharma and Mazmanian (2003, p. 102) commented that "sleep loss may be the final common pathway by which various putative risk factors produce psychosis in susceptible women." Sleep loss has been considered to be a significant risk factor for BD and in precipitating postpartum psychosis (Sharma & Mazmanian, 2003; Ross et al., 2005). It is also the most prominent early symptom of mania and a frequent early symptom of depression (Jackson et al., 2003).

The shift towards hypomania or mania may occur as early as within one day of lack of sleep, based on findings in a non-perinatal population (Bauer et al., 2006). Insomnia may be present in 42–100% of women who experience postpartum psychosis (Rohde & Marnerso, 1993; Hunt & Silverstone, 1995). Stabilizing mental health during this period may mitigate the effects of insomnia (Bilszta et al., 2010).

Bipolar disorder II

BD II is no longer thought to be a "milder" condition, because the instability of mood experienced by these individuals is typically accompanied by serious impairment in work and social functioning (American Psychiatric Association, 2013). Hypomania may not always cause impairment initially as it is associated with increased energy and productivity (Anderson et al., 2012). BD II is marked by repeated episodes of major depression alternating with brief periods of hypomania. Individuals with BD II tend to present with depressive symptoms, spend more time in the depressive phase of their illness, have greater chronicity of illness compared to BD I and present with high impulsivity (American Psychiatric Association, 2013). In clinical practice, it is often difficult to differentiate this period of elated mood from the normal period of euphoria following delivery. However, the manifestation of extreme elation with other hypomanic features observed in BD II women occurs between 9 and 20% of women after childbirth (Heron et al., 2009; Sharma et al., 2009). Sharma and Khan (2010) found that 57% of postpartum women with a diagnosis of Major Depressive Disorder (MDD) actually suffered from BD II or Bipolar Disorder Not Otherwise Specified. Misdiagnosis of BD II contributes to symptom exacerbation and prolonged illness trajectory, which can interfere with proper maternal attachment (Sharma et al., 2008). Early intervention and treatment are crucial in ensuring healthy mother-infant interaction, bonding and overall well-being of the family unit.

In a study by Baek and colleagues (2011), BD II was further differentiated from BD I by various characteristics. These included frequent depressive episodes and increased rapid cycling, seasonal variation, psychomotor agitation, suicidal ideation, higher comorbidities and substance use disorder. The prominent mood associated with BD II was one of higher irritability for shorter duration whereas presence of increased manic symptoms occurred for a longer period of time in BD I.

Screening

Since there is limited screening for BD in perinatal women, screening tools used in the general population, such as the Mood Disorder Questionnaire (Hirschfeld et al., 2000), have been utilized in clinical practice in some countries. Chessick and Dimidjian (2010) conducted a review of 11 self-report measures of BD and found that the Highs (Glover et al., 1994) appears to have specific relevance to the perinatal period; it is not a commonly used tool. Although not specific for BD, the Edinburgh Postnatal Depression Scale (Cox et al., 1987) is a commonly used instrument with cross-cultural validity to measure depressive symptoms. Optimal timing for screening women is at their first perinatal visit and shortly after delivery, as risk of a BD episode increases greatly in the postpartum. For those with a past personal history of BD, or a family history of the disease, using a screening tool can detect the level of vulnerability (Jones & Craddock, 2001).

It is important to screen for risk factors for BD, such as atypical symptoms of depression, hypomania, psychosis, early onset of mood symptoms, frequent mood episodes, poor treatment response, mixed or manic response to antidepressants and prior postpartum mood disorder. Screening is particularly helpful when recommended for women with comorbid disorders, such as substance use and anxiety disorders (Ranga Rama Krishnan, 2005; Perlis et al., 2006).

Comorbidity

Common comorbidities with BD include anxiety disorders, substance abuse, eating disorders, attention deficit disorder and certain medical conditions (Arnold, 2003; Kemp et al., 2010; McIntyre et al., 2007). The prevalence of most comorbid conditions differs between the sexes.

In a study by Merikangas and colleagues (2011), 76% of BD patients had at least one lifetime comorbid disorder, including anxiety, substance use, behavioral disorders and eating disorders. Among the anxiety disorders associated with BD, Sala and colleagues (2012) found that 51.5% had Generalized Anxiety Disorder, 47.8% had social anxiety disorder and 53.4% had panic disorder. Bipolar subjects were found to be younger and female, and had an earlier age at onset of illness (Ibiloglu & Caykoylu, 2011).

Another study reported that those with anxiety and BD had lower household income and presented with greater substance abuse and functional impairment

(Fracalanza et al., 2011). Generally, in clinical practice, comorbid BD and anxiety disorders tend to follow a complicated course and require skillfull psychopharmacological management.

There are studies suggesting that panic disorder is more commonly associated with BD in women than men (Arnold, 2003; Saunders et al., 2012). This comorbidity is clinically significant as patients with BD I and lifetime panic symptoms seem to have more depression, suicidal ideation and a six month longer time lag between acute treatment and achieving remission (Frank et al., 2002, Kilbane et al., 2009). Even though this comorbidity is common, it is often underdiagnosed or misdiagnosed (e.g., borderline, narcissistic or histrionic personality) leading to poorer treatment outcomes (Perugi & Akiskal, 2002).

When substance abuse complicates BD, treatment can be challenging, with complex presentation, resistance to treatment and high rates of suicide (Farren et al., 2012). In one study, bipolar women had four times the rate of alcohol use disorders and three times the rate of other substance use disorders than women from community-derived samples (Baldessano et al., 2005). BD and alcohol/substance use disorders may share some common characteristics in their genetic background, as well with neuroimaging and biochemical markers (Farren et al., 2012). Findings from a recent study suggest that intermittent stressors, mood episodes and occasional cocaine use may lead to chronicity and illness progression (Post & Kalivas, 2013).

The presence of eating disorder in BD patients is significantly associated with an earlier onset of the disease and an altered course of illness characterized by mixed episodes, greater frequency, rapid cycling and suicide attempts (McElroy et al., 2011). This comorbidity is associated with female gender, younger age, family history of mood disorders and substance abuse.

Findings from a recent meta-analysis showed that the relationship between attention deficit hyperactivity disorder among relatives of bipolar patients is significantly higher and appears to follow a bidirectional relationship with some degree of overlap (Faraone et al., 2012).

The mood symptoms in BD II may be particularly difficult to distinguish from the affective instability and impulsivity also found in borderline personality disorders (BPD) (Antoniadis et al., 2012; Perugi & Akiskal, 2002). However, consensus seems to favor the diagnosis of cyclothymic and BD II disorders over erratic and BPD (Ranga Rama Krishnan, 2005).

Bipolar patients with a comorbid personality disorder seem to have greater severity of residual mood symptoms, complex course of illness, frequent history of substance use disorder, use of more psychiatric drugs and a lower rate of current employment (George et al., 2003; Kay et al., 2002).

Medical conditions, including migraines, obesity and thyroid disease often accompany BD in women (Arnold, 2003; Baldassano et al., 2005; McIntyre et al., 2007). Comorbid rates for BD and migraine have been found to be 4.7–24.8% (Holland, Agius, & Zaman, 2011; McIntyre et al., 2006; Ortiz et al., 2010) compared to a rate of 10.3% in the general population (McIntyre et al., 2006). Migraine seems to be associated particularly with BD II (Ortiz et al., 2010), especially those with a positive family history.

Higher occurrence of BD and polycystic ovaries can be directly related through medication-induced obesity or a treatment effect (Burt & Rasgon, 2004; DiFlorio & Jones, 2010; Jiang et al., 2009). Some studies have reported that polycystic ovarian syndrome was linked to valproate use in bipolar patients, nearly 50% of whom presented with menstrual abnormalities and high levels of androgens (O'Donovan et al., 2002). This suggests a possible shared hypothalamic-pituitary-gonadal axis abnormality, which may also be indicative of shared genetic predisposition (Klipstein & Goldberg, 2006; Jiang et al., 2009).

The high prevalence of one or more comorbidity amongst patients with BD increases the complexity of the clinical treatment of women with BD.

Reproductive health

Distinct changes in hormones are markers of premenstrual, postpartum, and perimenopausal life cycles (see Chapter 8). These hormonal fluctuations appear to be linked to major depressive disorder and anxiety disorders, such as panic and generalized anxiety disorder (Eriksson et al., 2002; McKinlay et al., 1992) (see Chapter 19). Payne and colleagues (2007) found that 67.7% of bipolar disorder cohort reported premenstrual exacerbation in bipolar and unipolar depression, 20.9% had postpartum symptoms, and 26.4% experienced perimenopausal symptoms.

A history of premenstrual syndrome seems to be a strong predictor of perimenopausal symptoms (Binfa et al., 2004), even after adjusting for age, race, diagnosis of MDD and estradiol use (Freeman et al., 2004). Relatively few studies have examined the effect of perimenopause on BD, but the findings seem to indicate a general worsening of mood symptoms during this time (Freeman et al., 2002; Blehar et al., 1998; Sajatovic et al., 2006).

Preconception

Preconception counseling in a stable state is ideal (see Chapter 9); it provides an ideal opportunity to assist women with this decision-making process, inform them about the risks and benefits of their therapeutic options during pregnancy, and plan supports during the perinatal period (see also Chapter 9).

Benefits of pre-pregnancy consultation are multifold. It provides the opportunity to discuss treatment options and switch to a safer medication for pregnancy, decreasing the exposure of the fetus to multiple medications (Viguera et al., 2002). Women need to be informed about the high risk of relapse when discontinuing medication (Cohen & Nonacs, 2005) and this is a time when social support, such as family and friends, need to be involved (Frieder et al., 2008). In a study by Viguera and colleagues (2002), a reported 45% of women had been advised by health professionals not to conceive. Following their pre-pregnancy consultation, 63% of women tried to conceive, but 37% chose not to pursue pregnancy out of fear of adverse effects of medicines on fetal development (56%) and risk of relapse with medication cessation (50%).

Up to 49% of pregnancies in the general US population are unplanned (Finer & Zolna, 2011) and 50% of individuals with planned pregnancies will not have seen a healthcare provider prior to conception (American Academy of Neurology, 1998). By the time they present during the first trimester, the fetus has already been exposed to psychoactive medications (Yonkers et al., 2004; Galbally et al., 2010) (also see Chapter 9).

Genetic counseling can address patients' fears and educate them about disease inheritance. While the genetics of BD are not yet fully determined, it is clear that the offspring of individuals with this condition have an increased risk of psychiatric illness. The relative risk in individuals with a first-degree relative with BD has been reported to be 7–14 times higher than in those without (Mortensen et al., 2003; Wozniak et al., 2012). A maternal history of BD conferred a 12-fold relative risk, a paternal history a 15-fold greater risk and both parents a 113-fold greater risk than individuals without such a family history (Mortensen et al.,

2003). Other studies have also found that offspring of parents with a mental illness had a greater likelihood of an affective disorder (4-fold), any mental disorder (2.7-fold), and BD spectrum disorders (Birmaher et al., 2009; Lapalme et al., 1997). Such risk must, however, be discussed within the context of the relationship between genetic and environmental factors. Monozygotic twin studies show concordance rates greater than those of dizygotic twins, illustrating that while genetic factors are strong, environmental factors do influence the expression of this condition (Smoller & Finn, 2003).

Potential effects of untreated maternal bipolar disorder

As many as 51.2% of patients with BD in the United States might go untreated in a given one-year period (Wang et al., 2005). The literature on the effects of untreated maternal BD on the growing fetus and newborn child is evolving; however, the findings of the impact of untreated maternal depression suggest that this carries direct risks to the fetus and infant, as well as risks secondary to unhealthy maternal behaviors (Bonari et al., 2004).

Untreated maternal depression has been found to be related to negative expression and affect in infants, delays in infant growth, and a three-time increased risk of anxiety and depressive symptoms in later life (Avan et al., 2010; Weissman et al., 2006). Infants may also display more avoidant and disorganized attachment (Korja et al., 2008; Martins & Gaffan, 2000), which has been linked to internalizing and externalizing behavior problems in toddlers (Madigan et al., 2007; Trapolini et al., 2007). Some studies report that boys may be more adversely affected by prenatal and postnatal maternal depression compared to girls (Carter et al., 2001).

Higher cortisol levels in prenatally depressed women may be associated with negative growth development in the infant, such as delayed fetal growth, prematurity and impaired fetal brain development (Field & Diego, 2008; Van den Bergh et al., 2005; Weinstock, 2005). The infants of prenatally depressed women appear to show higher cortisol and lower dopamine and serotonin levels (Field et al., 2004).

In women with BD, acute episodes during pregnancy are of concern due to the risks of substance misuse, neglect of antenatal care, poor judgment, impulsive behavior, poor nutrition, increased risk of committing or being a victim of violence and the risk of self-harm, including suicide in major depression (Bonari et al., 2004; Finnerty, Levin, & Miller, 1996; Viguera et al., 2000). In the postpartum period, maternal recurrences can affect practical infant care and mother-infant attachment (Brockington, 2004; Vemuri & Williams, 2011) (also see Chapter 4). Postpartum psychosis carries the risk of neonaticide and infanticide, particularly in the early months; however, more research is needed to ascertain the exact risk factors for neonaticide and infanticide (Spinelli, 2001; Pearlstein et al., 2009; Flynn et al., 2007, 2013).

Bipolar disorder and pregnancy: pregnancy as a protective factor?

Overall, pregnancy may confer some protection for women (Grof et al., 2000); however, in most cases, this protection may not be enough to discontinue medication. Pregnancy is not likely to be protective for women with a refractory illness, early age of onset, multiple episodes and high relapse rate when unmedicated (Viguera et al., 2000; Viguera et al., 2007).

Paternal mood

Clinicians have recently gained awareness with regards to the effects of paternal psychopathology on parenting. Paternal psychiatric disorders have been shown to increase the likelihood of behavioral problems in the offspring not dissimilar to the effects of a mentally ill mother. Unwell fathers may be unable to support their partner in caring for their children (Dietz et al., 2009).

Very few studies have examined the prevalence of long-term paternal perinatal BD. Adolescents who have a parent with BD are up to 10 times more likely to develop BD themselves and 3–4 times more likely to develop other psychiatric disorders compared to those with parents without a mental illness (Henin et al., 2005; Hillegers et al., 2005). In one longitudinal follow-up study of fathers with depressive and BD spectrum episodes, Pinheiro and colleagues (2011) conducted mood assessments at 28–34 weeks of pregnancy, 30–60 days postpartum and at 12 months after childbirth. The results showed a mixture of depressive, mixed and hypomanic mood changes in fathers at different time points through the perinatal period. The prevalence of paternal depressive episodes overall was 5.0%, 4.5% and 4.3% respectively. Studies that

support the risk of paternal mood appear mostly to focus on depressive symptoms (Bradley & Slade, 2011). Specifically, boys may be at a greater risk than girls in terms of increased risk of behavioral rather than emotional difficulties. One relatively small study reported that father's depression at 8 weeks postpartum alone had negative effects and doubled the risk of behavioral and emotional problems in children at 3.5 years of age even after controlling for mother's depression (Ramchandani et al., 2005).

At our program, we provide individual and group educational sessions to mothers and fathers with regards to mental health during parenting and provide opportunities to discuss their own experiences and stresses (also see Chapter 4).

Management of bipolar disorder in pregnancy

Psychosocial interventions

An optimal therapeutic outcome is based on combining pharmacotherapy and psychotherapy, along with psychosocial interventions to aid in the recovery process.

Guidelines for BD tend to focus on pharmacotherapy, but also address adjunct and complementary therapies. The guidelines developed by the Canadian Network for Mood and Anxiety Treatments (CANMAT) for the management of patients with BD suggest that "although pharmacotherapy forms the cornerstone of management, utilization of adjunctive psychosocial treatments and incorporation of chronic disease management models involving a healthcare team are required for providing optimal management for patients with bipolar disorder" (Yatham et al., 2005).

Psychoeducation can affect the course of BD in a substantial way. It has been found to increase the time to recurrence of the illness and to reduce relapse rates (Colom et al., 2003; Swartz & Frank, 2001). In addition, psychoeducation has been shown to encourage patients to become actively involved in self-management, sleep regulation, avoidance of substance misuse and promote further collaboration among healthcare professionals (Yatham et al., 2005).

Adjunctive psychosocial therapies should be considered early on in treatment and can include psychoeducation, cognitive-behavioral therapy (CBT), interpersonal (IPT) and social rhythm therapy

(IPSRT) and family interventions. According to the CANMAT guidelines, CBT, used as an adjunctive therapy for BD, can improve functioning and adherence, as well as decreased relapses, mood fluctuations, need for medications and hospitalizations (Lam et al., 2000; Lam et al., 2003; Scott, 2003). Individual and/or group CBT may also have a role in patients with BD in improving compliance and increasing function and quality of life (Patelis-Siotis, 2001). IPT did not alter time to relapse, but significantly increased the duration of being euthymic and decreased the duration of depression (Lam et al., 2000; Lam et al., 2003; Scott, 2003). Family interventions have been associated with fewer relapses and hospitalizations and improvements in depressive symptoms and adherence with pharmacotherapy (Rea et al., 2003; Miklowitz et al., 2000; Miklowitz et al., 2003).

Psychosocial therapies for BD may be particularly helpful for the depressive phase of BD I and BD II. The UK National Institute for Health and Clinical Excellence (NICE) clinical management guidelines for antenatal and postnatal mental health also recommend brief psychological treatments (including counseling, CBT and IPT) for mild depressive symptoms in pregnant women with BD and combined medication and psychological treatments for moderate to severe depressive symptoms in this population (Tomson et al., 2007; NICE 2014).

In addition to psychotherapy, social support is a key factor in supporting women with BD during their perinatal period (Yonkers et al., 2004; Viguera, et al., 2002). Limited research has been undertaken on the effect of psychosocial therapies on families and partners of individuals with BD. In a study of patients with a major affective disorder or BD, married for 17 years, those who had psychoeducational marital intervention had improvements in adherence and overall function (but not symptoms), compared to individuals receiving medication only (Clarkin et al., 1998).

Yoga has been shown to be effective in both general and perinatal populations as an adjunct for severe mood disorders, as well as a monotherapy for mild depression (Field, 2011). While no studies to date have evaluated yoga as a treatment for BD, several plausible mechanisms of action through which yoga may exert its therapeutic effect on bipolar patients have been suggested. These include decrease in stress reactivity via regulation of the Hypothalamic-Pituitary-Adrenal axis, reduction of cortisol levels,

increase in Gamma-Aminobutyric Acid neuro-receptors, improved sleep efficiency and quality, and decreased rumination (Da Silva, Ravindran, & Ravindran, 2009). Yoga is a component in mindfulness-based cognitive therapy (MBCT), which involves meditation exercises, yoga and a therapeutic focus informed by the CBT framework. Recent studies show that MBCT is effective in bipolar patients as an adjunct to medication for reducing anxiety and depressive symptoms; improving emotional regulation, executive functioning, memory, ability to initiate and complete tasks; and increasing mindfulness (Williams et al., 2008; Ives-Deliperi et al., 2013; Stange et al., 2011; Deckersbach et al., 2012). However, larger and randomized controlled trials are needed to confirm its efficacy, and there is still a dearth in data for the pregnant and postpartum populations.

Pharmacotherapy principles of management

Experts recommend classifying all pregnant women with BD I as "high-risk" pregnancies (Viguera et al., 2011). A comprehensive and integrated approach to prenatal care of these high-risk cases has several elements (ACOG, 2008; Yonkers et al., 2004), including:

- maintaining the best possible control of BD;
- regular psychiatric monitoring by the mental healthcare provider;
- a multidisciplinary specialist team approach;
- addressing comorbid conditions;
- attending to self-care issues, such as diet, exercise, and sleep hygiene;
- avoiding substance use, including alcohol and cigarettes.

In order to ascertain the treatment options for each individual during pregnancy, key patient information requires knowledge of past history of BD, related and unrelated to pregnancy, as well as a family history of puerperal psychosis. Obtaining the medical history is also important to understand response to different agents and time to relapse (Jones & Craddock, 2001; Yonkers et al., 2004). The management of each patient must be decided on a case-by-case basis after evaluating the individual risk/benefit ratio. However, there are some general principles of management. Viguera and colleagues (2002) state that patients who have had one manic episode with rapid, total recovery with subsequent stability may be able to taper medication gradually prior to conception. A recognized drawback of this approach is the risk of relapse while awaiting conception. In an unplanned pregnancy, by the time conception is established, stopping certain medications may not be necessary if the period of greatest risk of fetal exposure has already passed. If medication is discontinued, it should be reinstituted if the patient becomes symptomatic, even during the first trimester. In women with brittle BD, with a history of numerous severe recurrences with potential risk of psychosis or suicidality, maintaining medication preconception and throughout pregnancy is typically recommended (Viguera et al., 2002; Yonkers et al., 2004). In clinical practice, however, medications with high teratogenic risk should be replaced with another mood stabilizer during preconception planning. Ideally, changing one mood stabilizer to another during pregnancy is best avoided to minimize fetal exposure to two sets of medication (see also Chapter 9).

The US Food and Drug Administration (FDA) has approved the use of some psychotropic agents in pregnant women. It is essential that the woman is stable prior to conception as pregnancy can escalate the prior symptomatology of the disorder. Once pregnant, careful monitoring and titrating is recommended. Medication is more difficult to titrate during childbearing as drug pharmacokinetics are affected by the physiological changes of pregnancy and delivery, particularly shifting fluid loads and altered drug clearance rates (Tomson et al., 2013). During parturition and the early postpartum period, the levels of some agents may increase rapidly with abrupt fluid losses; thus, intensive monitoring of maternal hydration status and drug levels is advised.

All psychotropic agents cross the placenta, and can affect fetal organ development/growth in utero and cause neonatal toxicity or withdrawal at birth in the absence of proper hydration (ACOG, 2008). Little is known about the impact of these drugs upon long-term behavior and development. There are specific periods of gestation during which drug exposure increases the risk of particular conditions, for example, exposure in weeks 3–8 can impact cardiac formation, weeks 6–9 can affect palate/lip formation, and up to day 32 can impact neural tube formation and closure (Starr & McMillan, 2011). Exposure in trimesters two and three has risks of low birth weight, preterm delivery, minor malformations and behavioral sequelae (Källén & Reis, 2012). Information on psychoactive drugs in pregnancy generally comes from retrospective cohort studies or case reports;

there are few less-biased prospective studies or randomized controlled trials due to practical and ethical reasons. Therefore, prescribing decisions are made with regards to different aspects of perinatal pharmacotherapy (see also Chapters 9 and 11).

Lithium

Fetal and neonatal effects. Lithium is the gold standard for mood stabilization in pregnant women with BD (Viguera et al., 2002; Vieta & Valenti, 2013) as it is not as teratogenic as once perceived (Yatham et al., 2013), with most exposed infants being born without abnormality. However, the risk of Ebstein's anomaly with lithium exposure continues to be a concern (Galbally et al., 2010). The rate of Ebstein's anomaly in infants exposed to lithium during gestation is estimated at 1 in 1000 compared to 1 in 20,000 in the general population. Due to this heightened risk, high-resolution ultrasound and fetal echocardiograph are recommended at 16–18 weeks of gestation for women taking lithium in trimester one (Gentile, 2012). Many clinicians prescribe atypical antipsychotics as mood stabilizers if patients do not respond to lithium. The use of novel antipsychotics as a first-line treatment has been recently recommended for mood stabilization by The American Congress of Obstetricians and Gynecologists (ACOG, 2008; Reis & Källén, 2008); however, caution is advised as research is sparse and their efficacy and tolerability profile will be confirmed in the future.

Lithium exposure during delivery has the potential of neonatal toxicity, with hallmarks of "floppy baby syndrome" including neonatal cyanosis and hypotonicity (Galbally, Snellen et al., 2010). Nephrogenic diabetes insipidus and neonatal hypothyroidism have also been reported (Sands & Bichet, 2006; Feingold & Brown, 2010). Fetal thyroid goiter infrequently occurs with lithium exposure during trimesters two and three (American Academy of Pediatrics: Committee on Drugs, 2000) and can complicate delivery. Increased birth weight (by a mean of 80 g, compared to controls) has been reported in neonates with trimester one exposure (Bodén et al., 2012). Long-term neurobehavioral and developmental effects from lithium exposure in utero have been researched in follow-up studies, with no consistent negative sequelae described (Kozma, 2005; Yonkers et al., 2004).

Lithium therapy during pregnancy and delivery. Due to the short half-life of lithium (8–10 h), dosing is recommended 3–4 times/day to maintain optimum steady state levels (Yonkers et al., 2004). Adequate hydration, particularly during concurrent medical illness, is important to avoid lithium toxicity. Maternal polyuria and polydypsia during pregnancy can be aggravated by lithium (Misri & Lusskin, 2004; Nivoli et al., 2011). Lithium levels should be monitored monthly, with increasing frequency as pregnancy progresses and delivery approaches. The required dose typically increases with advancing pregnancy, due to greater drug clearance (Misri & Lusskin, 2004; Gentile, 2012; Yonkers et al., 2004; Burt et al., 2010). There appears to be no consensus regarding lithium use prior to delivery, with some advocating maintenance of the same dose, and others suggesting slow tapering and complete discontinuation. This decision should be made by the treating clinician on an individual basis. Lithium is recommended to be withheld during prolonged labor (1–2 days if necessary) and restarted at preconception levels immediately after delivery (Newport et al., 2005; Bogen et al., 2012). This decision must be balanced against risk of maternal relapse in labor or thereafter. Preserving the patient's hydration status and intensive monitoring of maternal symptoms and lithium levels is recommended after delivery, because of the risk of toxicity or relapse during childbirth and the immediate postpartum (Gentile, 2012).

One-third of patients with BD do not respond to or tolerate lithium (AAP: Committee on Drugs, 2000) and may receive anticonvulsant therapy. The frequency of congenital anomalies remains high with anticonvulsant exposure (Gentile, 2010a; Gentile, 2010b).

Valproate

Fetal and neonatal effects. Valproate has the highest rate of fetal malformations at 8.7% as a single agent (Vajda et al., 2003). One of the primary concerns of valproate use in pregnancy is the 1–5% risk of neural tube defects (NTDs) (van Dijk et al., 2012). This dose-related risk coincides with the impact of drug exposure on days 17–30 of organogenesis. Polytherapy with carbamazepine can cause a rostral shift in the neural tube defect (Yonkers et al., 2004; van Dijk et al., 2012). Because valproate reduces folate levels (Linnebank et al., 2011), folic acid supplementation is recommended to reduce the risk of NTDs, although recommended amounts vary. Linnebank

et al. (2011) recommend 5 mg/day for epileptic women taking anticonvulsants, from preconception until the completion of trimester one at minimum, but the American Academy of Pediatrics (AAP) recommends 4 mg/day before pregnancy and 400 µg after (AAP: Committee on Drugs, 2000). Measuring vitamin B_{12} levels prior to folate administration is advised to rule out pernicious anemia (Linnebank et al., 2011). Prenatal testing for NTDs includes maternal serum α-fetoprotein, targeted ultrasound, and amniocentesis for α-fetoprotein levels.

DiLiberti et al. (1984) coined the term "fetal valproate syndrome" to describe the pattern of malformation of the "anticonvulsant face." It is unclear whether intrauterine growth restriction and intellectual disability form part of this syndrome (Yonkers et al., 2004). Neonatal toxicity with heart rate decelerations and symptoms of withdrawal, which include irritability, jitteriness, abnormal tone and feeding problems have been described from valproate administration in pregnant women with epilepsy (Ebbesen et al., 2000). Intrauterine growth restriction, hyperbilirubinemia, skeletal dysplasia and fetal/neonatal distress have also been linked to valproic acid (AAP: Committee on Drugs, 2000). Additionally, the fetus is at an increased risk of spina bifida, atrial septal defect, cleft palate, hypospadias, polydactyly and craniosynostosis (Vajda et al., 2013; Jentink et al., 2010). Studies have found a high recurrence risk (21.9%) of major congenital malformation for women with more than one child (Pennell et al., 2012; Campbell et al., 2013 and see also Chapter 11).

A 2006 study found that valproate clearance increases with concurrent oral contraception use (Galimberti et al., 2006). The FDA has also recently issued a warning against valproate for migraine headaches in pregnant women, noting potential risk of decreased IQ scores in children and increased risk for autism spectrum disorders, childhood autism and reduced cognition (Christensen et al., 2013; Meador et al., 2013). Therefore, the FDA has reclassified valproate from a category D to a category X medication. Due to the high risk of malformations caused by valproate, there is a trend to stop its use in pregnancy and choose atypical antipsychotics instead (Wisner et al., 2011; NICE 2014).

Valproate therapy during pregnancy and delivery. Intensive serum level monitoring is required as amounts can change over the course of pregnancy. The total daily dose is a greater contributing factor to major malformations than peak serum levels. Given the multiple problems associated with valproate use in pregnancy, in clinical practice balancing between adverse effects and maintaining euthymia in the mother is often complex.

Carbamazepine

Fetal and neonatal effects. Like many other psychotropic agents, carbamazepine crosses the placenta and fetal serum levels have been approximated at 44% of maternal levels (Pynnönen & Sillanpää, 1975; Pynnönen et al., 1977). Carbamazepine use in pregnancy carries a risk of NTDs reported as 0.2–1.0% after first trimester exposure, compared to a population rate of 0.03% (Wieck & Gregoire, 2009; Matlow & Koren, 2012). Therefore, as with valproate, folate supplementation is advised. Facial malformation or the "anticonvulsant face" from carbamazepine (as valproate) exposure can also occur, with midface hypoplasia, small nose, anteverted nostrils and a long upper lip (Holmes et al., 2000; Yonkers et al., 2004). A greater rate of major congenital anomalies (2.2–7.9%) and lower birth weight of about 250 g with trimester one carbamazepine exposure has been reported (Nguyen et al., 2009; Diav-Citrin et al., 2001). Cardiovascular malformations, hypospadiasis, craniofacial defects and fingernail hypoplasia have all been described (Nguyen et al., 2009). Carbamazepine exposure also increases the risk of microcephaly (Almgren et al., 2009; Viguera et al., 2002) and thalidomide-like phocomelia (Dursun et al., 2012). There is debate as to whether carbamazepine exposure increases the risk of neurodevelopmental impairment (Cummings et al., 2011; Matlow & Koren, 2012).

Carbamazepine therapy during pregnancy delivery. Clinicians treating pregnant women with carbamazepine must be aware that this agent can result in fetal vitamin K deficiency. This can affect midface development and lower levels of vitamin K dependent clotting factors (Yonkers et al., 2004; Holmes et al., 2005; Lippi & Franchini, 2011; Kaaja et al., 2002), risking neonatal bleeding including intracerebral hemorrhage (AAP: Committee on Drugs, 2000; Kumar et al., 2012). However, there is insufficient evidence to determine whether prenatal vitamin K supplementation reduces neonatal hemorrhagic complications (Harden et al., 2009). Carbamazepine can influence the efficacy of certain anticoagulant drugs (Bauler et al., 2012). The AAP advises maternal treatment with 10–20 mg/day oral vitamin K for the final month of pregnancy (AAP: Committee on Drugs, 2000) and 1 mg intramuscular vitamin K for neonates (Yonkers et al., 2004; Kumar et al., 2012).

It is also important to note that efficacy of the oral contraceptive pill (OCP) can by affected by medications used to treat BD. Carbamazepine is known to induce cytochrome p450, lowering OCP levels (Arnold, 2003).

Lamotrigine

Fetal and neonatal effects. Teratogenic risk with lamotrigine is found at doses exceeding 200 mg/day. The maximum recommended dosage for BD I is 400 mg (Nguyen et al., 2009; Moore & Aggarwal, 2012). The FDA recently issued a warning that women treated with lamotrigine during the first 3 months of pregnancy had an increased risk of cleft lip and cleft palate. While the relative risk of these malformations is high, the absolute risk is low, at 0.89% (Shor et al., 2007). Greater malformation rates have been described with polytherapy, particular with valproic acid (Cunnington et al., 2011). Information on intrauterine growth following lamotrigine exposure in utero has not been described. In a study of development at 1 year, no abnormalities were noted (Mackay et al., 1997).

Experts warn about hepatotoxicity and skin rash, which has occurred in adults receiving lamotrigine (Yonkers et al., 2004; Sedky et al., 2012). A number of studies have shown that lamotrigine levels decrease with concurrent use of combined hormonal contraception methods (Christensen et al., 2007; Herzog et al., 2009; Wegner et al., 2009). Progesterone-only contraceptives, however, have not been found to reduce lamotrigine serum levels (Reimers, Helde, & Brodtkorb, 2005).

Lamotrigine therapy during pregnancy and delivery. Lamotrigine clearance increases during pregnancy and decreases postpartum to preconception levels (Pennell et al., 2008). Changing lamotrigine clearance highlights the importance of monitoring drug levels and dosing over pregnancy and particularly in the immediate postpartum period.

Topiramate

Recent studies show that there is a 4.6% increased risk for major birth defects with topiramate exposure and that it may cause long-term behavioral and cognitive problems (Mølgaard-Nielsen & Hviid, 2011; Rihtman, Parush, & Ornoy, 2012). There is an established connection between topiramate exposure during the first trimester and cleft lip and palate (Margulis et al., 2012; Hernández-Diaz et al., 2012). Consequently, the FDA has issued a warning against its use in pregnancy and has reclassified it as a Pregnancy Category D drug. There is also a high recurrence risk (50%) of major congenital malformations for women with subsequent pregnancies (Campbell et al., 2013). One study found that topiramate crosses the placenta at almost 100%. Additional studies have shown a significant pregnancy-related increase in dose/concentration ratios of topiramate (Ohman et al., 2009). Topiramate may impact upon the contraceptive efficacy of the OCP by reducing ethinyl estradiol levels (Reddy, 2010).

First generation antipsychotics

Fetal and neonatal effects. First generation antipsychotics are recommended as first-line treatment for manic, hypomanic or mixed episodes. Haloperidol is recommended when newer injectible atypical antipsychotics are not available, as it has not been found to increase the risk of congenital anomalies compared to low potency phenothiazines (Diav-Citrin et al., 2005; Owen, 2011; Reis & Källén, 2008). Neonatal toxicity has been described in the context of both withdrawal and extra-pyramidal symptoms with conventional antipsychotics, but it is unclear whether this is due to the disease or to anticholinergic or antihistaminergic properties of these agents. In addition, fetuses exposed to first generation antipsychotics have a slightly higher risk of preterm birth (Lin et al., 2010). Neurobehavioral effects are unclear (Gentile, 2010b).

First generation antipsychotic therapy during pregnancy and delivery. First generation antipsychotics have previously had several applications in pregnant women with BD, particularly to manage acute manic episodes. Their use over lithium or anticonvulsants in pregnancy/first trimester has been advocated because of lower fetal risk. Moreover, these medications were chosen for women who were unmedicated during their pregnancy and became symptomatic (ACOG, 2008). Haloperidol appears both safe and effective for the pregnant woman and her fetus for manic, hypomanic, mixed episodes or mood elevated syndromes (Diav-Citrin et al., 2005; Owen, 2011).

Second generation or novel antipsychotics

Fetal and neonatal effects. Second generation antipsychotics are not associated with any greater risk of fetal abnormality (McCauley-Elsom et al., 2010). However, they may increase the risk of gestational metabolic complications and increased birth weight compared to first generation antipsychotics (Gentile, 2010a). Olanzapine is approved for use in acute mania, but limited data are available for this agent during pregnancy. The manufacturer's registry collected data prospectively ($N = 144$) and retrospectively ($N = 98$) on pregnant women taking olanzapine. No increase in malformation rates were detected (Einarson & Boskovic, 2009). The neonatal toxicity of olanzapine is currently unknown. Quetiapine was approved by the US FDA for treating acute mania but it has now been indicated for other disorders such as bipolar depression, schizophrenia, post-traumatic stress disorder, insomnia and depressive symptoms (Ribolsi, Magni, & Rubino, 2010; Byers et al., 2010; Tadger, et al, 2011; Coe & Hong, 2012). According to the manufacturers, 1.5% of pregnant women taking quetiapine reported congenital anomalies, with the majority of affected women having taken multiple medications during pregnancy. Risperidone is another novel antipsychotic used in BD treatment but data on its use in pregnancy is also limited. The manufacturer has confirmed that rates of major malformations are within rates for the general population, based on 68 cases with a known outcome (Einarson & Boskovic, 2009).

With regard to clozapine, a few case reports found no major malformations. The manufacturer's registry noted that of 523 babies exposed to clozapine in utero, 22 had unspecified malformations. White cell counts are required in infants of mothers on clozapine, as agranulocytosis can occur in adult patients receiving this medication (Lahdelma, 2012). Case reports have shown conflicting data that ziprasidone may be a possible cause of cleft palate (Ružić et al., 2009). Few studies have evaluated the safety of aripiprazole in pregnancy, but no adverse events have been reported thus far (Einarson & Boskovic, 2009).

Second generation antipsychotic therapy during pregnancy and delivery. Second generation antipsychotics are often prescribed in pregnancy and are preferable to lithium and anticonvulsants. Experts recommend close monitoring of blood pressure, blood sugar levels and weight increases in pregnant women taking olanzapine because data have linked it to weight gain, insulin resistance, gestational diabetes and preeclampsia (Yonkers et al., 2004). It is important to note that the prolactin-sparing qualities of some novel antipsychotics can lead to an increased risk of conception when changing between an older agent and a prolactin-sparing antipsychotic (Green et al., 2013).

Benzodiazepines

Benzodiazepines (BDPs) are not primary agents for the treatment of BD but are implemented to alleviate associated symptoms such as anxiety, agitation and sleeping difficulties (Yonkers et al., 2004). Pregnant women may also be exposed to BDPs when required for medical reasons such as preterm labor.

Fetal and neonatal effects. Teratogenic effects have not been described for lorazepam or clonazepam (which are most often used in BD). One study has found that diazepam may be associated with an increased risk for cleft lip/palate (Kjaer et al., 2007). Many women become unexpectedly pregnant on BDPs. Therefore, it is important to advise women on BDPs regarding the safety of these agents. Case-control studies show a small increased risk of the development of major malformations or oral cleft with BDP use (ACOG, 2008; Enato, Moretti, & Koren, 2011). A level two ultrasound is now recommended when BDPs are used in the first trimester to exclude visible oral cleft (ACOG, 2008), which can be corrected at birth. BDPs should only be used when necessary in the first trimester (Bellantuono et al., 2013). Cases of neonatal toxicity from BDP exposure in third trimester or at delivery have been reported (ACOG, 2008). Withdrawal symptoms (infant irritability, tremor, vomiting and diarrhea, hypertonicity and vigorous sucking) have also been reported from chronic maternal BDP use; however, another report of maternal clonazepam use for panic disorder did not report neonatal toxicity (Hudak et al., 2012; Yonkers et al., 2004). The risk of long-term developmental delay is unclear, as data are limited and existing studies have produced contradictory results (ACOG, 2008).

Benzodiazepine therapy during pregnancy and delivery. In pregnant women, high-potency BDPs may be the best option due to shorter half-life, decreased chance of sedation and reduced accumulation (Yonkers et al., 2004).

Electroconvulsive therapy

Once contraindicated in pregnancy, electroconvulsive therapy (ECT) now plays an important role in the management of acutely psychotic pregnant women with BD. ECT is considered a relatively safe and effective treatment (Nielsen & Damkier, 2012), and should be undertaken by a multidisciplinary team of obstetricians, anesthetists and psychiatrists. A number of studies also provide support for the benefits of ECT in the treatment of postpartum psychosis (Doucet et al., 2011). Recent studies report only transient side effects to postpartum women and no adverse effects for the infants who were breastfed (Babu, Thippeswamy, & Chandra, 2013). A 2009 review found 18 ECT-related maternal complications out of 339 mothers (5.3%), which included vaginal bleeding, uterine contractions and/or preterm labor. Preterm labor was found to be the most common complication (Anderson & Reti, 2009). Although evidence suggests that the use of ECT is safe and effective in women who require it urgently, caution should be exercised to prevent transient fetal effects including bradyarrhythmia. Maternal risks, which are infrequently experienced, can be minimized in the hands of expert obstetricians and anesthetists. Risks to the mother and fetus can also be minimized by adequate oxygenation, right hip elevation, and avoiding both atropine and hyperventilation (Yonkers et al., 2004).

Postpartum ECT risks are considered minimal, but breastfeeding is not recommended for several hours after the ECT because of co-administered pharmacotherapy (Focht & Kellner, 2012). There are important ethical issues when ECT is used in pregnant patients, as obtaining informed consent for a woman and her unborn child can be difficult if a patient's mental state adversely affects her understanding of the situation and capacity to consent to ECT. Furthermore, the physician is treating two patients and must consider the health of both the mother and the unborn child.

Management of bipolar disorder in the postpartum period

Treatment of postpartum psychosis

The acute treatment of postpartum psychosis typically involves hospital admission and antipsychotic medication. The excess risk of postpartum psychosis in women with BD means that experts recommend administering mood stabilizers with antipsychotics and the careful use of antidepressants because of the risk of rapid cycling (Chaudron & Pies 2003). Cohen and colleagues (1995) found that women with known BD who did not receive a mood stabilizer had 8.6 times greater relative risk of postpartum relapse in the first 3 months after childbirth than those who received pharmacotherapy (mostly lithium). Bergink and colleagues (2012) also found that postpartum pharmacotherapy reduced the rate of psychotic relapse in women with a history of postpartum psychosis, relative to control patients. The use of ECT in patients with acute postpartum psychosis is recommended in situations as previously discussed. A rising amount of data shows ECT as a safe and effective treatment option for postpartum psychosis (Focht & Kellner, 2012).

Breastfeeding and medication

For women with BD, the decision of whether or not to breastfeed is complex. The health benefits of breastfeeding for both mother and child are well-documented and publicly promoted. However, all psychotropic medications pass into the breastmilk and infant serum in varying amounts. Therefore, breastfeeding is decided on a case-by-case basis.

Numerous factors may influence a woman's decision whether or not to breastfeed. These include previous episodes, a family history of postpartum psychosis, the mother's desire to breastfeed, risks and benefits to the neonate, and maternal risks from breastfeeding (Chaudron, 2000). Breastfeeding involves sleep disruption throughout the night; generally, sleep deprivation is one of the triggers of inducing a manic episode. Therefore, many women give up nursing in order to maintain mood stability. Providing patients with information about the risks and benefits of breastfeeding and unknown risks such as long-term sequelae is advised (Chaudron & Jefferson, 2000). In women who choose to breastfeed and require mood stabilization, the principles governing drug administration are similar to those used in pregnancy, such as monotherapy where possible, using the lowest therapeutic dose and selecting agents based on the current condition and past responses to medication. (See also Chapter 11.)

Lithium. Postpartum lithium prophylaxis has been reported to decrease the relapse rate in women with BD from about 50% to 10% (Yatham et al.,

2005). Lithium should be administered to breastfeeding women with caution, as infant blood concentrations that are 11–56% of therapeutic levels have been reported (Viguera et al., 2007). Studies have found breastmilk lithium concentrations to be about 40% (range 24–72%) and infant levels to be 5–200% of maternal levels (Yatham et al., 2005; Burt & Rasgon, 2004; Yonkers et al., 2004; Ernst & Goldberg, 2002). If women do choose to breastfeed on lithium, lithium concentrations should be monitored closely in both the mother and baby. When it is not possible to measure infant levels, the mother should be advised to observe the baby and report to her healthcare provider when required. In these instances, whether to continue or discontinue breastfeeding will depend on the mother making an informed decision. The long-term impact of extended lithium exposure has not been determined, but limited data indicates no obvious developmental abnormalities (Grandjean & Aubry, 2009).

Anticonvulsants. Both valproic acid and carbamazepine were considered "usually compatible with breastfeeding" by the AAP: Committee on Drugs (2000). In the Reproductive Mental Health Program, our preference is to not use valproate or carbamazepine while breastfeeding due to negative data related to pregnancy.

Valproate. Valproate levels in breastmilk have been reported as 1–10% of maternal serum levels (Tettenborn, 2006; Pennell, 2003), with infant levels varying from undetectable to 40% of maternal levels (Tettenborn, 2006). No adverse effects were reported in several studies involving breastfed infants whose mothers received valproate for BD (Piontek et al., 2000; Wisner & Perel, 1998; Johannessen, Helde, & Brodtkorb, 2005). However, a case of thrombocytopenic purpura, anemia, and reticulocytosis has been described in a breastfed 3-month-old infant whose mother received valproic acid for epilepsy; these symptoms resolved with the cessation of breastfeeding (Stahl et al., 1997). Hepatotoxicity has been reported in children less than 24 months receiving valproate directly (not through breastmilk). In a 2010 study, the IQ of 3-year old children exposed to valproate from breastmilk was measured, and no long-term intelligence deficits were found (Meador et al., 2010). However, due to evidence regarding neurodevelopmental effects of in utero exposure to valproate (Vinten et al., 2005; Eriksson et al., 2005; Gaily et al., 2004; Adab et al., 2001), informed consent should include the possible neurodevelopmental effects from exposure in breastmilk.

Carbamazepine. Relatively high levels of carbamazepine are found in breastmilk, with reports ranging from 32–79% of maternal serum levels (Shimoyama, et al, 2000; Davanzo et al., 2013). Infant serum levels vary from 6 to 65% of maternal concentrations. Notably, in most cases exposure has occurred in utero (Stowe, 2007). Case reports also indicate transient infant hepatotoxicity (Frey et al., 2002).

Lamotrigine. Like other psychoactive agents, lamotrigine crosses over into the breastmilk. A large range of infant levels of lamotrigine from breastmilk exposure is noted due to the variability of studies. Case reports show infant serum levels at approximately 30% of maternal levels (Liporace, et al, 2004; Rubin, et al, 2004). Careful monitoring of infants for rashes is advised, as children receiving lamotrigine are at a heightened risk of life-threatening skin reactions (Guerrini et al., 2012). Another study has shown that exclusively breastfed infants would receive approximately 9% of the maternal weight-adjusted dosage (Page-Sharp et al., 2006). The AAP classifies lamotrigine as an agent of unknown effect, which may be of concern because of potentially therapeutic serum levels in infants (AAP: Committee on Drugs, 2000); therefore, lamotrigine is not recommended while breastfeeding.

Topiramate. In a study of five mother-infant pairs in women with epilepsy taking topiramate (who all concomitantly received either valproic acid or carbamazepine), three of the pairs were breastfed. Topiramate was found to be excreted into the breastmilk between 3–23% of the mother's weight-adjusted dose. Infant levels were about 10–20% of maternal serum levels and adverse effects were not reported in the infants (Ohman et al., 2002). These levels are confirmed by more recent studies (Froscher & Jurges, 2006). However, more data on this agent is warranted.

Antipsychotics

First generation antipsychotics. The AAP classifies numerous antipsychotics as having an "unknown" effect but which may be of concern in breastfed infants. The AAP also mentions the possible effect of decline in developmental scores with exposure to haloperidol and chlorprozamine through breastfeeding, and the potential for infant lethargy and

drowsiness, and maternal galactorrhea with chlorprozamine (AAP: Committee on Drugs, 2000). A review reported minimal adverse effects in infants exposed to high potency neuroleptics such as haloperidol, flupenthixol, zuclopenthixol and trifluoperazine in breastmilk, and a single case of drowsiness and lethargy in the infant as a result of chlorpromazine (Gentile, 2008). However, use of these agents is declining with the growth of second-generation antipsychotics.

Second generation or novel antipsychotics. The different side effect profile of atypical antipsychotics sometimes makes them more favored medical treatments in clinical practice when indicated. Information on these drugs in lactating women is scant, being limited to case reports. Clozapine is found in high concentrations in breastmilk and select cases have demonstrated that it may cause neurodevelopmental delay and other unwanted effects (Mendhekar, 2007; Dev & Krupp, 1995). Olanzapine appears to be safe in breastmilk exposure (Gilad et al., 2011), but exposure during pregnancy can lead to a high birth weight (Babu et al., 2010). Data on risperidone is still quite scarce. In a study of two breastfed infants whose mothers took risperidone, the maternal milk/plasma concentration ratio was ≤0.5 and the relative infant dose ranged from 2.3% to 4.7% of the maternal weight-adjusted dose; the drug was undetectable in the infant serum and no adverse effects were described (Ilett et al., 2004). A similar study found that the infant would receive 0.84% of the maternal dose and 3.46% from risperidone metabolites (Hill et al., 2000). Another case study reported no adverse reactions from risperidone exposure during lactation (Ratnayake & Libretto, 2002). Quetiapine has a favorable risk/benefit profile due to its low levels in infant serum (0.09–0.43% of the weight-adjusted maternal dose) (Gentile, 2008; Lee et al., 2004; Rampono et al., 2007). A study by Misri et al. (2006), where breastfeeding mothers were taking quetiapine along with other antipsychotics, suggested slight or mild neurodevelopmental delay in infants exposed to quetiapine in lactation. Nonetheless, dosages less than 75 mg/day are likely undetectable in breastmilk. Although these very limited data suggest olanzapine, risperidone and clozapine may be used in nursing women, the nursing infant should be monitored when indicated.

Benzodiazepines. The primary role of BDPs in the postpartum period is alleviation of anxiety, agitation, panic and sleeping difficulties. Adverse effects from BDPs with no active metabolites (e.g., loraze-pam and clonazepam) have not been reported, but diazepam has been linked to neonatal sedation in one case report (Yonkers et al., 2004). A 2012 study of 124 mothers, found central nervous system depression in 1.6% of infants exposed to BDPs in breastmilk (Kelly et al., 2012). The AAP classifies diazepam, lorazepam, midazolam, temazepam and several other anxiolytics as having an unknown effect on breastfed infants, but which may be of concern, particularly if administered for extended periods (AAP: Committee on Drugs, 2000). BDPs should be used only when indicated while breastfeeding and the main concern is with-drawal in the infant.

Conclusions

The reproductive lifecycle of a woman with BD is dynamic. There are mental health concerns that arise with each phase—whether mania or depression. Phys-icians require a flexible outlook and a keen awareness of the issues pertinent to each stage so that their therapeutic approach can shift as women transition from each phase. During the childbearing era, women with BD face specific risks, particularly illness exacer-bation. For some individuals, this period may be their first presentation of the disorder.

1. BD affects women during their childbearing years, therefore has implications for both the mother and baby given the chronic and disruptive nature of the illness.
2. Pregnancy planning, postpartum prophylaxis and intensive monitoring by a multidisciplinary team that includes links between psychiatrists, obstetricians and pediatricians is recommended in the treatment of patients with BD in pregnancy and the postpartum.
3. Each case must be individually analyzed from a risk/benefit perspective and management planned accordingly.
4. Pharmacotherapy is challenging, but with proper preconception counseling and ongoing monitoring during pregnancy and the postpartum, the risks to the mother and baby can be minimized.

References

ACOG Committee on Practice Bulletins (2008). Use of psychiatric medications during pregnancy and lactation. *Obstetrics & Gynecology*, 111, 1001–1020.

Adab, N., Jacoby, A., Smith, D., et al. (2001). Additional educational needs in children born to mothers with epilepsy. *Journal of Neurology, Neurosurgery & Psychiatry*, 70, 15–21.

Almgren, M., Källén, B., and Lavebratt, C. (2009). Population-based study of antiepileptic drug exposure in utero—Influence on head circumference in newborns. *Seizure*, 18, 672–675.

American Academy of Neurology. (1998). Practice parameter: Management issues for women with epilepsy (summary statement): Report of the Quality Standards Subcommittee of the American Academy of Neurology. *Neurology*, 51, 944–948.

American Academy of Pediatrics: Committee on Drugs (2000). Use of psychoactive medication during pregnancy and possible effects on the fetus and newborn. *Pediatrics*, 105, 880–887.

American Psychiatric Association. (2013). *Diagnostic and Statistical Manual of Mental Disorders* (5th ed.). Arlington, VA: American Psychiatric Publishing.

Anderson, E. L. and Reti, I. M. (2009). ECT in pregnancy: A review of the literature from 1941 to 2007. *Psychosomatic Medicine*, 71, 235–242.

Anderson, I. M., Haddad, P. M., and Scott, J. (2012). Bipolar disorder. *British Medical Journal*, 345, e8505.

Antoniadis, D., Samakouri, M., and Livaditis, M. (2012). The association of bipolar spectrum disorders and borderline personality disorder. *Psychiatric Quarterly*, 83, 449–465.

Arnold, L. M. (2003). Gender differences in bipolar disorder. *Psychiatric Clinics of North America*, 26, 595–620.

Avan, B., Richter, L. M., Ramchandani, et al. (2010). Maternal postnatal depression and children's growth and behaviour during the early years of life: Exploring the interaction between physical and mental health. *Archives of Disease in Childhood*, 95, 690–695.

Babu, G. N., Desai, G., Tippeswamy, H., et al. (2010). Birth weight and use of olanzapine in pregnancy: A prospective comparative study. *Journal of Clinical Psychopharmacology*, 30, 331–332.

Babu, G. N., Thippeswamy, H., and Chandra, P. S. (2013). Use of electroconvulsive therapy (ECT) in postpartum psychosis—a naturalistic prospective study. *Archives of Women's Mental Health*, 16, 247–251.

Baek, J. H., Park, D. Y., Choi, et al. (2011). Differences between bipolar I and bipolar II disorders in clinical features, comorbidity, and family history. *Journal of Affective Disorders*, 131, 59–67.

Baldassano, C. F., Marangell, L. B., Gyulai, L., et al. (2005). Gender differences in bipolar disorder: Retrospective data from the first 500 STEP-BD participants. *Bipolar Disorders*, 7, 465–470.

Baldessarini, R. J., Bolzani, L., Cruz, N., et al. (2010). Onset-age of bipolar disorders at six international sites. *Journal of Affective Disorders*, 121, 143–146.

Bauer, M., Grof, P., Rasgon, et al. (2006). Temporal relation between sleep and mood in patients with bipolar disorder. *Bipolar Disorders*, 8, 160–167.

Bauler, S., Janoly-Dumenil, A., Sancho, P. O., et al. (2012). Effect of carbamazepine on fluindione's anticoagulant activity: A case report. *Thérapie*, 67, 488–489.

Bellantuono, C., Tofani, S., Di Sciascio, G., et al. (2013). Benzodiazepine exposure in pregnancy and risk of major malformations: A critical overview. *General Hospital Psychiatry*, 35, 3–8.

Bergink, V., Bouvy, P. F., Vervoort, J. S., et al. (2012). Prevention of postpartum psychosis and mania in women at high risk. *American Journal of Psychiatry*, 169, 609–615.

Bilszta, J. L., Meyer, D., and Buist, A. E. (2010). Bipolar affective disorder in the postnatal period: Investigating the role of sleep. *Bipolar Disorders*, 12, 568–578.

Binfa, L., Castelo-Branco, C., Blümel, J. E., et al. (2004). Influence of psychosocial factors on climacteric symptoms. *Maturitas*, 48, 425–431.

Birmaher, B., Axelson, D., Monk, K., et al. (2009). Lifetime psychiatric disorders in school-aged offspring of parents with bipolar disorder: The Pittsburgh Bipolar Offspring study. *Archives of General Psychiatry*, 66, 287–296.

Blehar, M. C., DePaulo Jr., J. R., Gershon, E. S., et al. (1998). Women with bipolar disorder: Findings from the NIMH genetics initiative sample. *Psychopharmacology Bulletin*, 34, 239–243.

Bodén, R., Lundgren, M., Brandt, L., et al. (2012). Risks of adverse pregnancy and birth outcomes in women treated or not treated with mood stabilisers for bipolar disorder: Population based cohort study. *British Medical Journal*, 345, e7085.

Bogen, D. L., Sit, D., Genovese, A., et al. (2012). Three cases of lithium exposure and exclusive breastfeeding. *Archives of Women's Mental Health*, 15, 69–72.

Bonari, L., Pinto, N., Ahn, E., et al. (2004). Perinatal risks of untreated depression during pregnancy. *Canadian Journal of Psychiatry*, 49, 726–735.

Bradley, R. and Slade, P. (2011). A review of mental health problems in fathers following the birth of a child. *Journal of Reproductive and Infant Psychology*, 29, 19–42.

Brockington, I. (2004). Postpartum psychiatric disorders. *Lancet*, 363, 303–310.

Burt, V. K. and Rasgon, N. (2004). Special considerations in treating bipolar disorder in women. *Bipolar Disorders*, 6, 2–13.

Burt, V. K., Bernstein, C., Rosenstein, W. S., et al. (2010). Bipolar disorder and pregnancy: Maintaining psychiatric stability in the real world of obstetric and psychiatric complications. *American Journal of Psychiatry*, 167, 892–897.

Byers, M. G., Allison, K. M., Wendel, C. S., et al. (2010). Prazosin versus quetiapine for nighttime posttraumatic stress disorder symptoms in veterans: An assessment of long-term comparative effectiveness and safety. *Journal of Clinical Psychopharmacology*, 30, 225–229.

Campbell, E., Devenney, E., Morrow, J., et al. (2013). Recurrence risk of congenital malformations in infants exposed to antiepileptic drugs in utero. *Epilepsia*, 54, 165–171.

Carter, A. S., Garrity-Rokous, F. E., Chazan-Cohen, R., et al. (2001). Maternal depression and comorbidity: Predicting early parenting, attachment security, and toddler social-emotional problems and competencies. *Journal of the American Academy of Child and Adolescent Psychiatry*, 40, 18–26.

Chaudron, J. H. and Pies, R. W. (2003). The relationship between postpartum psychosis and bipolar disorder: A review. *Journal of Clinical Psychiatry*, 64, 1284–1292.

Chaudron, L. H. (2000). When and how to use mood stabilizers during breastfeeding. *Primary Care Update for Obstetricians and Gynaecologists*, 7, 113–117.

Chaudron, L. H. and Jefferson, J. W. (2000). Mood stabilizers during breastfeeding: A review. *Journal of Clinical Psychiatry*, 61, 79–90.

Chessick, C. A. and Dimidjian, S. (2010). Screening for bipolar disorder during pregnancy and the postpartum period. *Archives of Women's Mental Health*, 13, 233–248.

Christensen, J., Gronborg, T. K., and Sorensen, M. J. (2013). Prenatal valproate exposure and risk of autism spectrum disorders and childhood autism. *JAMA*, 309, 1696–1703.

Christensen, J., Petrenaite, V., Atterman, J., et al. (2007). Oral contraceptives induce lamotrigine metabolism: Evidence from a double-blind, placebo-controlled trial. *Epilepsia*, 48, 484–489.

Clarkin. J. F., Carpenter, D., Hull, J., et al. (1998). Effects of psychoeducational intervention for married patients with bipolar disorder and their spouses. *Psychiatric Services*, 49, 531–553.

Coe, H. V. and Hong, I. S. (2012). Safety of low doses of quetiapine when used for insomnia. *The Annals of Pharmacotherapy*, 46, 718–722.

Cohen, L. S. and Nonacs, R. M. (Eds.) (2005). In J. M. Oldham and R. M. Nonacs (Series Eds.), *Review of Psychiatry: Vol. 24. Mood and Anxiety Disorders During Pregnancy and Postpartum*. Arlington, VA: American Psychiatric Publishing.

Cohen, L. S., Sichel, D. A., Robertson, L. M., et al. (1995). Postpartum prophylaxis for women with bipolar disorder. *American Journal of Psychiatry*, 152, 1641–1645.

Colom, F., Vieta, E., Reinares, M., et al. (2003). Psychoeducation efficacy in bipolar disorders: Beyond compliance enhancement. *The Journal of Clinical Psychiatry*, 64, 1101–1105.

Cox, J. L., Holden, J. M., and Sagovsky, R. (1987). Detection of postnatal depression. Development of the 10-item Edinburgh Postnatal Depression Scale. *British Journal of Psychiatry*, 150, 782–786.

Cummings, C., Stewart, M., Stevenson, M., et al. (2011). Neurodevelopment of children exposed in utero to lamotrigine, sodium valproate and carbamazepine. *Archives of Disease in Childhood*, 96, 643–647.

Cunnington, M. C., Weil, J. G., Messenheimer, J. A., et al. (2011). Final results from 18 years of the International Lamotrigine Pregnancy Registry. *Neurology*, 76, 1817–1823.

Da Silva, T. L., Ravindran, L. N., and Ravindran, A. V. (2009). Yoga in the treatment of mood and anxiety disorders: A review. *Asian Journal of Psychiatry*, 2, 6–16.

Davanzo, R., Dal Bo, S., Bua, J., et al. (2013). Antiepileptic drugs and breastfeeding. *Italian Journal of Pediatrics*, 39, 1–11.

Deckersbach, T., Hölzel, B. K., Eisner, L. R., et al. (2012). Mindfulness-based cognitive therapy for nonremitted patients with bipolar disorder. *CNS Neuroscience & Therapeutics*, 18, 133–141.

Dev, V. J. and Krupp, P. (1995). Adverse event profile and safety of clozapine. *Reviews in Contemporary Pharmacotherapy*, 6, 197–208.

Diav-Citrin, O., Shechtman, S., Arnon, J., et al. (2001). Is carbamazepine teratogenic? A prospective controlled study of 210 pregnancies. *Neurology*, 57, 321–324.

Diav-Citrin, O., Shechtman, S., Ornoy, S., et al. (2005). Safety of haloperidol and penfluridol in pregnancy: A multicenter, prospective, controlled study. *The Journal of Clinical Psychiatry*, 66, 317–322.

Dietz, L. J., Jennings, K. D., Kelley, S. A., et al. (2009). Maternal depression, paternal psychopathology, and toddlers' behavior problems. *Journal of Clinical Child & Adolescent Psychology*, 38, 48–61.

DiFlorio, A. and Jones, I. (2010). Is sex important? Gender differences in bipolar disorder. *International Review of Psychiatry*, 22, 437–452.

DiLiberti, J. H., Farndon, P. A., Dennis, N. R., et al. (1984). The fetal valproate syndrome. *American Journal of Medical Genetics*, 19, 473–481.

Doucet, S., Jones, I., Letourneau, N., et al. (2011). Interventions for the prevention and treatment of postpartum psychosis: A systematic review. *Archives of Women's Mental Health*, 14, 89–98.

Dursun, A., Karadag, N., Karagöl, B., et al. (2012). Carbamazepine use in pregnancy and coincidental thalidomide-like phocomelia in a newborn. *Journal of Obstetrics & Gynaecology*, 32, 488–489.

Ebbesen, F., Joergensen, A., Hoseth, E., et al. (2000). Neonatal hypoglycaemia and withdrawal symptoms after exposure in utero to valproate. *Archives of Disease in Childhood Fetal and Neonatal Edition*, 83, F124–F129.

Einarson, A. and Boskovic, R. (2009). Use and safety of antipsychotic drugs during pregnancy. *Journal of Psychiatric Practice*, 15, 183–192.

Enato, E., Moretti, M., and Koren, G. (2011). The fetal safety of benzodiazepines: An updated meta-analysis. *Journal of Obstetrics and Gynaecology Canada*, 33, 46.

Eriksson, K., Viinikainen, K., Mönkkönen, A., et al. (2005). Children exposed to valproate in utero—population based evaluation of risks and confounding factors for long-term neurocognitive development. *Epilepsy Research*, 65, 189–200.

Eriksson, E., Andersch, B., Ho, H. P., et al. (2002). Diagnosis and treatment of premenstrual dysphoria. *Journal of Clinical Psychiatry*, 63(Suppl. 7), 16–23.

Ernst, C. L. and Goldberg, J. F. (2002). The reproductive safety profile of mood stabilizers, atypical antipsychotics, and broad-spectrum psychotropics. *Journal of Clinical Psychiatry*, 63(Suppl. 4), 42–55.

Eros, E., Czeizel, A. E., Rockenbauer, M., et al. (2002). A population-based case–control teratologic study of nitrazepam, medazepam, tofisopam, alprazolum and clonazepam treatment during pregnancy. *European Journal of Obstetrics & Gynecology and Reproductive Biology*, 101, 147–154.

Faraone, S. V., Biederman, J., and Wozniak, J. (2012). Examining the comorbidity between attention deficit hyperactivity disorder and bipolar I disorder: A meta-analysis of family genetic studies. *American Journal of Psychiatry*, 169, 1256–1266.

Farren, C. K., Hill, K. P., and Weiss, R. D. (2012). Bipolar disorder and alcohol use disorder: A review. *Current Psychiatry Reports*, 14, 659–666.

Feingold, S. B. and Brown, R. S. (2010). Neonatal thyroid function. *NeoReviews*, 11, e640–e646.

Field, T. (2011). Yoga clinical research review. *Complementary Therapies in Clinical Practice*, 17, 1–8.

Field, T. and Diego, M. (2008). Cortisol: The culprit prenatal stress variable. *International Journal of Neuroscience*, 118, 1181–1205.

Field, T., Diego, M., Dieter, J., et al. (2004). Prenatal depression effects on the fetus and the newborn. *Infant Behavior and Development*, 27, 216–229.

Finer, L. B. and Zolna, M. R. (2011). Unintended pregnancy in the United States: Incidence and disparities, 2006. *Contraception*, 84, 478–485.

Finnerty, M., Levin, Z., and Miller, L. J. (1996). Acute manic episodes in pregnancy. *American Journal of Psychiatry*, 153, 261–263.

Flynn, S., Shaw, J., Abel, K. M. (2007) Homicide of infants: a cross-sectional study. *Journal of Clinical Psychiatry*, 68, 1501–1509.

Flynn, S. M., Shaw, J., Abel, K. M. (2013). Filicide: mental illness in those who kill their children. *PLoS ONE*, 8(4), DOI:10.1371/journal.pone.0058981

Focht, A., and Kellner, C. (2012). Electroconvulsive therapy (ECT) in the treatment of postpartum psychosis. *The Journal of Electroconvulsive Therapy*, 28, 31–33.

Fracalanza, K. A., McCabe, R. E., Taylor, V. H., et al. (2011). Bipolar disorder comorbidity in anxiety disorders: Relationship to demographic profile, symptom severity, and functional impairment. *The European Journal of Psychiatry*, 25, 223–233.

Frank. E., Cyranowski, I. M., Rucci, P., et al. (2002). Clinical significance of lifetime panic spectrum symptoms in the treatment of patients with bipolar l disorder. *Archives of General Psychiatry*, 59, 905–911.

Freeman, E. W., Sammel, M. D., Rinaudo, P. J., et al. (2004). Premenstrual syndrome as a predictor of menopausal symptoms. *Obstetrics & Gynecology*, 103, 960–966.

Freeman, M. P., Smith, K. W., Freeman. S. A., et al. (2002). The impact of reproductive events on the course of bipolar disorder in women. *Journal of Clinical Psychiatry*, 63, 284–287.

Frey, B., Braegger, C. P., and Ghelfi, D. (2002). Neonatal cholestatic hepatitis from carbamazepine exposure during pregnancy and breast feeding. *The Annals of Pharmacotherapy*, 36, 644–647.

Frieder, A., Dunlop, A. L., Culpepper, L., et al. (2008). The clinical content of preconception care: Women with psychiatric conditions. *American Journal of Obstetrics and Gynecology*, 199, S328–S332.

Froscher, W. and Jurges, U. (2006). Topiramate used during breast feeding. *Aktuelle Neurologie*, 33, 215–217.

Gaily, E., Kantola-Sorsa, E., Hiilesmaa, V., et al. (2004). Normal intelligence in children with prenatal exposure to carbamazepine. *Neurology*, 62, 28–32.

Galbally, M., Roberts, M., and Buist, A. (2010). Mood stabilizers in pregnancy: A systematic review. *Australian and New Zealand Journal of Psychiatry*, 44, 967–977.

Galbally, M., Snellen, M., Walker, S., et al. (2010). Management of antipsychotic and mood stabilizer medication in pregnancy: Recommendations for antenatal care. *Australian and New Zealand Journal of Psychiatry*, 44, 99–108.

Galimberti, C. A., Mazzucchelli, I., Arbasino, C., et al. (2006). Increased apparent oral clearance of valproic acid during intake of combined contraceptive steroids in women with epilepsy. *Epilepsia*, 47, 1569–1572.

Gentile, S. (2008). Infant safety with antipsychotic therapy in breast-feeding: A systematic review. *The Journal of Clinical Psychiatry*, 69, 666–673.

Gentile, S. (2010a). Antipsychotic therapy during early and late pregnancy: A systematic review. *Schizophrenia Bulletin*, 36, 518–544.

Gentile, S. (2010b). Neurodevelopmental effects of prenatal exposure to psychotropic medications. *Depression and Anxiety*, 27, 675–686.

Gentile, S. (2012). Lithium in pregnancy: The need to treat, the duty to ensure safety. *Expert Opinion on Drug Safety*, 11, 425–437.

George, E.L., Miklowitz, D.J., Richards, J. A., et al. (2003). The comorbidity of bipolar disorder and axis II personality disorders: Prevalence and clinical correlates. *Bipolar Disorders*, 5, 115–122.

Gilad, O., Merlob, P., Stahl, B., et al. (2011). Outcome of infants exposed to olanzapine during breastfeeding. *Breastfeeding Medicine*, 6, 55–58.

Glover, V., Liddle, P., Taylor, A., et al. (1994). Mild hypomania (the highs) can be a feature of the first postpartum week. Association with later depression. *The British Journal of Psychiatry*, 164, 517–521.

Goldberg, J. F. and Ernst, C. L. (2002). The economic and social burden of bipolar disorder: A review. In M. Maj, H. S. Akisal, J. J. Lopez-Ibor, et al. (Series Eds.), *Bipolar Disorder*, Vol. 5 (pp. 441–467). Chichester, UK: Wiley.

Grandjean, E. M., & Aubry, J. M. (2009). Lithium: updated human knowledge using an evidence-based approach. *CNS Drugs*, 23(5), 397–418.

Green, L., Vais, A., and Harding, K. (2013). Preconception care for women with mental health conditions. *British Journal of Hospital Medicine*, 74, 319–321.

Grof, P., Robbins, W., Alda, M., et al. (2000). Protective effect of pregnancy in women with lithium-responsive bipolar disorder. *Journal of Affective Disorders*, 61, 31–39.

Guerrini, R., Zaccara, G., la Marca, G., et al. (2012). Safety and tolerability of antiepileptic drug treatment in children with epilepsy. *Drug Safety*, 35, 519–533.

Harden, C. L., Pennell, P. B., Koppel, B. S., et al. (2009). Practice Parameter update: Management issues for women with epilepsy—focus on pregnancy (an evidence-based review): Vitamin K, folic acid, blood levels, and breastfeeding. *Neurology*, 73, 142–149.

Hendrick, V., Altshuler, L. L., Gitlin, M. J. et al. (2000). Gender and bipolar illness. *Journal of Clinical Psychiatry*, 61, 393–396.

Henin, A., Biederman, J., Mick, E., et al. (2005). Psychopathology in the offspring of parents with bipolar disorder: A controlled study. *Biological Psychiatry*, 58, 554–561.

Hernández-Díaz, S., Smith, C. R., Shen, A., et al. (2012). Comparative safety of antiepileptic drugs during pregnancy. *Neurology*, 78, 1692–1699.

Heron, J., Haque, S., Oyebode, F., et al. (2009). A longitudinal study of hypomania and depression symptoms in pregnancy and the postpartum period. *Bipolar Disorders*, 11, 410–417.

Herzog, A. G., Blum, A. S., Farina, E. L., et al. (2009). Valproate and lamotrigine level variation with menstrual cycle phase and oral contraceptive use. *Neurology*, 72, 911–914.

Hill, R. C., McIvor, R. J., Wojnar-Horton, R. E., et al. (2000). Risperidone distribution and excretion into human milk: Case report and estimated infant exposure during breast-feeding. *Journal of Clinical Psychopharmacology*, 20, 285–286.

Hillegers, M. H., Reichart, C. G., Wals, M., et al. (2005). Five-year prospective outcome of psychopathology in the adolescent offspring of bipolar parents. *Bipolar Disorders*, 7, 344–350.

Hirschfeld, R. M., Williams, J. B., Spitzer, R. L., et al. (2000). Development and validation of a screening instrument for bipolar spectrum disorder: The Mood Disorder Questionnaire. *American Journal of Psychiatry*, 157, 1873–1875.

Holland, J., Agius, M., and Zaman, R. (2011). Prevalence of co-morbid bipolar disorder and migraine in a regional hospital psychiatric outpatient department. *Psychiatria Danubina*, 23(Suppl. 1), S23–S24.

Holmes, L. B., Adams, J., Coull, B., et al. (2000). Anticonvulsant face: Association with cognitive dysfunction. *Pediatric Research*, 47(Suppl.), 82A.

Holmes, L. B., Coull, B. A., Dorfman, J., et al. (2005). The correlation of deficits in IQ with midface and digit hypoplasia in children exposed in utero to anticonvulsant drugs. *The Journal of Pediatrics*, 146, 118–122.

Hudak, M. L., Tan, R. C., Frattarelli, D. A., et al. (2012). Neonatal drug withdrawal. *Pediatrics*, 129, e540–e560.

Hunt, N. and Silverstone, T. (1995). Does puerperal illness distinguish a subgroup of bipolar patients? *Journal of Affective Disorders*, 34, 101–107.

Ibiloglu, A. O. and Caykoylu, A. (2011). The comorbidity of anxiety disorders in bipolar I and bipolar II patients among Turkish population. *Journal of Anxiety Disorders*, 25, 661–667.

Ilett, K. F., Hackett, L. P., Kristensen, J. H., Vaddadi, K. S., Gardiner, S. J., & Begg, E. J. (2004). Transfer of risperidone and 9-hydroxyrisperidone into human milk. *Annals of Pharmacotherapy*, 38(2), 273–276.

Ives-Deliperi, V. L., Howells, F., Stein, D. J., et al. (2013). The effects of mindfulness-based cognitive therapy in patients with bipolar disorder: A controlled functional MRI investigation. *Journal of Affective Disorders*, 150, 1152.

Jackson, A., Cavanagh, J., and Scott, J. (2003). A systematic review of manic and depressive prodromes. *Journal of Affective Disorders*, 74, 209–217.

Jentink, J., Loane, M. A., Dolk, H., et al. (2010). Valproic acid monotherapy in pregnancy and major congenital malformations. *New England Journal of Medicine*, 362, 2185–2193.

Jiang, B., Kenna, H. A., and Rasgon, N. L. (2009). Genetic overlap between polycystic ovary syndrome and bipolar disorder: The endophenotype hypothesis. *Medical Hypotheses*, 73, 996–1004.

Johannessen, S. I., Helde, G., and Brodtkorb, E. (2005). Levetiracetam concentrations in serum and in breast milk at birth and during lactation. *Epilepsia*, 46, 775–777.

Jones, I. and Craddock, N. (2001). Familiality of the puerperal trigger in bipolar disorder: Results of a family study. *American Journal of Psychiatry*, 158, 913–917.

Kaaja, E., Kaaja, R., Matila, R., et al. (2002). Enzyme-inducing antiepileptic drugs in pregnancy and the risk of bleeding in the neonate. *Neurology*, 58, 549–553.

Källén, B. and Reis, M. (2012). Neonatal complications after maternal concomitant use of SSRI and other central nervous system active drugs during the second or third trimester of pregnancy. *Journal of Clinical Psychopharmacology*, 32, 608–614.

Kay, J. H., Altshuler, L. L., Ventura, J., et al. (2002). Impact of axis II comorbidity on the course of bipolar illness in men: A retrospective chart review. *Bipolar Disorders*, 4, 237–242.

Kelly, L. E., Poon, S., Madadi, P., et al. (2012). Neonatal benzodiazepines exposure during breastfeeding. *The Journal of Pediatrics*, 161, 448–451.

Kemp, D. E., Gao, K., Chan, P. K., et al. (2010). Medical comorbidity in bipolar disorder: Relationship between illnesses of the endocrine/metabolic system and treatment outcome. *Bipolar Disorders*, 12, 404–413.

Kendell, R. E., Chalmers, J. C., and Platz, C. (1987). Epidemiology of puerperal psychoses. *The British Journal of Psychiatry*, 150, 662–673.

Kilbane, E. J., Gokbayrak, N. S., Galynker I., et al. (2009). A review of panic and suicide in bipolar disorder: Does comorbidity increase risk? *Journal of Affective Disorders*, 115, 1–10.

Kjaer, D., Horvath-Puhó, E., Christensen, J., Vestergaard, M., Czeizel, A. E., Sørensen, H. T., & Olsen, J. (2007). Use of phenytoin, phenobarbital, or diazepam during pregnancy and risk of congenital abnormalities: a case-time-control study. *Pharmacoepidemiology and Drug Safety*, 16(2), 181–188.

Klipstein, K. G. and Goldberg, J. F. (2006). Screening for bipolar disorder in women with polycystic ovary syndrome: A pilot study. *Journal of Affective Disorders*, 91, 205–209.

Korja, R., Savonlahti, E., Ahlqvist-Bjorkroth, S., et al. (2008). Maternal depression is associated with mother-infant interaction in preterm infants. *Acta Paediatrica*, 97, 724–730.

Kozma, C. (2005). Neonatal toxicity and transient neurodevelopmental deficits following prenatal exposure to lithium: Another clinical report and a review of the literature. *American Journal of Medical Genetics Part A*, 132, 441–444.

Kumar, S., Mohanty, B. B., Agrawal, D., et al. (2012). Antiepileptics and pregnancy: A review. *International Journal of Current Research and Review*, 4, 132–143.

Kupka, R. W., Luckenbaugh, D. A., Post, R. M., et al. (2005). Comparison of rapid-cycling and non-rapid-cycling bipolar disorder based on prospective mood ratings in 539 outpatients. *American Journal of Psychiatry*, 162, 1273–1280.

Lahdelma, L. (2012). Clozapine/neuropsychotherapeutics: Agranulocytosis: 7 case reports. *Reactions*, 1420, 20.

Lam, D. H., Bright, J., Jones, S., et al. (2000). Cognitive therapy for bipolar illness—a pilot study of relapse prevention. *Cognitive Therapy and Research*, 24, 503–520.

Lam, D. H., Watkins, E. R., Hayward, P., et al. (2003). A randomized controlled study of cognitive therapy for relapse prevention for bipolar affective disorder: Outcome of the first year. *Archives of General Psychiatry*, 60, 145–152.

Lapalme, M., Hodgins, S. and LaRoche, C. (1997). Children of parents with bipolar disorder: A metaanalysis of risk for mental disorders. *Canadian Journal of Psychiatry*, 42, 623–631.

Lee, A., Giesbrecht, E., Dunn, E., et al. (2004). Excretion of quetiapine in breast milk. *The American Journal of Psychiatry*, 161, 1715–1716.

Lin, H. C., Chen, I. J., Chen, Y. H. et al. (2010). Maternal schizophrenia and pregnancy outcome: Does the use of antipsychotics make a difference? *Schizophrenia Research*, 116, 55–60.

Linnebank, M., Moskau, S., Semmler, A., et al. (2011). Antiepileptic drugs interact with folate and vitamin B12 serum levels. *Annals of Neurology*, 69, 352–359.

Liporace, J., Kao, A., and D'Abreu, A. (2004). Concerns regarding lamotrigine and breast-feeding. *Epilepsy & Behavior*, 5, 102–105.

Lippi, G. and Franchini, M. (2011). Vitamin K in neonates: Facts and myths. *Blood Transfusion*, 9, 4–9.

Mackay, F. J., Wilton, L. V., Pearce, G. L., et al. (1997). Safety of long-term lamotrigine in epilepsy. *Epilepsia*, 38, 881–886.

Madigan, S., Moran, G., Schuengel, C., et al. (2007). Unresolved maternal attachment representations, disrupted maternal behavior and disorganized attachment in infancy: Links to toddler behavior problems. *Journal of Child Psychology and Psychiatry and Allied Disciplines*, 48, 1042–1050.

Margulis, A. V., Mitchell, A. A., Gilboa, S. M., et al. (2012). Use of topiramate in pregnancy and risk of oral clefts. *American Journal of Obstetrics & Gynecology*, 207, 405.e1–405.e7.

Martins, C. and Gaffan, E. A. (2000). Effects of early maternal depression on patterns of infant-mother attachment: A meta-analytic investigation. *Journal of Child Psychology and Psychiatry and Allied Disciplines*, 41, 737–746.

Matlow, J. and Koren, G. (2012). Is carbamazepine safe to take during pregnancy? *Canadian Family Physician*, 58, 163–164.

McCauley-Elsom, K., Gurvich, C., Elsom, S. J., et al. (2010). Antipsychotics in pregnancy. *Journal of Psychiatric and Mental Health Nursing*, 17, 97–104.

McElroy, S. L., Frye, M. A., Hellemann, G., et al. (2011). Prevalence and correlates of eating disorders in 875 patients with bipolar disorder. *Journal of Affective Disorders*, 128, 191–198.

McElroy, S. L., Altshuler, L. L., Suppes, T., et al. (2001). Axis I psychiatric comorbidity and its relationship to historical illness variables in 288 patients with bipolar disorder. *American Journal of Psychiatry*, 158, 420–426.

McIntyre, R. S., Konarski, J. Z., Wilkins, K., et al. (2006). The prevalence and impact of migraine headache in bipolar disorder: Results from the Canadian Community Health Survey. *Headache: The Journal of Head and Face Pain*, 46, 973–982.

McIntyre, R. S., Soczynska, J. K., Beyer, J. L., et al. (2007). Medical comorbidity in bipolar disorder:

Reprioritizing unmet needs. *Current Opinion in Psychiatry*, 20, 406–416.

McKinlay, S. M., Brambilla, D. J., and Posner, J. G. (1992). The normal menopause transition. *The American Journal of Human Biology*, 4, 37–46.

Meador, K. J., Baker, G. A., Browning, N., et al. (2010). Effects of breastfeeding in children of women taking antiepileptic drugs. *Neurology*, 75, 1954–1960.

Meador, K. J., Baker, G. A., Browning, N., et al. (2013). Fetal antiepileptic drug exposure and cognitive outcomes at age 6 years (NEAD study): A prospective observational study. *The Lancet Neurology*, 12, 244–252.

Mendhekar, D. N. (2007). Possible delayed speech acquisition with clozapine therapy during pregnancy and lactation. *The Journal of Neuropsychiatry and Clinical Neurosciences*, 19, 196–197.

Merikangas, K. R., Akiskal, H. S., Angst, J., et al. (2007). Lifetime and 12-month prevalence of bipolar spectrum disorder in the National Comorbidity Survey replication. *Archives of General Psychiatry*, 64, 543–552.

Merikangas, K. R., Jin, R., He, J. P., et al. (2011). Prevalence and correlates of bipolar spectrum disorder in the world mental health survey initiative. *Archives of General Psychiatry*, 68, 241–251.

Miklowitz, D. J., George, E. L., Richards, J. A., et al. (2003). A randomized study of family-focused psychoeducation and pharmacotherapy in the outpatient management of bipolar disorder. *Archives of General Psychiatry*, 60, 904–912.

Miklowitz, D. J., Simoneau, T. L., George, E. L., et al. (2000). Family-focused treatment of bipolar disorder: 1-year effects of a psychoeducational program in conjunction with pharmacotherapy. *Biological Psychiatry*, 48, 582–592.

Misri, S. and Lusskin, S. I. (2004). Postpartum mood disorders. In B. D. Rose (Ed.), *UpToDate.*

Misri, S., Corral, M., Wardrop, A. A., et al. (2006). Quetiapine augmentation in lactation: A series of case reports. *Journal of Clinical Psychopharmacology*, 26, 508–511.

Mølgaard-Nielsen, D. and Hviid, A. (2011). Newer-generation antiepileptic drugs and the risk of major birth defects. *JAMA*, 305, 1996.

Moore, J. L. and Aggarwal, P. (2012). Lamotrigine use in pregnancy. *Expert Opinion on Pharmacotherapy*, 13, 1213–1216.

Mortensen, P. B., Pedersen, C. B., Melbye, M., et al. (2003). Individual and familial risk factors for bipolar affective disorders in Denmark. *Archives of General Psychiatry*, 60, 1209–1215.

Munk-Olsen, T., Laursen, T. M., Meltzer-Brody, S., et al. (2012). Psychiatric disorders with postpartum onset: Possible early manifestations of bipolar affective disorders. *Archives of General Psychiatry*, 69, 428.

Nassir Ghaemi, S., Miller, C.J., Berv, D.A., et al. (2005). Sensitivity and specificity of a new bipolar spectrum diagnostic scale. *Journal of Affective Disorders*, 84, 273–77.

Newport, D. J., Viguera, A. C., Beach, A. J., et al. (2005). Lithium placental passage and obstetrical outcome: Implications for clinical management during late pregnancy. *American Journal of Psychiatry*, 162, 2162–2170.

Nguyen, H. T., Sharma, V., and McIntyre, R. S. (2009). Teratogenesis associated with antibipolar agents. *Advances in Therapy*, 26, 281–294.

Nielsen, R. E. and Damkier, P. (2012). Pharmacological treatment of unipolar depression during pregnancy and breast-feeding:

A clinical overview. *Nordic Journal of Psychiatry*, 66, 159–166.

Nivoli, A., Pacchiarotti, I., Rosa, A. R., et al. (2011). Gender differences in a cohort study of 604 bipolar patients: The role of predominant polarity. *Journal of Affective Disorders*, 133, 443–449.

O'Donovan, C., Kusumakar, V., Graves, G. R. et al. (2002). Menstrual abnormalities and polycystic ovary syndrome in women taking valproate for bipolar mood disorder. *The Journal of Clinical Psychiatry*, 63, 322–330.

Ohman, I., Sabers, A., de Flon, P., et al. (2009). Pharmacokinetics of topiramate during pregnancy. *Epilepsy Research*, 87, 124–129.

Ohman, I., Vitols, S., Luef, G., et al. (2002). Topiramate kinetics during delivery, lactation, and in the neonate: Preliminary observations. *Epilepsia*, 43, 1157–1160.

Ortiz, A., Cervantes, P., Zlotnik, G., et al. (2010). Cross-prevalence of migraine and bipolar disorder. *Bipolar Disorders*, 12, 397–403.

Owen, J. A. (2011). Psychopharmacology. In Levenson, J. L. (Ed.). *The American Psychiatric Publishing Textbook of Psychosomatic Medicine: Psychiatric Care of the Medically Ill* (pp. 957–1020). Washington, DC: American Psychiatric Publishing.

Page-Sharp, M., Kristensen, J. H., Hackett, L. P., et al. (2006). Transfer of lamotrigine into breast milk. *The Annals of Pharmacotherapy*, 40, 1470–1471.

Patelis-Siotis, I. (2001). Cognitive-behavioral therapy: Applications for the management of bipolar disorder. *Bipolar Disorders*, 3, 1–10.

Payne, J. L., Roy, P. S., Murphy-Eberenz, K., et al. (2007). Reproductive cycle-associated mood symptoms in women with major depression and bipolar disorder. *Journal of Affective Disorders*, 99, 221–229.

Pearlstein, T., Howard, M., Salisbury, A., et al. (2009). Postpartum depression. *American Journal of Obstetrics and Gynecology*, 200, 357–364.

Pennell, P. B. (2003). Antiepileptic drug pharmacokinetics during pregnancy and lactation. *Neurology*, 61(6 Suppl. 2), S35–S42.

Pennell, P. B., Klein, A. M., Browning, N., et al. (2012). Differential effects of antiepileptic drugs on neonatal outcomes. *Epilepsy & Behavior*, 24, 449–456.

Pennell, P. B., Peng, L., Newport, D. J., et al. (2008). Lamotrigine in pregnancy: Clearance, therapeutic drug monitoring, and seizure frequency. *Neurology*, 70, 2130–2136.

Perlis, R. H., Ostacher, M. J., Patel, J. K., et al. (2006). Predictors of recurrence in bipolar disorder: Primary outcomes from the Systematic Treatment Enhancement Program for Bipolar Disorder (STEP-BD). *FOCUS: The Journal of Lifelong Learning in Psychiatry*, 4, 553–561.

Perugi, G. and Akiskal, H. S. (2002). The soft bipolar spectrum redefined: Focus on the cyclothymic, anxious-sensitive, impulse-dyscontrol, and binge-eating connection in bipolar II and related conditions. *Psychiatric Clinics of North America*, 25, 713–737.

Pfuhlmann, B., Stoeber, G., and Beckmann, H. (2002). Postpartum psychoses: Prognosis, risk factors, and treatment. *Current Psychiatry Reports*, 4, 185–190.

Pinheiro, K.A.T., Coelho, F.M.C., Quevedo, L. Á., et al. (2011). Paternal postpartum mood: Bipolar episodes? *Revista Brasileira de Psiquiatria*, 33, 283–286.

Piontek, C. M., Baab, S., Peindl, K. S., et al. (2000). Serum valproate levels in 6 breastfeeding mother-infant pairs. *The Journal of Clinical Psychiatry*, 61, 170–172.

Porter, T. and Gavin, H. (2010). Infanticide and neonaticide: A review of 40 years of research literature on incidence and causes. *Trauma, Violence, & Abuse*, 11, 99–112.

Post, R. M. and Kalivas, P. (2013). Bipolar disorder and substance misuse: Pathological and therapeutic implications of their comorbidity and cross-sensitisation. *The British Journal of Psychiatry*, 202, 172–176.

Pynnönen, S. and Sillanpää, M. (1975). Carbamazepine and mother's milk. *The Lancet*, 306, 563.

Pynnönen, S., Kanto, J., Sillanpää, M., et al. (1977). Carbamazepine: Placental transport, tissue concentrations in foetus and newborn, and level in milk. *Acta Pharmacologica et Toxicologica*, 41, 244–253.

Ramchandani, P., Stein, A., Evans, J., et al. (2005). Paternal depression in the postnatal period and child development: A prospective population study. *The Lancet*, 365, 2201–2205.

Rampono, J., Kristensen, J. H., Ilett, K. F., et al. (2007). Quetiapine and breast feeding. *The Annals of Pharmacotherapy*, 41, 711–714.

Ranga Rama Krishnan, K. (2005). Psychiatric and medical comorbidities of bipolar disorder. *Psychosomatic Medicine*, 67, 1–8.

Ratnayake, T. and Libretto, S. E. (2002). No complications with risperidone treatment before and throughout pregnancy and during the nursing period. *Journal of Clinical Psychiatry*, 63, 76–77.

Rea, M. M., Tompson, M. C., Miklowitz, D. J., et al. (2003). Family-focused treatment versus individual treatment for bipolar disorder: Results of a randomized clinical trial. *Journal of Consulting and Clinical Psychology*, 71, 482–492.

Reddy, D. S. (2010). Clinical pharmacokinetic interactions between antiepileptic drugs and hormonal contraceptives. *Expert Review of Clinical Pharmacology*, 3, 183–192.

Reimers, A., Helde, G., and Brodtkorb, E. (2005). Ethinyl estradiol, not progestogens, reduces lamotrigine serum concentrations. *Epilepsia*, 46, 1414–1417.

Reis, M. and Källén, B. (2008). Maternal use of antipsychotics in early pregnancy and delivery outcome. *Journal of Clinical Psychopharmacology*, 28, 279–288.

Ribolsi, M., Magni, V., and Rubino, I.A. (2010). Quetiapine fumarate for schizophrenia and bipolar disorder in young patients. *Drugs Today*, 46, 581–587.

Rihtman, T., Parush, S., and Ornoy, A. (2012). Preliminary findings of the developmental effects of in utero exposure to topiramate. *Reproductive Toxicology*, 34, 308–311.

Rohde, A. and Marneros, A. (1993). Postpartum psychoses: Onset and long-term course. *Psychopathology*, 26, 203–209.

Ross, L. E., Murray, B. J., and Steiner, M. (2005). Sleep and perinatal mood disorders: A critical review. *Journal of Psychiatry and Neuroscience*, 30, 247–256.

Rubin, E. T., Lee, A., and Ito, S. (2004). When breastfeeding mothers need CNS-acting drugs. *The Canadian Journal of Clinical Pharmacology*, 11, e257–e266.

Ružić, K., Dadić-Hero, E., Knez, R., et al. (2009). Pregnancy and atypical antipsychotics. *Psychiatria Danubina*, 21, 368–370.

Sajatovic, M., Friedman, S. H., Schuermeyer, I. N., et al. (2006). Menopause knowledge and subjective experience among peri- and postmenopausal women with bipolar disorder, schizophrenia and major depression. *The Journal of*

Nervous and Mental Disease, 194, 173–178.

Sala, R., Goldstein, B. I., Morcillo, C., et al. (2012). Course of comorbid anxiety disorders among adults with bipolar disorder in the US population. *Journal of Psychiatric Research*, 46, 865–872.

Sands, J. M. and Bichet, D. G. (2006). Nephrogenic diabetes insipidus. *Annals of Internal Medicine*, 144, 186–194.

Saunders, E. F., Fitzgerald, K. D., Zhang, P., et al. (2012). Clinical features of bipolar disorder comorbid with anxiety disorders differ between men and women. *Depression and Anxiety*, 29, 739–746.

Scott, J. (2003). Group psychoeducation reduces recurrence and hospital admission in people with bipolar disorder. *Evidence-Based Mental Health*, 6, 115.

Sedky, K., Nazir, R., Joshi, A., et al. (2012). Which psychotropic medications induce hepatotoxicity? *General Hospital Psychiatry*, 34, 53–61.

Sharma, V. (2009). Management of bipolar II disorder during pregnancy and the postpartum period-Motherisk update 2008. *The Canadian Journal of Clinical Pharmacology*, 16, e33–e41.

Sharma, V., Burt, V., and Ritchie, H. (2009). Bipolar II postpartum depression: Detection, diagnosis, and treatment. *American Journal of Psychiatry* 166, 1217–1221.

Sharma, V. and Khan, M. (2010). Identification of bipolar disorder in women with postpartum depression. *Bipolar Disorders*, 12, 335–340.

Sharma, V., Khan, M., Corpse, C., et al. (2008). Missed bipolarity and psychiatric comorbidity in women with postpartum depression. *Bipolar Disorders*, 10, 742–747.

Sharma, V. and Mazmanian, D. (2003). Sleep loss and postpartum

psychosis. *Bipolar Disorders*, 5, 98–105.

Sharma, V., Smith, A., and Khan, M. (2004). The relationship between duration of labour, time of delivery, and puerperal psychosis. *Journal of Affective Disorders*, 83, 215–220.

Shimoyama, R., Ohkubo, T., and Sugawara, K. (2000). Monitoring of carbamazepine and carbamazepine 10, 11-epoxide in breast milk and plasma by high-performance liquid chromatography. *Annals of Clinical Biochemistry*, 37, 210–215.

Shor, S., Koren, G., and Nulman, I. (2007). Teratogenicity of lamotrigine. *Canadian Family Physician*, 53, 1007–1009.

Sit, D., Rothschild, A. J., and Wisner, K. L. (2006). A review of postpartum psychosis. *Journal of Women's Health*, 15, 352–368.

Smoller, J. W. and Finn, C. T. (2003). Family, twin, and adoption studies of bipolar disorder. *American Journal of Medical Genetics Part C*, 123C, 48–58.

Spinelli, M. G. (2001). A systematic investigation of 16 cases of neonaticide. *American Journal of Psychiatry*, 158, 811–813.

Stahl, M. M., Neiderud, J., and Vinge, E. (1997). Thrombocytopenic purpura and anemia in a breast-fed infant whose mother was treated with valproic acid. *Journal of Pediatrics*, 130, 1001–1003.

Stange, J. P., Eisner, L. R., Hölzel, B. K., et al. (2011). Mindfulness-based cognitive therapy for bipolar disorder: Effects on cognitive functioning. *Journal of Psychiatric Practice*, 17, 410–419.

Starr, C. and McMillan, B. (2011). *Human biology* (9th ed.). Belmont, CA: Cengage Learning.

Stowe, Z. N. (2007). The use of mood stabilizers during breastfeeding. *The Journal of Clinical Psychiatry*, 68 (Suppl. 9), 22–28.

Suominen, K., Mantere, O., Valtonen, H., et al. (2009). Gender differences in bipolar disorder type I and II.

Acta Psychiatrica Scandinavica, 120, 464–473.

Swartz, H. A. and Frank, E. (2001). Psychotherapy for bipolar depression: A phase-specific treatment strategy? *Bipolar Disorders*, 3, 11–22.

Tadger, S., Paleacu, D., and Barak, Y. (2011). Quetiapine augmentation of antidepressant treatment in elderly patients suffering from depressive symptoms: A retrospective chart review. *Archives of Gerontology and Geriatrics*, 53, 104–105.

Tettenborn, B. (2006). Management of epilepsy in women of childbearing age. *CNS Drugs*, 20, 373–387.

Tomson, D., Pilling, S., Blake, F., et al. (2007). *Antenatal and postnatal mental health: Clinical management and service guidance (NICE Clinical Guideline No. 45)*. Manchester: National Institute for Health and Clinical Excellence. Available at: www.nice.org.uk/nicemedia/live/11004/30433/30433.pdf (Accessed December 1, 2013).

Tomson, T., Landmark, C. J., and Battino, D. (2013). Antiepileptic drug treatment in pregnancy: Changes in drug disposition and their clinical implications. *Epilepsia*, 54, 405.

Trapolini, T., McMahon, C. A., and Ungerer, J. A. (2007). The effect of maternal depression and marital adjustment on young children's internalizing and externalizing behaviour problems. *Child: Care, Health and Development*, 33, 794–803.

Vajda, F. J. E., O'Brien, T.J., Graham, J., et al. (2013). Associations between particular types of fetal malformation and antiepileptic drug exposure in utero. *Acta Neurologica Scandinavica*, 4, 228–234.

Vajda, F. J. E., O'Brien, T. J., Hitchcock, A., et al. (2003). The Australian registry of anti-epileptic drugs in pregnancy: Experience after 30 months. *Journal of Clinical Neuroscience*, 10, 543–549.

Valdimarsdóttir, U., Hultman, C. M., Harlow, B., et al. (2009). Psychotic illness in first-time mothers with no previous psychiatric hospitalizations: A population-based study. *PLoS Medicine*, 6, e1000013.

Van den Bergh, B. R., Mulder, E. J., Mennes, M., et al. (2005). Antenatal maternal anxiety and stress and the neurobehavioral development of the fetus and child: Links and possible mechanisms: A review. *Neuroscience & Biobehavioral Reviews*, 29, 237–258.

van Dijk, M. H., Bulk, S., van Oppen, A.C.C., et al. (2012). 1508 spectrum of neural tube defects after prenatal antiepileptic drug exposure: Extensive case series. *Archives of Disease in Childhood*, 97(Suppl. 2), A427–A428.

Vemuri, M. and Williams, K. (2011). Treating bipolar disorder during pregnancy: Optimal outcomes require careful preconception planning, medication risk/benefit analysis. *Current Psychiatry*, 10, 58–66.

Vieta, E. and Morralla, C. (2010). Prevalence of mixed mania using 3 definitions. *Journal of Affective Disorders*, 125, 61–73.

Vieta, E. and Valentí, M. (2013). Pharmacological management of bipolar depression: Acute treatment, maintenance, and prophylaxis. *CNS Drugs*, 27, 515–529.

Viguera, A. C., Baldessarini, R. J., and Tondo, L. (2001). Response to lithium maintenance treatment in bipolar disorders: Comparison of women and men. *Bipolar Disorders*, 3, 245–252.

Viguera, A. C., Cohen, L. S., Baldessarini, R. J., et al. (2002). Managing bipolar disorder during pregnancy: Weighing the risks and benefits. *Canadian Journal of Psychiatry*, 47, 426–436.

Viguera, A. C., Cohen, L. S., Bouffard, S., et al. (2002). Reproductive decisions by women with bipolar disorder after prepregnancy psychiatric consultation. *American Journal of Psychiatry*, 159, 2102–2104.

Viguera, A. C., Newport, D., Ritchie, J., et al. (2007). Lithium in breast milk and nursing infants: Clinical implications. *American Journal of Psychiatry*, 164, 342–345.

Viguera, A. C., Nonacs, R., Cohen, L. S., et al. (2000). Risk of recurrence of bipolar disorder in pregnant and nonpregnant women after discontinuing lithium maintenance. *American Journal of Psychiatry*, 157, 179–184.

Viguera, A. C., Tondo, L., Koukopoulos, A. E., et al. (2011). Episodes of mood disorders in 2,252 pregnancies and postpartum periods. *American Journal of Psychiatry*, 168, 1179–1185.

Viguera, A., Whitfield, T., Baldessarini, R., et al. (2007). Risk of recurrence in women with bipolar disorder during pregnancy: Prospective study of mood stabilizer discontinuation. *American Journal of Psychiatry*, 164, 1817–1824.

Vinten, J., Adab, N., Kini, U., et al. (2005). Neuropsychological effects of exposure to anticonvulsant medication in utero. *Neurology*, 64, 949–954.

Wang, P. S., Lane, M., Olfson, M., et al. (2005). Twelve-month use of mental health services in the United States: Results from the National Comorbidity Survey Replication. *Archives of General Psychiatry*, 62, 629–640.

Wegner, I., Edelbroek, P. M., Bulk, S., et al. (2009). Lamotrigine kinetics within the menstrual cycle, after menopause, and with oral contraceptives. *Neurology*, 73, 1388–1393.

Weinstock, M. (2005). The potential influence of maternal stress hormones on development and mental health of the offspring. *Brain, Behavior, and Immunity*, 19, 296–308.

Weissman, M. M., Wickramaratne, P., Nomura, Y., et al. (2006). Offspring of depressed parents: 20 years later. *American Journal of Psychiatry*, 163, 1001–1008.

Wieck, A. and Gregoire, A. (2009). Pharmacological management and ECT in childbearing women with psychiatric disorders. *Psychiatry*, 8, 33–37.

Williams, J. M. G., Alatiq, Y., Crane, C., et al. (2008). Mindfulness-based cognitive therapy (MBCT) in bipolar disorder: Preliminary evaluation of immediate effects on between-episode functioning. *Journal of Affective Disorders*, 107, 275–279.

Wisner, K. L., Leckman-Westin, E., Finnerty, M., et al. (2011). Valproate prescription prevalence among women of childbearing age. *Psychiatric Services*, 62, 218–220.

Wisner, K. L. and Perel, J. M. (1998). Serum levels of valproate and carbamazepine in breastfeeding mother–infant pairs. *Journal of Clinical Psychopharmacology*, 18, 167–169.

Wozniak, J., Faraone, S. V., Martelon, M., et al. (2012). Further evidence for robust familiality of pediatric bipolar I disorder: Results from a very large controlled family study of pediatric bipolar I disorder and a meta-analysis. *The Journal of Clinical Psychiatry*, 73, 1328–1334.

Yang, A. C., Yang, C. H., Hong, C. J., et al. (2013). Effects of age, sex, index admission, and predominant polarity on the seasonality of acute admissions for bipolar disorder: A population-based study. *Chronobiology International*, 30, 478–485.

Yatham, L. N., Kennedy, S. H., O'Donovan, C., et al. (2005). Canadian Network for Mood and Anxiety Treatments

(CANMAT) guidelines for the management of patients with bipolar disorder: Consensus and controversies. *Bipolar Disorders*, 7(Suppl. 3), 5–69.

Yatham, L. N., Kennedy, S. H., Parikh, S. V., et al. (2013).

Canadian Network for Mood and Anxiety Treatments (CANMAT) and International Society for Bipolar Disorders (ISBD) collaborative update of CANMAT guidelines for the management of patients with bipolar disorder:

Update 2013. *Bipolar Disorders*, 15, 1–44.

Yonkers, K. A., Wisner, K.L., Stowe, Z., et al. (2004). Management of bipolar disorder during pregnancy and the postpartum period. *American Journal of Psychiatry*, 161, 608–620.

Chapter 22

Women and schizophrenia

Kathryn M. Abel, Jill M. Goldstein, Nicky Stanley and David J. Castle

Introduction

Schizophrenia is a major psychiatric disorder, which is thought to be neurodevelopmental in origin. It manifests as a syndrome of disorders of thinking, perception, affect and behavior (ICD F20–29). So-called productive or positive symptoms include delusions (culturally unexplained false beliefs), hallucinations (perceptions in the absence of sensory stimuli from outside) and disorders of the form of thought making people appear incoherent when they speak. Such features are particularly associated with first onset illness and with acute relapses; these are most likely to be modeled by drug-induced schizophrenia-like episodes and are also most responsive to antipsychotic medications. Other, more difficult to treat features include disorders of thinking and processing information: the so-called cognitive and negative symptoms. Poor motivation, loss of volition, blunting of affect, as well as poverty of thought, speech and actions and difficulty learning new skills and planning are all part of the negative symptom cluster.

Schizophrenia is relatively rare with a lifetime prevalence risk of 5–10 per 1,000. The incidence is also low (0.5 %) in a population per annum, but because it tends to have onset in early adulthood and last a lifetime, its prevalence is greater than disorders such as multiple sclerosis and motor neuron disease. It is significantly more common in men than in women overall (1.4:1) (McGrath, et al., 2004). Symptoms usually start in adolescence or young adulthood with approximately one-third making complete recovery, a third showing complete or partial resolution between acute episodes with substantial disability and a third severe, persistent disability (Emsley, et al., 2007). Such early life onset means that schizophrenia is linked to chronic disability with profound effects throughout people's lives. Each relapse significantly increases the risk of chronicity, as well as worsening personal, social and occupational functioning (Wiersma, et al. 1998; Wiersma, et al., 2000). This means that, for most women, the illness starts just as they develop reproductive maturity and they remain unwell throughout most of their reproductive lives. Most first episodes resolve with medication (Emsley, et al., 2007). However, risk of relapse is linked to nonadherence with antipsychotic treatment, substance misuse, carers' critical comments and poor premorbid adjustment (Alvarez-Jimenez, et al., 2012). There is high prevalence of comorbid problems. In women, compared to their well, age-matched population counterpart, these are particularly likely to include substance and alcohol misuse, obesity, smoking and physical health problems such as hypertension, cardiovascular disease and diabetes (Buckley, et al., 2009; Wildgust and Beary, 2010).

Whether and how women and men with schizophrenia differ is highly significant for etiological understanding and clinical outcomes (Castle et al., 1995; Moldin, 2000). Following an overview of schizophrenia epidemiology, we consider how gender and age at onset may determine premorbid functioning, course of disease and outcome. We shall particularly consider how sex and gender differences in schizophrenia may be expressions of sex differences in healthy brain development and how this might influence gender differences in the social effects on disease risk and course. Finally, we consider women with schizophrenia in the context of their lives as mothers and partners, particularly paying attention to the longer-term outcomes and needs of their children. Treatment for women with schizophrenia is the subject of a separate chapter (Chapter 23). Very late onset

Comprehensive Women's Mental Health, ed. David J. Castle and Kathryn M. Abel. Published by Cambridge University Press.
© Cambridge University Press 2016.

schizophrenia-like psychosis ("late paraphrenia") is covered in Chapter 24.

Incidence and prevalence of schizophrenia in women

Disease incidence provides a measure of how many new cases are expected to occur in a given population over a given period of observation. This may be particularly important in disorders like schizophrenia that are effectively groups of symptoms making up syndromes where up to a third of new cases do not develop into chronic illness (Jablensky et al., 2000). Gradients in the incidence of a disorder across time and place can provide powerful clues to help unravel etiology. However, variations in incidence are also well described within or between various populations. This implies that etiological or risk factors are not uniformly distributed. Sex differences in the incidence, or prevalence, presentation and outcome of illnesses represents an important boundary between risk groups (Jablensky, 2003).

Sex difference in incidence or prevalence of schizophrenia may depend on the stringency of the diagnostic criteria applied: the broader the criteria the less significant are the sex differences in incidence or prevalence (Castle et al., 1993, 1995; Goldstein, 1995; Morgan et al., 2008). Recent meta-analysis identified a mean ratio of male:female schizophrenia incidence of 1.42 (95% CI 1.30, 1.56) and also found evidence of significantly lower estimates for less restrictive criteria (Aleman, 2003). However, all ratio estimates from different types of study (including for methodologically rigorous studies, those using DSM III-R/IV or ICD criteria, those before 1980) lay between 1.27 and 1.54 and significantly exceeded 1.0. The review of McGrath and colleagues (2008) found a median ratio of 1.40 (10th & 90th centiles 0.9, 2.4).

Most psychiatrists believe that women have a later onset of schizophrenia and a better course of illness than men and that these two phenomena are related to one another, that is, a worse illness subtype occurs earlier and therefore accounts for the worse prognosis in men; or, later illness onset in women represents a less aggressive illness and allows for better outcome. To a great extent the epidemiological literature encourages such views. Incidence rate ratios tell of rates of disease within specified time frames. They do not reflect the interactions seen in some studies between disease age-of-onset and gender. Whilst

the rate ratio curve for incidence is normally distributed, the curves for age-at-onset are not. Men show a modal incidence in their early twenties and perhaps a second peak around middle age. Women also show modal onset in their early 20s, but this is a lower frequency, somewhat broader mode and is followed by a more pronounced peak in middle age than men (see Figure 22.1) (Leung & Chue, 2000; Hambrecht et al., 1992; Häfner et al., 1993; Drake et al., 2015). Thus, there is a switch from male predominance in incidence during the early 20s to female predominance in incidence at older ages. Using admixture analysis of a relatively small case register sample of incident cases, Castle and colleagues (1993) suggested that the early modal onset of non-affective psychosis lies at 21–22 years in both women and men, whereas there are secondary underlying curves with modes at ~36 years in men and ~39 years in women; women alone have a third mode of onset in their early 60s.

Sex and age-at-onset differences in the clinical presentation and course of non-affective psychosis are key biomarkers and may provide important clues to the etiology of the disorder. However, conclusions from this literature have been unclear because of small sample sizes, lack of follow up or the bias inherent in nonincident samples (e.g., Goldstein & Link, 1988; Thara & Rajkumar, 1992; Castle et al., 1993; Vazquez-Barquero et al., 1996; Roy et al., 2001). More recently, one of the largest samples to date (n=537) of first episode schizophrenia (i.e., two incident samples combined [Lewis et al., 2002]) aged 10–65 was examined for differences in presentation and course of disorder over a 12–18 month follow-up period (Drake et al., 2015). Admixture analysis suggested underlying distributions with modes in the early 20s and mid 40s for each sex. Men predominated under 43 years and women over 43 (Figure 22.1).

Using the 10 countries WHO cohort, Susser & Wanderling (1994) examined incidence of schizophrenia in women and men presenting with non-affective remitting psychosis (NARP) and looked at variation by setting, that is, developing versus developed countries and rural versus urban settings. They reported that the annual incidence of NARP per 10,000 people in women was approximately double that in men in the developing-country setting: 0.878 versus 0.486, respectively (P=.07); in the industrialized-country setting, 0.104 versus 0.040, respectively (P=.04). In the developing-country setting, the incidence was about 10-fold that in the industrialized-country setting

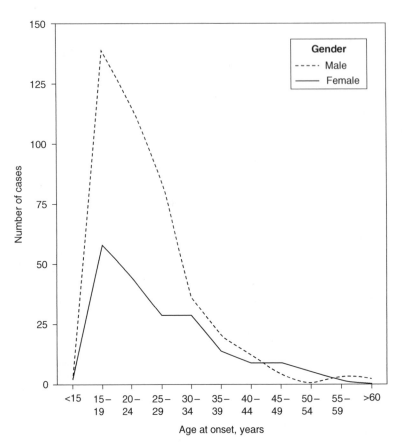

Figure 22.1 Incidence of Schizophrenia

for both sexes: men, 0.486 versus 0.040, respectively (P<.001); women, 0.878 versus 0.104, respectively (P<.001). This was an unexpected finding as the cases came from the original 10-countries study, which found incidence was similar in developed and developing countries, but prevalence was lower in developing nations.

Prevalence studies are also influenced by diagnostic criteria, as well as case ascertainment methods; sample selection; availability of, and access to, appropriate treatments; response to treatment and the burden of disease-maintaining, rather than disease risk factors within the environment. Saha et al. (2005) undertook a comprehensive systematic review and concluded that, in contrast to sex differences in schizophrenia incidence, there was no significant sex difference in prevalence. This was the case for combined point, period and lifetime estimates where median values ranged from 3.3–7.2 per 1000 persons. This was surprising given the clear sex difference in incidence and the consistently reported differences in course and prognosis of illness for women and men,

both of which predict greater male prevalence. Recent reviews (McGrath et al., 2008) and well-designed population studies (e.g., Perälä et al., 2007) suggest the overall prevalence of schizophrenia in women is equal to that in men, suggesting that women remain at risk of new onset illness across their lifetimes and possibly that once ill, they tend to survive longer than men with schizophrenia.

Presentation and course of illness in women

Symptom expression at presentation has important implications for a number of reasons, such as determining treatment regimens and understanding course of illness. Gender differences in clinical presentation and course have been reported as broadly consistent in different countries and cultures (Hambrecht et al., 1992; Goldstein, 1997; Harrison et al., 2001). One of the largest and most comprehensive epidemiological, population-based samples is from the National "Low Prevalence" study from Australia (Morgan et al.,

2008). This is an incident sample that includes 1,090 new cases of psychotic disorder: at presentation, women were more likely to have depressive symptoms and less likely to show negative symptoms. Women may also have higher levels of depressive symptoms than men throughout disease progression (Goldstein & Link, 1988; Castle et al., 1993). The prominence of affective symptoms in mentally ill women overall may represent the likelihood that women are more likely to express affective symptoms than men overall, and therefore sex differences in symptom expression in schizophrenia may be related to gender differences per se (in illness expression) rather than schizophrenia per se (Flor-Henry, 1983; see also Chapter 19).

During first illness episodes, levels of negative symptoms are generally lower in women (Vazquez-Barquero et al., 1996; Leung & Chue, 2000; Morgan et al., 2008), but this is not always found to be the case (e.g., Salokangas' first contact sample aged 15–44 [Salokangas, 1997a,b] and the ABC cohort [Hafner et al., 1993]). *Specific* positive symptoms such as paranoia or persecutory delusions (e.g., Goldstein and Link, 1988; Goldstein, 1997; Hambrecht et al., 1992) and auditory hallucinations (Tien, 1991; Rector & Seeman, 1992) have been found to be higher in women in some studies. However, the Australian Low Prevalence study (Morgan et al., 2008) suggested that if positive symptoms were defined as an overall score, women presented with as many positive symptoms overall as did men.

However, the problem with prevalence data is that they may be less reliable for determining symptom burden at true illness onset. Drake et al. (2015) addressed this using a large first-episode sample. Consistent with previous studies, they reported that early onset women showed worse overall PANSS (Positive and Negative Syndrome Scale) scores (negative and cognitive symptoms) than later onset cases and that women showed significantly worse depression-anxiety scores. Overall, independent of age at onset, women presented with fewer negative symptoms and more mood symptoms. The association of older age at onset with fewer negative and cognitive symptoms at presentation among women was also consistent with other findings (e.g., Sartorius et al., 1986; Morgan et al., 2008; Grossman et al., 2008). Paranoid symptoms may be more severe in women with older onset than men with older onset (e.g., Castle et al., 1993; Häfner et al., 1993).

In most studies, women with schizophrenia have a better prognosis over 2–10 years than men for many measures (e.g., Angermayer et al., 1990; Jablensky et al., 1992; Häfner et al., 1993; Robinson et al., 1999); though some studies, often smaller ones, find no differences (e.g., McCreadie et al., 1989; Rajkumar & Thara, 1989; and see Angermeyer et al., 1990) and studies that control for premorbid adjustment and baseline symptoms often find these mediate outcome, especially social measures (e.g., Salokangas, 1997b). In general, earlier age of illness onset predicts worse negative and disorganization symptoms and a more malign symptomatic course (e.g., Jablensky et al., 1992; Morgan et al., 2008; Grossman et al., 2008), albeit Selten's (2007) group did not find this to be the case in a sample restricted to presentations under age 55.

The relationships between age at first presentation, duration of illness, symptoms and gender are complex. Thus, some suggest there are minimal differences between women and men with schizophrenia in familial cases (see Leung & Chue, 2000) or after adjustment for premorbid function (Jablensky & Cole, 1997). In keeping with this complexity, Drake and colleagues (2015) found that although age of onset and sex predicted presenting symptoms, neither predicted medium-term deficit, psychotic, cognitive/disorganized, excitement and dysphoric symptom outcomes after adjusting for baseline scores.

To summarize, at onset, older age and affective symptoms predict better course in women in most studies. Young onset, negative and disorganized symptoms predict worse short- and medium-term outcomes and are less associated with women. In clinical practice, symptoms at presentation still have a role as reliable and obvious indicators of likely course in women (and men). Illness course over the first two years also appears to mediate the effect of sex on long-term outcomes (Harrison et al., 2001), so after this stage, illness history may be a better guide than demography.

The brain in women with schizophrenia

As a neurodevelopmental disorder, it is likely that schizophrenia originates during fetal and early postnatal life and therefore it is also likely that sex differences in early differentiation of the brain during fetal and early postnatal life are key in understanding sex differences in schizophrenia (Goldstein and Walder, 2006). This premise has support from animal studies demonstrating brain abnormalities and behavioral consequences, depending on the timing of the insult during fetal and early postnatal brain development, for female compared with male animals (Goldman et al., 1974; Grimm and Frieder, 1985). Human studies are also consonant with the animal literature (Rantakallio and Wendt, 1985; Goldstein et al., 2014).

Early studies of sex differences in structural brain abnormalities in schizophrenia generally found less pervasive brain abnormalities than men with schizophrenia, although not wholly consistent (Nopoulos, Flaum et al., 1997). (Nopoulos, et al., 1997). More recent work reports region-specific structural brain abnormalities in women with schizophrenia. Some studies have reported smaller volumes of heteromodal association areas among women with schizophrenia than men (e.g., dorsolateral prefrontal cortex and superior temporal gyrus [STG] and orbital prefrontal cortex). Others found smaller volumes of STG in men, and similar abnormalities in women and men in dorsolateral prefrontal cortex (Gur, et al. 2000). Studies have demonstrated varied differences between women with schizophrenia compared with their healthy controls, depending on the prefrontal region assessed (e.g., Gur, et al. 2000; Goldstein, et al. 2002) and inconsistencies across studies may be, in part, due to methodological and sample size differences.

Goldstein and colleagues (2002) reported that structural brain abnormalities occur in nonpsychotic offspring of parents with schizophrenia in a number of brain regions found to be normally sexually dimorphic, and differentially abnormal in adult women and men with schizophrenia. Szeszko et al. (2002) also provided evidence for differential sex effects in brain abnormalities during the premorbid period using MRI and neuropsychological tests in first episode patients. That study reported an association between anterior hippocampal volume and executive and motor functioning in male patients, which was not present in women. First episode studies have been important in taking account of the differing age at onset and treatment exposures between the sexes (see Drake et al. 2015).

There has been an increase in work on sex differences in the brain in schizophrenia over the past 5 years. Earlier studies of sex differences in brain abnormalities in schizophrenia focused primarily on analyses of gray matter volumes. However, emerging literature on sex differences in white matter tracts has been possible with the development of diffusion tensor imaging (DTI) (Kunimatsu, et al., 2012; Savadjiev, et al., 2013). Additionally, the field has become more accepting of the importance of sex differences in schizophrenia and thus increasing

numbers of functional brain imaging studies are characterizing sex differences in prefrontal cortical functions in more refined ways (i.e., as brain-clinical phenotypes), (Elsabagh, et al., 2009; Jimenez, et al., 2010; Abbs, et al., 2011; Mendrek, et al., 2011). The role of estradiol and genes in understanding these sex differences is also being explored (Elsabagh, et al., 2009; Irle, et al., 2011; Chen, et al., 2014).

Recent structural analyses of white matter found sex-dependent orbitofrontal white matter density and sulcogyral patterns were related to symptomatology (Uehara-Aoyama, et al., 2011; Joshi, et al., 2012) and an increased diffusion coefficient in the anterior cingulum bundle in men with schizophrenia versus male controls related to negative symptoms that was not found in women with schizophrenia (Kunimatsu, et al. 2012). However, an increased diffusion coefficient in right anterior cingulum and left fornix was found in women with schizophrenia compared with female controls and not between schizophrenia and control males (Kunimatsu, et al. 2012), suggesting a more complex pattern of sex-dependent findings when laterality was taken into account.

Structural findings have continued to underscore sex differences in hippocampal volume, but extended this by considering duration of illness: reduced hippocampal size in men with schizophrenia compared with women did not progress with illness duration, but reduced hippocampal size was found only in women with schizophrenia with long illness duration (Irle, et al., 2011). In a more refined structural analysis of networks of brain regions associated with particular functional domains, covariances of brain regions implicated in verbal memory circuitry (hippocampus, inferior parietal, dorsolateral prefrontal [DLPFC] and anterior cingulate cortices) were consistent with greater abnormalities in associations of hippocampus with anterior cingulate gyrus and DLPFC, and between inferior parietal cortex and prefrontal cortex, with better verbal memory performance in females with schizophrenia than males (Abbs, et al. 2011).

However, not all studies have been consistent. Two studies of early-onset schizophrenia (Thormodsen, et al., 2013; Weisinger, et al., 2013) reported a lack of structural abnormalities by sex in cortical thickness (Thormodsen, et al., 2013; Weisinger, et al., 2013) and insula volume (Shepherd, et al., 2012). Also, in childhood-onset schizophrenia (COS), the hippocampus, caudate, amygdala, thalamus, putamen and pallidum were not found to be sexually divergent (Weisinger, et al., 2013). Lack of sex differences in early onset or COS is consistent with the lack of sex differences in incidence of COS suggesting other factors (e.g., gonadal hormones); genes may "override" mechanisms usually regulating sex differences in brain development.

Methodological variation may contribute to the inconsistencies in results. Most studies are small; a particular concern in studies with unbalanced sex ratios (e.g., Uehara-Aoyama, et al., 2011; Joshi, et al., 2012); many studies represent a mix of adult and early-onset samples (Savadjiev, et al., 2013; Thormodsen, et al., 2013; Weisinger, et al., 2013) including a wide range of illness duration. These factors have been found to influence the direction of sex-dependent effects, for example hippocampal size (Irle, et al., 2011; Weisinger, et al., 2013) and sex-dependent effects on fronto-parietal working memory related brain activity in schizophrenia (Elsabagh, et al., 2009). In addition, analyses have not necessarily compared women and men directly, reporting sex-stratified results alone (Kunimatsu, et al., 2012). This may explain the failure to replicate sex-dependent findings in the corpus callosum (Kunimatsu, et al., 2012; Savadjiev, et al., 2013). Finally, when additional clinical phenotyping (such as negative and positive symptomatology) has been included, sex differences in brain-clinical phenotypes have emerged (Mendrek, et al., 2011; Uehara-Aoyama, et al., 2011; Kunimatsu, et al., 2012; Manuseva, et al., 2012).

Functional studies demonstrating sex differences in brain abnormalities have included electrophysiological event-related potential (ERP). Overall, studies reported lower amplitudes in all four components (P100, N170, N250, P300) in men with schizophrenia compared with women (Lee, et al., 2010; Jung, et al., 2012); with respect to N170 and N250, findings corresponded to source activities in superior temporal gyrus, middle temporal gyrus, insula and inferior frontal gyrus (Jung, et al., 2012). Further, when depressive symptoms in schizophrenia were examined, there was a positive association between depression and early perceptual processing in response to novel stimuli in men and later processing stage abnormalities associated with parietal activity in women (Sumich, et al., 2014). Significantly greater QEEG beta-type amplitudes over left central, temporal, parietal and occipital regions and theta frequencies over left frontal and temporal regions have been reported

in women with schizophrenia compared with men with schizophrenia and correlated with greater symptomatology (Manuseva, et al., 2012). These findings underscore the importance of brain-clinical phenotyping in characterizing sex-dependent functional brain abnormalities in schizophrenia.

This is also highlighted by functional fMRI studies of specific cognitive and emotional tasks in schizophrenia. In general, fMRI tasks of visual-spatial ability (mental rotation; Jimenez, et al., 2010), object location memory (Shipman, et al., 2009) and phonemic dichotic listening (Hahn, et al., 2011) demonstrate better performance and fewer brain activity deficits in women than men with schizophrenia. However, in a standard n-back fMRI task of working memory, duration of illness further influenced sex-dependent effects on fronto-parietal working memory activity with reduced DLPFC and inferior parietal cortices in men and reduced inferior frontal and superior temporal gyri activity in women (Elsabagh, et al., 2009). Sex differences in visuospatial performance and pattern of brain activation comparing schizophrenia patients with controls suggested a diagnosis-by-sex interaction in accuracy and reaction time. Thus, men with schizophrenia performed significantly worse on a 3-D mental rotation task with brain activity deficits in precuneus, prefrontal and parietal cortex (Jimenez, et al., 2010). Women with schizophrenia perform better on object-location tasks, but there was a significant interaction of sex by diagnosis for object-exchange and object-shifting tasks, with no sex differences on delayed-recognition tasks (Shipman, et al., 2009).

Brain activity associated with emotional stimuli also varied by sex, dependent on hormonal responses (Goldstein, et al., 2015) and symptomatology (Mendrek, et al., 2011). Using a visual stress challenge (negative affective stimuli versus neutral stimuli) while uniquely collecting blood throughout functional magnetic resonance imaging (fMRI), males with psychosis (schizophrenia and bipolar psychosis) showed *hyper*activity across all hypothesized stress response regions, including hypothalamus and anterior cingulate cortex, whereas females showed *hyper*activity only in hippocampus and amygdala *and hypo*activity in orbital and medial prefrontal cortices. Hypercortisolemia was associated with hyperactivity in prefrontal cortices in men and hypoactivity in prefrontal cortices in women with psychoses. Findings suggested disruptions in neural-hormone associations in response to stress are sex-dependent in psychosis, particularly in prefrontal cortex, a finding that was shared with schizophrenia and bipolar psychoses (Goldstein, et al., 2015). In an alternative strategy for eliciting emotion response circuitry, during exposure to sad versus neutral film excerpts, there was an inverse correlation between positive symptoms and activity in hippocampus and parietal and occipital cortices among women, while men with schizophrenia exhibited prefrontal, temporal and anterior cingulate cortices and caudate and cerebellum deficits that were positively correlated with negative symptoms (Mendrek, et al., 2011).

Sex differences in brain-clinical phenotypes also vary by genotype (Zhang, et al., 2011; Radulescu, et al., 2013). Some of these genes have been implicated in glutamatergic and dopamine pathways (Martins-de-Souza, et al., 2010; O'Tuathaigh, et al., 2010; von Wilmsdorff, et al., 2010; Bychkov, et al., 2011; Holley, et al., 2013; Bertholet, et al., 2014; Chen, et al., 2014). Using a genetic knock-out (KO) mouse model of a dopamine-pathway signaling gene, greater deficits were reported in male KOs compared with female KOs in locomotion and the striatum, but this could be reversed with 17β-estradiol (Chen, et al., 2014). These studies suggest that genes, hormones and clinical presentation should all be considered as we refine our understanding of sex differences in brain abnormalities in schizophrenia.

Gonadal hormones and symptoms in women with schizophrenia

The majority of women develop psychotic illnesses like schizophrenia in early adulthood. This coincides with the development of a mature (adult) hypothalamic-gonadal axis. Here, we consider a range of ways in which the reproductive and stress axes may influence an illness like schizophrenia in women. First, there is some evidence that psychotic symptomatology varies with menstrual phase, such that higher symptom levels have been associated with lower estrogen levels (Endo et al., 1978; Huber et al., 2004; Bergemann et al., 2002). In addition, low estrogen phases of the menstrual cycle have also been associated with higher rates of hospital admission (Huber et al., 2004) and with poorer cognitive performance, in particular verbal and spatial memory, and perceptual-motor speed (Hoff et al., 2001). Second, disruptions in a number of endocrine axes, whatever the cause, are unlikely to be specific to schizophrenia, but they may have important consequences for the nature and course of cognitive and other functional deficits in the disease process. Third, during episodes of relapse and worsening psychosis, women with schizophrenia may be more likely to lead chaotic lifestyles, with poor nutrition and self-care. This may also coincide with oligo- or amenorrhea. It is clear that many women with schizophrenia suffer menstrual disruption over varied lengths of time.

Fourthly, prolonged amenorrhea, oligomenorrhea or hypo-estrogenemia is associated with a wide array of premature aging effects. Thus, severe mental illness such as schizophrenia may be associated with an increased risk of fracture, especially osteoporotic fracture and especially in young women, and in those treated with prolactin-raising agents (Abel et al., 2007). Finally, although evidence of the beneficial effects of adjunct estrogen therapy in schizophrenia for women is relatively weak (see Chapter 23 for a detailed account), clinicians caring for women with schizophrenia should include menstrual and reproductive health checks as part of routine care planning.

Women with schizophrenia as mothers

Chapter 4 of this book considers broader issues relating to women as mothers. Here, we consider some particular difficulties for women with schizophrenia and their children. Women with a mental illness who become pregnant represent a high-risk group of mothers, not only because the mental illness may be more likely to recur or worsen following childbirth (see later in chapter), but also because they are more likely to be exposed (and to expose their fetus) to a range of adverse circumstances. We may say that mothers with mental illness have relatively poor "maternal condition." This means greater risk of poor antenatal care, poor nutrition, use of prescribed medications, illicit drugs and alcohol, greater likelihood of smoking and of continuing to smoke through pregnancy and fewer positive benefits available from material and emotional supports (Abel et al., 2005).

Much recent attention has been paid to concerns about fetal exposure to psychotropic medication during pregnancy (Abel, 2013). However, the risks of relapse for women with schizophrenia off medication during pregnancy are likely to be considerable and to expose the mother-to-be and her fetus to increased anxiety and stress, which itself is associated with a range of obstetric complications, such as prematurity. The experiences of pregnant women with severe mental illness is covered in more detail in Chapter 10. Undoubtedly, far more research is required in this area and should include examination of differences across countries and cultures.

Parenting infants and preschool children is a stressful occupation, and missed sleep and raised levels of anxiety together with the isolation and emotional demands experienced in the early stages of infants' lives can combine to precipitate or exacerbate periods of illness. Long-term mental illness can leave mothers without the support of a long-term relationship and relationships generally may be fractured and characterized by violence or abuse. Ill mothers are also far more likely to lose custody of their child after delivery, fear of which may exacerbate psychotic symptomatology during pregnancy and/or pregnancy-related anxiety (Abel et al., 2005). Mothers diagnosed with schizophrenia may be subject to high levels of scrutiny and monitoring from social services and these interventions are often experienced as hostile and threatening. Nearly all the mothers with severe mental illness interviewed by Stanley et al. (2003) reported fears that they might lose their children as a result of their mental health problems and a third of these women noted that such fears had restricted their willingness to seek help; as one interviewee remarked: "that's why I won't always ask for help. I'm worried that they will come and take them off me."

Children whose mothers suffer with schizophrenia can be exposed to a variety of parenting problems including inconsistency and lack of predictability; emotional inaccessibility and unresponsiveness; and role reversal, which may involve inappropriate expectations on children and overinvolvement, where children are incorporated into paranoid or threatening delusions (Falkov, 2013). Such delusions may indicate a high level of risk for the child. However, an Irish study (Somers, 2007) of 37 children, aged 8–16, who were living with a parent with schizophrenia found no differences between the sample children and the matched controls in terms of physical health, positive family feelings, friendships, hobbies and household tasks. However, children with a parent with schizophrenia were less likely to have contact with relatives, were more likely to miss school and were more likely to have behavioral problems and "strange behavior" or mental health problems. The majority of sample children evinced an acute

awareness of the stigma associated with mental illness and saw it as something that had to be kept hidden. It is clear that social isolation and social attitudes are heavily implicated in the impact of parental mental illness on children.

The risks to children of mothers with schizophrenia continue throughout their lives (Bee, et al., 2013; Bee, et al., 2014) although the level of risk may vary as levels of mental illness fluctuate. Generally, the study of this vulnerable group has been considered as "high-risk research" and has focused on the quantification of genetic risk. However, as noted earlier, many key social and environmental effects require consideration in the poor outcomes of these children. Thus, as discussed in Chapter 9, the pregnancies of women with schizophrenia are more likely to be unplanned, unwanted or a result of coerced sexual encounters than those of women in the general population.

Few epidemiological studies have assessed the parenting outcomes for mothers with serious mental illness. Kumar et al. (1995) reported on a small case-series of women admitted to a single UK mother-and-baby unit and suggested that mothers with schizophrenia had the poorest outcome, with 50% being separated from their babies at discharge. One follow-up study of women with postpartum psychosis found that they were more likely to experience further psychiatric episodes than mothers with non-psychotic affective disorders, endangering the relationship between mother and child further (Videbech & Gouliaev, 1995). In the largest reported sample, Salmon et al. (2003) described clinical and parenting outcomes in 1,081 joint mother-baby admissions (mean age 30 years), including 224 women with schizophrenia, 155 with bipolar disorder and 409 with non-psychotic depression. Poor outcomes were associated with a diagnosis of schizophrenia, behavioral disturbance, low social class, psychiatric illness in the woman's partner and the absence of a good relationship with a partner. More detailed analysis of an overlapping UK mother-baby sample of 1,153 consecutive admissions (n=239 schizophrenia; n=693 affective disorder) suggested that mothers with schizophrenia were characterized by staff as having more complex clinical and psychosocial problems, and were considerably more likely to have a range of poor parenting outcomes compared to mothers with affective disorder (Abel et al., 2005). Only half of the mothers with schizophrenia were discharged home to care for their infants without any level of formal supervision by the social services, in contrast to the great majority of mothers with affective disorders (91% and 80% for unipolar depression and bipolar disorder respectively). Successful parenting was related, in part, to stability within the family, and access to financial and social resources. Thus, mothers with schizophrenia who have better parenting outcomes may be protected by certain factors such as supportive marital and other relationships, and higher social class.

How the expression of severe mental illness is mediated by life course experiences is critical to understanding the intimate nexus between genetic and environmental predictors of outcome for children of parents with mental illness. This includes not only prenatal exposures but also rearing environment and exposure to stressors and adversity. Animal models demonstrate that the experience of deprived rearing environments can permanently change gene expression (Meaney and Szyf, 2005) and chronically alter vital homeostatic systems (Pryce, et al., 2004).

There is evidence that children of mothers with severe mental illness such as schizophrenia experience a significantly poorer child rearing environment than those of well mothers, with children of depressed mothers somewhere in between (Goodman 1987; Donatelli, et al., 2010). Weintraub (1987) also reported that families of children of a parent with schizophrenia functioned significantly worse than those with well parents. However, in their study (Weintraub, 1987) families with a parent with affective psychosis did not differ from those with a parent with schizophrenia, while in contrast, in the New England Family Studies high-risk design, children of parents with affective psychosis fared better than those with parents with schizophrenia (Donatelli, et al., 2010). In the Rochester high-risk sample of children of women with schizophrenia, low socioeconomic status and maternal illness chronicity were more important predictors of early outcomes of children to age 4 years than maternal diagnosis per se (Sameroff, et al., 1987). When long-term outcomes were examined, high-risk children who go on to develop severe mental illnesses themselves reported poorer relationships with their parents than those who do not (Burman, et al., 1987). Far more translational research is needed to identify modifiable risk factors for high-risk children, so that appropriate interventions can be developed and implemented for both mother and child across the developmental life course, commencing in the antenatal period.

Conclusions

There is clear evidence that women show differences in the incidence, course and outcome of schizophrenia. It is also likely that normal differences in brain development inform sex-differentiated brain abnormalities in schizophrenia. These may be initiated during fetal and early postnatal development, but are also likely to be influenced by gender differences in psychosocial experience and exposures that occur throughout life. Such differences are likely to be non-specific and may pertain in other mental disorders. The differences described are relevant to clinical outcomes including women's responses to treatment and susceptibility to adverse events. Government health policy in the UK and elsewhere has embraced gender and sex as key determinants of health, service need and therefore of service planning (UK Department of Health 2002). Recognizing ways in which the needs of people with severe mental illness like schizophrenia differ as a result of their sex and gender provides an important opportunity to deliver high quality, patient-centered care and the prospect of better clinical and psychosocial outcomes.

References

Abbs, B., L. Liang, et al. (2011). Covariance modeling of MRI brain volumes in memory circuitry in schizophrenia: Sex differences are critical. *NeuroImage* 56(4): 1865–1874.

Abel, K. M., Allin, M. A., van Amelsvoort. T., Hemsley. D., Geyer, M. A. (2007). The indirect serotonergic agonist d-fenfluramine and prepulse inhibition in healthy men. *Neuropharmacology* 52: 1088–1094.

Abel, K. M., Svensson, A., Dal, H., Dalman, C., Susser, E., Rai, D., Idring, S., Magnusson, C. (2013). Deviance fetal growth and autism spectrum disorder. *American Journal of Psychiatry* 170:391–398.

Abel, K. M., Webb, R., Salmon, M., Wan, M. W., Appleby, L. (2005). Prevalence and predictors of parenting outcomes in a cohort of mothers with schizophrenia admitted for joint mother and baby psychiatric care in England. *Journal of Clinical Psychiatry* 66: 781–789.

Aleman, A., Kahn, R. S., Selten, J. P. (2003). Sex differences in the risk of schizophrenia: evidence from meta-analysis. *Archives of General Psychiatry*, 60 (6) 565–571.

Alvarez-Jimenez, M., A. Priede, et al. (2012). Risk factors for relapse following treatment for first episode psychosis: A systematic review and meta-analysis of longitudinal studies. *Schizophrenia Research* 139: 116–128.

Angermeyer. M. C., Kühn, L., Goldstein, J. M. (1990). Gender and the course of schizophrenia: Differences in treated outcomes. *Schizophrenia Bulletin* 16: 293–307.

Bee, P., Berzins, K., Calam, R., Pryjmachuk, S., Abel, K. M. (2013). Defining quality of life in the children of parents with severe mental illness: A preliminary stakeholder-led model. *PLOS One*, 8(9), doi: 10.1371/journal. pone.0073739

Bee, P., Bower, P., Byford, S., Churchill, R., Calam, R., Stallard, P., Pryjmachuk, S., Berzins, K., Cary, M., Wan, J., Abel K. (2014). The clinical-effectiveness, cost-effectiveness and acceptability of community-based interventions aimed at improving or maintaining quality of life in children of parents with serious mental illness; a systematic evidence synthesis. *Health Technology Assessment*, 18(8), doi: 10.3310/hta18080

Bergemann, N., Parzer, P., Nagl, I., Salbach, B., Runnebaum, B., Mundt, Ch., Resch. F. (2002). Acute psychiatric admission and menstrual cycle phase in women with schizophrenia. *Archives of Women's Mental Health* 5 119–126.

Bertholet, L., C. Meunier, et al. (2014). Sex biased spatial strategies relying on the integration of multimodal cues in a rat model of schizophrenia: Impairment in predicting future context? *Behavioural Brain Research* 262: 109–117.

Buckley, P. F., B. J. Miller, et al. (2009). Psychiatric comorbidities and schizophrenia. *Schizophrenia Bulletin* 35: 383–402.

Burman, B., S. A. Mednick, et al. (1987). Children at high risk for schizophrenia: Parent and offspring perceptions of family relationships. *Journal of Abnormal Psychology* 96(4): 364–366.

Bychkov, E., M. R. Ahmed, et al. (2011). Sex differences in the activity of signalling pathways and expression of G-protein-coupled receptor kinases in the neonatal ventral hippocampal lesion model of schizophrenia. *The International Journal of Neuropsychopharmacology / Official Scientific Journal of the Collegium Internationale Neuropsychopharmacologicum* 14(1): 1–15.

Castle, D. J., Abel, K. M., Takei, N., Murray, R. M. (1995). Gender differences in schizophrenia: Hormonal effect or subtypes? *Schizophrenia Bulletin*, 21:1–12.

Castle, D. J., Wessley, S., Murray, R. M. (1993). Sex and schizophrenia: Effects of diagnostic stringency, and associations with premorbid variables. *British Journal of Psychiatry* 93(162) 658–664.

Chen, Y. W., H. Y. Kao, et al. (2014). A sex- and region-specific role of akt1 in the modulation of methamphetamine-induced hyperlocomotion and striatal neuronal activity: Implications in schizophrenia and methamphetamine-induced psychosis. *Schizophrenia Bulletin* 40(2): 388–398.

Donatelli, J. L., Seidman, L. J., Goldstein, J. M., Tsuang, M. T., Buka, S. L. (2010) Children of parents with affective and non-affective psychoses: A longitudinal study of behavior problems. *American Journal of Psychiatry* 167(11):1331–1338.

Drake, R., Addington, J., Viswanathan, A., Lewis, S., Cotter, J., Yung, A., Abel, K. (2015). How age and gender predict illness course in a first-episode non-affective psychosis

cohort. *Journal of Clinical Psychiatry*, eScholarID:252717.

Elsabagh, S., P. Premkumar, et al. (2009). A longer duration of schizophrenic illness has sex-specific associations within the working memory neural network in schizophrenia. *Behavioural Brain Research* 201(1): 41–47.

Emsley, R., J. Rabinowitz, et al. (2007). Remission in early psychosis: Rates, predictors, and clinical and functional outcome correlates. *Schizophrenia Research* 89: 129–139.

Endo, M., Daiguji, M., Asano, Y., Yamashita, I., Takahashi. S. (1978). Periodic psychosis recurring in association with menstrual cycle. *Journal of Clinical Psychiatry* 39: 456–466.

Falkov, A. (2013). *The Family Model Handbook: An integrated approach to supporting mentally ill parents and their children.* Teddington: Pavilion.

Flor-Henry, P. The influence of gender on psychopathology. (1983). In: Flor-Henry, P. (ed.), *Cerebral Basis of Psychopathology* (Chapter 5, pp. 97–116). Littleton, MA: Wright-PSG Inc.

Goldman, P. S., Crawford, H. T., Stokes, L. P., Galkin, T. W., Rosvold, H. E. (1974). Sex-dependent behavioral effects of cerebral cortical lesions in the developing rhesus monkey. *Science*, 186: 540–542.

Goldstein J. M. (1997). Sex differences in schizophrenia: Epidemiology, genetics, and the brain. *Internat'l Rev Psychiatry: The Neuropsychiatry of Schizophrenia.* 9: 399–408. G. D. Pearlson, P. R. Slavney (eds.).

Goldstein J. M. (1995). The impact of gender on understanding the epidemiology of schizophrenia: A critical review. In: Seeman, M. V. (ed.), *Gender and psychopathology* (pp. 159–199). Washington DC: American Psychiatric Association Press.

Goldstein, J. M,, S. Cherkerzian, et al. (2014). Prenatal maternal immune disruption and sex-dependent risk for psychoses. *Psychological Medicine* 44(15):3249-3261.

Goldstein, J. M., K. Lancaster, et al. (2015) Sex differences, hormones, and fMRI stress response circuitry deficits in psychoses. *Psychiatry Research* 232(3):226-236.

Goldstein, J. M., Link, B. G. (1988). Gender and the expression of schizophrenia. *J Psychiatry Research*, 22: 141–155.

Goldstein, J. M., L. J. Seidman, et al. (2001). Normal sexual dimorphism of the adult human brain assessed by in vivo magnetic resonance imaging. *Cerebral Cortex* 11(6): 490–497.

Goldstein, J. M., L. J. Seidman, et al. (2002). Impact of normal sexual dimorphisms on sex differences in structural brain abnormalities in schizophrenia assessed by magnetic resonance imaging. *Archives of General Psychiatry* 59(2): 154–164.

Goldstein, J. M., Walder, D. (2006). *Sex differences in schizophrenia: The case for developmental origins and etiological implications.* United Kingdom: Oxford University Press.

Goodman, S. (1987). Emory University project on children of disturbed parents. *Schizophrenia Bulletin* 13: 411–422.

Grimm, V. E., Frieder, B. (1985). Differential vulnerability of male and female rats to the timing of various perinatal insults. *International Journal of Neuroscience*, 27, 155–64.

Grossman L. S., Harrow, M., Rosen, C., Faull, R., Strauss, G. P. (2008). Sex differences in schizophrenia and other psychotic disorders: A 20-year longitudinal study of psychosis and recovery. *Comprehensive Psychiatry*, 49(6), 523–529.

Gur, R. E., P. E. Cowell, et al. (2000). Reduced dorsal and orbital prefrontal gray matter volumes in schizophrenia. *Archives of General Psychiatry* 57(8): 761–768.

Häfner, H., Maurer, K., Loffler, W., Riecher-Rössler, A. (1993). The influence of age and sex on the onset and early course of schizophrenia. *British Journal of Psychiatry*, 162, 80–86.

Hahn, C., A. H. Neuhaus, et al. (2011). Smoking reduces language lateralization: A dichotic listening study with control participants and schizophrenia patients. *Brain and Cognition* 76(2): 300–309.

Hambrecht, M., Maurer. K., Häfner, H., Sartorius, N. (1992). Transnational stability of gender differences in schizophrenia. *Eur Arch Psychiatr & Neurol Sci*, 242, 6–12.

Harrison, G., K. Hopper, et al. (2001). Recovery from psychotic illness: a 15- and 25-year international follow-up study. *British Journal of Psychiatry* 178, 506–17.

Hoff A. L., Kremen, W. S. (2001). Association of estrogen levels with neuropsychological performance in women with schizophrenia. *American Journal of Psychiatry* 158(7): 1134–1139.

Holley, S. M., E. A. Wang, et al. (2013). Frontal cortical synaptic communication is abnormal in Disc1 genetic mouse models of schizophrenia. *Schizophrenia Research* 146(1–3): 264–272.

Huber, T. J., Borsutzky, M., Schneider, U., Emrich, H. M. (2004). Psychotic disorders and gonadal function: Evidence supporting the estrogen hypothesis. *Acta Psychiatrica Scandinavica* 109: 269–274.

Irle, E., C. Lange, et al. (2011). Hippocampal size in women but not men with schizophrenia relates to disorder duration. *Psychiatry Research* 192(3): 133–139.

Jablensky, A. (2003). Schizophrenia: the epidemiological horizon. In: Hirsch, S. R. and Weinberger, D. R. (eds.), *Schizophrenia* (pp. 203–231). Oxford: Blackwell Science.

Jablensky A., Cole, S. W. (1997). Is the earlier age at onset of schizophrenia in males a confounded finding? Results from a cross-cultural investigation. *British Journal of Psychiatry*, 170, 234–240.

Jablensky, A., McGrath, J., Herrman, H., Castle, D., Gureje, O., Evans, A., Carr, V., Morgan, V., Korten, A., Harvey, C. (2000). Psychotic disorders in urban areas: An overview of the study on low prevalence disorders. *Australian and New Zealand Journal of Psychiatry*, 34:221–236.

Jablensky, A., Sartorius, N., Ernberg, E., Anker, M., Korten, A., Cooper, J. E., Day, R., Bertelsen, A. (1992). Schizophrenia: Manifestations, incidence and course in different cultures. A World Health Organization ten country study. *Psychological Medicine* Monograph, Suppl 20.

Jimenez, J. A., A. Mancini-Marie, et al. (2010). Disturbed sexual dimorphism of brain activation during mental rotation in schizophrenia. *Schizophrenia Research* 122(1–3): 53–62.

Joshi, D., S. J. Fung, et al. (2012). Higher gamma-aminobutyric acid neuron density in the white matter of orbital frontal cortex in schizophrenia. *Biological Psychiatry* 72(9): 725–733.

Jung, H. T., D. W. Kim, et al. (2012). Reduced source activity of event-related potentials for affective facial pictures in schizophrenia patients. *Schizophrenia Research* 136(1–3): 150–159.

Kumar, R., Marks, M., Platz, C., Yoshida, K. (1995). Clinical survey of a psychiatric mother and baby unit: characteristics of 100 consecutive admissions. *Journal of Affective Disorders* 33(1): 11–22.

Kunimatsu, N., S. Aoki, et al. (2012). Tract-specific analysis of white matter integrity disruption in schizophrenia. *Psychiatry Research* 201(2): 136–143.

Lee, S. H., E. Y. Kim, et al. (2010). Event-related potential patterns and gender effects underlying facial affect processing in schizophrenia patients. *Neuroscience Research* 67(2):172–180.

Leung, A., Chue, P. (2000). Sex differences in schizophrenia, a review of the literature. *Acta Psychiatrica Scandinavica, Supplementum* 40: 3–38.

Lewis, S., N. Tarrier, et al.(2002). Randomised controlled trial of cognitive-behavioural therapy in early schizophrenia: acute-phase outcomes. *British Journal of Psychiatry*, Suppl. 43: s91–7.

Manuseva, N., A. Novotni, et al. (2012). Some QEEG parameters and gender differences in schizophrenia patients. *Psychiatr Danub* 24(1): 51–56.

Martins-de-Souza, D., A. Schmitt, et al. (2010). Sex-specific proteome differences in the anterior cingulate cortex of schizophrenia. *Journal of Psychiatric Research* 44(14): 989–991.

McCreadie, R. G., D. Wiles, et al. (1989). The Scottish first episode schizophrenia study. *VII. Two-year follow-up. Scottish Schizophrenia Research Group. Acta Psychiatrica Scandinavica* 80, 597–602.

McGrath, J., Saha, S., Chant, D., Welham, J. (2008). Schizophrenia: A concise overview of incidence, prevalence, and mortality. *Epidemiologic Reviews*. 30:67–76.

McGrath, J., S. Saha, et al. (2004). A systematic review of the incidence of schizophrenia: the distribution of rates and the influence of sex, urbanicity, migrant status and methodology. *BMC Medicine* 2(13).

Meaney, M. J., Szyf, M. (2005). Maternal care as a model for experience-dependent chromatin plasticity? *Trends in Neurosciences* 28: 456–463.

Mendrek, A., J. Jiménez, et al. (2011). Correlations between sadness-induced cerebral activations and schizophrenia symptoms: An fMRI study of sex differences. *European Psychiatry* 26(5): 320–326.

Moldin, S. O. (2000). Gender and schizophrenia: An overview. In: Frank, E. (Ed.), *Gender and its effects on psychopathology* (pp. 169–186). Washington, DC: American Psychiatric Press, Inc.

Morgan, V. A., Castle, D. J., Jablensky, A. V. (2008). Do women express and experience psychosis differently from men? Epidemiological evidence from the Australian National Study of Low Prevalence (Psychotic) Disorders. *Australian & New Zealand Journal of Psychiatry*, 42(1):74–82.

Nopoulos, P., M. Flaum, et al. (1997). Sex differences in brain morphology in schizophrenia. *American Journal of Psychiatry* 154(12): 1648–1654.

O'Tuathaigh, C. M., M. Harte, et al. (2010). Schizophrenia-related endophenotypes in heterozygous neuregulin-1 'knockout' mice. *European Journal of Neuroscience* 31(2): 349–358.

Perälä, J., J. Suvisaari, et al. (2007). Lifetime prevalence of psychotic and bipolar I disorders in a general population. *Archives of General Psychiatry* 64(1):19–28. doi:10.1001/archpsyc.64.1.19.

Pryce, C. R., A. C. Dettling, et al. (2004). Deprivation of parenting disrupts development of homeostatic and reward systems in marmoset monkey offspring. *Biological Psychiatry* 56: 72–79.

Radulescu, E., F. Sambataro, et al. (2013). Effect of schizophrenia risk-associated alleles in SREB2 (GPR85) on functional MRI phenotypes in healthy volunteers. *Neuropsychopharmacology* 38(2): 341–349.

Rajkumar, S., Thara, R. (1989). Factors affecting relapse in schizophrenia. *Schizophrenia Research* 2:403–9.

Rantakallio, P., von Wendt, L. (1985). Trauma to the nervous system and its sequelae in a one-year birth cohort followed up to the age of 14 years. *Journal of Epidemiology & Community Health* 39(4):353–356.

Rector, N. A., Seeman, M. V. (1992). Auditory hallucinations in women and men. *Schizophrenia Research* 7: 233–236.

Robinson, D., M. G. Woerner, et al. (1999). Predictors of relapse following response from a first episode of schizophrenia or schizoaffective disorder. *Archives of General Psychiatry* 56, 241–247.

Roy, M. A., Maziade, M., Labbé, A., Mérette, C. (2001). Male gender is associated with deficit schizophrenia: a meta-analysis *Schizophrenia Research* 47 (2–3), 141–147.

Saha, S., Chant, D., Welham, J., McGrath, J. (2005). A systematic review of the prevalence of schizophrenia. *PLoS Med* 2: e141.

Salmon, M., Abel, K. M., Cordingly, L., Friedman, T., Appleby, L. (2003). Clinical and parenting skills outcomes following joint mother-baby psychiatric admission. *Australian and New Zealand Journal of Psychiatry* 37(5):556–562.

Salokangas, R.K.R. (1997a). Living situation, social network and outcome in schizophrenia: A five-year prospective follow-up study. *Acta Psychiatrica Scandanavica* 96: 459–468.

Salokangas, R.K.R. (1997b). Structure of schizophrenic symptomatology and its changes over time: Prospective factor analytical study. *Acta Psychiatrica Scandanavica* 95, 32–39.

Sameroff, A., R. Seifer, et al. (1987). Early indicators of developmental risk: Rochester longitudinal study. *Schizophrenia Bulletin* 13: 383–394.

Sartorius, N., Jablensky, A., Korten, A., Ernberg, G., Anker, M., Cooper, J. E., Day, R. (1986). Early manifestations and first-contact incidence of schizophrenia in different cultures. A preliminary report on the initial evaluation phase of the WHO Collaborative Study on determinants of outcome of severe mental disorders. *Psychological Medicine* 16(4):909–928.

Savadjiev, P., T. J. Whitford, et al. (2013). Sexually Dimorphic White Matter Geometry Abnormalities in Adolescent Onset Schizophrenia. *Cerebral Cortex* 24(5): 1389–1396.

Schulz, K. M., H. A. Molenda-Figueira, et al. (2009). Back to the future: The organizational-activational hypothesis adapted to puberty and adolescence. *Hormones and Behavior* 55(5): 597–604.

Selten, J. P., Veen, N. D., Hoek, H. W., Laan, W., Schols, D., van der Tweel, I., Feller, W., Kahn, R. S. (2007). Early course of schizophrenia in a representative Dutch incidence cohort. *Schizophrenia Research* 97(1–3): 79–87.

Shepherd, A. M., S. L. Matheson, et al. (2012). Systematic meta-analysis of insula volume in schizophrenia. *Biological Psychiatry* 72(9): 775–784.

Shipman, S. L., E. K. Baker, et al. (2009). Absence of established sex differences in patients with schizophrenia on a two-dimensional object array task. *Psychiatry Research* 166(2–3): 158–165.

Somers, V. (2007). Schizophrenia: The impact of parental illness on children. *British Journal of Social Work* 37: 1319–1334.

Stanley, N., Penhale, B., Rioran, D., Barbour, R. S., Holdern, S. (2003). *Child Protection and Mental Health Services: Interprofessional responses to the needs of mothers*. Bristol: Policy Press.

Sumich, A., A. P. Anilkumar, et al. (2014). Sex specific event-related potential (ERP) correlates of depression in schizophrenia. *Psychiatr Danub* 26(1): 27–33.

Susser, E., Wanderling, J. (1994). Epidemiology of nonaffective acute remitting psychosis: sex and sociocultural setting. *Archives of General Psychiatry* 51:294–301.

Szeszko, P. R., Strous, R. D., Goldman, R. S., Ashtari, M., Knuth, K. H., Lieberman, J. A., Bilder, R. M. (2002). Neuropsychological correlates of hippocampal volumes in patients experiencing a first episode of schizophrenia. *American Journal of Psychiatry* 159(2): 217–226.

Thara. R., Rajkumar, S. (1992). Gender differences in schizophrenia. Results of a follow-up study from India. *Schizophrenia Research* 7(1):65–70.

Thormodsen, R., L. M. Rimol, et al. (2013). Age-related cortical thickness differences in adolescents with early-onset schizophrenia compared with healthy adolescents. *Psychiatry Research* 214(3): 190–196.

Tien, A. Y. (1991). Distributions of hallucinations in the population. *Psychological Medicine* 26, 203–208.

Uehara-Aoyama, K., M. Nakamura, et al. (2011). Sexually dimorphic distribution of orbitofrontal sulcogyral pattern in schizophrenia. *Psychiatry and Clinical Neurosciences* 65(5): 483–489.

UK Department of Health (2002). Into the Mainstream. http://webarchive .nationalarchives.gov.uk/+/www.dh .gov.uk/en/Consultations/ Closedconsultations/DH_4075478 (accessed October 10, 2015).

Vazquez-Barquero, J. L., Cuesta Nunez, M. J., Herrera Castanedo, S., Diez Manrique, J. F., Pardo, G., Dunn, G. (1996). Sociodemographic and clinical variables as predictors of the diagnostic characteristics of first episodes of schizophrenia. *Acta Psychiatrica Scandinavica* 94(3):149–155.

Videbech, P., Gouliaev, G. (1995). First admission with puerperal psychosis: 7-14 years of follow-up. *Acta Psychiatrica Scandinavica* 91(3):167–173.

von Wilmsdorff, M., U. Sprick, et al. (2010). Sex-dependent behavioral effects and morphological changes in the hippocampus after prenatal invasive interventions in rats: Implications for animal models of schizophrenia. *Clinics (Sao Paulo)* 65(2): 209–219.

Walsh, D., Wiersma, D. (2001). Recovery from psychotic illness: A 15- and 25-year international follow-up study. *British Journal of Psychiatry* 178, 506–517.

Weintraub, S. (1987). Risk factors in schizophrenia: The Stony Brook high-risk project. *Schizophrenia Bulletin* 13: 439–450.

Weisinger, B., D. Greenstein, et al. (2013). Lack of gender influence on cortical and subcortical gray matter development in childhood-onset schizophrenia. *Schizophrenia Bulletin* 39(1): 52–58.

Wiersma, D., F. J. Nienhuis, et al. (1998). Natural course of schizophrenic disorders: A 15-year follow up of a Dutch incidence cohort. *Schizophrenia Bulletin* 24: 75–85.

Wiersma, D., J. Wanderline, et al. (2000). Social disability in schizophrenia: Its development and prediction over 15 years in incidence cohorts in six European centres. *Psychological Medicine* 30: 1155–1167.

Wildgust, H. J., Beary, M. (2010). Are there modifiable risk factors which will reduce the excess mortality in schizophrenia? *Journal of Psychopharmacology* 24(4 Suppl): 37–50.

Zhang, F., Q. Chen, et al. (2011). Evidence of sex-modulated association of ZNF804A with schizophrenia. *Biological Psychiatry* 69(10): 914–917.

Chapter

23

Treating women with schizophrenia

Shubulade Smith and Fiona Gaughran

Introduction

The management of schizophrenia has largely been conceptualized around men. This may be partly because schizophrenia is more common in men, except in later life when the prevalence in women rises (see Chapter 22). Also, the illness, especially its behavioral consequences, is often more severe in men than women, with the prognosis for many women being better, which means that clinicians, especially those working in acute, forensic or inpatient settings see male patients more frequently.

However, the evidence relating to treatment of schizophrenia in men cannot be replicated wholesale in the management of women with the illness. Women with schizophrenia have more comorbid affective symptoms, which may affect presentation, accuracy of diagnosis, treatment choice and prognosis (Leung and Chue 2000). Management of schizophrenia in women needs to take into account that they are more likely to be carers of children and relatives. Also, women with schizophrenia are more likely to have been abused (sexually, emotionally and physically) (Bonoldi et al. 2013), which can affect both treatment and outcomes. Finally, many of the treatments and management of the side effects of these have been developed with men in mind (Merkatz and Junod 1994), or based on evidence from a predominantly male sample; it is of huge importance that women are underrepresented in clinical trials because of the risk of pregnancy.

Women are thus likely to be at a disadvantage when it comes to informed, evidence-based schizophrenia treatment, whilst clinicians' "default" choices are more likely to be informed by evidence from responses in males. This chapter aims to enable the practitioner to provide treatments tailored more towards the many different and multifactorial needs of their female patients and thereby provide safer, more effective and efficacious solutions to treating their schizophrenia.

Biology

Female physiology differs significantly from that of males and this affects the way in which women process medications. The response of any individual to a given medication partly relates to the effectiveness of the drug for that person's condition, but is also greatly affected by how much of that drug is available to them, that is, how well it is absorbed into and eliminated from the body. This is impacted by age, ethnicity and gender as well as individual factors.

Absorption and bioavailability
Gastric emptying

The majority of medications are administered in oral form, with the intestine being the main site of drug absorption. Because gastric emptying is slower in women, they absorb antipsychotics more slowly and, if tested, show lower peak levels of antipsychotic than expected if male reference ranges are used (Bennink et al. 1998, Lorena et al. 2004). Women also have lower concentrations of gastric acid than men, which theoretically may slow the absorption of acidic compounds such as phenothiazines. In practice, absorption is greatly affected by the speed of gastric emptying and also by the presence of other substances that change gastric pH such as proton pump inhibitors.

Distribution

The total blood volume in women is smaller than in men, meaning that there is less volume available for a

---

Comprehensive Women's Mental Health, ed. David J. Castle and Kathryn M. Abel. Published by Cambridge University Press.
© Cambridge University Press 2016.

drug to be distributed. However, men have more lean muscle mass and less body fat than women, with young adult women having, on average, 15% more body fat than their male counterparts. Antipsychotic medications are lipophilic, so readily enter the body fat. With the more fat-soluble compounds, such as many depot antipsychotics, this results in greater distribution of antipsychotic in a woman's body compared with a man for the same dose of drug. Over time, more depot antipsychotic will accumulate in a woman compared with a man. This implies that women may need a longer interval between depot doses than a man to reduce the side effect burden (Smith 2010).

This effect is magnified in women of South Asian or Chinese origin. People from these ethnic groups have a higher body fat to lean mass ratio than other groups. Thus, women of South Asian heritage are more likely to experience antipsychotic accumulation than both South Asian men and men and women of other ethnic groups (Lear et al. 2007, 2009).

Metabolism

Intra-individual differences in antipsychotic metabolism account for much of the variability in drug response. The bulk of drug breakdown takes place in the liver, largely through the cytochrome P450 (CYP450) enzyme system. All antipsychotic medications are metabolized by the CYP450 system, which is dominated by three main pathways – CYP1A2, CYP2D6 and CYP3A4 (see Table 23.1). Genetic variations in CYP450 enzymes govern the rate of drug metabolism, and both gender and ethnic differences have been found. Men generally have higher CYP1A2 activity compared with women, while the reverse is

the case for CYP3A4 activity (Anthony & Berg 2002, Wolbold et al. 2003, Scandlyn et al. 2008).

The role of the drug transporter P-glycoprotein is also relevant. This is the main transporter of substrates across the intra- and extracellular membrane and men have more than twice as much of this as women in their hepatocytes. This results in lower levels of drug in the serum of women because more drug substrate is bound to this protein carrier (Meibohm et al. 2002, Fleeman et al. 2010).

A number of psychotropic and non-psychotropic medications, as well as naturally occurring substances, interfere with CYP metabolism by either inhibiting or inducing the enzymes. The ability of medications such as antidepressants and mood stabilizers to induce or inhibit CYP enzymes is particularly relevant in women because women are prescribed more of these drugs than men. Many selective serotonin reuptake inhibitor (SSRI) antidepressants are inhibitors of the CYP2D6. Fluoxetine and paroxetine are potent inhibitors, while fluvoxamine, sertraline and citalopram are weak inhibitors. Co-prescription of these drugs will exert a considerable influence on the metabolism of those antipsychotics that are substrates for this system, such as risperidone, clozapine and olanzapine. These drugs are more likely to accumulate when given concomitantly with certain SSRIs, increasing the risk of side effects and toxicity. As women with serious mental illness (SMI) are more likely to be receiving concomitant antidepressants, they are more likely to be exposed to this possibility.

The CYP enzymes, such as CYP1A2 and 3A4, are also affected by diet. Ethnicity and gender influence dietary choices. This is most likely to be of relevance when treating women with protein-rich diets

Table 23.1 Cytochrome P450 Enzymes, Antipsychotic Substrates, Inhibitors and Inducers

Enzyme	Substrate	Inhibitor	Inducer
CYP1A2	Clozapine, haloperidol, olanzapine	Fluvoxamine, grapefruit juice, antibiotics	Carbamazepine, Smoking, brassica vegetables
CYP2D6	Aripiprazole, chlorpromazine, clozapine, haloperidol, olanzapine, perphenazine, risperidone, thioridazine, zuclopenthixol	Bupropion, fluoxetine, paroxetine, citalopram, duloxetin, fluvoxamine, fluphenazine, moclobemide, chlorpromazine, haloperidol, perphenazine, propranolol, antibiotics	
CYP3A4	Aripiprazole, clozapine, haloperidol, quetiapine, risperidone, sertindole, ziprasidone, lurasidone	Fluoxetine, fluvoxamine, olanzapine, nefazodone, grapefruit juice, erythromycin, ketoconazole, St John's Wort	Carbamazepine, St John's Wort

and South Asian women who have adapted to a more protein-rich Western diet, as this results in faster metabolism of drugs in this population (Alvares 1976).

The hydrocarbons in tobacco smoke act as enzyme inducers and, given that a large proportion of people with SMI smoke, this has implications for drug metabolism and response. Smokers taking clozapine or olanzapine have lower plasma levels of the drug than non-smokers taking the same dose as the hydrocarbons in cigarette smoke induce CYP1A2, accelerating breakdown of the dibenzodiazepines; (Tang et al. 2007, Lane et al. 1999). The rates of smoking in the general population vary considerably by gender, although it is not clear if the same effect is seen in men and women with psychosis. In terms of attitudes to smoking, although there are no major gender differences in smokers with psychosis regarding reasons for smoking/quitting or smoking outcomes, female smokers with psychosis are more likely than males to report that they smoke to prevent weight gain. Therefore, in practice, it will help to focus specifically on weight in helping women smokers with psychosis to quit (Filia et al., 2014).

Renal clearance

Women have a lower glomerular filtration rate, renal tubular secretion and reabsorption than men, which means that the elimination of antipsychotics is slower in women than in men. This further increases the likelihood of drug accumulation within the body.

The multiple factors that affect drug handling in women are not simply countered by dosing on a mg/kg basis as multiple mechanisms underlie the gender-based pharmacokinetic differences. Thus, a man of the same weight will clear a drug quicker and have lower plasma levels than a woman; for example, men clear olanzapine 38% faster than women. Women are therefore at greater risk of a range of adverse drug reactions from antipsychotics because the drug stays in the body for longer (Smith 2010). The main factors influencing adverse effects are pharmacodynamic and are related to the receptor binding profiles of these drugs. For antipsychotic receptor binding profiles and related adverse effects see Tables 23.2 and 23.3.

Medication treatment response

Antipsychotic drugs are the mainstay of the medical treatment of people with schizophrenia. However, women with schizophrenia on average have a slightly

Table 23.2 Receptor-binding and commonly associated adverse effects

Receptor type	Side effect
D_2	Neurological – extrapyramidal, EPS (acute dystonia, TD, parkinsonism, akathisia) Hormonal – prolactin elevation, weight gain, sexual and reproductive dysfunction
M_1	Dry mouth, constipation, urinary retention, blurred vision, ↑HR, cognitive deficits, sexual dysfunction
H_1	Sedation, weight gain, dizziness
$α_1$	Orthostatic hypotension, ↑QTc
$α_2$	Anesthesia, hypotension, cardiac effects
$5HT_{2A}$	?anti-EPS
$5HT_{2C}$	Satiety

later age of onset (although see Chapter 22), complicated reproductive and hormonal considerations, frequent affective symptoms and a greater likelihood of prior or ongoing victimization This is related to a common requirement for concomitant antidepressant and mood stabilizing medications, as well as being more likely to be co-prescribed hormonal preparations such as the combined oral contraceptive pill and hormone replacement therapy.

Even where antipsychotics are prescribed alone, there are considerable gender differences that should be borne in mind when prescribing. For example, for the same dose of clozapine or olanzapine, women will achieve much higher blood levels than men. They are likely to start showing a therapeutic response at a lower dose than men; if the dose is not modified to take account of gender, it may well lead to a much higher rate of side effects (Salokangas 2004, Tang et al. 2007b, Usall et al. 2007).

Adverse reactions to medication

There are two situations whereby women may experience adverse drug reactions. One, as alluded to earlier, is where the plasma levels of the medication are higher than intended by virtue of gender, leading to a greater likelihood of dose-related side effects.

The other type of side effect is where the effect is either specific to, or amplified in, women. An obvious example is drugs where there is a risk of teratogenicity

Table 23.3 Receptor binding profiles of different antipsychotic medications

	Haloperidol	Clozapine	Olanzapine	Quetiapine	Risperidone	Paliperidone	Amisulpride	Aripiprazole*	Lurasidone	Zotepine	Ziprasidone
D_2	+++	+	+++	+	+++	+++	+++	+++	+++	+++	+++
M_1	neg	+++	+++	+++	neg	neg	neg	+	neg	+++	neg
H_1	+	+++	+++	+++	+++	+++	neg	++	neg	+++	++
α_1	+++	+++	+++	+++	+++	++	neg	+++	+	+++	+++
α_2	+	+++	++	+	+++	++	+	+++	+	++	++
$5HT_{2A}$	+	+++	+++	++	+++	+++	neg	+++	+++	+++	+++
$5HT_{2C}$	neg	+++	+++	+	+++	++	neg	+++	+	+++	+++

Receptor binding affinity +++ = strong, ++ = moderate, += weak, neg = negligible effect,
*Partial agonist

in women of childbearing age. This is dealt with in Chapter 11 of this book. Many psychotropic medications affect the reproductive cycle or female sexual function, and may increase the risk of disorders that are more common in women in the general population, such as osteoporosis.

Antipsychotics

There are no specific antipsychotics used preferentially in women rather than men, but it should be noted that women are more at risk of the hormonal and metabolic side effects of antipsychotic medication, with men being more likely to suffer with the neurological side effects of these medications (Van Os 1999, Christodoulou & Kalaitzi 2005, Zhang et al. 2009). There is some limited evidence that women may experience a greater side effect burden with the newer second generation antipsychotics (SGAs), in particular clozapine and olanzapine, which is most likely related to the effects of these drugs on metabolic parameters (Aichhorn 2006).

Hyperprolactinemia

The most common cause of amenorrhea in women with psychosis is not pregnancy, but rather antipsychotic induced hyperprolactinemia – although for safety's sake, the old medical school adage, "every woman is pregnant until proven otherwise" still applies. The antipsychotic most at fault here are those with strong affinity to the dopamine D2 receptor, especially amisulpride, risperidone and paliperidone. As dopamine is the main prolactin inhibitory factor, antagonism of this receptor may cause a large and clinically meaningful rise in prolactin. This can result in amenorrhea, galactorrhea, enlarged breasts, and, in the longer term, an increased risk of osteoporosis and fractures (Abel et al. 2008; Inder & Castle, 2011). Up to 75% of women taking prolactin-raising medications (those with significant D2 blocking effects) experience hyperprolactinemia (Smith et al. 2002, Wieck & Haddad 2003).

The use of antipsychotic medication is commonly associated with sexual dysfunction (in both women and men). However, because of the complex nature of female sexuality, the significant negative impact on women's sexual function of antipsychotic medication may be missed. Studies indicate that antipsychotic-related sexual dysfunction is more common in women than men with up to 90% of women taking antipsychotics experiencing sexual dysfunction (MacDonald et al. 2003). Unlike with men (for whom there are multiple underlying mechanisms driving sexual dysfunction), the main cause of sexual dysfunction in women taking antipsychotic medication is hyperprolactinemia (Smith et al. 2002, Harley et al. 2010). Low libido is often the first sign of antipsychotic-induced hyperprolactinemia, but this symptom must be directly inquired about as patients are unlikely to report it spontaneously (Smith 2002, Baggaley 2008).

Hyperprolactinemia is not the only cause of amenorrhea or oligomenorrhea in women with severe mental illness. The use of the mood stabilizer sodium valproate not only results in a far greater risk of teratogenicity than other anticonvulsants, but also confers a risk of polycystic ovarian syndrome (PCOS), which adds to cardiac risk in the longer term (Wild et al. 2010, Hillman et al. 2014). Given the shortened life expectancy already experienced by people with psychosis, this additive risk is a substantial concern. The anti-diabetic drug metformin has been shown not just to help reduce weight, but also to improve amenorrhea in women with schizophrenia (Wu et al., 2012).

Cardiovascular risk and metabolic syndrome

There is increasing evidence that in addition to being at risk of hormonally mediated side effects of psychotropic medications, women are at greater risk of the metabolic adverse effects of these drugs. The CATIE study found that 51% of women taking antipsychotic medication had metabolic syndrome compared with 36% of men (McEvoy et al 2005). The NIHR funded IMPaCT (IMProving health and ReduCing subsTance Use in Psychosis) program in the UK found very high rates of central obesity, most marked in women (personal communication, Gaughran et al. 2013). Given the greater diabetes hazard ratio in women, that is, that women are more likely to develop diabetes complications and die from the cardiovascular disease related to their diabetes, this represents a major physical health burden for women. It is therefore incumbent upon prescribers to ensure that they choose antipsychotic medications that are less likely to worsen the cardiovascular status of women in the long term. This could help to improve the shortened life expectancy seen in this group.

Table 23.2 shows the side effects associated with different antipsychotic medications. It is apparent from this which medications are most likely to be troublesome in women and prescribers can use this information to tailor the medication to the individual in order to minimize the risk of short- and long-term side effects.

Other psychotropics used in the treatment of women with schizophrenia and psychotic disorders

Antidepressants – Depression is common in schizophrenia with prevalence rates estimated at 40% or more (Wassink et al. 1999, Micallef et al. 2006). Women with schizophrenia are more likely to have an affective component to their illness (Tang 2007b, Martin-Reyes 2011). Generally, women are more likely to be treated for depression than men, which may partly be due to differences in health-seeking behavior between the sexes. A recent study found that depression and psychotic depression were common amongst a group of women and men with schizophrenia, yet only one-third of the sample had received antidepressants. They recommended that prescribers could significantly improve the prognostic outcomes for their patients if they regularly reviewed depressive symptomatology and their prescribing practices (Nejtek et al. 2012).

There are no specific antidepressant medications which are felt to be more advantageous in women than men with schizophrenia, but it should be remembered that the SSRI medications may interfere with hepatic metabolism in a way that is likely to differentially affect women by interfering with antipsychotic metabolism, and that they may cause sexual dysfunction thus adding to any sexual dysfunction problems caused by co-prescribed antipsychotic medication (see Table 23.1).

Hypnotics (benzodiazepines and antihistamines) – Although not in and of themselves treatments for schizophrenia, these drugs are often used in the acute stages of treatment to manage agitation, anxiety and disturbed behavior. Benzodiazepines are both overprescribed to, and overused by, women and those of advancing age (Simoni-Wastila 2004). However, despite benzodiazepine use in schizophrenia being common, women with schizophrenia appear no more likely to receive these drugs than men with schizophrenia (Xiang et al. 2012). Antihistamines are often used instead of benzodiazepines as sedatives because they have a far lower addiction potential.

These drugs are relatively safe and there are no significant gender differences in their handling; the main consideration should be that prescribers might consider using these rather than the more addictive benzodiazepines where possible, given that one-third of people are likely to continue benzodiazepines for 8 years or more after initial prescription and more recently benzodiazepine use has been linked with a significant increase in mortality (van Hulten et al. 2003, Weich et al. 2014).

Mood stabilizers

Schizophrenia in women often has an affective component and therefore, it should be expected that women with schizophrenia are often given concomitant mood stabilizing medications. With this in mind, prescribers should be aware of, and be cautious about, the following.

Sodium valproate – The significant adverse effects associated with sodium valproate have a disproportionate effect on women. This is dealt with in Chapter 21, but in brief, sodium valproate is associated with menstrual abnormalities and PCOS, and has a high risk of teratogenicity in the fetus. Therefore, great care should be given to ensuring it is not given to sexually active, reproductively able women. If there is no alternative to valproate, robust contraception plus folate is essential.

Lithium – Lithium use is well-known to be associated with thyroid abnormalities, in particular, goiter, hypothyroidism, hyperthyroidism and autoimmune thyroiditis. Lithium-associated thyroid dysregulation occurs more frequently in women (Bauer et al. 2014, Ozerdem et al. 2014) and therefore monitoring of thyroid function (serum thyroid stimulating hormone, free thyroid hormones – T3 and T4, and thyroid autoantibodies) and clinical assessment of thyroid size should be undertaken at initiation of lithium and annually.

There is evidence that over time lithium gradually reduces glomerular filtration rate (GFR), that is, it can compromise renal function. GFR has been estimated to decrease by 0.64ml/min (95% CI = 0.38 to 0.90, $p = 0.00$) for each year of lithium treatment (Bocchetta et al. 2013). This has disproportionately negative effects on women who already have slower GFRs than men. In a recent study, women treated with lithium not only had lower GFR to begin with but also had a higher rate of reduction in GFR. They were more likely to have an eGFR <60ml/min, which indicates chronic kidney disease stage 3–5 (Bocchetta et al. 2013). This means that lithium is more likely to be associated with renal disease in women.

In addition, lithium is exquisitely sensitive to changes in fluid balance, which are more likely to occur around the menstrual cycle. This can affect the volume of distribution of lithium, which has a narrow therapeutic range. Therefore prescribers must be vigilant and ensure adequate monitoring when prescribing to women.

Treatment resistance

Although there is evidence that women are more likely to respond to antipsychotic treatment than men, it might be assumed that those women who are treatment resistant have a particularly unusual form of schizophrenia. However, there is no evidence that women who are treatment resistant are more difficult to treat than men (Mortimer et al. 2010, Teo et al. 2013). In fact, of 153 sequential admissions to a specialist tertiary psychosis unit in the UK, 86 were male and 67 female (Sarker et al. 2014). Nonetheless, treatment resistance occurs in approximately 30% of women and the differences in the underlying etiology and pathogenesis of schizophrenia in women have been exploited when trying to explore ways of improving outcome in treatment resistance.

The putative neuroprotective effects of estrogen have been linked to the later onset of schizophrenia in women. However, the relationship between gender, age at onset and symptomatology is complex and covered in detail in this book elsewhere (see Chapter 22). Certainly, at a receptor level, estrogen exerts an effect on central indices of dopaminergic function (Chavez et al. 2010) and it has been proposed to act as a neuroleptic by inhibiting dopamine-mediated psychotic symptoms (Seeman, 1996). Therefore, the exploration of estrogen as a therapy for schizophrenia seems quite logical. However, to date, the evidence that estrogen acts to reduce schizophrenia risk or psychotic symptom severity directly is weak. One open-study, added 100 μg per day of transdermal estradiol for 28 days as adjunctive treatment in 102 women with refractory psychosis and reported label improvements in Positive and Negative Syndrome Scale (PANSS) scores and cognition when compared with antipsychotic medication alone (Kulkarni et al. 2008). However,

these were driven by changes in affective symptom scores. The same group also piloted the adjuvant use of the selective estrogen receptor modulator (SERM), raloxifene, finding an effect with 120 mg (usual maximum dose is 60mg) over 12 weeks in postmenopausal women with schizophrenia. The addition of raloxifene resulted in significant improvements in psychopathology (Kulkarni et al., 2010). These studies require independent replication before estrogen or SERMs can be advocated for the treatment of women with schizophrenia. Their use also needs to be balanced against potential side effects.

It is possible that hormonal modulators may at least partially be acting on the affective dimensions of schizophrenia. Estrogen is well known as a potent modulator of mood and of cognitive inhibitory processes (see Chapter 8). The estrogen receptor antagonist tamoxifen, best known for its use in breast cancer, has also been shown to have efficacy in reducing manic symptoms; it is believed that this related to its action as a protein C kinase inhibitor, although the antimanic properties of tamoxifen have not been fully elucidated (Zarate et al. 2007; Armani et al. 2014).

Psychological treatments for schizophrenia

Over the years there have been a number of psychological interventions that have been trialed in schizophrenia. Psychodynamic psychotherapy, client-centered, supportive and insight-oriented psychotherapy and behavioral modification techniques (token economy) once found favor, but lack a robust empirical evidence base as effective treatments for schizophrenia (Bellack 1986, Scott et al. 1995, Dickerson et al. 2005, Rosenbaum et al. 2012). Psychoeducation, family therapy, assertive community treatment, cognitive remediation therapy and cognitive behavioral therapy (CBT) have all been shown to be useful in schizophrenia, including treatment-resistant schizophrenia. A recent Cochrane review found that psychoeducation can reduce relapse, re-admission, length of stay and enhance medication adherence (Xia et al. 2011). Family therapy and assertive community treatment can help prevent psychotic relapse and re-hospitalization; however, they have little effect on specific positive and negative symptoms of schizophrenia, overall social functioning and employment. Social skills training helps to improve social skills, but has no clear effect on symptoms, relapse prevention or employment (Bustillo et al. 2001, Giron et al. 2010). Supportive employment programs have been found to improve the chances of gaining competitive employment (Huxley et al. 2000). Cognitive remediation therapy was designed to treat cognitive problems that affect social functioning and is effective in people with schizophrenia who are stable when combined with psychiatric rehabilitation (Wykes et al. 2007).

The most robust evidence for psychosocial treatment exists for CBT. A number of studies, including large meta-analyses have found that CBT is effective for schizophrenia and psychosis. The National Institute for Clinical Excellence (NICE) concluded that CBT is effective in reducing symptom severity in schizophrenia and that this therapy should be offered to everyone with psychosis as an adjunctive treatment as standard (Sensky et al. 2000, Wykes et al. 2003, Garety et al. 2008).

All psychosocial interventions have been found to work as adjuncts to pharmacotherapy. Despite the benefits of these treatments, there is little evidence that one modality is superior to another. Jones et al. (2012) found that there was no significant difference between the effects of CBT and other psychological therapies in schizophrenia including psychoeducation, supportive psychotherapy, counseling, family therapy and cognitive remediation therapy when systematic biases were taken into account. There is no evidence of a gender difference in response to CBT, or other psychosocial therapies. However, as women are known to favor psychological therapies, it is presumed that these are forms of treatment that they may be more likely to adhere to. Adherence to treatment (of whatever modality) is more likely to be associated with a better outcome in any disorder, including schizophrenia.

Social considerations when treating women with schizophrenia

Recreational drugs

Schizophrenia and psychosis are closely related to substance misuse. Up to 50% of people with schizophrenia use substances at some point in their lives (Buckley et al. 2009). Although women are less likely to use cannabis in general, and specifically high-potency cannabis, those who do may be more likely

to have a younger age of onset of psychosis and a worse outcome (Di Forti et al., 2014; Donoghue et al. 2014), suggesting that cannabis misuse may have a disproportionately negative effect on women compared to men with psychosis.

Cocaine and crack may be used more frequently by women with psychosis compared with women in the general population. These women are already at higher risk of physical health problems, in particular cardiovascular problems, and therefore there should be careful inquiry into substance misuse during psychiatric history taking. Women who use stimulant recreational drugs should be considered at high risk for the development of cardiovascular disease and monitored accordingly. Women with schizophrenia who misuse substances experience more victimization and medical illness than their male counterparts (Brunette and Drake 1997, DiNitto et al. 2002). This has implications for the type of input these women might benefit from, with an emphasis on psychological treatment of their substance use disorder including work around victimization. In addition, close attention should be paid to monitoring their physical health.

More recently "legal highs" have been associated with worsening in mental health (Lally et al. 2013). As yet there is little information about any gender differences in response/adverse effects of these drugs. The UK government is considering legislation to regulate these drugs as they have been associated with an increasing number of deaths.

Women with schizophrenia as carers

Most care for schizophrenia now takes place outside of institutional settings. This places a greater responsibility on family members to provide support and this role may disproportionately fall to women. Taking up a caregiving role is more common in some Black and Minority Ethnic groups (Guada et al. 2009). When examining the gender aspects of treating schizophrenia, paying attention to the needs of the women in the family is integral to the development of the package of care.

In a UK study, over 70% of women who underwent Mental Health Act assessments had dependent children (Hatfield et al. 1997). This means that psychiatrists who usually advocate for their patients may find themselves having to work with someone whose illness interferes with their ability to parent their child adequately. At any point that the welfare of a child is at risk, the primary duty is to the child and safeguarding concerns should be raised. Working with the parent and enabling and enhancing their recovery is the primary step in helping them to care for their child. The interested reader is also referred to Chapter 3 of this book.

Sexual health

The importance of including contraceptive advice to both women and men as part of routine care in schizophrenia cannot be overstated. There is an excess of unplanned pregnancies, although people with schizophrenia have lower fertility rates than controls (Bundy et al. 2011; Seeman and Ross 2011). As in the general population, choice of hormonal, non-hormonal or barrier contraception will depend on clinical factors such as age, smoking history and the presence or absence of other factors such as obesity, diabetes, migraine, cardiovascular disease or a family history of breast cancer. It is incumbent on prescribers to check for interactions that may reduce the effectiveness of hormonal contraception used. Women may prefer the convenience of long-acting contraceptive methods, such as intrauterine contraceptive devices, progesterone depots or tubal ligation. Discussions should include the importance of adding barrier methods of contraception. Advice about sexually transmitted infections should also be provided (Seeman and Ross 2011).

Service delivery

Single sex environments

Since 1997, UK government policy has been that inpatient units should be single sex, requiring strict demarcations between female and male inpatient areas. In the UK, the Care Quality Commission (CQC) reported that 77% of women in inpatient psychiatric settings were not in a designated single-sex ward, 16% did not have access to a designated single-sex toilet and bathing facilities, and 39% did not have access to a designated single-sex lounge area/day space. This is of particular importance to women with schizophrenia as they have been found to be at disproportionate risk of exploitation, especially sexual exploitation. The risk of male staff members abusing vulnerable female inpatients will be reduced by the

stringent checks that are carried out in most mainstream work environments in the UK and other Western countries. Being on a single-sex ward will not eliminate sexual harassment, but it should help to reduce the rate of inappropriate sexual attention for most people. Of note, Mezey et al. (2005) found that women in single-sex units reported intimidation, threats and abuse by other women, though they were less vulnerable to sexual abuse and exploitation and serious physical assault.

There is evidence that services are not adequately equipped to deal with women with schizophrenia. Researchers have questioned whether services are geared up to meet the needs of women with schizophrenia, given that a series of studies found marked differences in the service received by women and men. As a group, women had been in contact with services longer, received less intensive input than men for their condition, and the service had been less responsive to their changing needs (Perkins & Rowland 1991).

Sociocultural aspects of treatment are dealt with elsewhere in this book (see Chapter 2). However, it is worth emphasizing that cultural expectations may interfere with accessing treatment. Families may regard mental illness as taboo and therefore not seek out treatment or delay seeking treatment. Given the widely varying attitudes towards mental illness that exist throughout all societies, it is important to ascertain the particular cultural mores of an individual by asking them and those close to them.

Conclusions

Women present with schizophrenia differently to men. When treating a woman with schizophrenia, it is important to remember that she is more likely to respond more quickly to medication, but may suffer more from certain side effects. She may be particularly affected by hormonal and metabolic adverse effects – which may in turn be associated with shorter life span. Women are also more likely to be negatively affected by the adverse and interactive effects of adjunctive medication for affective symptoms. Although there is no evidence that women respond better to psychosocial treatments, the benefit in schizophrenia is such that women should be offered these to ensure optimal outcome. Throughout treatment, it should be borne in mind that women with schizophrenia are more likely to be parents or carers, more likely to have been subjected to abuse during childhood, and more likely to be victimized as adults. To compound this, services are generally primarily set up to look after the needs of men rather than women. Prescribers should seek to offer "female-friendly" medication and treatment providers should consciously develop services able to meet the complex needs of women with schizophrenia.

References

Abel, K., Heathlie, H. F., Howard, L. M., & Webb, R. T. (2008). "Sex- and age-specific incidence of fractures in mental illness: a historical population-based cohort study." *J Clin Psychiatry*, 69(9), 1398–1404.

Aichhorn, W., et al. (2006). "Second-generation antipsychotics: is there evidence for sex differences in pharmacokinetic and adverse effect profiles?" *Drug Saf* 29(7): 587–598.

Alvares, A. P., et al. (1976). "Interactions between nutritional factors and drug biotransformations in man." *Proc Natl Acad Sci U S A*, 73(7), 2501–2504.

Anthony, M., & Berg, M. J. (2002). "Biologic and molecular mechanisms for sex differences in pharmacokinetics, pharmacodynamics, and pharmacogenetics: Part I." *J Womens Health Gend Based Med*, 11(7), 601–615.

Armani, F., et al. (2014). "Tamoxifen use for the management of mania: a review of current preclinical evidence." *Psychopharmacology (Berl)* 231(4): 639–649.

Baggaley, M. (2008). "Sexual dysfunction in schizophrenia: focus on recent evidence." *Hum Psychopharmacol* 23(3): 201–209.

Bajaj, N., et al. (2010). "Dependence and psychosis with 4-methylmethcathinone (mephedrone) use." *BMJ Case Rep* 2010.

Bauer, M., et al. (2014). "Role of lithium augmentation in the management of major depressive disorder." *CNS Drugs* 28(4), 331–342.

Bellack, A. S., & Mueser, K. T. (1986). "A comprehensive treatment program for schizophrenia and chronic mental illness." *Community Ment Health J* 22(3), 175–189.

Bennink, R., et al. (1998). "Comparison of total and compartmental gastric emptying and antral motility between healthy men and women." *Eur J Nucl Med* 25(9): 1293–1299.

Bocchetta, A., et al. (2013). "Duration of lithium treatment is a risk factor for reduced glomerular function: a cross-sectional study." *BMC Med* 11: 33.

Bonoldi, I., et al. (2013). "Prevalence of self-reported childhood abuse in psychosis: a meta-analysis of retrospective studies." *Psychiatry Res* 210(1): 8–15.

Brabban, A., et al. (2009). "Predictors of outcome in brief cognitive behavior therapy for schizophrenia." *Schizophr Bull* 35(5): 859–864.

Brunette, M. F. and R. E. Drake (1997). "Gender differences in patients with schizophrenia and substance abuse." *Compr Psychiatry* 38(2): 109–116.

Buckley, P. F., Miller, B. J., Lehrer, D. S., & Castle, D. J. (2009). "Psychiatric comorbidities and schizophrenia." *Schizophr Bull* 35(2): 383–402.

Bundy, H., et al. (2011). "A systematic review and meta-analysis of the fertility of patients with schizophrenia and their unaffected relatives." *Acta Psychiatr Scand* 123(2): 98–106.

Bustillo, J., et al. (2001). "The psychosocial treatment of schizophrenia: an update." *Am J Psychiatry* 158(2): 163–175.

Chavez, C., et al. (2010). "The effect of estrogen on dopamine and serotonin receptor and transporter levels in the brain: an autoradiography study." *Brain Res* 1321: 51–59.

Christodoulou, C. and C. Kalaitzi (2005). "Antipsychotic drug-induced acute laryngeal dystonia: two case reports and a mini review." *J Psychopharmacol* 19(3): 307–311.

Dickerson, F. B., et al. (2005). "The token economy for schizophrenia: review of the literature and recommendations for future research." *Schizophr Res* 75(2–3), 405–416.

Di Forti M., et al. (2014). "Daily use, especially of high-potency cannabis, drives the earlier onset of psychosis in cannabis users." *Schizophr Bull* 40(6): 1509–1517.

DiNitto, D. M., et al. (2002). "Gender differences in dually-diagnosed clients receiving chemical dependency treatment." *J Psychoactive Drugs* 34(1): 105–117.

Donoghue, K., et al. (2014). "Cannabis use, gender and age of onset of schizophrenia: Data from the ÆSOP study." *Psychiatry Res* 215(3):528–532. doi: 10.1016/j.psychres.2013.12.038. Epub 2014 Jan 4.

Filia, S. L., et al. (2014). "Gender differences in characteristics and outcomes of smokers diagnosed with psychosis participating in a smoking cessation intervention." *Psychiatry Res* 215(3): 586–593.

Fleeman, N., et al. (2011). "Cytochrome P450 testing for prescribing antipsychotics in adults with schizophrenia: systematic review and meta-analyses." *Pharmacogenomics J* 11(1), 1–14.

Garety, P. A., et al. (2008). "Cognitive-behavioural therapy and family intervention for relapse prevention and symptom reduction in psychosis: randomised controlled trial." *Br J Psychiatry* 192(6): 412–423.

Gaughran, F., et al. (2013). "Improving physical health and reducing substance use in psychosis–randomised control trial (IMPACT RCT): study protocol for a cluster randomised controlled trial." *BMC Psychiatry* 13: 263.

Giron, M., et al. (2010). "Efficacy and effectiveness of individual family intervention on social and clinical functioning and family burden in severe schizophrenia: a 2-year randomized controlled study." *Psychol Med* 40(1): 73–84.

Guada, J., et al. (2009). "The relationships among perceived criticism, family contact, and consumer clinical and psychosocial functioning for African-American consumers with schizophrenia." *Community Ment Health J* 45(2): 106–116.

Harley, E. W., et al. (2010). "Sexual problems in schizophrenia: prevalence and characteristics. A cross sectional survey." *Soc Psychiatry Psychiatr Epidemiol* 45(7): 759–766.

Hatfield, B., Huxley, P., Mohamad, H. (1997). "Social factors and compulsory detention of psychiatric patients in the UK. The role of the approved social worker in the 1983 Mental Health Act." *International Journal of Law and Psychiatry* 20: 389–397.

Hillman, J. K., et al. (2014). "Black women with polycystic ovary syndrome (PCOS) have increased risk for metabolic syndrome and cardiovascular disease compared with white women without PCOS." *Fertil Steril* 101(2): 530–535.

Huxley, N. A., et al. (2000). "Psychosocial treatments in schizophrenia: a review of the past 20 years." *J Nerv Ment Dis* 188(4): 187–201.

Inder, W. and D. Castle (2011) "Antipsychotic-induced hyperprolactinaemia." *Australian*

and *New Zealand Journal of Psychiatry* 45: 830–837.

Jones, C., et al. (2012). "Cognitive behaviour therapy versus other psychosocial treatments for schizophrenia." *Cochrane Database Syst Rev* 4, CD008712.

Kulkarni, J., et al. (2008). "Estrogen in severe mental illness: a potential new treatment approach." *Arch Gen Psychiatry* 65(8): 955–960.

Kulkarni, J., et al. (2010). "Piloting the effective therapeutic dose of adjunctive selective estrogen receptor modulator treatment in postmenopausal women with schizophrenia." *Psychoneuroendocrinology* 35(8): 1142–1147.

Lally, J., Higaya, E., Nisar, Z., Bainbridge, E., Hallahan, B. (2013). "Prevalence study of head shop drug usage in mental health services." *The Psychiatrist* 37:44–48, doi:10.1192/pb.bp.111.038315

Lane, H. Y., et al. (1999). "Effects of gender and age on plasma levels of clozapine and its metabolites: analyzed by critical statistics." *J Clin Psychiatry* 60(1): 36–40.

Lear, S. A., et al. (2007). "Visceral adipose tissue accumulation differs according to ethnic background: results of the Multicultural Community Health Assessment Trial (M-CHAT)." *Am J Clin Nutr* 86(2): 353–359.

Lear, S. A., et al. (2009). "Ethnic variation in fat and lean body mass and the association with insulin resistance." *J Clin Endocrinol Metab* 94(12): 4696–4702.

Leung, A. and P. Chue (2000). "Sex differences in schizophrenia, a review of the literature." *Acta Psychiatr Scand Suppl* 401: 3–38.

Lorena, S. L., et al. (2004). "Gastric emptying and intragastric distribution of a solid meal in functional dyspepsia: influence of gender and anxiety." *J Clin Gastroenterol* 38(3): 230–236.

Macdonald, S., et al. (2003). "Nithsdale Schizophrenia Surveys 24: sexual dysfunction. Case-control study." *Br J Psychiatry* 182: 50–56.

Martin-Reyes, M., et al. (2011). "Depressive symptoms evaluated by the Calgary Depression Scale for Schizophrenia (CDSS): genetic vulnerability and sex effects." *Psychiatry Res* 189(1): 55–61.

Merkatz, R.,B., and Junod, S.W., (1994). "Historical background of changes in FDA policy on the study and evaluation of drugs in women." *Acad Med* 69: 703–707.

McEvoy, J. P., et al. (2005). "Prevalence of the metabolic syndrome in patients with schizophrenia: baseline results from the Clinical Antipsychotic Trials of Intervention Effectiveness (CATIE) schizophrenia trial and comparison with national estimates from NHANES III." *Schizophr Res* 80(1): 19–32.

Meibohm, B., et al. (2002). "How important are gender differences in pharmacokinetics?" *Clin Pharmacokinet* 41(5), 329–342.

Meyer, J. M., et al. (2005). "The Clinical Antipsychotic Trials Of Intervention Effectiveness (CATIE) Schizophrenia Trial: clinical comparison of subgroups with and without the metabolic syndrome." *Schizophr Res* 80(1): 9–18.

Mezey, G., et al. (2005). "Safety of women in mixed-sex and single-sex medium secure units: staff and patient perceptions." *Br J Psychiatry* 187, 579–582.

Micallef, J., et al. (2006). "Use of antidepressant drugs in schizophrenic patients with depression." *Encephale* 32(2 Pt 1): 263–269.

Mortimer, A. M., et al. (2010). "Clozapine for treatment-resistant schizophrenia: National Institute of Clinical Excellence (NICE) guidance in the real world." *Clin Schizophr Relat Psychoses* 4(1): 49–55.

Nejtek, V. A., et al. (2012). "Race- and gender-related differences in clinical characteristics and quality of life among outpatients with psychotic disorders." *J Psychiatr Pract* 18(5): 329–337.

Ozerdem, A., et al. (2014). "Female vulnerability for thyroid function abnormality in bipolar disorder: role of lithium treatment." *Bipolar Disord* 16(1): 72–82.

Perkins, R. & Rowland, L. (1991). "Sex differences in service usage in long-term psychiatric care are women adequately served?" *Br J Psychiatry Suppl* (10): 75–79.

Rosenbaum, B., et al. (2012). "Supportive psychodynamic psychotherapy versus treatment as usual for first-episode psychosis: two-year outcome." *Psychiatry* 75(4): 331–341.

Salokangas, R. K. (2004). "Gender and the use of neuroleptics in schizophrenia." *Schizophr Res* 66(1): 41–49.

Scandlyn, M. J., et al. (2008). "Sex-specific differences in CYP450 isoforms in humans." *Expert Opin Drug Metab Toxicol* 4(4): 413–424.

Scott, J. E., & Dixon, L. B. (1995). "Psychological interventions for schizophrenia." *Schizophr Bull* 21(4), 621–630.

Seeman, M. V. (1996). "The role of estrogen in schizophrenia." *J Psychiatry Neurosci* 21(2), 123–127.

Seeman, M. V. (2012). "Menstrual exacerbation of schizophrenia symptoms." *Acta Psychiatr Scand* 125(5): 363–371.

Seeman, M. V. and R. Ross (2011). "Prescribing contraceptives for women with schizophrenia." *J Psychiatr Pract* 17(4): 258–269.

Sensky, T., et al. (2000). "A randomized controlled trial of cognitive-behavioral therapy for persistent symptoms in schizophrenia resistant to medication." *Arch Gen Psychiatry* 57(2): 165–172.

Simoni-Wastila, L., et al. (2004). "A retrospective data analysis of the impact of the New York triplicate prescription program on benzodiazepine use in medicaid patients with chronic psychiatric and neurologic disorders." *Clin Ther* 26(2): 322–336.

Simoni-Wastila, L. and G. Strickler (2004). "Risk factors associated with problem use of prescription drugs." *Am J Public Health* 94(2): 266–268.

Smith, S. (2010). "Gender differences in antipsychotic prescribing." *Int Rev Psychiatry* 22(5): 472–484.

Smith, S. M., et al. (2002). "Sexual dysfunction in patients taking conventional antipsychotic medication." *Br J Psychiatry* 181: 49–55.

Tang, C. S., et al. (2007a). "Gender differences in characteristics of Chinese treatment-seeking problem gamblers." *J Gambl Stud* 23(2): 145–156.

Tang, Y. L., et al. (2007b). "Gender, age, smoking behaviour and plasma clozapine concentrations in 193 Chinese inpatients with schizophrenia." *Br J Clin Pharmacol* 64(1): 49–56.

Teo, C., et al. (2013). "The role of ethnicity in treatment refractory schizophrenia." *Compr Psychiatry* 54(2): 167–172.

Usall, J., et al. (2007). "Gender differences in response to antipsychotic treatment in outpatients with schizophrenia." *Psychiatry Res* 153(3): 225–231.

van Hulten, R., et al. (2003). "Comparing patterns of long-term benzodiazepine use between a Dutch and a Swedish community." *Pharmacoepidemiol Drug Saf* 12(1): 49–53.

van Os, J., et al. (1999). "Tardive dyskinesia in psychosis: are women really more at risk? UK700 Group." *Acta Psychiatr Scand* 99(4): 288–293.

Wassink, T. H., et al. (1999). "Prevalence of depressive symptoms early in the course of schizophrenia." *Am J Psychiatry* 156(2): 315–316.

Weich, S., et al. (2014). "Effect of anxiolytic and hypnotic drug prescriptions on mortality hazards: retrospective cohort study." *BMJ*, 348, g1996.

Wieck, A. and P. M. Haddad (2003). "Antipsychotic-induced hyperprolactinaemia in women: pathophysiology, severity and consequences. Selective literature review." *Br J Psychiatry* 182: 199–204.

Wild, R. A., et al. (2010). "Assessment of cardiovascular risk and prevention of cardiovascular disease in women with the polycystic ovary syndrome: a consensus statement by the Androgen Excess and Polycystic Ovary Syndrome (AE-PCOS) Society." *J Clin Endocrinol Metab* 95(5): 2038–2049.

Wolbold, R., et al. (2003). "Sex is a major determinant of CYP3A4 expression in human liver." *Hepatology* 38(4), 978–988.

Wu, R. R., et al. (2012). "Metformin for treatment of antipsychotic-induced amenorrhea and weight gain in women with first-episode schizophrenia: a double-blind, randomized, placebo-controlled study." *Am J Psychiatry* 169(8): 813–821.

Wykes, T., et al. (2007). "Cognitive remediation therapy in schizophrenia: randomised controlled trial." *Br J Psychiatry* 190, 421–427.

Wykes, T., et al. (2003). "Are the effects of cognitive remediation therapy (CRT) durable? Results from an exploratory trial in schizophrenia." *Schizophr Res* 61(2–3), 163–174.

Wykes, T., et al. (2011). "A meta-analysis of cognitive remediation for schizophrenia: methodology and effect sizes." *Am J Psychiatry* 168(5): 472–485.

Xia, J., Merinder, L. B., & Belgamwar, M. R. (2011). "Psychoeducation for schizophrenia." *Cochrane Database Syst Rev*(6): CD002831.

Xiang, Y. T., et al. (2012). "Adjunctive mood stabilizer and benzodiazepine use in older Asian patients with schizophrenia, 2001–2009." *Pharmacopsychiatry* 45(6): 217–222.

Zarate, C. A., Jr., et al. (2007). "Efficacy of a protein kinase C inhibitor (tamoxifen) in the treatment of acute mania: a pilot study." *Bipolar Disord* 9(6): 561–570.

Zhang, X. Y., et al. (2009). "Gender differences in the prevalence, risk and clinical correlates of tardive dyskinesia in Chinese schizophrenia." *Psychopharmacology (Berl)* 205(4): 647–654.

Chapter 24

Psychotic disorders in women in later life

Eleanor Curran, Nicola T. Lautenschlager and David J. Castle

Introduction

The clinical picture of a cognitively intact elderly woman – living alone, hearing impaired and always having been a little suspicious – developing new and florid delusions and hallucinations of someone in her home is familiar to most clinicians practicing in psychiatry of old age. The health, social and economic implications of the aging population are increasingly recognized across the globe (e.g., Australian Institute of Health and Welfare, 2013; Institute of Ageing, Oxford, UK). Yet, the phenomenon of psychosis occurring for the first time in older people in the absence of mood disorder, dementia or other apparent neurological cause remains understudied and enigmatic.

Research on this topic is bedeviled by the generic problems facing studies of people with psychotic illness and is further hampered by problems inherent in studying older persons. Heterogeneous populations, inconsistent definitions of caseness and reliance on syndromes that likely reflect multiple underlying pathophysiologies exemplify the former. Frequent presence of comorbidity, difficulties with enrollment and retention in research studies and limitations in collateral history exemplify the latter (Michelet, et al., 2014). Examination of this "gap" in the psychiatric literature suggests that social stigma, pessimistic attitudes towards treatment expectations and an overall lack of clinical data compound the difficulties in conducting research in this domain (Jeste, et al., 1999a).

Notwithstanding, the available data suggest that first presentation of a non-affective psychotic disorder in later life is not rare (Castle & Murray, 1993; Harris & Jeste, 1988; Kohler et al., 2007; Rodriguez-Ferrera et al., 2004; van Os et al., 1995; Meesters et al., 2012). This chapter presents a summary of the current state of knowledge about first presentation of "functional," non-affective psychotic symptoms in the elderly. We focus on the preponderance of women in those experiencing these symptoms and the implications for hypotheses of etiology and development of effective management strategies.

History and nosology

There remains much controversy in the literature about age cutoffs and terminology for the definition of "late onset" non-affective psychoses. Kraepelin first described these symptoms as the (rare) later onset of "dementia praecox." Manfred Bleuler subsequently coined the term "late onset schizophrenia" in delineating a subtype of schizophrenia that begins after 40 years of age. He noted some differences from earlier onset illness, particularly with respect to course and outcome. German-speaking psychiatry subsequently focused on the question of whether this group represents a subtype of schizophrenia or is a discrete illness (e.g., Riecher-Rossler, 1999).

English-speaking psychiatric researchers and clinicians were, in contrast, influenced by the studies of Roth and Kay in the United Kingdom in the 1950s and 1960s (Kay & Roth, 1961). They demarcated a group with onset of psychosis after the age of 60 in the absence of cognitive decline, for whom they coined the label "late paraphrenia"; however, they did not argue that they represented a discrete diagnostic entity (Roth & Kay, 1998). These historical factors remain, at least in part, responsible for the heterogeneity of study populations.

The term "very-late-onset-schizophrenia-like-psychosis" (or VLOS) was adopted and defined by the International Late-Onset Schizophrenia Group

---

Comprehensive Women's Mental Health, ed. David J. Castle and Kathryn M. Abel. Published by Cambridge University Press.
© Cambridge University Press 2016.

in 2000 (Howard et al., 2000). VLOS refers to patients first presenting after 60 years of age with symptoms satisfying recognized diagnostic criteria for schizophrenia. The definition specifically acknowledges that heterogeneity is inherent in schizophrenia at any age (and more so at the extremes of life) and that presentation with such symptoms late in life may reflect different etiological factors to early onset schizophrenia (EOS) (Howard et al., 2000). Those people presenting for the first time between 40 and 60 years of age were classified as experiencing "late-onset schizophrenia" (LOS) (Howard et al., 2000). Despite an understandable degree of arbitrariness in the specific age-cutoff, the concept is based on epidemiological evidence (Castle & Murray, 1993; van Os et al., 1995) and has face validity (Howard et al., 2000).

The VLOS demarcation allows for exploration of a "tighter" group that appears relatively distinct and that this chapter considers. It implies separation from EOS and LOS, and accumulating data suggest a divergent etiology. However, many authors continue to employ different age and diagnostic boundaries. Due to the paucity of available data specific to VLOS, pooled samples and some older studies of "late paraphrenia" samples are also considered where appropriate.

Epidemiology

The epidemiological data on VLOS are notoriously difficult to interpret and comparison across studies is fraught (Castle, 2005; Minnett et al., 2013). Many studies included only inpatients. Methods for ascertaining and excluding neurodegenerative illness in particular, but also other physical illness that could cause psychotic symptoms, are infrequently documented and often inadequate. Given these challenges, the available data must be interpreted with caution.

Population-based studies of people over 60 or 65 years of age, living in the community, have reported 12-month prevalence rates for VLOS of between 0.1% and 1.6% (Keith et al., 1991; Kua, 1992; Copeland et al., 1992; Copeland et al.,1998). Some authors have suggested higher rates, albeit with somewhat wider definitions of caseness (Skoog, 1993; Christenson & Blazer, 1984). The Epidemiological Catchment Area (ECA) study, from the United States, suggested a rate of 0.3% (Keith et al., 1991). However, the ECA study has been criticized for reliance on lay interviewers and questionable validity of the diagnostic instrument used (Regier, 2000).

Another approach has been to focus on the proportion of clinical samples of individuals first presenting with psychotic symptoms in later life. These prevalence estimates, again, vary widely (Castle & Murray, 1993; Harris & Jeste, 1988; Meesters et al., 2012; Girard & Simard, 2008; Alici-Evcimen et al., 2003; Castle et al., 1997; Mitford et al., 2010): from 0.7% in a recent study of first admissions with psychotic symptoms in Canada (Girard & Simard, 2008), to 16% of all community contacts for non-affective psychosis in the Camberwell Cumulative Psychiatric Case Register sample (Castle et al., 1997). The wide range is likely to reflect a combination of methodological factors. Underestimation in inpatient samples is thought to be particularly significant in studies of older people with psychosis as a high proportion of older onset patients can be managed in the community (Regier, 2000; Alici-Evcimen et al., 2003; Mitford et al., 2010; Henderson & Kay, 1997; Hassett, 1999). Non-random non-response due to paranoid symptoms and poor service access is common (Henderson & Kay, 1997). Again, diagnostic criteria likely account for a large degree of variability: studies with lower rates tend to have applied strict diagnostic criteria for schizophrenia specifically, while studies with higher reported rates tend to use broader definitions of caseness (Harris & Jeste, 1988; Castle et al., 1997; Mitford et al., 2010). For example, the Camberwell group report that 11.1% of their VLOS group met criteria for delusional disorder and only just over half met strict DSM-III criteria for schizophrenia (Castle et al., 1997). Similarly, Mitford et al. (2010) used data from all first psychosis presentations to a psychiatry service in Northumberland: 23% were 65 years or over, of whom 43% received a schizophrenia spectrum diagnosis but only 12% received a schizophrenia diagnosis.

There is more convergence for incidence data. A recent prospective study of first presentations fulfilling DSM-IV criteria for schizophrenia reported an incidence rate of 8 per 100,000 person years in people over 65 (Bogren et al., 2010). This is slightly lower than earlier studies. An incidence of 12.6 per 100,000 person years was noted in the Camberwell Register Study (Castle & Murray, 1993); van Os et al. (1995) examined "non-organic, non-affective psychosis" and reported an incidence of 10 per 100,000 person years for people between 60 and 65, with an 11% increase in incidence for every 5 years of age after that. Highlighting the effects of diagnostic parameters, Holden (1987) prospectively estimated annual rates of late paraphrenia between 17 and 24 per 100,000 in an elderly population, dependent upon whether or not cases with "organic" contributors were included.

Rates of psychotic *symptoms* in the elderly are much higher than those estimated specifically for non-organic psychotic disorders, with most attributable to cognitive impairment and dementia. Henderson et al. (1998) reported point prevalence of 5.7% for any psychotic symptom in persons living in the community and of 24.2% in persons living in supported accommodation, from a sample of individuals over 70 years old. Among those who were cognitively intact, the rates were 3.8% in the community and 7.9% in supported accommodation, respectively (total population prevalence of 4.3%). Paranoid ideation was found in 2.6% of community dwelling cognitively intact people in another sample (Forsell & Henderson, 1998).

Like VLOS, the rate of psychotic symptoms appears to increase with increasing age: 12-month prevalence rates of up to 7.4% have been reported in "old old," non-demented and community dwelling groups (van Os et al., 1995; Ostling & Skoog, 2002). However, the proportion of these likely secondary to "functional" illness, or to VLOS specifically, decreases at the same time, making the data difficult to interpret. Again, most authors note that underreporting and non-random non-response probably means these rates are underestimates. Adding to the difficulty, studies tend to use differential cutoffs on cognitive screening instruments (e.g., a Mini-Mental State Examination [MMSE] score of 24) to dichotomize psychotic symptoms as secondary to cognitive impairment, or to VLOS (Hasset, 2005). The MMSE is a rather crude measure of cognition and lacks sensitivity in identifying early, minor cognitive impairment or very mild dementia. Thus, incidence appears to increase with age, although this relationship is complex and may be particularly influenced by cognition and gender (Castle et al., 1997; Bogren et al., 2010).

Risk factors

Established risk factors for EOS are, generally, less prevalent in VLOS. Confirming family history in elderly patients may be challenging but there appears consensus that genetic factors are less prominent in later onset compared to early onset illness. People experiencing psychosis late in life appear to be no more likely than people with EOS or healthy controls to have a family history of any psychiatric disorder,

with the possible exception of depression, where findings have not been consistent (Harris & Jeste, 1988; Castle, et al., 1997; Henderson & Kay, 1997; Howard, et al., 1997; Jeste, et al., 1995; Brodaty, et al., 1999). Further, genetic risk appears to differentiate early from late onset illness: family history of schizophrenia is significantly greater in the former group (Harris & Jeste, 1988; Castle, et al., 1997; Brodaty, et al., 1999; Brunelle, et al., 2013).

While compelling evidence for a late-life psychotic illness that runs in families is lacking, data are emerging that genetic predisposition may have a role in determining age of onset and phenomenology in the wider population of people with schizophrenia, notwithstanding that none of these studies has focused on the over 60 group specifically (Hamshere, et al., 2011; van der Werf, et al., 2012). Of particular interest, the CCR5 32-bp deletion allele and the rs2734830 polymorphism of the DRD2 gene and the 1bp deletion allele of the dopa decarboxylase gene have been associated with a later age of onset (Hamshere, et al., 2011; Voisey, et al., 2012; Rasmussen, et al., 2006; Borglum, et al., 2001). However, see Chapter 20 for evidence of the influence of life stressors on mild cognitive decline and dementia risk.

Obstetric complications are established risk factors for EOS but have not shown a strong association with LOS or VLOS (Castle, et al., 1997). Indeed, an inverse linear correlation has been found between age of onset of psychosis and a history of obstetric complications (Verdoux, et al., 1997).

Adverse life experiences and migrant status, thought to be "lesser" risk factors in EOS have, conversely, demonstrated an association with VLOS. Increasing data suggest that negative life experiences may increase risk for VLOS, particularly severe trauma and cumulative adverse experiences resulting in post-traumatic stress disorder (Brunelle, et al., 2012; Reulbach, et al., 2007; Giblin, et al., 2004). Other authors have focused on the nature of the trauma and noted higher risk associations with trauma that is stigmatizing or discriminating, or which identifies the individual as an outsider (Fuchs, 1999a, b). It has been suggested that these experiences interact with attitudes, behaviors and interpersonal factors to increase vulnerability to subsequent psychosis. A series of studies from the Mile End and Maudsley hospitals in the UK have reported an increased incidence in migrant, particularly African-Caribbean born populations compared with the local born, with the association particularly evident in men (Reeves, et al., 2002, 2001; Mitter, et al., 2004, 2005).

Studies of premorbid personality in VLOS consistently report premorbid personalities that are anxious, "odd and eccentric," paranoid, quarrelsome and dictatorial (Kay & Roth, 1961; Fuchs, 1999a; Herbert & Jacobson, 1967; Almeida, et al., 1992). Up to 70% of cases have been noted to exhibit significant paranoid or schizoid personality traits (Brunelle, et al., 2013). Using the five-factor model of personality, Hassett (1999) reported VLOS patients to be more conscientious and less neurotic, extroverted and open than their healthy peers. A more recent study explored characteristic cognitive schemata, reporting a tendency to put the needs and wishes of others before their own (other directedness), a tendency to avoid the experience and expression of spontaneous emotions and needs (over vigilance), and lower overall morale (Giblin, et al., 2004). The effects of illness, however, are difficult to exclude. A qualitative study (of very small numbers) also identified a solitary premorbid coping style as common in patients with diagnosed VLOS (Quin, et al., 2009).

These premorbid personality traits and discriminating or traumatic social experiences may feed into other sociodemographic associations, particularly social isolation (Giblin, et al., 2004; Forsell, 2000) and relatively poor premorbid interpersonal functioning but relatively good occupational functioning (Castle, et al., 1997; Brodaty, et al., 1999; Forsell, 2000). However, a recent review of cohort studies was not able to confirm these findings (Brunelle, et al., 2012). Of note, social isolation can be a consequence of psychosis and of aging and its status as a risk factor for, or consequence of, psychotic symptoms remains unclear (Brunelle, et al., 2012, 2013). Similarly, the oft-quoted finding that premorbid functioning is better in VLOS than in those with an earlier onset of illness is problematic because people with later onset illness by definition have a much longer "illness-free" period in which to accomplish themselves.

Whether sensory impairment is greater in VLOS patients similarly remains debated. Studies have shown an excess of corrected and/or uncorrected impairments, particularly of severe, conductive hearing impairment (Almeida, et al., 1992; Cooper & Curry, 1976; Prager & Jeste, 1993). However, cumulative results from longitudinal studies contradict these findings (Hassett, 1999; Brunelle, et al., 2012; Brodaty, et al., 1999). Caution in interpreting any association

is also urged on the basis of high rates of sensory impairment in non-psychotic elderly people and the low base rates of the disorder (Hassett, 2002). Perhaps the greatest implication of the findings is for treatment, given the potential for sensory impairment to exacerbate social isolation and poor outcomes, and the increased likelihood that people with psychosis have impairments that remain insufficiently corrected.

Little data are available on the physical health status of VLOS sufferers, in part because it usually relies on self-report. What data there are, not surprisingly, suggest that VLOS is associated with poor general health (Holden, 1987; Brunelle, et al., 2012; Barak, et al., 2002), but causal direction has not been established. In a sample of people with an onset of schizophrenia after 50 years of age, "soft" neurological signs were found at the same rate as in persons with earlier onset of illness (Sachdev, et al., 1999). Cardiovascular risk factors are more commonly found in VLOS sufferers premorbidly. While requiring replication, the finding was not noted for a LOS group and may differentiate between the two (van der Heijden, et al., 2010).

Similarly, exploration of premorbid cognitive function is difficult because of the exclusion, by definition, of people with significant cognitive impairment from studies of VLOS.

Gender and VLOS

Older studies reported a female excess of between 3:1 and 45:2 (Almeida, et al., 1992) in VLOS, though most were within the more modest range of 6:1 – 10:1 (Harris & Jeste, 1988). More recent studies have also reported a less pronounced female excess, generally between 2:1 and 6:1 (Castle & Murray, 1993; Meesters, et al., 2012; Girard & Simard, 2008; Alici-Evcimen, et al., 2003; Castle, et al., 1997; Mitford, et al., 2010). Diagnostic boundaries and age cutoffs affect the magnitude of the gender difference, but not its existence. Recent studies of schizophrenia throughout the lifespan have also reported that female gender is associated with later onset of illness (Bogren, et al., 2010; van der Werf, et al., 2012; Hafner, et al., 1998).

Urging caution, neither a recent review of risk factors for VLOS nor a prospective study of patients between 60 and 65 found any difference in gender-specific rates (Brunelle, et al., 2012; Kohler, et al., 2007). Earlier, van Os and colleagues (1995) noted that the increasing incidence with age was stronger for men than women. Some authors have also found that the ratio of women to men is the same in early and late onset populations (Brodaty, et al., 1999; Huang & Zhang, 2009). Others have noted that the effect of gender diminishes or disappears when only cognitively intact elderly are included (Holden, 1987; Henderson, et al., 1998), as genetic risk increases (Abel, et al., 2010) and in migrant populations in the UK (Mitter, et al., 2004). These findings suggest confounding for at least some of the excess seen.

Looking at the possible effect of gender more closely, there is good support for an incidence curve for women with three peaks that can crudely be described as early, mid and late life (after 60) (Castle & Murray, 1993). The first peak is less prominent for women than men; the mid-life peak is greater in women than in men; and the late-life peak is almost exclusively female (Castle & Murray, 1993; Castle, 1999). Efforts to understand the mechanisms behind the gender effect in late life psychosis have been limited and focused on biological, rather than social or environmental effects.

Some authors highlight differential patterns of D2 receptor loss: namely, that men begin with an excess of D2 receptors but lose them faster, leaving older women with a relative excess and, consequently, increased risk of psychosis (Castle, 1999). While this hypothesis has prima facie merit, well-designed, prospective, population-based studies are lacking. Sex-differentiated epigenetic effects following environmental exposures over a lifetime may also play a role although no research has explored this in LOS or VLOS (see Chapter 5).

The estrogen hypothesis of schizophrenia appears insufficient to explain the third peak in incidence in women. The hypothesis posits that menopause results in a loss of protection from the neuromodulatory effects of estrogen on several neurotransmitter systems implicated in schizophrenia (Kulkarni, 1997; Riecher-Rossler, et al., 1994; Hafner, et al., 1998; Seeman, 1999). However, menopause is complete in most women by 50 and a reduction in estrogen levels begins at the age of 35, that is, 25 years before 60. Menopause is a universal experience for women, yet psychosis occurs in only a small proportion. Also, an etiological theory based on declining estrogen levels cannot account for late onset illness in at least some men. Finally, studies of exogenous estrogen have been conspicuous in failing to show a substantial preventative or treatment effect in schizophrenia (Castle, 1999; Riecher-Rossler, et al., 1994; see Chapter 8 on hormones and women).

The small amount of available data regarding social or environmental factors includes some interesting early findings. While the large majority of the incidence data are from clinical settings and may not apply to community samples, one population-based study found no gender difference in rates of generalized persecutory ideation (Christenson & Blazer, 1984). Other authors have noted that male patients, initially seen as inpatients, were significantly more likely than their female counterparts to be lost to follow-up (Reeves, et al., 2002), and are less likely to have severe or florid symptomatology (Kohler, et al., 2009). Thus, some of the reported female excess may be related to differential patterns of help-seeking or otherwise coming to the attention of health services. This is consistent with the wider literature in aged populations and health care access (Galdas, et al., 2005).

Differences in life expectancy have been examined and are not likely to be sufficient to explain the female excess in VLOS (Howard, 1999). However, social factors that also have differential gender patterns may, in turn, result in higher rates of other potential risk factors in women. For example, longer life expectancy, when combined with lifetime differences in earnings and workforce participation, may lead to greater social disadvantage, social isolation, decreased access to functional supports and poorer general health for women (O'Rand, 1996; see Chapter 1). An association with VLOS has been shown for some of these (see earlier). The effects of such factors on cognitive functioning and its rate of decline are currently of great interest to researchers and may also be significant in the context of VLOS (Sheffield & Peek, 2009; Nguyen, et al., 2008; Fratiglioni, et al., 2004).

There may also be a more direct relationship between Alzheimer's disease (AD), or other neuropsychiatric conditions with a clear preponderance of women, and VLOS. Early AD can certainly present with behavioral and psychological symptoms (BPSD), including psychotic symptoms (Di Iulio, et al., 2010; Geda, et al., 2013; Rosenberg, et al., 2013). The relationship between VLOS and neuropsychiatric syndromes of cognitive impairment remains an active area of research, with relatively short follow-up periods and inconsistent data (Holden, 1987; Brodaty, et al., 2003; Palmer, et al., 2003; Korner, et al., 2009a,

2009b). Gender-based rates of subsequent dementia diagnosis in VLOS cohorts are generally not reported. In spite of this, a recent case-linkage study has shown that people with VLOS have a risk of subsequently developing dementia 2 to 3 times greater than the general population (Korner, et al., 2009b). Some authors have specifically hypothesised that VLOS might represent a prodromal state for AD or dementia more generally (Brodaty, et al., 2003; Korner, et al., 2009b). Moreover, clinicopathological data has recently shown that elderly women with onset of psychotic symptoms after 40 years of age (i.e., encompassing both the LOS and VLOS groups) have neuro-pathological changes indicative of possible AD more frequently than their male counterparts (Casanova, et al., 2002). Thus, some of the excess of females in VLOS may also reflect the misclassification of some people with early dementia or mild cognitive impairment and a prodromal state of dementia, and the preponderance of women in both. It may also suggest that women are more likely than men to experience neuropsychiatric symptoms as the presenting feature of cognitive decline, at least early in its course. The reasons for this are beyond the scope of this chapter, but are likely to reflect a combination of biological and social vulnerability factors. While speculative, these conjectures demonstrate the lack of data or understanding around this patient group and therefore the need for caution when drawing conclusions.

Clinical presentation

The literature on clinical presentation in VLOS is expanding. While exceptions remain, recent data generally supports earlier observations from the late-paraphrenia literature, namely, that these patients present rather differently to those with earlier onset illness (Almeida, et al., 1992; Barak, et al., 2002; Howard, et al., 1994). An absence of affective blunting and apathy differentiated LOS from VLOS in a retrospective chart review comparing the two groups (Girard & Simard, 2008), although these and other authors have disputed the dictum that formal thought disorder and negative symptoms are absent in the latter group (Girard & Simard, 2008; Brunelle, et al., 2013; Mason, et al., 2013). Earlier work showed that the only symptoms *not* significantly different between a VLOS and EOS group were bizarre delusions, delusional perceptions and delusions of reference: formal thought disorder, passivity phenomena,

thought interference and negative symptoms were all significantly more common in the EOS group; persecutory delusions (especially very organized ones) and auditory hallucinations were more common the VLOS group (Castle, et al., 1997; also see Drake, et al., 2015).

The nature of some delusions appears to have some specificity. Thus, in one study, 93% of VLOS patients had persecutory delusions and up to half of them had "partition delusions" (Castle et al., 1997). Long associated with psychosis in the elderly and rare in younger populations, these are a false belief that persons, objects, gases or radiation can pass through an objectively unpassable barrier (Howard, 1992). They have been differentiated from delusions seen in dementia on the basis of complexity and bizarreness (Henderson & Kay, 1997).

People with VLOS are also particularly likely to experience hallucinations, including in multiple modalities (Girard & Simard, 2008; Alici-Evcimen, et al., 2003; Castle, et al., 1997; Howard, et al., 1994; Yasuda, et al., 2013). Hallucinations of some kind are almost ubiquitous in the condition (Girard & Simard, 2008).

There is less agreement regarding neuropsychological profile and course, and most data combine LOS with VLOS cases. Some have argued that cognitive impairment in such cases is consistent with that seen in EOS, with differences from healthy controls in executive and general cognitive function in particular (Jeste, et al., 1995; Almeida, et al., 1999). A review, pooling VLOS with LOS data but reporting an average age of onset for the group over 60, suggested some sparing of cognitive dysfunction in those with later onset (Rajji, et al., 2009). The impairment seen is generally thought to be distinguishable from that of AD in severity of cognitive impairment and in its course (Howard, 1999; Levy, et al., 1987; Lagodka & Robert, 2009). One study, examining course over 3 years in a group with onset after 45 years of age, found that cognitive impairments progressed less than in AD and so much more slowly as to be considered essentially static (Palmer, et al., 2003). By contrast, Hymas (1989), in a 3-year follow-up study of patients with late paraphrenia, suggested that there was slow and subtle but clear decline in cognition from a baseline that was already different to controls at illness onset. He noted the decline continued despite symptomatic improvement but rarely reached diagnostic threshold for dementia.

Recent data also suggests a mixed picture. As noted, some authors have reported substantial increases in risk of subsequent dementia (Ostling & Skoog, 2002; Korner, et al., 2009a, 2009b), and even specifically AD (Brodaty, et al., 2003), compared with healthy, age-matched controls when extended follow-up periods are conducted. Girard and colleagues (2011) found that their sample of patients with psychosis beginning after 50 years of age were overall not significantly different to controls when age and education were taken into account. However, they had significantly more executive dysfunction than a comparison group of age-matched patients with EOS and 20% met diagnostic criteria for dementia, in comparison with 5.0% of an EOS group. Two relatively recent reviews of the topic concluded that there was evidence of progressive cognitive decline, particularly with a longer disease duration (Lagodka & Robert, 2009; Reeves & Brister, 2008). However, they highlighted that most studies did not separate data on the LOS and VLOS groups, and that there were no studies comparing types of dementia where psychotic symptoms are common, particularly dementia with Lewy Bodies (DLB) (Lagodka & Robert, 2009).

A neurodegenerative process?

The aforementioned data regarding relative risk of subsequent dementia and neuropsychological functioning speaks to an increasing consensus that VLOS may have, in part at least, a neurodegenerative basis, in contrast to the neurodevelopmental hypothesis now generally accepted for EOS (Howard, et al., 2000; Brunelle, et al., 2013; Lagodka & Robert, 2009; Reeves & Brister, 2008).

Neuronal loss or damage per se, particularly subcortical lesions, are certainly known to be associated with psychotic symptoms (Forstl, 1994). Barak (2002) included brain computed tomography (CTB) findings in his sample of 21 patients with onset of illness after 70 years and reported more pronounced cerebellar atrophy and a trend towards higher ventricle to brain volume ratios (VBR) in comparison with age-matched patients with EOS.

Structural CTB and magnetic resonance imaging (MRI) data from pooled samples (with either lower age cutoffs or heterogeneous diagnoses) have also shown enlarged VBR compared with healthy controls (Levy, et al., 1987; Miller & Lesser, 1988; Howard, 2001; Rabins, et al., 2000; Pearlson, 1999) and

sometimes with aged-matched EOS patients (Corey-Bloom, et al., 1995). Using MRI, an excess of deep white matter lesions (WML) has been noted (Miller & Lesser, 1988; Sachdev & Brodaty, 1999), but this finding was not subsequently confirmed when cerebrovascular risk factors were taken into consideration (Howard, et al., 1995; Rivkin, et al., 2000; Symonds, et al., 1997). Volumetric studies have shown larger thalamic volumes in VLOS compared with EOS (Corey-Bloom, et al., 1995) but failed to show any evidence of frontal lobe, hippocampus, amygdala or basal ganglia size abnormalities distinct from those seen in EOS (Sachdev, et al., 1999; Rabins, et al., 2000; Howard, et al., 1995). Further, an MRI study of 27 patients with illness onset after 50 years of age (Sachdev, et al., 1999) showed no reduction in cerebellar volume, in contrast to the aforementioned study by Barak (2002).

Functional imaging using single photon emission computed tomography (SPECT) has suggested that frontal and/or temporal hypoperfusion is common in VLOS and may show a different pattern to that seen in EOS (Miller, et al., 1992; Sachdev, et al., 1997; Dupont, et al., 1994). This aligns with epidemiological findings of increased cardiovascular risk factors in psychiatric disorders with late life onset (van der Heijden, et al., 2010). However, diffusion tensor imaging (DTI) studies have suggested that frontal and cortical tracts are intact (Jones, et al., 2005).

Interpretation of neuroimaging data in LOS and VLOS is challenging. Many studies, particularly earlier ones, did not control for cerebrovascular (or other) risk factors for neurological abnormality; comparison groups are extremely variable and may not be optimal controls; and sample sizes are mostly very small.

Turning to neuropathological studies, Casanova (2002) found changes indicative of AD pathology (extensive neurofibrillary tangles) in women with VLOS, but neither they nor other researchers found that the overall proportion of AD-associated changes differ significantly from controls (Bozikas, et al., 2002). However, there is some evidence of other neuritic changes that suggest a "restricted limbic tauopathy" resulting in very slowly progressing neurodegeneration (Casanova, et al., 2002). Similar findings of fronto-temporal-dementia-like neuropathology were seen in a small study of people who developed psychotic symptoms after 50 years of age (Velakoulis, et al., 2009).

Other authors have countered that the biological abnormalities detected are also seen in elderly people *without* psychotic symptoms. Therefore, they may be vulnerability factors, but must be accompanied by other "mediating" processes for psychosis to manifest in certain people but not in others. These processes may be psychosocial and may be long-standing or aging-related (Hasset, 1997, 2002, 2005; Quin, et al., 2009; Smeets-Janssen, et al., 2013).

Hassett (1997) suggested that premorbid personality style may be important in negotiating the normal developmental crises that Erikson postulated were central to old age, namely, ego-integrity versus despair. Ego-integrity refers to an ability to synthesize and reflect on one's life experiences and accept them. Failure to do so can lead to a sense of meaninglessness or despair (Erikson & Erikson, 1998). Current or cumulative threats to one's self-concept could interfere with this process by leading to an abnormal, specifically externalizing, attributional style as a defense. The findings of premorbid personality and cognitive schema abnormalities in people who subsequently develop psychosis in old age support the view that such factors may be a mediating process by which the biological changes of aging or the abnormalities noted earlier may result in psychosis.

Another hypothesis to gain some support is that aging itself can act as a threat to one's self-concept, as well as confer vulnerability due to biological changes. In those with a personality-based tendency to externalize responsibility and control over their internal experiences or who have theory of mind deficits, this could lead to a perception of the outside world as threatening. Combined with diminished executive functioning or other cognitive deficits that may impair reality testing, this perceptual bias could become paranoia (Aguera-Ortiz, et al., 1999; Moore, et al., 2006). Empirical support for this is limited. One group found that people with VLOS displayed more mentalizing errors than healthy controls but less than in EOS, supporting this theory (Moore, et al., 2006). By contrast, another study demonstrated no difference in "actual" and "other" self concepts (a proxy for beliefs about how others see us) between healthy elderly people and those with VLOS (McCulloch, et al., 2006).

Differential diagnosis

As noted, dementia is by far the most common cause of psychotic symptoms in elderly people, occurring in up to 50% of patients at some point (Brunelle, et al., 2013). They can develop at any stage of a dementing illness, including as the presenting symptoms, and are associated with both cortical and subcortical dementias (Mintzer & Targum, 2003). AD remains the most common type of dementia in the Western world, but psychotic symptoms are particularly associated with DLB, in which complex, dream-like visual hallucinations are a defining feature. They also commonly occur in fronto-temporal dementia, Huntington's Disease and in dementia associated with Parkinson's Disease (Mintzer & Targum, 2003). There is some argument that hallucinations, which may not require intact cortical functioning, can continue to occur relatively later in the course of dementia than delusions (Forstl, et al., 1994).

Other organic causes for psychotic symptoms are significantly more common in aged than younger patients. These can include specific cerebral lesions or delirium due to infectious, metabolic or other medical problems. Urinary tract infections, electrolyte abnormalities, constipation and pain are all commonly implicated (Hasset, 2005).

Intoxication or withdrawal, from either prescribed or illicit substances, can also trigger psychotic symptoms (Thirthalli, et al., 2010). Of the prescribed medications, those with anticholinergic side effects are particularly problematic, as are sedating medications such as benzodiazepines and opiate analgesics. Alcohol use and dependence is not uncommon in the elderly and, particularly if excessive use has been present for a long time, can result in neurotoxicity. Wernicke-Korsakoff syndrome arises from thiamine depletion in people with chronic alcohol dependence. It is thought to be significantly underdiagnosed and frequently does not present with the classical triad of opthalmoplegia, ataxia and confusion (Sechi & Serra, 2007). Psychosis in the setting of chronic alcohol use, particularly if this has recently stopped because of hospitalization, should prompt consideration of alcohol withdrawal and Wernicke-Korsakoff syndrome.

Anti-NMDA receptor and limbic encephalitis, both frequently but not universally occurring as a paraneoplastic syndrome, are also increasingly recognized (Titulaer, et al., 2013; Ganerod, et al., 2010; Chapman & Vause, 2011). While neurological symptoms are common, subacute onset of psychosis and memory impairment can be presenting symptoms (Boylan, 2000). Teratomas, small cell lung carcinoma and lymphoma are particularly associated.

The presence of Parkinsonian features, complex partial seizures or distal symmetrical sensory impairment (e.g., gait abnormalities) should heighten suspicion, as should prodromal viral illness or headaches, seizures or systemic symptoms of malignancy, such as weight loss (Boylan, 2000). The course can be stable, progressive or remit with treatment of any associated tumor and/or with use of other therapies such as immunoglobulin, plasma exchange or corticosteroids (Titulaer, et al., 2013).

Charles Bonnet syndrome refers to the experience of visual hallucinations, with full insight, in individuals with visual impairment. Similar experiences can occur with sensory impairment in other modalities, albeit less commonly. Quite common, however, are misinterpretations of others' actions in the setting of sensory impairment, particularly if there is associated cognitive decline.

Finally, it is imperative to note that older persons can experience isolated psychotic symptoms in the absence of illness. Relatively common scenarios for this include hallucinations of a lost loved one during bereavement and hallucinations or illusions suggesting an intruder. As older persons are probably more likely to experience bereavement, and to feel vulnerable due to frailty and social isolation, such experiences are understandably more frequent.

In terms of other psychiatric syndromes, affective disorders, EOS and delusional disorder are the most common differential diagnoses. Affective disorders must be considered, particularly as older people are more likely to develop psychotic symptoms during an episode of depression than younger people (Brunelle, et al., 2013). Moreover, they may not present with an overtly depressed affect, as in so-called pseudodementia; delusions are usually mood congruent. Most older people with schizophrenia will have developed the illness early in their adult life. While they usually have a history of multiple hospital admissions and chronic psychiatric care, they may have been relatively free of positive symptoms for some time or have avoided contact with health services.

Delusional disorder was often included in samples of people with late paraphrenia and is sometimes difficult to distinguish from VLOS. It also occurs more commonly in the elderly (Brunelle, et al., 2013). Classically, it presents with a single, mostly non-bizarre, delusion. However, over time this frequently becomes extremely detailed, systematized and incorporates new experiences into a delusional interpretation. Hallucinations related to this delusional kernel can also occur, albeit are not prominent.

Treatment

Prior to instituting management, careful investigation of differential diagnoses, particularly organic causes, is vital. History, examination and investigations should also consider issues for immediate and longer-term management, including evidence of malnutrition, dehydration or other neglect; evidence of falls, functional decline or unsafe decision making that may necessitate later assessment of capacity (which should be delayed until acute symptoms have been treated).

Like EOS, antipsychotic medication is the mainstay of treatment for VLOS, despite a paucity of randomized controlled trial evidence. Indeed, a recent Cochrane review noted that no trial-based evidence was available to inform treatment guidelines (Essali & Ali, 2012).

Second-generation medications are now usually preferred, given the reduced likelihood of extrapyramidal side effects (EPSE). This is particularly pertinent to those with VLOS as older persons have consistently been shown to be at greater risk of tardive dyskinesia (TD) than their younger counterparts, even with relatively short-term treatment and low doses (Fabbrini, et al., 2001; Jeste, et al., 1995; 1999b). There is limited evidence suggesting that second-generation medications may be less likely to cause TD (Jeste, et al., 1999c). Unfortunately, there is also now clear evidence for significant metabolic side effects from some of these medications, both secondary to and independent of antipsychotic-induced weight gain (Kelly, et al., 2010; Rummel-Kluge, et al., 2010). In people with dementia, both first- and second-generation antipsychotics have also shown an increased risk of stroke (Schneider, et al., 2005). Given the high prevalence of metabolic and cardiovascular comorbidities in the VLOS population, the risk of adverse outcomes from antipsychotic medication is not insignificant and appropriate discussions, monitoring and primary and secondary prevention measures must be undertaken.

Similarly, the risk of falls is substantially increased with prescription of sedating medication, especially those that may also cause or exacerbate postural hypotension, such as olanzapine or clozapine, and particularly when that occurs in an unfamiliar environment and when there may be agitation, restlessness or fear. The literature regarding falls-associated morbidity and mortality is extensive and any sedating medication should only be prescribed with extreme care and careful monitoring (Reeves & Brister, 2008; Woolcott, et al., 2009).

As in most prescribing for older persons, antipsychotic medication should be commenced at low doses and increased very slowly, in small increments. Although most available data is from pooled samples, there is consistent evidence that lower doses of antipsychotics are required in older persons to achieve symptom amelioration. The international consensus group suggested that doses as low as 1/10 those used in younger populations may be sufficient in VLOS (Howard, et al., 2000).

Given the suspicion of a neurodegenerative basis for VLOS, there are reasonable theoretical grounds for the use of cognitive-enhancing medications, namely, cholinesterase inhibitors or memantine. However, to our knowledge, there is no evidence to date for their effectiveness for psychotic symptoms in this population. There is some evidence for effective treatment of associated cognitive impairment (Brunelle, et al., 2013).

Benzodiazepines are still commonly used as a short-term medication for associated agitation, insomnia and anxiety. While long-term prescription is strongly discouraged and associated with significant risk (particularly of falls), careful, short-term use can be appropriate.

Clearly, the longer-term success of pharmacological management depends upon effective prevention and/or treatment of side effects and optimizing adherence. Patients with VLOS may be particularly likely to be lost to follow-up (Reeves, et al., 2002) and people with a chronic psychotic illness are known to be particularly prone to poor medication adherence (Brunelle, et al., 2013). Some authorities advocate the use of depot medication and a community psychiatric nurse to support outpatient treatment (Howard & Levy, 1992). Psychiatric and medical comorbidities, particularly the advent of dementia or of a post-psychosis depression, can also significantly worsen outcome and individuals should be monitored for their emergence.

There is very limited literature regarding psychological treatments specifically for VLOS patients (Aguera-Ortiz, et al., 1999). There is, however, an increasing evidence base for psychotherapies for older

people with psychiatric illness in general, demonstrating that older people can both participate in and benefit from psychological therapy. Group-based schema-focused therapy has been shown to be effective in treatment of depression in older people (Kindynis, et al., 2013). Cognitive Behavioral Social Skills Training (CBSST) is a CBT-based group intervention for elderly people with schizophrenia. It focuses on challenging beliefs that are thought to interfere with treatment in this population and improving skill development and retention through behavioral technique practice. Evidence currently supports it as associated with development of more adaptive coping skills and improved social functioning, which importantly appears to be maintained after the intervention is withdrawn (Granholm, et al., 2007).

Various other models of psychosocial rehabilitation, ranging from detailed, manualized programs to a socially stimulating group also appear to have beneficial effects for functioning and continued independent living. Some form of regular social interaction appears to be key (Brunelle, et al., 2013).

Prognosis

Historically, symptomatic outcomes for VLOS have been thought of as better than for EOS (Almeida, et al., 1992), but recent data suggest that partial symptomatic improvement, rather than complete, is the general rule and that symptomatic remission may be no more common than in EOS (Meesters, et al., 2012; Alici-Evcimen, et al., 2003; Brodaty, et al., 2003; Howard & Levy, 1992). Hospitalization, however, does appear shorter than for younger adults and a single admission is common (Alici-Evcimen, et al., 2003). Of note, improvement appears to be both greater and more common with the use of second-generation antipsychotic medications (Barak, et al., 2002; Brunelle, et al., 2013).

Functional impairment, even in those who do not develop dementia, does appear to persist, although this may be relatively mild in most and less severe than that seen in EOS or identified dementia with psychotic symptoms (Kohler, et al., 2009; Brodaty, et al., 2003; Mazeh, et al., 2005; Rabins & Lavrisha, 2003). While some patients will require residential care, this appears to be mostly related to the extent of cognitive impairment and is usually avoidable (Mazeh, et al., 2005). Mortality, as expected, is higher and has a different pattern to that in schizophrenia with a younger onset, but is lower than in dementia. In one follow-up study, suicide accounted for 71% of deaths in people with EOS, whereas circulatory system failure caused half of those in VLOS (Kohler, et al., 2009).

Conclusions

VLOS remains an elusive entity, despite its clinical familiarity. This is in part due to a scarcity of specific data. The case for further research is clear,

particularly given the public health implications for the aging population. It does seem likely that this is an illness that clinically presents predominantly in women, probably through multiple mechanisms. Etiological and clinical heterogeneity are also likely but it appears that a neurodegenerative process is at play for at least some people. Finally, patients can respond well to comprehensive, integrated management plans that consider psychosocial rehabilitation and avoid the pessimism and paternalism that has historically influenced psychiatric care for older people.

References

Abel, K. M., Drake, R., & Goldstein, J. M. (2010). Sex differences in schizophrenia. *International Review Psychiatry*, 22 (5), 417–428.

Aguera-Ortiz, L., & Reneses-Prieto, B. (1999). The place of non-biological treatments. In R. Howard, P. Rabins, & D. Castle (eds.), *Late Onset Schizophrenia* (pp. 233–260). Guildford, UK: Wrightson Biomedical Publishing Ltd.

Alici-Evcimen, Y., Ertan, T., & Eker, E. (2003). Case series with late-onset psychosis hospitalized in a geriatric psychiatry unit in Turkey: experience in 9 years. *International Psychogeriatrics*, 15 (1), 69–72.

Almeida, O. (1999). The neuropsychology of schizophrenia in late life. In R. Howard, P. Rabins, & D. Castle (eds.), *Late Onset Schzophrenia* (pp. 181–190). Guildford, UK: Wrightson Biomedical Publishing Ltd.

Almeida, O., Howard, R., Forstl, H., Derrick, M., & Levy, R. (1992). Late paraphrenia: a review. *International Journal of Geriatric Psychiatry*, 7, 543–548.

Australian Institute of Health and Welfare. (2013). *Australia's Welfare 2013*. Canberra: Australian Institute of Health and Welfare.

Barak, Y., Aizenberg, D., Mirecki, I., Mazeh, D., & Achiron, A. (2002). Very-late-onset schizophrenia-like

psychosis: clinical and imaging characteristics in comparison with elderly patients with schizophrenia. *Journal of Nervous and Mental Diseases*, 190, 733–736.

Bogren, M., Mattisson, C., Isberg, P. E., Munk-Jorgensen, P., & Nettelbladt, P. (2010). Incidence of psychotic disorders in the 50 year follow-up of the Lundby population. *Australian and New Zealand Journal of Psychiatry*, 44, 31–39.

Borglum, A. D., Hampson, M., Kjeldsen, T. E., Muir, W., Murray, V., Ewald, H., et al. (2001). Dopa decarboxylase genotypes may influence age at onset of schizophrenia. *Molecular Psychiatry*, 6, 712–717.

Boylan, L. (2000). Limbic encephalitis and late-onset psychosis. *The American Journal of Psychiatry*, 157, 1343–1344.

Bozikas, V. P., Kovari, E., Bouras, C., & Karavatos, A. (2002). Neurofibrillary tangles in elderly pateints with late onset schizophrenia. *Neuroscience Letters*, 324, 109–112.

Brodaty, H., Sachdev, P., Koschera, A., Monk, D., & Cullen, B. (2003). Long-term outcome of late-onset schizophrenia: 5 year follow-up study. *British Journal of Psychiatry*, 183, 213–219.

Brodaty, H., Sachdev, P., Rose, N., Rylands, K., & Prenter, L. (1999). Schizophrenia with onset after age 50 years. I: Phenomenology and risk

factors. *British Journal of Psychiatry*, 175, 410–415.

Brunelle, S., Cole, M. G., & Elie, M. (2012). Risk factors for the late-onset psychoses: a systematic review of cohort studies. *International Journal of Geriatric Psychiatry*, 27, 240–252.

Brunelle, S., Vahia, I., & Jeste, D. (2013). Late-onset schizophrenia. In T. Dening & A. Thomas (eds.), *Oxford Textbook of Old Age Psychiatry* (pp. 603–20). New York, NY: Oxford University Press.

Casanova, M. F., Stevens, J. R., Brown, R., Royston, C., & Bruton, C. (2002). Disentangling the pathology of schizophrenia and paraphrenia. *Acta Neuropathologica*, 103, 313–320.

Castle, D. (2005). Epidemiology of late onset schizophrenia. In A. Hassett, D. Ames, & E. Chiu, *Psychosis in the elderly.* (pp. 18–27). Andover, UK: Taylor and Francis Group.

Castle, D. (1999). Gender and age at onset in schizophrenia. In R. Howard, P. Rabins, & D. Castle (eds.), *Late Onset Schizophrenia* (pp. 147–64). Guildford, UK: Wrightson Biomedical Publishing Ltd.

Castle, D. J., & Murray, R. M. (1993). The epidemiology of late-onset schizophrenia. *Shizophrenia Bulletin*, 19, 288–294.

Castle, D. J., Wessely, S., Howard, R., & Murray, R. M. (1997). Schizophrenia with onset at the extremes of adult life. *International*

Journal of Geriatric Psychiatry, 12, 712–717.

Chapman, M. R., & Vause, H. E. (2011). Anti-NMDA receptor encephalitis: diagnosis, psychiatric presentation and treatment. *American Journal of Psychiatry*, 168, 245–251.

Christenson, R., & Blazer, D. (1984). Epidemiology of persecutory ideation in an elderly population in the community. *American Journal of Psychiatry*, 141, 1088–1091.

Cooper, A., & Curry, A. (1976). The pathology of deafness in the paranoid and affective psychoses of later life. *Journal of Psychosomatic Research*, 20, 97–105.

Copeland, J., Davidson, I., Dewey, M., Gilmore, C., Larkin, B., & McWilliam, C. (1992). Alzheimer's disease, other dementias, depression and pseudo-dementia: prevalence, incidence and three-year outcomes. *British Journal of Psychiatry*, 161, 230–239.

Copeland, J., Dewey, M., Scott, A., Gilmore, C., Larkin, B., & Cleave, N. (1998). Schizophrenia and delusional disorder in older age: community prevalence, incidence comorbidity and outcome. *Schizophrenia Bulletin*, 24, 153–161.

Corey-Bloom, J., Jernigan, T., Archibald, S., Harris, M., & Jeste, D. (1995). Quantitative magnetic resonance imaging of the brain in late-life schizophrenia. *American Journal of Psychiatry*, 152, 447–449.

Davey, D. A. (2014). Alzheimer's disease and vascular dementia: one potentially preventable and modifiable disease. Part I: Pathology, diagnosis and screening. *Neurodegenerative Disease Management*, 4, 253–259.

Di Iulio, F., Palmer, K., Blundo, C., Casini, A., Gianni, W., Caltagirone, C., et al. (2010). Occurrence of neuropsychiatric symptoms and psychiatric disorders in mild Alzheimer's disease and mild cognitive impairment subtypes.

International Psychogeriatrics, 22, 629–640.

Dupont, R. M., Lehr, P. P., Lamoureaux, G., Halpern, S., Harris, M. J., & Jeste, D. V. (1994). Preliminary report: cerebral blood flow abnormalities in older schizophrenic patients. *Psychiatry Research*, 55, 121–130.

Erikson, E., & Erikson, J. (1998). Major stages in psychosocial development. In E. Erikson, & J. Erikson, *The Life Cycle Completed* (pp. 55–66). New York, NY: W.W. Norton and Company.

Essali, A., & Ali, G. (2012). Antipsychotic drug treatment for elderly people with late-onset schizophrenia. *Cochrane Database of Systematic Reviews*, 2.

Fabbrini, G., Barbanti, P., & Aurilia, C. (2001). Tardive dyskinesias in teh elderly. *International Journal of Geriatric Psychiatry*, 16 (S1), S19–S23.

Forsell, Y. (2000). Predictors for depression, anxiety and psychotic symptoms in a very elderly population: data from a 3 year follow-up study. *Social Psychiatry and Psychiatric Epidemiology*, 35, 259–263.

Forsell, Y., & Henderson, A. S. (1998). Epidemiology of paranoid symptoms in an elderly population. *British Journal of Psychiatry*, 172, 429–432.

Forstl, H. (1994). The short history of focal brain degeneration. *The Canadian Journal of Neurological Sciences*, 21, 78.

Forstl, H., Burns, A., Levy, R., & Cairns, N. (1994). Neuropathological correlates of psychotic phenomena in confirmed Alzheimer's disease. *British Journal of Psychiatry*, 165 (1), 53–59.

Fratiglioni, L., Paillard-Borg, S., & Winblad, B. (2004). An active and socially integrated lifestyle in late life might protect againsta dementia. *Lancet Neurology*, 3, 343–353.

Fuchs, T. (1999a). Life events in late paraphrenia and depression. *Psychopathology*, 32, 60–69.

Fuchs, T. (1999b). Patterns of relation and premorbid personality in late paraphrenia and depression. *Psychopathology*, 32, 70–80.

Galdas, P., Cheater, F., & Marshall, P. (2005). Men and health help-seeking behaviour: literature review. *Journal of Advanced Nursing*, 49, 616–623.

Ganerod, J., Ambrose, H., & Davies, N. (2010). Causes o fencephalitis and differences in their presentation in England: a multicentre, population based prospective study. *Lancet Infectious Diseases*, 10, 835–844.

Geda, Y., Schneider, L., Gitlin, L., Miller, D., Smith, G., Bell, J., et al. (2013). Neuropsychiatric symptoms in Alzheimer's disease: past progress and anticipation of the future. *Alzheimer's Dementia*, 9, 602–608.

Giblin, S., Clare, L., Livingston, G., & Howard, R. (2004). Psychosocial correlates of late-onset psychosis: life experiences, cognitive schemas and attitudes to ageing. *International Journal of Geriatric Psychiatry*, 19, 611–623.

Girard, C., & Simard, M. (2008). Clinical characterisation of late- and very late-onset first psychotic episode in psychiatric inpatients. *American Journal of Geriatric Psychiatry*, 16, 478–487.

Girard, C., Sirnard, M., Noiseux, R., Laplante, L., Dugas, M., Rousseau, F., et al. (2011). Late-onset-psychosis: cognition. *International Psychogeriatrics*, 23, 1301–1316.

Granholm, E., McQuaid, J., McClure, F., Link, P., Perivoliotis, D., Gottlieb, J., et al. (2007). Randomized controlled trial of cognitive behavioural social skills training for older people with schizophrenia: 12-month follow-up. *The Journal of Clinical Psychiatry*, 68, 730–737.

Hafner, H., Maurer, K., Loffler, W., van der Heiden, W., Munk-Jorgensen,

P., Hambrecht, M., et al. (1998). The ABC schizophrenia study: a preliminary overview of the results. *Social Psychiatry and Psychiatric Epidemiology*, 33, 380–386.

Hafner, H., van der Heiden, W., Behrens, S., Gattaz, W., Hambrecht, M., Loffler, W., et al. (1998). Causes and consequences of the gender difference in age at onset of schizophrenia. *Schizophrenia Bulletin*, 24, 99–113.

Hamshere, M. L., Holmans, P. A., McCarthy, G. M., Jones, L. A., Murphy, K. C., Sanders, R. D., et al. (2011). Phenotype evaluation and genomewide linkage study of clinical variables in schizophrenia. *American Journal of Medical Genetics Part B. Neuropsychiatric Genetics*, 156B, 929–940.

Harris, M. J., & Jeste, D. V. (1988). Late-onset schizophrenia: an overview. *Schizophrenia Bulletin*, 14 (1), 39–55.

Hasset, A. (2005). Defining psychotic disorders in an aging population. In A. Hassett, D. Ames, & E. Chiu (eds.), *Psychosis in the elderly* (pp. 8–17). Andover, UK: Taylor and Francis.

Hassett, A. (2002). Schizophrenia and delusional disorders with onset in later life. *Revista Brasileira de Psiquiatria*, 24 (S1), 81–88.

Hassett, A. (1999). A descriptive study of first presentation psychosis in old age. *Australian and New Zealand Journal of Psychiatry*, 33, 814–824.

Hassett, A. (1997). The case for a psychological perspective on late-onset psychosis. *Australian and New Zealand Journal of Psychiatry*, 31, 68–75.

Henderson, A. S., & Kay, D. W. (1997). The epidemiology of functional psychosises of late onset. *European Archieves of Psychiatry and Clinical Neuroscience*, 247, 176–189.

Henderson, A. S., Korten, A. E., Levings, C., Jorm, A. F., Christensen, H., Jacomb, P. A., et al. (1998). Psychotic symptoms in the elderly: a prospective study in a population sample. *International Journal of Geriatric Psychiatry*, 13, 484–492.

Herbert, M. E., & Jacobson, S. (1967). Late Paraphrenia. *British Journal of Psychiatry*, 113, 461–469.

Holden, N. (1987). Late paraphrenia or the paraphrenias? A descriptive study with a 10 year follow-up. *British Journal of Psychiatry*, 150, 635–639.

Howard, R. (2001). Late-onset schizophrenia and very late-onset schizophrenia-like psychosis. *Reviews in Clinical Gerontology*, 11, 337–352.

Howard, R. (1999). Schizophrenia-like psychosis with onset in late life. In R. Howard, P. Rabins, & D. Castle (eds.), *Late Onset Schizophrenia* (pp. 127–138). Guildford, UK: Wrightson Biomedical Publishing Ltd.

Howard, R. (1992). Permeable walls, floors, ceilings and doors. Partition delusions in late paraphrenia. . *International Journal of Geriatric Psychiatry*, 7, 719–724.

Howard, R., Almeida, O., & Levy, R. (1994). Phenomenology, demography and diagnosis in late paraphrenia. *Psychological Medicine*, 24, 397–410.

Howard, R. J., Graham, C., Sham, P., Dennehey, J., Castle, D. J., Levy, R., et al. (1997). A controlled family study of late-onset non-affective psychosis (late paraphrenia). *British Journal of Psychiatry*, 170, 511–514.

Howard, R., & Levy, R. (1992). Which factors affect treatment response in late paraphrenia? *International Journal of Geriatric Psychiatry*, 7, 667–672.

Howard, R., Mellers, J., Petty, R., Bonner, D., Menon, R., Almeida, O., et al. (1995). Magnetic resonance imaging volumetric measurements of the superior temporal gyrus, hippocampus, parahippocampal gyrus, frontal and temporal lobes in late paraphrenia. *Psychological Medicine*, 25, 495–503.

Howard, R., Rabins, P. V., Seeman, M. V., & Jeste, D. (2001). Letter to the editor; Dr Howard and colleagues reply. *American Journal of Psychiatry*, 158, 1335–1336.

Howard, R., Rabins, P. V., Seeman, M. V., & Jeste, D. V. (2000). Late-onset schizophrenia and very-late-onset schizophrenia-like psychosis: an international consensus. The International Late-Onset Schizophrenia Group. *American Journal of Psychiatry*, 157, 172–178.

Huang, C., & Zhang, Y. (2009). Clinical diffrences between late-onset and early-onset chronically hospitalized elderly schizophrenic patients in Taiwan. *International Journal of Geriatric Psychiatry*, 24, 1166–1172.

Hymas, N., Naguib, M., & Levy, R. (1989). Late paraphrenia – a follow-up study. *International Journal of Geriatric Psychiatry*, 4, 23–29.

Jeste, D. V., Alexopoulos, G. S., Bartels, S. J., Cummings, J. L., Gallo, J. J., Gottlieb, G. L., et al. (1999a). Consensus statement on the upcoming crisis in geriatric mental health: research agenda for the next two decades. *Archives of General Psychiatry*, 56, 848–853.

Jeste, D. V., Caligiuri, M. P., Paulsen, J. S., Heaton, R. K., Lacro, J. P., Harris, M. J., et al. (1995). Risk of tardive dyskinesia in older patients. A prospective ongitudinal study of 266 outpatients. *Archives of General Psychiatry*, 52, 756–765.

Jeste, D. V., Harris, M. J., Krull, A., Kuck, J., McAdams, L. A., & Heaton, R. (1995). Clinical and neuropsychological characteristics of patients with late-onset schizophrenia. *American Journal of Psychiatry*, 152, 722–30.

Jeste, D. V., Lacro, J. P., Bailey, A., et al. (1999b). Lower incidence of tardive dyskinesia with risperidone compared with haloperidol in older patients. *Journal of the American Geriatrics Society*, 47, 716–719.

Jeste, D. V., Lacro, J. P., Palmer, B., Rockwell, E., Harris, M. J., & Caligiuri, M. P. (1999c). Incidence of tardive dyskinesia in early stages of low-dose treatment with typical neuroleptics in older patients. *American Journal of Psychiatry*, 156, 309–311.

Jin, H., Shih, P. A., Golshah, S., Mudaliar, S., Henry, R., Glorioso, D. K., et al. (2013). Comparison of longer-term safety and effectiveness of four atypical antipsychotics in patients over age 40: a trial using equipoise-stratified randomization. *The Journal of Clinical Psychiatry*, 74, 10–18.

Jones, D. K., Catani, M., Pierpaoli, C., Reeves, S., Shergill, S., et al. (2005). A diffusion tensor magnetic resonance imaging study of frontal cortex connections in very-late-onset schizophrenia-like psychosis. *American Journal of Geriatric Psychiatry*, 13, 1092–1099.

Kay, D. W., & Roth, M. (1961). Environmental and hereditary factors in the schizophrenias of age ("late paraphrenia") and their bearing on the general problem of causation in schizophrenia. . *The Journal of Mental Science*, 107, 649–686.

Keith, S., Regier, D., & Rae, D. (1991). Schizophrenic disorders. In L. Robins, & D. Regier (eds.), *Psychiatric Disorders in America* (pp. 33–52). New York, NY: The Free Press.

Kelly, D. L., McMahon, R. P., Liu, F., Love, R., Wehring, H. J., Shim, J. C., et al. (2010). Cardiovascular disease mortality in patients with chronic schizophrenia treated with clozapine: a retrospective cohort study. *The Journal of Clinical Psychiatry*, 71, 304–311.

Kindynis, S., Burlacu, S., Louville, P., & Limosin, F. (2013). Effect of schema-focused therapy on depression, anxiety and maladaptive cognitive schemas in the elderly. *L'Encephale*, 39, 393–400.

Kohler, S., van der Werf, M., Hart, B., Morrison, G., McCreadie, R., Kirkpatrick, B., et al. (2009). Evidence that better outcome of psychosis in women is reversed with increasing age of onset: a population based 5 year follow-up study. *Schizophrenia Research*, 113, 226–232.

Kohler, S., van OS, J., de Graaf, R., Vollebergh, W., Verhey, F., & Krabbendam, L. (2007). Psychosis risk as a function of age at onset: a comparison between early- and late-onset psychosis in a general population sample. *Social Psychiatry and Psychiatric Epidemiology*, 42, 288–294.

Korner, A., Lopez, A. G., Lauritzen, L., Andersen, P. K., & Kessing, L. V. (2009a). Acute and transient psychosis in old age and the subsequent risk of dementia: a nationwide register-based study. *International Journal of Geriatric Psychiatry*, 24, 62–68.

Korner, A., Lopez, A., Lauritzen, L., Andersen, P., Kessing, L. (2009b). Late and very-late first-contact schizophrenia and the risk of dementia-a nationwide register based study. *International Journal of Geriatric Psychiatry*, 24, 61–67.

Kua, E. A. (1992). Community study of mental disorders in elderly Singaporean Chinese using the GMS-AGECAT package. *Australian and New Zealand Journal of Psychiatry*, 26, 502–506.

Kulkarni, J. (1997). Women and schizophrenia: a review. *Australian and New Zealand Journal of Psychiatry*, 31(1): 46–56.

Lagodka, A., & Robert, P. (2009). Is late-onset schizophrenia related to neurodegenerative processes? A review of literature. . *L'Encephale*, 35, 386–393.

Levy, R., Naguib, M., & Hymas, N. (1987). Late paraphrenia. *British Journal of Psychiatry*, 151, 702.

Mason, O., Stott, J., & Sweeting, R. (2013). Dimensions of positive symptoms in late versus early onset psychosis. *International Psychogeriatrics*, 25, 397–410.

Mazeh, D., Zemishlani, C., Aizenberg, D., & Barak, Y. (2005). Patients with very-late-onset schizophrenia-like psychosis: a follow-up study. *American Journal of Geriatric Psychiatry*, 13, 417–419.

McCulloch, Y., Clare, L., Howard, R., & Peters, E. (2006). Psychological processes underlying delusional thinking in late-onset psychosis: a preliminary investigation. *International Journal of Geriatric Psychiatry*, 21, 768–777.

Meesters, P. D., de Haan, L., Comijs, H. C., Stek, M. L., Smeets-Janssen, M. M., & Weeda, M. R. (2012). Schizophrenia spectrum disorders in later life: prevalence and distribution of age at onset and sex in a dutch catchment area. *American Journal of Geriatric Psychiatry*, 20, 18–28.

Michelet, M., Lund, A., & Sveen, U. (2014). Strategies to recruit and retain older adults in intervention studies: a quantitative comparative study. *Archives of Gerontology & Geriatrics*, 59, 25–31.

Miller, B. L., & Lesser, I. M. (1988). Late-life psychosis and modern neuroimaging. *Psychiatric Clinics of North America*, 11, 337–352.

Miller, B. L., Lesser, I. M., Mena, I., & et al. (1992). Regional cerebral blood flow in late-life-onset psychosis. *Neuropsychiatry, Neuropsychology and Behavioural Neurology*, 5, 132–137.

Minnett, T., Blossom, S., & Brayne, C. (2013). Epidemiology of old age psychiatry: an overview of concepts and main studies. In T. Dening, & A. Thomas, *Oxford Textbook of Old Age Psychiatry*. New York, NY: Oxford University Press.

Mintzer, J., & Targum, S. (2003). Psychosis in elderly patients: classification and pharmacotherapy. *Journal of Geriatric Psychiatry and Neurology*, 16 (4), 199–206.

333

Mitford, E., Reay, R., McCabe, K., Paxton, R., & Turkington, D. (2010). Ageism in first episode psychosis. *International Journal of Geriatric Psychiatry*, 25, 1112–1118.

Mitter, P., Krishnan, S., Bell, P., Stewart, R., & Howard, R. (2004). The effect of ethnicity and gender on first-contact rates for schizophrenia-like psychosis in Bangladeshi, Black and White elders in Tower Hamlets, London. *International Journal of Geriatric Psychiatry*, 19, 286–290.

Mitter, P., Reeves, S., Romero-Rubiales, F., Bell, P., Stewart, R., & Howard, R. (2005). Migrant status, age, gender and social isolation in very-late-onset schizophrenia-like psychosis. *International Journal of Geriatric Psychiatry*, 20, 1046–1051.

Moore, R., Blackwood, N., Corcoran, R., Rowse, G., Kinderman, P., Bentall, R., et al. (2006). Misunderstanding the intentions of others: an exploratory study of the cognitive etiology of persecutory delusions in very late-onset schizophrenia-like psychosis. *American Journal of Geriatric Psychiatry*, 14, 410–418.

Nguyen, C. T., Couture, M. C., Alvarado, B. E., & Zununegui, M. V. (2008). Life course socioeconomic disadvantage and cognitive function among the elderly population of seven capitals in Latin America and the Caribbean. *Journal of Aging and Health*, 20 (3), 347–362.

O'Rand, A. M. (1996). The precious and the precocious: understanding cumulative disadvantage and cumulative advantage over the life course. *Gerontologist*, 36, 230–238.

Ostling, S., & Skoog, I. (2002). Psychotic symptoms and paranoid ideation in a non-demented population based sample of the very old. *Archives of General Psychiatry*, 59 (1), 53–59.

Palmer, B. W., Bondi, M. W., Twamley, E. W., Thal, L., Golshan, S., & Jeste, D. V. (2003). Are late-onset schizophrenia spectrum disorders neurodegenerative conditions? Annual rates of change on two dementia measures. *Journal of Neuropsychiatry and Clinical Neurosciences*, 15, 45–52.

Pearlson, G. (1999). Brain imaging in late onset schizophrenia. In R. Howard, P. Rabins, & D. Castle (eds.), *Late Onset Schizophrenia* (pp. 191–204). Guildford, UK: Wrightson Biomedical Publishing Ltd.

Prager, S., & Jeste, D. V. (1993). Sensory impairment in late-life schizophrenia. *Schizophrenia Bulletin*, 19, 755–772.

Quin, R. C., Clare, L., Ryan, P., & Jackson, M. (2009). 'Not of this world': the subjective experience of late-onset psychosis. *Aging and Mental Health*, 13, 779–787.

Rabins, P., Aylward, e., Holroyd, S., & Pearlson, G. (2000). MRI findings differentiate between late-onset schizophrenia and late-life mood disorder. *International Journal of Geriatric Psychiatry*, 15, 954–960.

Rabins, P., & Lavrisha, M. (2003). Long-term follow-up and phenomenologic differences distinguish among late-onset schizophrenia, late-life depression and progressive dementia. *American Journal of Geriatric Psychiatry*, 11, 589–594.

Rajji, T., Ismail, Z., & Mulsant, B. (2009). Age at onset and cognition in schizophrenia: meta-analysis. *British Journal of Psychiatry*, 195, 286–293.

Rasmussen, H. B., Timm, S., Wang, A. G., Soeby, K., Lublin, H., Fenger, M., et al. (2006). Association between the CCR5 32-bp deletion allele and late onset of schizophrenia. *American Journal of Psychiatry*, 163 (3), 507–511.

Reeves, R., & Brister, J. (2008). Psychosis in late life: emerging issues. *Journal of Psychosocial Nursing and Mental Health Services*, 46, 45–52.

Reeves, S., Sauer, J., Stewart, R., Granger, A., & Howard, R. (2001). Increased first-contact rates for very-late-onset schizophrenia-like psychosis in African and Carribean born elders. *British Journal of Psychiatry*, 179, 172–174.

Reeves, S., Stewart, R., & Howard, R. (2002). Service contact and psychopathology in very-late-onset schizophrenia: the effects of gender and ethnicity. *International Journal of Geriatric Psychiatry*, 17, 473–479.

Regier, D. (2000). Community diagnosis counts. *Archives of General Psychiatry*, 57, 223–224.

Reulbach, U., Bleich, S., Biermann, T., Pfahlberg, A., & Sperling, W. (2007). Late-onset schizophrenia in child survivors of the Holocaust. *Journal of Nervous and Mental Disease*, 195, 315–319.

Riecher-Rossler, A. (1999). Late onset schizophrenia: The German concept and literature. In R. Howard, P. Rabins, & D. Castle, *Late Onset Schizophrenia* (pp. 3–16). Guildford, UK: Wrightson Biomedical Publishing Ltd.

Riecher-Rossler, A., Hafner, H., Dutsch-Strobel, A., Oster, M., Stumbaum, M., van Gulick-Bailer, M., et al. (1994). Further evidence for a specific role of estradiol in schizophrenia? *Biological Psychiatry*, 36, 492–494.

Riecher-Rossler, A., Hafner, H., Stumbaum, M., Maurer, K., & Schmidt, R. (1994). Can estradiol modulate schizophrenic symptomatology? *Schizophrenia Bulletin*, 20, 203–214.

Rivkin, P., Kraut, M., Barta, P., Anthony, J., Arria, A. M., & Pearlson, G. (2000). White matter hyperintensity volume in late-onset and early-onset schizophrenia. *International Journal of Geriatric Psychiatry*, 15, 1085–1089.

Rodriguez-Ferrera, S., Vassilas, C. A., & Haque, S. (2004). Older people with schizophrenia: a community study in a rural catchment area. *International Journal of Geriatric Psychiatry*, 19, 1181–1187.

Rosenberg, P. B., Mielke, M. M., Appleby, B. S., Oh, E. S., Geda, Y. E., & Lyketos, C. G. (2013). The association of neuropsychiatric symptoms in MCI with incident dementia and Alzheimer's disease. *American Journal of Geriatric Psychiatry*, 21, 685–695.

Roth, M., & Kay, D. W. (1998). Late paraphrenia: a variant of schizophrenia manifest in late life or an organic clinical syndrome? A review of recent evidence. *International Journal of Geriatric Psychiatry*, 13, 775–784.

Rummel-Kluge, C., Komossa, K., Schwarz, S., Hunger , H., Schmid, F., Lobos, C. A., et al. (2010). Head-to-head comparisons of metabolic side-effects of second generation antipsychotics in the treatment of schizophrenia: a systematic review and meta-analysis. *Schizophrenia Research*, 123, 225–233.

Sachdev, P., & Brodaty, H. (1999). Quantitative study of signal hyperintensities on T2-weighted magnetic resonance imaging in late-onset schizophrenia. *American Journal of Psychiatry*, 156, 1958–1967.

Sachdev, P., Brodaty, H., Rose, N., & Cathcart, S. (1999). Schizophrenia with onset after age 50 years. II: Neurological, neuropsychological and MRI investigation. *British Journal of Psychiatry*, 175, 416–421.

Sachdev, P., Brodaty, H., Rose, N., & Haindl, W. (1997). Regional cerebral blood flow in late-onset schizophrenia: a SPECT study using 99mTc-HMPAO. *Schizophrenia Research*, 27, 105–117.

Schneider, J. A., Arvanitakis, Z., Bang, W., & Bennett, D. A. (2007). Mixed brain pathologies account for most dementia cases in community-dwelling older persons. *Neurology*, 69, 2197–2204.

Schneider, L. S., Dagerman, K. S., & Insel, P. (2005). Risk of death with atypical antipsychotic drug treatment for dementia: meta-analysis of randomized placebo-controlled trials. *JAMA*, 294, 1934–1943.

Sechi, G., & Serra, A. (2007). Wernicke's encephalopathy: new clinical settings and recent advances in diagnosis and management. *Lancet Neurology*, 6, 442–455.

Seeman, M. (1999). Oestrogens and psychosis. In M. Howard, P. Rabins, & D. Castle, *Late Onset Schizophrenia* (pp. 165–180). Guildford, UK: Wrightson Biomedical Publishing Ltd.

Sheffield, K., & Peek, M. K. (2009). Neighborhood context and cognitive decline in older Mexican Americans: results from the Hispanic established populations for epidemiologic studies of the elderly. *American Journal of Epidemiology*, 169, 1092–1101.

Skoog, I. (1993). The prevalence of psychotic, depressive and anxiety syndromes in demented and non-demented 85-year-olds. *International Journal of Geriatric Psychiatry*, 8, 247–53.

Smeets-Janssen, M. J., Meesters, P. D., Comijs, H. C., Eikelenboom, P., Smit, J. H., de Haan, L., et al. (2013). Theory of mind differences in older patients with early-onset and late-onset paranoid schizophrenia. *International Journal of Geriatric Psychiatry*, 28, 1141–1146.

Symonds, L. L., Olichney, J. M., Jernigan, T. L., Corey-Bloom, J., Healy, J. F., & Jeste, D. V. (1997). Lack of clinically significant gross structural abnormalities in MRIs of older patients with schizophrenia and related psychoses. *Journal Neuropsychiatry and Clinical Neurosciences*, 9, 251–258.

Thirthalli, J., Benegal, V., & Gangadhar, B. (2010). Substance induced psychosis. In P. Sachdev, & M. Keshavan, *Secondary Schizophrenia*. New York, NY: Cambridge University Press.

Titulaer, M., McCracken, L., Gabilondo, I., Armangue, T., Glaser, C., Iizuka, T., et al. (2013). Treatment and prognostic factors for long-term outcome in patients with anti-NMDA receptor encephalitis: an observational cohort study. *Lancet Neurology*, 12, 157–165.

van der Heijden, F. M., Zeebregts, C. J., & Reijnen, M. M. (2010). Does extracranial arterial pathology play a role in late-onset psychiatric disorders? *Cognitive Behaviour and Neurology*, 23, 147–151.

van der Werf, M., Kohler, S., Verkaaik, M., Verhey, F., van Os, J., et al. (2012). Cognitive functioning and age at onset in non-affective psychotic disorders. *Acta Psychiatrica Scandinavica*, 126, 274–281.

van Os, J., Howard, R., Takei, N., & Murray, R. M. (1995). Increasing age is a risk factor for psychosis in the elderly. *Social Psychiatry and Psychiatric Epidemiology*, 30 (4), 161–164.

Velakoulis, D., Walterfang, M., Mocellin, R., Pantelis, C., Dean, B., & McLean, C. (2009). Abnormal hippocampal distribution of TDP-43 in patients with late-onset psychosis. *Australian and New Zealand Journal of Psychiatry*, 43, 739–745.

Verdoux, H., Geddes, J.R., Takei, N., Lawrie, S.M., Bovet, P., Eagles, J.M., et al. (1997) Obstetric complications and age at onset in schizophrenia: an international collaborative meta-analysis of individual patient data. *American Journal of Psychiatry*, 154, 1220–1227.

Voisey, J., Swagell, C. D., Hughes, I. P., Lawford, B. R., Young, R. M., & Morris, C. P. (2012). A novel DRD2 single-nucleotide polymorphism analysis. *Genetic Testing and Molecular Biomarkers*, 16, 77–81.

Woolcott, J. C., Richardson, K. J., Wiens, M. O., Patel, B., Marin, J., Kahn, K. M., et al. (2009). Meta-analysis of the impact of nine medication classes on falls in elderly persons. *Archives of Internal Medicine*, 169, 1952–1960.

Yasuda, M., Kobayashi, T., Kato, S., & Kishi, K. (2013). Clinical features of late-onset schizophrenia in Japan: comparison with early-onset cases. *Psychogeriatrics*, 13, 244–249.

Dementia in women

Cynthia A. Munro and Susan W. Lehmann

Dementia, by definition, is a decline in cognitive functioning from a previously higher level, in the presence of clear consciousness (i.e., not due to delirium) and is associated with impairment in functioning. As such, it can be rapid or slow in onset, and can be progressive or static in the cognitive impairment that ensues. Dementia has numerous causes, including traumatic brain injury, psychiatric illness (e.g., depression), vascular disease (e.g., stroke), vitamin deficiency, certain toxins, anoxia and neurodegenerative disease. The largest risk factor for dementia is advancing age, and among the elderly, dementia disproportionately affects women. This chapter reviews neurodegenerative dementia in late life and focuses on women.

Epidemiology

In 2013, an estimated 44.35 million individuals worldwide were living with dementia. This number is expected to double every 20 years, with between 115 and 135 million individuals living with dementia by 2050 (Prince et al., 2013; Alzheimer Disease International, 2013). The prevalence of dementia increases with advancing age, affecting an estimated 25% of individuals by age 85 (Ferri et al., 2005).

The sex difference in dementia prevalence also increases with advancing age; roughly 5% of men and an almost equal percentage of women between ages 71–80 are diagnosed with dementia; after age 80, almost 28% of women and over 17% of men develop dementia (Plassman, et al., 2007).

The type of dementia appears to account for the sex difference in prevalence rates. Among individuals older than 65 years of age, the most common cause of dementia is Alzheimer disease (AD), accounting for about 70% of cases (Alzheimer's Association, 2011). Defined neuropathologically by the presence of intraneuronal neurofibrillary tangles, extracellular amyloid plaques, and neuronal cell death, AD disproportionately affects women. Two-thirds of patients with AD are women (www.alz.org/downloads/facts_figures_2012.pdf) and after age 80, the proportion of women with the disease (21%) is almost twice that of men (12%; Plassman et al., 2007). Although women generally live longer than men, women's increased longevity is not sufficient to explain the 1.5 times greater likelihood of developing AD (Gao et al., 1998). Although the reasons why women are at greater risk than men for developing AD are not well understood, one possible explanation is that the disease appears to cause a more rapid global cognitive decline in women than it does in men (Ito et al., 2011). Sex differences in disease progression are supported by the fact that men are more likely than women to be diagnosed with mild cognitive impairment (MCI; Katz et al., 2012; Petersen et al., 2010), a condition that is often considered a prodrome of AD.

Vascular dementia, resulting from small vessel disease, a series of strokes, or a single stroke, is widely considered the second most common cause of late-life dementia, and estimated to account for around 20% of cases (e.g. Jellinger, 2013; Plassman et al., 2007). In contrast to the sex differences in the prevalence of AD, vascular dementia is equally prevalent in women and men, affecting 2–3% of each sex over age 70 years (Plassman, et al., 2007). Of studies that do find a sex difference in the prevalence of vascular dementia, a greater proportion of men than women are reported to be affected (e.g., Kalaria et al., 2008).

The hallmark pathologic feature of Lewy body dementia is the presence of Lewy bodies in the

Comprehensive Women's Mental Health, ed. David J. Castle and Kathryn M. Abel. Published by Cambridge University Press.
© Cambridge University Press 2016.

cortical and subcortical regions of the brain. Lewy body dementia is the third-most common type of dementia and has been estimated to account for 10–20% of cases of late-life dementia (Weisman et al., 2007; Oda et al., 2009). Because of the relatively recent development of diagnostic criteria for Lewy body dementia, estimates of its prevalence are not as consistent as those for other dementias. In general, Lewy body disease is more common in men than women, with a four-fold incidence rate excess in men after age 70 in one North American study (Savica et al., 2013), and a smaller sex difference (with an incidence of 121/100,000 in men compared to 107/100,000 in women) noted in a French cohort (Perez et al., 2010). In a large autopsy series of patients seen in dementia research centers in the United States, patients with Lewy bodies were significantly more likely to be male, with an odds ratio of roughly 2.9 (Nelson et al., 2010).

Parkinson's disease (PD) is characterized by loss of dopaminergic neurons in the substantia nigra and the presence of Lewy bodies in the cytoplasm of neurons in subcortical regions with accompanying gliosis. The prevalence of PD increases with advancing age, ranging from 40.5 per 100,000 individuals between ages 40–49 years to 1,903 per 100,000 individuals aged 80 years and older (Pringsheim et al., 2014). There is a consistently greater prevalence of PD in men (1,057 per 100,000) than in women (794 per 100,000) across all geographic regions (Pringsheim et al., 2014). Similarly, many studies find a higher incidence of PD in men, with a male:female ratio of 1.5–2.0:1 (Twelves et al., 2003). The mechanisms underlying sex differences in PD are unknown. Women's higher estrogen levels, which lead to increased striatal dopamine, have been proposed as potentially related to sex differences in this disease (Haaxma et al., 2007).

Frontotemporal dementia (FTD), defined by neurodegeneration in the frontal and temporal lobes, typically has an earlier age of onset than other forms of dementia, often becoming manifest in the 50s or 60s. Consequently, roughly 60% of individuals with FTD are between ages 56 and 64 years, and the disease is as common as AD in those younger than 65 years. The estimated point prevalence of FTD is 15–22/100,000, with an annual incidence of 2.7–4.1/100,000 (Onyike & Diehl-Schmid, 2013). Because FTD is a heterogeneous disorder with several known genetic factors and other as-yet-unidentified causes, reports of the sex distribution of this disease vary widely. In one study, for example, the ratio of cases in men compared to women was 14:3 (Ratnavalli et al., 2002),

whereas other studies found a females excess, with a ratio of 1:3 (Bernardi et al., 2012; Gilberti et al., 2012).

Taken together, epidemiological studies reveal that age is a risk factor for all leading causes of dementia in late life and that AD accounts for the majority of cases of dementia. Most types of dementia are either equally prevalent in women and men, or are slightly more prevalent in men, with the notable exception of AD. Not only does AD affect many more women than men, the risk of developing this disease is greater in women than in men.

Clinical presentation

Because dementia caused by neurodegenerative disease is characterized by insidious onset, it often goes undetected until well into the course of the disease. This is particularly true in patients with AD, who are often able to maintain social skills, typically have little insight into their cognitive decline and can appear unimpaired in casual conversation. Unless cognition is specifically assessed, their disease is likely to be overlooked in its early stages. Indeed, studies consistently find that many cases of dementia are not recognized in primary care settings (e.g., Valcour et al., 2000). One meta-analysis of physician accuracy in diagnosing cognitive impairment indicated that approximately one in four cases of dementia, and approximately half of cases of mild cognitive impairment or mild dementia, remain undetected in primary care (Mitchell et al., 2011). Of particular concern are older individuals who live alone, in whom both physicians and knowledgeable informants are less likely to detect dementia compared to persons with dementia living with others (Lehmann et al., 2010). Thus, being aware of the prevalence of dementia among older people and of some of the ways in which it may present may aid earlier detection and diagnosis as well as life planning.

Impairment of memory for recent events is among the earliest symptoms of dementia. Although individuals with dementia may be able to converse about recent events in general, their memory impairment may cause them to repeat questions or stories, forget appointments, or lose their belongings. Because normal aging is associated with cognitive changes, including general slowing of information processing, increased difficulty with multitasking, and mild impairment of episodic memory (Glisky, 2007), it can be difficult to determine whether a memory complaint indicates disease or simply an awareness of the gradual inefficiency in encoding new information that normally accompanies advancing age. For this reason, family members are often better informants about a person's functioning than is the individual him- or herself, as he or she may lack insight or be overly sensitive to cognitive failures due to excessive worry.

Deficient access to semantic information, manifest as word-finding difficulties, is also a common early symptom of dementia, and of AD in particular. As with memory difficulties, occasional difficulty thinking of a particular word becomes more common with normal aging. Pathological word-finding difficulties, however, occur with greater frequency in individuals with dementia and can lead to vague speech (words devoid of content) and interfere with the ability to communicate meaningful information effectively.

Personality changes in the absence of frank cognitive impairment can be an early symptom of dementia. In patients with FTD, for example, family members sometimes report marked changes affecting food preferences, judgment or interest in others. Individuals with FTD frequently exhibit disinhibited and impulsive behaviors and may curse or demonstrate uncharacteristic sexual impropriety in social situations. The patient, in contrast, is not likely to be aware of these changes.

Neuropsychiatric disturbances commonly occur in the course of a dementing illness (Steinberg et al., 2006). They include depression and anxiety, psychotic symptoms such as hallucinations, paranoia, or delusions, irritability and sleep disturbances. In general, the severity of the behavioral disturbance is related to the severity of dementia (Majic et al., 2012). Although symptoms vary widely, some aspects of the clinical presentation of dementia differ in women compared to men. In patients with dementia living in residential care facilities, staff ratings indicated that women and men differed on 7 of 39 behaviors and symptoms (Lövheim et al., 2009). Women were more often depressed, whereas men were more often aggressive and engaged in inappropriate ("regressive") behaviours. No sex differences in passiveness (lack of spontaneous speech, initiative and/or cooperation with staff) or hallucinations were found.

Specific dementing illnesses can manifest different symptoms in women compared to men. Among patients with AD seen in outpatient clinics, caregivers' ratings indicated that women were more reclusive, were more emotionally labile, and tended to hoard and refuse help, as well as display inappropriate laughter or crying more frequently than men.

Men, in contrast, exhibited behaviors more indicative of psychomotor changes (apathy, pacing) and vegetative changes such as excessive eating and sleeping (Ott et al., 1996).

Very few studies have explored sex differences in the clinical presentation of vascular dementia. In a Chinese cohort of 467 patients with vascular dementia, Xing and colleagues (2012) found that among patients with mild vascular dementia, women were rated by caregivers to be more likely than men to have delusions, hallucinations and depression. In moderate to severe vascular dementia, men were more likely than women to manifest apathy. These findings suggest that, compared to men, women have more neuropsychiatric symptoms in mild vascular dementia, whereas in more severe cases, only apathy distinguishes women from men.

Women with PD have been shown to be diagnosed later than men with PD (51.3 vs. 53.4 years; Haaxma et al., 2007). At disease onset, women are reported to have more dyskinesias, whilst men have more rigidity, possibly related to medication use (Accolla et al., 2007). Abnormal sleep behaviors may be less common in women than in men with PD (Ozekmekçi et al., 2005), although results from one study found no sex difference in the prevalence of sleep disturbance in patients with PD, but reported that men had more violent behaviors during sleep than women did (Bjørnarå et al., 2013).

Studies of Lewy body dementia typically control for sex rather than compare women and men. For this reason, there are not sufficient findings to comment on whether sex differences exist in the clinical presentation of this disease. Similarly, research on FTD has not yielded reports of sex differences in its clinical presentation.

Risk factors for dementia

Because treatments for dementia are limited, efforts aimed at identifying risk factors have received increasing research attention. This line of work has implicated numerous risk factors, many of which pertain to general health status (e.g., obesity, high blood pressure at midlife, diabetes mellitus all increase risk), lifestyle (e.g., smoking increases risk; moderate alcohol consumption decreases risk), or demographic factors (e.g., higher socioeconomic status reduces risk) and have been found to be salient for both women and men. Several factors, however, have been shown to pose differential risks in women and men.

Education. The protective effect of higher education on dementia risk has been hypothesized to be related to "cognitive reserve" (Satz et al., 1993). That is, the brains of individuals with higher cognitive abilities prior to onset of dementia can withstand more disease before overall functioning is affected. The association between education and dementia-related death appears to be particularly relevant for women. In a meta-analysis of 11 prospective studies that included over 85,000 individuals in the United Kingdom, Russ and colleagues (2013) found that leaving full-time education at an earlier age increased the risk of dementia death in women but not in men, even after controlling for occupational social class and other common risk behaviors and comorbidities. Similarly, an Italian study found education to reduce the risk of dementia in women but not in men (Noale et al., 2013).

Diet. Lifestyle choices, including diet, have received much research attention as a potentially modifiable factor in dementia risk. Although most studies in this area have not revealed differential effects in women and men, findings from one study suggest that fruit and vegetable consumption is protective in women only. In a cohort of Swedish twins discordant for dementia in (in particular AD), greater consumption of fruit and vegetables during mid-life reduced the risk of dementia and AD 30 years later in women, but not in men (Hughes et al., 2010). This risk was reduced even further in women with angina, supporting the idea that improved vascular health is the mechanism by which a healthier diet is protective against the development of dementia in women.

Sex hormones. The relationship between sex hormones and dementia is complex and different studies have produced conflicting findings. A number of studies provided support for the notion that increased exposure to estrogens (endogenous estradiol) reduced the risk of dementia in women. Studies comparing women with higher versus lower lifetime exposures to endogenous or hormone supplements make up a large portion of the findings.

Parity. Several studies have shown that having children increases the likelihood of developing AD in women but not men (Colucci et al., 2006), and is positively correlated with AD neuropathology in women but not men (Beeri et al., 2009). Similarly, a series of studies revealed that women with a greater number of pregnancies have a higher risk of developing AD and/or a younger age of onset (Colucci et al.,

2006; Sobow et al., 2004). The association between parity and age of AD onset appears confined to women without the APOE4 allele as it was not observed in women with the APOE4 allele in one study (Corbo et al., 2007), suggesting fertility is an independent risk factor for AD in women.

Hysterectomy. Women who have undergone hysterectomy have an increased risk of early-onset dementia (Phung et al., 2010), and this risk is increased with younger age of hysterectomy (Rocca et al., 2012; Phung et al., 2010). Furthermore, the combined results from two cohort studies (in the United States and Denmark) indicated that extent of gynecological surgery was associated with a stepwise increase in the risk of dementia. Specifically, women who had hysterectomy were at increased risk of cognitive impairment or dementia. The risk was further increased in women who had undergone hysterectomy with unilateral oophorectomy, and even further increased in women who had undergone hysterectomy with bilateral oophorectomy (Rocca et al., 2012).

Hormone replacement therapy. Whether hormone replacement therapy should be offered to women who are experiencing symptoms of menopause is a topic of controversy. Many early observational studies found a protective association between "ever-use" hormone therapy in women and dementia in later life (Hogervorst et al., 2000; LeBlanc et al, 2001). Results from a large, randomized, placebo-controlled trial of hormone replacement therapy in postmenopausal women (age 65–79 years) with no history of hormone replacement therapy prior to age 65 showed that the risk of dementia (not just AD) was doubled in women receiving combined hormone (estrogen + progesterone) therapy, but hormone supplementation did not reduce the risk for developing mild cognitive impairment (Shumaker et al., 2003). Moreover, hormone replacement therapy also increased risk for breast cancer, stroke and cardiovascular disease (Grady et al., 2002; Writing Group, 2002). Since initial results of that study were published, a meta-analysis of all double-blind, placebo-controlled trials studying the effects of estrogen replacement therapy or hormone therapy on cognitive functioning confirmed that neither estrogen alone nor estrogen combined with a progestagen prevented cognitive decline in postmenopausal woman (Lethaby et al., 2008).

One study reported smaller hippocampal volumes in women who received hormonal therapy (Shumaker et al., 2003), leading the researchers to postulate that the cognitive impairment seen in hormonally treated women may be mediated by brain atrophy, rather than ischemic brain changes (Espeland et al., 2009). However, studies focused on exposure to HRT of younger, perimenopausal women converge in support of the "critical window" hypothesis such that hormone replacement therapy confined to perimenopause, rather than later in life, actually *decreases* the risk of dementia later in life (Whitmer et al., 2011; Shao et al., 2012).

Stress. Environmental stress can impair cognition, particularly memory (see Lupien et al., 2005, for a review). While the mechanisms underlying these effects are not well understood, the extent to which stressors impair cognition appears to be related to the degree of an individual's cortisol response to stress, rather than the experience of stress itself (Takahashi et al., 2004; Wolf et al., 2001).

Cortisol response to stress. One meta-analysis of 45 studies found that the effect of age on the cortisol response to a pharmacologic or psychological challenge was 3-fold higher in women than in men (Otte et al., 2005). Importantly, effect sizes did not differ in studies that controlled for sex hormone variations in women (e.g., standardizing menstrual cycles, excluding women on oral contraceptives or hormone replacement therapy) compared to those that did not, suggesting that sex hormones do not alter the effect of aging on the stress response in women. In line with this finding, studies have shown that acute psychosocial stressors are associated with memory impairment in elderly women but not in elderly men (Almela et al., 2011; Wolf et al., 1998).

Neuroticism. The propensity to perceive situations as negative or stressful, termed *neuroticism*, has been shown to increase the risk for dementia in several studies. In a 35-year longitudinal study of women, Johansson and colleagues (2010) found that reports of "frequent/chronic" stressors during mid-life increased the risk of AD at follow-up. Similarly, a recent meta-analysis of five prospective studies (Terraccino et al., 2014) reported that individuals in the top quartile of "distress proneness" (high scores on neuroticism) had a three-fold increased risk of AD. Sex differences in neuroticism are consistently reported across the world, with women scoring higher than men (Lynn & Martin, 1997), and the magnitude of the difference remains constant across the adult age span (Chapman et al., 2007; Costa et al., 2001).

These findings suggest that, even if neuroticism increases the risk equally in women and men, the fact that women tend to score higher on neuroticism may place them at differential risk.

Stressful life events. Given that stress can impair cognition and increase risk for AD, it is notable that one of life's most stressful events – death of a spouse – is much more common in older women than in older men. From ages 75–84, 55% of women and 18% of men have lost a spouse to death. After age 85, 72% of women and 35% of men have been widowed (U.S. Census Bureau, 2006). Widowhood during midlife increases the risk of cognitive impairment and AD in those who never remarry, and the risk is even greater among those with APOE4 allele (Håkansson, 2009). Of note, a recent 25-year follow-up study found that death of a spouse did not increase the risk of dementia, but women who lost a partner had a temporary decline in executive functioning during the first 2 years after their husbands' deaths compared with women who were still married (Vidarsdottir et al., 2014). To the extent that elderly individuals are vulnerable to stress-induced cognitive decline or AD, women might be expected to be at particular risk for dementia compared to men simply by virtue of being much more likely to experience death of a spouse (see Munro, 2014, for a review).

Mild Cognitive Impairment (MCI). MCI is a term used to describe a heterogeneous condition in individuals who have cognitive deficits at an intermediate stage between normal aging and dementia. Individuals with MCI have subjective memory complaints and score lower on objective memory testing than cognitively normal older adults, but the cognitive changes of MCI do not cause impairment in overall functioning. MCI may also be considered a risk factor for dementia; roughly 6–10% of individuals with MCI progress to dementia each year, but some will show improvement in cognitive functioning or will remain stable without progression to dementia (Petersen et al., 2010). Some studies have reported differences in incidence rates of MCI between women and men and risk factors for MCI may differ in women and men as well. In one community study, higher rates of MCI in younger men were associated with higher rates of cardiovascular disease and higher homocysteine levels compared with women, whereas lower rates of MCI in women correlated with better physical fitness and lower homocysteine levels (Sachdev, 2012).

Depression. Late-life depression can be mistaken for dementia. Many older patients with depression develop reversible impairment in executive functioning with cognitive slowing, and often these changes are more prominent than changes in mood (Butters et al., 2004). In addition, depression is frequently an early symptom of dementia, in both AD and vascular dementia (Alexopoulos, et al., 1997; Ownby et al., 2006). A large retrospective cohort study of over 13,000 patients found that individuals with late-life depressive symptoms showed a two-fold increase in risk of AD, whereas those with midlife and late-life depression had a greater than three-fold increase in risk of vascular dementia (Barnes et al., 2012). A longitudinal study of 436 healthy older women reported that those with significant depressive symptoms at baseline were more likely to become impaired on cognitive testing during a 7-year follow-up period (Rosenberg et al., 2010). Depression is twice as common in women than it is in men from puberty through mid-life, and continues to be more prevalent among women through early old age. These findings suggest that not only is recognition and treatment of late-life depression important in improving quality of life and functioning, it may also help prevent cognitive decline, especially for women.

Treatment approaches

Management of dementia requires a multifaceted approach. To date, there are no disease-modifying medications that prevent or cure dementia. The mainstay of pharmacologic treatment for individuals who have dementia involves cholinesterase inhibitor medications, which include donepezil, galantamine and rivastigmine, as well as memantine, which is an N-methyl-D-aspartate receptor antagonist. Individuals with dementia are particularly vulnerable to the further cognition-impairing effects of anticholinergic medications and such medications should be minimized in all patients with dementia (Bishara and Harwood, 2014). There are no known sex differences in response to these pharmacologic agents.

Reduction of risk factors is still the key approach to prevention of dementia and management of cognitive impairment. Among potential factors associated with reduced dementia risk, physical exercise has the most consistent empirical support (Ahlskog et al., 2011), and may be more beneficial for women than for men. A study of women who had vascular disease

and coronary risk factors found that those who engaged in regular physical activity, including walking, had lower rates of cognitive decline over a 5-year follow-up period (Vercambre et al., 2011). Results from a randomized, controlled trial of aerobic exercise in patients with MCI found that 6 months of aerobic exercise resulted in improvements on multiple tests of executive functioning in women but not in men (Baker et al., 2010). These findings suggest that the potential cognitive benefits of aerobic exercise should be considered, particularly in women who are at risk for dementia.

Caregiving

Aside from the fact that more women than men develop dementia, women are also disproportionately affected by virtue of being caregivers to others with dementia (see also Chapter 3). In the United States, 65–75% of caregivers are women (National Alliance for Caregiving, 2009). In Europe, almost 70% of caregivers for patients with AD are women, with the overwhelming majority being either the spouse or child of the patient (Haro et al., 2014). Among children, many fewer sons than daughters or daughters-in-law take on the caregiver role for patients with dementia (Pinquart & Sörensen, 2011).

Caregiving is associated with significant health risks. Not only are caregivers less likely to engage in preventative health behaviors (Schulz et al., 1997), they may also have decreased immune responses (Kiecolt-Glaser et al., 1996), a nearly two-fold increased risk of cardiovascular disease (Capistrant et al, 2011), slower wound healing (Kiecolt-Glaser et al., 1995) and poor sleep quality (Cupidi et al., 2012). Being an elderly caregiver was first demonstrated to be an independent risk factor for mortality over 15 years ago (Shultz & Beach 1999). Since then, the reasons underlying this increased risk have been examined. In a study of women-only caregivers (Fredman et al., 2010), increased rates of mortality were observed only in women who reported greater perceived stress; caregivers reporting low stress had no increase in mortality. Other studies have recorded similar results, suggesting that it is not the act of caregiving *per se*, but rather the degree of perceived stress and/or other factors that underlie the increased mortality associated with caregiving (Brown et al., 2009).

Physicians need to be aware that caregiving has potential negative health consequences and should screen caregivers to assess for stress affecting emotional and/or physical well-being. Results from numerous studies indicate that interventions that improve caregiver health focus on caregiver stress reduction and include referral for medical day care, in-home assistance and respite care services. Caregivers also benefit from education about strategies to enable them to manage difficult behaviors presented by the individual with dementia (Nehen and Hermann, 2014). The reader is referred to Chapter 3 for a broader discussion of women as caregivers.

Conclusion

Although age is the biggest risk factor for developing dementia, women are disproportionately affected by late-life dementia, and are at greater risk than men for AD, the most common cause of dementia. Not only do some aspects of the clinical presentation of various dementias differ by sex, but several risk factors for dementia have differential effects in women compared to men. Because women constitute the majority of informal caregivers for patients with dementia, the stressors associated with caregiving represent additional risks to women's health. Studies reporting sex differences in the prevalence rates of dementia and in symptom presentation have been largely descriptive in nature. To date, the reasons behind these reported differences remain unclear. A better understanding of the mechanisms underlying differences between women and men in the development of dementia will be important for future research, as well as for clinicians and patients. Given that several environmental and lifestyle factors seem to pose an increased risk for dementia in women, recognizing the complexity of women's lives with a view toward identifying ways of reducing the risk for dementia is an important aspect of women's health care.

References

Accolla, E., Caputo, E., Cogiamanian F., et al. (2007). Gender differences in patients with Parkinson's disease treated with subthalamic deep brain stimulation. *Movement Disorders*, 22, 1150–1156.

Ahlskog, J. E., Geda Y. E., Graff-Radford, N. R., et al. (2011). Physical exercise as a preventive or disease-modifying treatment dementia and brain aging. *Mayo Clinic Proceedings*, 86, 876–884.

Alexopoulos, G. S., Meyers, B. S., Young, R. C., et al., (1997). "Vascular depression" hypothesis. *Archives of General Psychiatry*, 54, 915–922. doi:10.1001/archpsyc.1997.01830220033006.

Almela, M., Hidalgo, V., Villada, C., et al. (2011). Salivary alpha-amylase response to acute psychosocial stress: The impact of age. *Biological Psychology*, 87, 421–429. doi: 10.1016/j.biopsycho.2011.05.008.

Alzheimer's Association. (2011). Alzheimer's Association report: 2011 Alzheimer's disease facts and figures. *Alzheimer's & Dementia*, 7, 208–244.

Alzheimer Disease International. (2013). The Global Impact of Dementia 2013-2050. www.alz.co.uk/research/GlobalImpactDementia2013.pdf.

Baker, L. D., Frank, L. L., Foster-Schubert, K., et al. (2010). Effects of aerobic exercise on mild cognitive impairment: A controlled trial. *Archives of Neurology*, 67, 71–79.

Barnes, D. E., Yaffe, K. and Byers. A. L. (2012). Midlife vs. late-life depressive symptoms and risk of dementia: Differential effects for Alzheimer disease and vascular dementia. *Archives of General Psychiatry*, 69, 493–498. doi:10.1001/archgenpsychiatry.2011.1481.

Beeri, M. S., Rapp, M., Schmeidler, J., et al. (2009). Number of children is associated with neuropathology of Alzheimer's disease in women. *Neurobiology of Aging*, 30(8), 1184–1191.

Bernardi,L., Frangipane, F., Smirne, N., et al. (2012). Epidemiology and genetics of frontotemporal dementia: a door-to-door survey in southern Italy. *Neurobiology of Aging*, 33, 2948.e1–2948.e10. doi: 10.1016/j.neurobiolaging.2012.06.017. Epub Jul 20, 2012.

Bishara, D. and Harwood, D. (2014). Safe prescribing of physical health medication in patients with dementia. *International Journal of Geriatric Psychiatry*, Aug 4. doi: 10.1002/gps.4163. [Epub ahead of print].

Bjørnarå, K. A., Dietrichs, E. and Toft, M. (2013). REM sleep behavior disorder in Parkinson's disease–is there a gender difference? *Parkinsonism and Related Disorders*, 19, 120–122. doi: 10.1016/j.parkreldis.2012.05.027.

Brown, S. L., Smith, D. M., Schulz, R., et al. (2009). Caregiving behavior is associated with decreased mortality risk. *Psychological Science*, 20, 488–494. doi: 10.1111/j.1467-9280.2009.02323.x. Epub Mar 20, 2009.

Butters, M. A., Whyte, E. M., Nebes, R. D., et al. (2004). The nature and determinants of neuropsychological functioning in late-life depression. *Archives of General Psychiatry*, 61, 587–595. doi:10.1001/archpsyc.61.6.587.

Capistrant, D. B., Moon, J. R., Berkman, L. F., et al. (2011). Current and long-term spousal caregiving and onset of cardiovascular disease. *Journal of Epidemiology and Community Health*, 66, 951–956. doi:10.1136/jech-2011-200040.

Chapman, B. P., Duberstein, P. R., Sörensen, S., et al. (2007). Gender differences in five factor model personality traits in an elderly cohort: Extension of robust and surprising findings to an older generation. *Personality and Individual Differences*, 43, 1594–1603.

Colucci, M., Cammarata, S., Assini, A., et al. (2006). The number of pregnancies is a risk factor for Alzheimer's disease. *European Journal of Neurology*, 13, 1374–1347.

Corbo, R. M., Gambina, G., Ulizzi, L., et al. (2007). Combined effect of apolipoprotein e genotype and past fertility on age at onset of Alzheimer's disease in women. *Dementia and Geriatric Cognitive Disorders*, 24, 82–85.

Costa, P., Terracciano, A. and McCrae, R. R. (2001). Gender differences in personality traits across cultures: Robust and surprising findings. *Journal of Personality and Social Psychology*, 81(2), 322–331.

Cupidi, C., Realmuto, S., Lo Coco, G., et al. (2012). Sleep quality in caregivers of patients with Alzheimer's disease and Parkinson's disease and its relationship to quality of life. *International Psychogeriatrics*, 24, 1827–1835.

Espeland, M.A., Tindle, H.A., Bushnell, C.A., et al. (2009). Brain volumes, cognitive impairment, and conjugated equine estrogens. *Journal of Gerontology: Biological Sciences*, 64, 1243–1250.

Ferri, C.P., Prince, M., Brayne, C., et al. (2005). Global prevalence of dementia: a Delphi consensus study. *The Lancet*, 366, 2112–112L.

Fredman, L., Cauley, J. A., Hochberg, M., et al. (2010). Mortality associated with caregiving, general stress, and caregiving-related stress in elderly women: results of caregiver-study of osteoporotic fractures. *Journal of the American Geriatrics Society*, 58, 937–943. doi: 10.1111/j.1532-5415.2010.02808.x. Epub Mar 30, 2010.

Gao, S., Hendrie, H. C., Hall, K. S., et al. (1998). The relationships between age, sex, and the incidence of dementia and Alzheimer disease: a meta-analysis. *Archives of General Psychiatry*, 55, 809–815.

Gilberti, N., Turla, M., Alberici, A., et al. (2012). Prevalence of frontotemporal lobar degeneration in an isolated population: the Vallecamonica study. *Neurological Sciences*, 33, 899–904. doi: 10.1007/s10072-011-0865-0.

Glisky, E. L. (2007). Changes in cognitive function in human aging. In *Brain Aging: Models, Methods and Mechanisms*. Edited by Riddle, D. R. Boca Raton, FL: CRC Press.

Grady, D., Herrington, D., Bittner, V., et al. (2002). Cardiovascular disease outcomes during 6.8 years of hormone therapy. *JAMA*, 288, 49–57.

Haaxma, C.A., Bloem, B.R., Borm, G.F., et al. (2007). Gender differences in Parkinson's disease. *Journal of Neurological and Neurosurgical Psychiatry*, 78, 819–824.

Håkansson, K., Rovio, S., Helkala, E.L., et al. (2009). Association between mid-life marital status and cognitive function in later life: Population based cohort study. *British Medical Journal*, 339, b2462. doi: 10.1136/bmj.b2462.

Haro J. M., Kahle-Wrobleski, K., Bruno, G., et al. (2014). Analysis of burden in caregivers of people with Alzheimer's disease using self-report and supervision hours. *Journal of Nutrition, Health, & Aging*, 18, 677–684. doi: 10.1007/s12603-014-0036-0.

Hogervorst, E., Williams, J., Budge, M., et al. (2000). The nature of the effect of female gonadal hormone replacement therapy on cognitive function in post-menopausal women: a meta-analysis. *Neuroscience*, 101, 485–512.

Hughes, T. F., Andel, R., Small, B. J., et al. (2010). See comment in PubMed Commons belowMidlife fruit and vegetable consumption and risk of dementia in later life in Swedish twins. *American Journal of Geriatric Psychiatry*, 18, 413–420. doi: 10.1097/JGP.0b013e3181c65250.

Ito, K., Corrigan, B., Zhao, Q., et al. (2011). Disease progression model for cognitive deterioration from Alzheimer's Disease Neuroimaging Initiative database. *Alzheimer's and Dementia*, 7, 151–160. doi: 10.1016/j.jalz.2010.03.018.

Jellinger, K. A. (2013). Pathology and pathogenesis of vascular cognitive impairment-a critical update. *Frontiers in Aging and Neuroscience*, 5, 17. doi: 10.3389/fnagi.2013.00017.

Johansson, L., Guo, X., Waern, M., et al. (2010). Midlife psychological stress and risk of dementia: A 35-year longitudinal population study. *Brain*, 133(Pt 8), 2217–2224. doi: 10.1093/brain/awq116.

Kalaria, R. N., Maestre, G. E. Arizaga, R., et al. (2008). Alzheimer's disease and vascular dementia in developing countries: Prevalence, management, and risk factors. *Lancet Neurology*, 7, 812–826.

Katz, M. J., Lipton, R. B., Hall, C. B., et al. (2012). Age-specific and sex-specific prevalence and incidence of mild cognitive impairment, dementia, and Alzheimer dementia in blacks and whites: a report from the Einstein Aging Study. *Alzheimer Disease and Associated Disorders*, 26, 335–343. doi: 10.1097/WAD.0b013e31823dbcfc.

Kiecolt-Glaser, J. K., Glaser, R., Gravenstein, S., et al. (1996). Chronic stress alters the immune response to influenza virus vaccine in older adults. *Proceedings of the National Academy of Science*, 93, 3043–3047.

Kiecolt-Glaser, J. K., Marucha, P. T., Malarkey, W. B., et al. (1995). Slowing of wound healing by psychological stress. *Lancet*, 346, 1194–1196.

LeBlanc, E. S., Janowsky, J., Chan, B.K.S., et al. (2001). Hormone replacement therapy and cognition: Systematic review and metaanalysis. *JAMA*, 285, 1489–1499.

Lehmann, S. W., Black, B. S., Shore, A., et al. (2010). Living alone with dementia: lack of awareness adds to functional and cognitive vulnerabilities. *International Psychogeriatrics*, 22, 778–784. doi: 10.1017/S1041610209991529

Lethaby, A., Hogervorst, E., Richards, M., et al. (2008). Hormone replacement therapy for cognitive function in postmenopausal women. *Cochrane Database Systematic Reviews*, 1: CD003122. doi: 10.1002/14651858.CD003122. pub2.

Lövheim, H., Sandman, P. O., Karlsson, S., et al. (2009). Sex differences in the prevalence of behavioral and psychological symptoms of dementia. *International Psychogeriatrics*, 21, 469–475.

Lupien, S. J., Fiocco, A., Wan, N., et al. (2005). Stress hormones and human memory function across the lifespan. *Psychoneuroendocrinology*, 30, 225–242.

Lynn, R. and Martin, T. (1997). Gender differences in extraversion, neuroticism, and psychoticism in 37 nations. *The Journal of Social Psychology*, 137, 369–373.

Majic, T., Pluta, J. P., Mell, T., et al. (2012). Correlates of agitation and depression in nursing home residents with dementia. *International Psychogeriatrics*, 24, 1779–1789.

Mitchell, A. J., Meader, N. and Pentzek, M. (2011). Clinical recognition of dementia and cognitive impairment in primary care: A meta-analysis of physician accuracy. *Acta Psychiatry Scandanavia*, 124, 165–183.

Munro, C. A. (2014). Sex differences in Alzheimer's disease risk: Are we looking at the wrong hormones? *International Psychogeriatrics*, 26,1579–1584. doi:10.1017/S1041610214001549

National Alliance for Caregiving (2009). *Caregiving in the U.S.* Retrieved November 2, 2010, from www.caregiving.org/data/Caregiving_in_the_US_2009_full_report.pdf.

Nehen, N-G. and Hermann, D. M. (2014). Supporting dementia patients and their caregivers in daily life challenges: review of physical, cognitive, and psychosocial rehabilitation studies. *European Journal of Neurology*, Aug 7. doi: 10.1111/ene.12535. [Epub ahead of print]

Nelson, P. T., Jicha, G. A., Kryscio, R. J., et al. (2010). Low sensitivity in clinical diagnoses of dementia with Lewy bodies. *Journal of Neurology*, 257(3), 359–366.

Noale, M., Limongi, F., Zambon, S., et al. (2013). Incidence of dementia: evidence for an effect modification by gender. The ILSA Study. *International Psychogeriatrics*, 25, 1867–1876. doi: 10.1007/s00415-010-5630-4.

Oda, H., Yamamoto, Y. and Maeda, K. (2009). Neurospsychological profile of dementia with Lewy bodies. *Psychogeriatrics*, 9, 85–90.

Onyike, C. U. and Diehl-Schmid, J. (2013). The epidemiology of frontotemporal dementia. *International Review of Psychiatry*, 25, 130–137. doi: 10.3109/09540261.2013.776523.

Ott, B. R., Tate, C. A., Gordon, N. M., et al. (1996). Gender differences in the behavioral manifestations of Alzheimer's disease. *Journal of the American Geriatrics Society*, 44, 583–587.

Otte, C., Hart, S., Neylan, T. C., et al. (2005). A meta-analysis of cortisol response to challenge in human aging: importance of gender. *Psychoneuroendocrinology*, 30, 80–91.

Ownby, R. L., Crocco, E., Acevedo, A., et al. (2006). Depression and risk for Alzheimer disease: Systematic review, meta-analysis, and metaregression analysis. *Archives of General Psychiatry*, 63, 530–538.

Ozekmekçi, S., Apaydin, H. and Kiliç, E. (2005). Clinical features of 35 patients with Parkinson's disease displaying REM behavior disorder. *Clinical Neurology and Neurosurgery*, 107, 306–309.

Perez, F., Helmer, C., Dartigues, J. F., et al. (2010). A 15-year population-based cohort study of the incidence of Parkinson's disease and dementia with Lewy bodies in an elderly French cohort. *Journal of Neurological and Neurosurgical Psychiatry*, 81, 742–746. doi:10.1136/jnnp.2009.189142.

Petersen, R. C., Roberts, R. O., Knopman, D. S., et al. (2010). Prevalence of mild cognitive impairment is higher in men: The Mayo Clinic Study of Aging. *Neurology*, 75, 889–897. doi: 10.1212/WNL.0b013e3181f11d85.

Phung, T. K., Waltoft, B. L., Laursen, T. M., et al. (2010). Hysterectomy, oophorectomy and risk of dementia: a nationwide historical cohort study. *Dementia and Geriatric Cognitive Disorders*, 30, 43–50. doi: 10.1159/000314681.

Pinquart, M. and Sörensen, S. (2011). Spouses, adult children, and children-in-law as caregivers of older adults: A meta-analytic comparison. *Psychology and Aging*, 26, 1–14.

Plassman, B. L., Langa, K. M., Fisher, G. G., et al. (2007). Prevalence of dementia in the United States: The aging, demographics, and memory Study. *Neuroepidemiology*, 29, 125–132.

Prince, M., Bryce, R., Albanese, E., et al. (2013). The global prevalence of dementia: A systematic review and metaanalysis. *Alzheimer's & Dementia*, 9, 63–75.

Pringsheim, T., Jette, N., Frolkis, A., et al. (2014). The prevalence of Parkinson disease: A systematic review and meta-analysis. *Movement Disorders*, Jun 28. doi: 10.1002/mds.25945. [Epub ahead of print].

Ratnavalli, E., Brayne, C., Dawson, K., et al. (2002). The prevalence of frontotemporal dementia. *Neurology*, 58, 1615–1621.

Rocca, W. A., Grossardt, B. R., Shuster, L. T., et al. (2012). Hysterectomy, oophorectomy, estrogen, and the risk of dementia. *Neurodegenerative Disorders*, 10, 175–178. doi: 10.1159/000334764.

Rosenberg, P. B., Mielke, M. M., Xue, Q. L., et al. (2010). Depressive symptoms predict incident cognitive impairment in cognitive healthy older women. *American Journal of Geriatric Psychiatry*, 18, 204–211. doi: 10.1097/ JGP.0b013e3181c53487.

Russ, T. C., Stamatakis, E., Hamer, M., et al. (2013). Socioeconomic status as a risk factor for dementia death: Individual participant meta-analysis of 86 508 women and men from the UK. *British Journal of Psychiatry*, 203, 10–17. doi: 10.1192/bjp. bp.112.119479.

Sachdev, P. S., Lipnicki, D. M., Crawford, J., et al. (2012). Risk profiles for mild cognitive impairment vary by age and xex: The Sydney Memory and Ageing Study. *The American Journal of Geriatric Psychiatry*, 20(10), 854–865. doi:10.1097/ JGP.0b013e31825461b0.

Satz, P. (1993). Brain reserve capacity on symptom onset after brain injury: A formulation and review of evidence for threshold theory. *Neuropsychology*, 7, 273–295.

Savica, R., Grossardt, B. R., Bower, J. H., et al. (2013). Incidence of dementia with Lewy bodies and Parkinson disease dementia. *JAMA Neurology*, 70, 1396–1402. doi: 10.1001/jamaneurol.2013.3579.

Schulz, R., Newsom, J., Mittelmark, M., et al. (1997). Health effects of caregiving: The Caregiver Health Effects Study: An ancillary study of The Cardiovascular Health Study. *Annals of Behavioral Medicine*, 19, 110–116.

Schulz, R. and Beach, S. R. (1999). Caregiving as a risk factor for mortality. *JAMA*, 282, 2215–2219.

Shao, H., Breitner, J. C., Whitmer, R. A., et al. (2012). Hormone therapy and Alzheimer disease dementia: New findings from the Cache County Study. *Neurology*, 79, 1846–1852. doi: 10.1212/ WNL.0b013e318271f823.

Shumaker, S. A., Legault, C., Rapp, S., et al. (2003). Estrogen plus progestin and the incidence of dementia and mild cognitive impairment in postmenopausal women: The women's health initiative memory study: A randomized controlled trial. *JAMA*, 289, 2651–2662. doi:10.1001/jama.289.20.2651.

Sobow, T. and Kloszewska, I. (2004). Parity, number of pregnancies, and the age of onset of Alzheimer's disease. *Journal of Neuropsychiatry and Clinical Neurosciences*, 16(1), 120–121.

Steinberg, M., Corcoran, C., Tschanz, J. T., et al. (2006). Risk factors for neuropsychiatric symptoms in dementia: the Cache County Study. *International Journal of Geriatric Psychiatry*, 21, 824–830.

Takahashi, T., Ikeda, K., Ishikawa, M., et al. (2004). Social stress-induced cortisol elevation acutely impairs social memory in humans. *Neuroscience Letters*, 363, 125–130.

Terracciano, A., Sutin, A. R., An, Y., O'Brien, R. J., Ferrucci, L., Zonderman, A. B. and Resnick, S. M. (2014). Personality and risk of Alzheimer's disease: New data and meta-analysis. *Alzheimer's and Dementia*, 10(2), 179–186. doi: 10.1016/j.jalz.2013.03.002.

Twelves, D., Perkins, K.S.M. and Counsell, C. (2003). Systematic review of incidence studies of Parkinson's disease. *Movement Disorders*, 18, 19–31.

Valcour, V. G., Masaki, K. H., Curb, J. D., et al. (2000). The detection of dementia in the primary care setting. *Archives of Internal Medicine*, 160, 2964–2968. doi:10.1001/archinte.160.19.2964.

Vercambre, M. N., Grodstein, F., Manson, J. E., et al. (2011). Physical activity and cognition in women with vascular conditions. *Archives of Internal Medicine*, 171, 1258–1259.

Vidarsdottir, H., Fang, F., Chang, M., et al. (2014). Spousal loss and cognitive function in later life: A 25-year follow-up in the AGES-Reykjavik Study. *American Journal of Epidemiology*, 179, 674–683.

Wassertheil-Smoller, S., Hendrix, S., Limacher, M., et al. (2003). Effect of estrogen plus progestin on stroke in postmenopausal women: The Women's Health Initiative: A randomized trial. *JAMA*, 289, 2673–2684. doi:10.1001/ jama.289.20.2673.

Weisman, D. and McKeith, I. (2007). Dementia with Lewy bodies. *Seminars in Neurology*, 27, 42–47.

Whitmer, R. A., Quesenberry, C. P., Zhou, J., et al. (2011). Timing of hormone therapy and dementia: the critical window theory revisited. *Annals of Neurology*, 69, 163–169. doi: 10.1002/ana.22239. Epub Nov 12, 2010.

Wolf, O. T., Schommer, N. C., Hellhammer, D. H., et al. (2001). The relationship between stress-induced cortisol levels and memory differs between women and men. *Psychoneuroendocrinology*, 26, 711–720.

Wolf, O. T., Kudielka, B. M., Hellhammer, D. H., et al. (1998). Opposing effects of DHEA replacement in elderly subjects on declarative memory and attention after exposure to a laboratory stressor. *Psychoneuroendocrinology*, 23, 617–629.

Writing Group for the Women's Health Initiative Investigators (2002). Risks and benefits of estrogen plus progestin in healthy postmenopausal women: Principal results from the Women's Health Initiative randomized controlled trial. *JAMA*, 288, 321–333.

Xing, Y., Wei, C., Chu, C., et al. (2012). Stage-specific gender differences in cognitive and neuropsychiatric manifestations of vascular dementia. *American Journal of Alzheimer's Disease and Other Dementias*, 27, 433–438. doi: 10.1177/ 1533317512454712.

Index

Printed in the United States
by Baker & Taylor Publisher Services